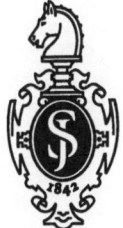

A.H. Cruickshank and E.W. Benbow

Pathology of the Pancreas

Second Edition

With 276 figures

Springer
London Berlin Heidelberg New York
Paris Tokyo Hong Kong
Barcelona Budapest

Alan H. Cruickshank
The Old House
28 North Road
Grassendale Park
Liverpool L19 0LR

Emyr W. Benbow
Department of Pathology
The Medical School, University of Manchester
Oxford Road
Manchester M13 9PT

Front cover illustration: see Fig. 6.6 (page 96)

ISBN-13: 978-1-4471-3007-9 2nd edition. Springer-Verlag Berlin Heidelberg New York

British Library Cataloguing in Publication Data
Cruickshank, Alan H.
  Pathology of the Pancreas. – 2 Rev. ed
  I. Title   II. Benbow, Emyr W.
  616.3707
  ISBN-13: 978-1-4471-3007-9   e-ISBN-13: 978-1-4471-3005-5
  DOI: 10.1007/978-1-4471-3005-5
Library of Congress Cataloging-in-Publication Data
Cruickshank, Alan H.
  Pathology of the pancreas / A.H. Cruickshank and E.W. Benbow. – 2nd ed.
    p.   cm.
  Includes bibliographical references and index.
  ISBN 3–540–19923–3 (alk. paper)
  1. Pancreas – Diseases.   2. Pancreas – Histopathology,   I. Benbow, E.W. (Emyr W.), 1952– II. Title.
  [DNLM: 1. Pancreatic Diseases.   2. Pancreas – pathology.   WI 800
  C955p 1955]
  RC857.4.C78   1995
  616.3'7 – dc20
  DNLM/DLC
  for Library of Congress   95–33

Typeset by EXPO Holdings, Malaysia
Printed by Henry Ling, The Dorset Press, Dorchester, England
28/3830-543210 Printed on acid-free paper

To our wives

Preface to the First Edition

The recent advances in the techniques for imaging the pancreas without surgical intervention have reduced the inaccessibility of the pancreas. However, although certain lesions of the pancreas can now be recognised and localised without an operation, the pathology of the pancreas remains to be more thoroughly investigated. Moreover, the almost unrelated exocrine and endocrine functions of the pancreas have led to the management of different pancreatic diseases by different groups of specialists, while the effects of primarily non-pancreatic diseases upon the pancreas have tended to escape recognition. Even in the autopsy room the pancreas is often inadequately examined, and autolysis may make microscopic examination unrewarding. This book is an attempt by a general histopathologist to make available some of his experience of the various aspects of pancreatic disease that he has encountered during his working career.

My interest in the pathology of the pancreas was aroused while working with Prof. Arnold Rice Rich of the Johns Hopkins Hospital, Baltimore. Rich himself, in his earlier work, had continued the tradition, begun in the same department of pathology by Opie, of carrying out morbid anatomical and experimental studies on pancreatic disease. Rich later became more involved in work on tuberculosis and on the collagen diseases but his interest in disease of the pancreas persisted and the work he allotted to me included an experimental study of chemically induced diabetes mellitus.

After my return to England I spent the next 30 years as a member of the Department of Pathology at the University of Liverpool. There much of my time was occupied with teaching, with routine surgical pathology and with many autopsies upon patients that had died in the Liverpool Royal Infirmary and in Newsham General Hospital. I also had to perform a share of the autopsies carried out for the Liverpool City Coroner. It was during these years that most of the material for this book was collected: retirement provided an opportunity to review and select from the accumulated material. It was Mr. Michael Jackson of the Springer-Verlag organisation who suggested that the book should be written, and it was he also who then provided the encouragement and stimulation without which the book would never have been finished.

I am particularly grateful to Prof. Donald Heath of the Department of Pathology at the University of Liverpool for allowing me, although no longer a member of his staff, to use the facilities of his department, and for giving me access to the records and the material stored in the department. The assistance of the department's photographic staff has been invaluable, and I am indebted to Mr. Alan J. Williams for all but a few of the photographs and photomicrographs that I have used. I am grateful also to Mr. John Massey who willingly undertook the work of recutting and staining sections from old blocks of tissue.

Dr. John Bouton of the Department of Pathology at Alder Hey Children's Hospital, Liverpool, allowed me to use his records and Miss Catherine D. M. McDougall of his department provided sections and electron micrographs. Dr. D. R. Clark, now in the Department of Pathology, Launceston General Hospital, Tasmania, carried out many of the post-mortem pancreatograms and Dr. Mavis McConnell of the Liverpool Regional Cancer Registry provided records and follow-up information about cases of pancreatic cancer. Many colleagues provided specimens or case records and such material has been acknowledged in the text or in the figure legends. Dr. Anne Clark of the Diabetes Research Laboratories of the Nuffield Department of Clinical Medicine, the University of Oxford, generously provided material and advice for the chapter on the pancreatic lesions associated with diabetes and I am most grateful to her. I am obliged to Mrs. G. C. Pattinson, Mrs. Alison Rimmer and to Miss Collette Youd for having typed the manuscript and also to the staff of the library of the Liverpool Medical Institution for much assistance with the literature.

Liverpool, February 1986   A. H. Cruickshank

Preface to the Second Edition

As the senior author of the second edition of Pathology of the Pancreas I must begin by stating that I had expected the edition that appeared in 1986 to be the only edition and to be my swan song. Thus it was with some dismay that I received an invitation from the late Michael Jackson to begin work on a second edition, and it was only when Michael Jackson suggested that I should find a co-author that my reluctance to undertake the job was overcome.

It was at a meeting of the North West branch of the Association of Clinical Pathologists that Emyr Benbow and I found we had a common interest in generalised cryptococcal infections, a case of which he had presented at the meeting. Better acquaintance showed that there were other topics in pathology that interested both of us and that pathology of the pancreas was such a topic. Until then, Emyr Benbow's main interest had been in the field of pulmonary and cardiovascular pathology but, as a lecturer in pathology in the University of Manchester, he had been influenced by Dr. Joan Braganza's enthusiasm for the investigation of pancreatic disease, and had been particularly intrigued when Dr. Braganza's ideas on pathogenesis had helped explain an autopsy case where acute pancreatitis had occurred simultaneously in both pancreases in a patient generously endowed with two! We met Michael Jackson and, with his approval, we agreed to start work.

Initial progress was slow for each revised or re-written chapter was read by both of us and our written comments on what we had read were nearly as long as the chapter that they concerned. This method of working, however, allowed our meetings, when they could be arranged, to be more social and convivial rather than scholastic. Time went by but eventually we decided that we must finish and after some terminal haste our typescript was submitted. In the meantime Michael Jackson had died, and the task of stimulating and encouraging us had been taken over by Dr. Gerald Graham, but he retired about the time we finished writing and Dr. Andrew Colborne was just taking over as Medical Editor when our typescript was delivered.

The preliminary editing of our efforts was entrusted to Dr. Margaret Carver and we are grateful to her for the correction of our many mistakes and omissions. We found her rigorous requirements for detail in our references to be more exacting than anything either of us had met before but we appreciate the hard work she did in clarifying and tightening our sentences, and in making our choice of words more genteel.

As in the case of the first edition, we are much obliged to Mr. Alan Williams for his photography, and the senior author wishes to thank Mrs. B. N. Ridley and Miss Gaynor Southern for typing his manuscript.

Liverpool, March 1995   A. H. Cruickshank

Contents

1 The Normal Pancreas

The Greek anatomists of the Alexandrian school of medicine that flourished about 300 BC were familiar with the pancreas and were probably responsible for naming this organ, whose name means "all flesh". The word they used for "flesh" was the word for animal meat used for food, which suggests that at that time the pancreas, still one of the organs prized as "sweetbread", may have been a delicacy. Andreas Vesalius in his famous work *On the Fabric of the Human Body*, published in 1543, differentiated between the pancreas and the mesenteric lymph nodes but some confusion about the distinction appears to have persisted for almost a century after that time. In 1642 Wirsung identified, in man, the pancreatic duct that still bears his name. In 1775 Santorini published an illustration of an accessory duct; such a duct is now usually called the duct of Santorini, although the historical researches of Stern (1986) have shown that at least seven earlier anatomists were already aware of the existence of an accessory pancreatic duct.

Descriptions of the shape, position and connections of the pancreas are provided in all the commonly used textbooks of anatomy. This large gland, whose endocrine component, the islets of Langerhans, is not normally recognisable with the naked eye, lies more or less transversely on the posterior abdominal wall in the epigastric and left hypochondriac regions of the abdomen. Although there is no anatomical division between the three regions of the gland, it is described as consisting of a head, body and a tail. The head, which lies in the loop of the duodenum, and the body are retroperitoneal and lie behind the lesser sac of the peritoneum. The tail turns forwards in the lienorenal ligament to reach the hilum of the spleen. The relationship to the lesser sac of the peritoneum is of particular importance in relation to the formation of the pancreatic pseudocysts that may follow inflammation of, or injury to, the pancreas. A groove on the posterior surface of the pancreas is regarded as the neck or dividing line between the head and the body. There is no such landmark between the body and tail of the pancreas. The groove between the head and the body accommodates the terminal part of the superior mesenteric vein and the beginning of the portal vein. The splenic vein runs from left to right from the hilum of the spleen to join the superior mesenteric vein behind the neck of the pancreas to form the portal vein. Its course is behind the pancreas, close to the upper border of the pancreas. It is intimately attached to the posterior surface of the pancreas but it forms no sulcus in the gland. The close relationship of the splenic and portal veins to the pancreas makes them vulnerable to invasion by cancer of the pancreas and attachment of a cancer to the wall of the portal vein may be decisive in determining the resectability or otherwise of a pancreatic tumour. The superior mesenteric artery, like the superior mesenteric vein, passes behind the neck of the pancreas and the presence of these vessels seems to be associated, at least in some pancreases, with a marked alteration in the pattern of the ducts in the region of the neck of the pancreas (Figs 1.1–1.3). An expansion of the head of the pancreas extends to the left along the upper border of the third part of the duodenum and forms the uncinate process, and, although the superior mesenteric blood vessels pass behind the neck of the pancreas, they pass in front of the uncinate process.

The anterior surfaces of the head and body of the pancreas have a serous peritoneal covering but there is no peritoneal covering posteriorly and the pos-

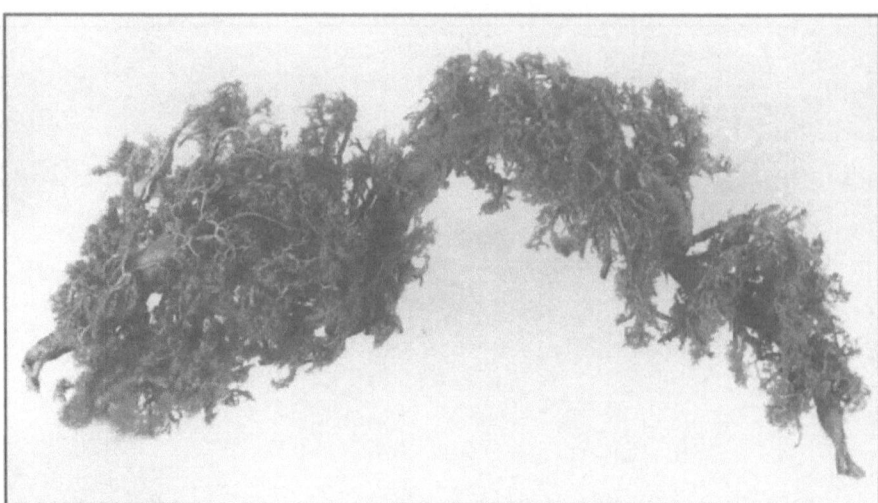

Fig. 1.1. A cast of the ducts of a normal pancreas obtained by the method of Berman et al. (1960). The absence of ducts in the region that is in contact with the superior mesenteric vessels is a common finding.

terior surface of the gland is in contact with the aorta, the left renal vessels, the left crus of the diaphragm, the left adrenal gland and the upper pole of the left kidney, as well as with the retroperitoneal lymph nodes and nerve fibres and ganglia. Any of the latter structures may be invaded by extending cancers of the pancreas.

It is in the region of the head, however, that the anatomical arrangements are of particular importance in relation to pancreatic disease. The lower 3–5 cm of the common bile duct run in a groove in the posterior surface of the head of the pancreas and may seem to be embedded in the pancreatic tissue. In all but a very few of the cases of the latter type, however, the duct lies in a cleft in the pancreas and is overlapped by pancreatic tissue that does not,

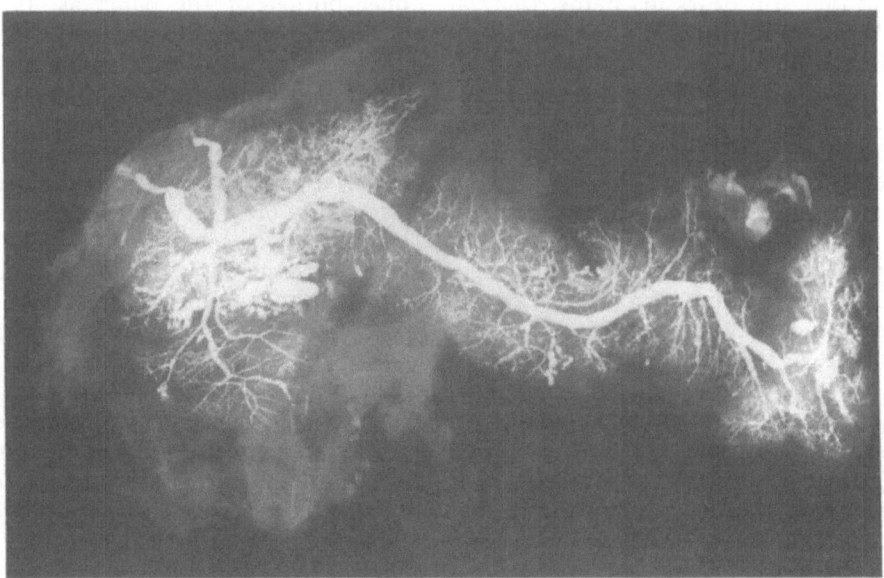

Fig. 1.2. A radiograph of the ducts of the pancreas after injection of barium sulphate, in a woman aged 73. An accessory pancreatic duct is present and the "cysts" noted by Kreel and Sandin (1973) are well marked in the head. There are filling defects in the vicinity of the superior mesenteric vessels and also towards the tail in the vicinity of a calcified aneurysm of the splenic artery. The subject had diabetes mellitus and there was marked general arteriosclerosis with gangrene on the left foot. The immediate cause of death was pulmonary tuberculosis.

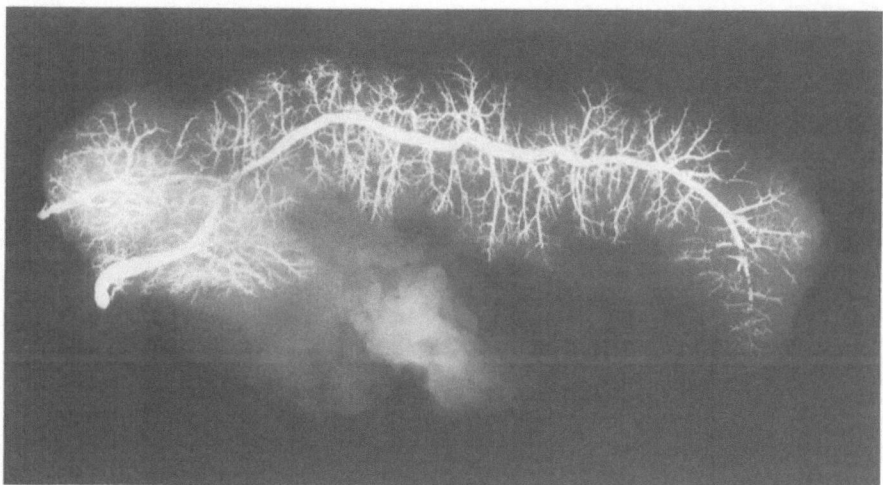

Fig. 1.3. Radiograph of the pancreatic ducts injected with barium sulphate. An accessory duct is present and there is apparent stenosis of the main duct near the neck of the pancreas.

however, prevent the cleft from being recognised by palpation (Lytle 1959–1960). In such cases the duct can usually be exposed through a plane of cleavage between the overlapping pancreatic tissue and the back of the head of the pancreas. This makes it unnecessary to cut through glandular tissue. The bile duct usually passes down close to, or runs in direct contact with, the left border of the second part of the duodenum, but it may be as much as 2 cm from the duodenal wall before it begins to incline to the right to reach, and then pass through, the wall of the second part of the duodenum. Its progress to the right may be in a straight line, or in a gentle curve, or, less commonly, it may turn towards the duodenum almost at a right angle. In any of the variants of its course in the region of the head of the pancreas, the common bile duct is liable to be invaded when carcinoma develops in the head of the pancreas, with consequent obstructive jaundice.

The Duct System of the Pancreas

The relationship between the common bile duct and the usual termination of the main pancreatic duct and its variants, has long been of importance in that reflux of bile or duodenal contents into the duct system of the pancreas might or might not be possible under the anatomical circumstances in any given patient. Now the advent of pancreatography, especially of endoscopic retrograde pancreatography, has given clinical importance to the details of the anatomy of the pancreatic ducts.

The results of early studies of the pancreatic ducts, including those of Wirsung (1642) and of Santorini (1775), were reviewed by Baldwin in 1911. Nearly all of Baldwin's own results, obtained in all but a few cases by dissection of the pancreases of 100 embalmed anatomical cadavers, have since, in general, been confirmed by methods that depended more upon injection methods than upon tracing the ducts by dissection.

The Main Pancreatic Duct

As was noted by Baldwin, the main duct is formed in the tail of the gland by the convergence of a number of small duct radicles that have no characteristic arrangement. It then passes to the right towards the head of the gland, running nearer to the dorsal and superior surfaces of the gland than to the ventral and inferior surfaces. In the body of the gland it receives tributaries that join it more or less at right angles, the tributaries from opposite sides alternating in the sites of their junctions. In the head of the gland the main duct inclines sharply downwards and backwards with the convexity towards the right, coming nearer to the posterior surface of the gland. At the level of the major duodenal papilla the duct then usually runs almost horizontally to the right and joins the posterior aspect of the common bile duct to form with it a common orifice upon the major duodenal papilla. In the head of the gland the tributaries of the duct are irregular both in their arrangement and in the angles of their junctions with the main duct; variants in the course of the main duct as it passes through the head of the gland

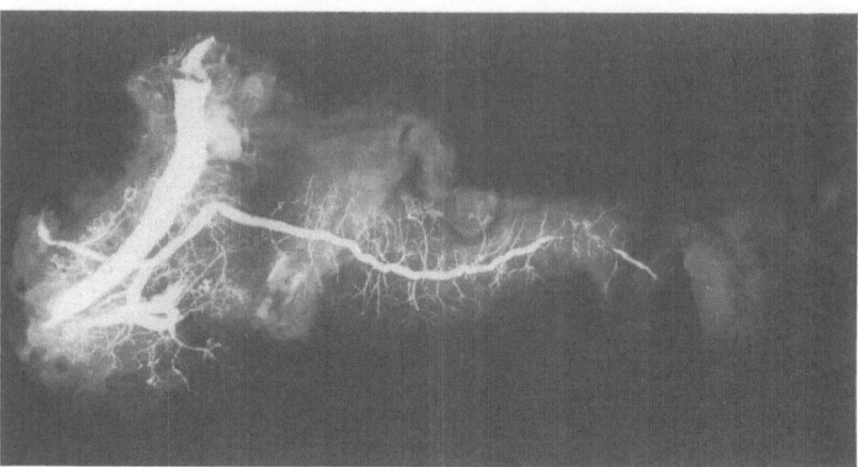

Fig. 1.4. Radiograph of the common bile duct and the pancreatic ducts after injection with barium sulphate. An accessory duct that communicates with the main duct is present and the main duct forms a complete loop in the head of the gland. The pancreas was obtained post-mortem from a woman aged 60, who died of a ruptured aneurysm of the right middle cerebral artery.

are relatively common, and the formation of a common orifice with the bile duct is by no means invariable. In cases of the latter type, the common bile duct and the main pancreatic duct each end on the major duodenal papilla, having been separated by a septum right up to their termination. Baldwin (1911) found that 22% of his cases were of this type, Rienhoff and Pickrell (1945) found that in 24% of their 250 dissections there was no junction of the pancreatic and bile ducts, while Singh (1956) found that, in 30 of the 100 dissections he carried out, the two ducts remained separate. Thus by investigations that relied mainly upon dissection, it was shown that between 20% and 30% of cases may have separate biliary and pancreatic orifices on the duodenal papilla. In Millbourn's studies, however (Millbourn 1950), in which he used injection methods followed by radiography, it was only exceptionally (about one in 20 cases) that there were separate entrances. Somewhat similar results were obtained by Berman et al. (1960), who made vinyl acetate casts of the ducts of pancreases obtained at routine post-mortem examinations and then digested away the glandular tissue. They found that in only 6.2% of their 130 specimens did the main pancreatic duct (duct of Wirsung) and the common bile duct open independently into the duodenum. Such variations in the results obtained by different workers make it clear that there must be many cases in which it is difficult to discriminate between a common orifice and two ducts that open separately but close together. A substantial length of the common channel is relatively uncommon, occurring in only 6.2% of cases according to Berman et al. In such a channel, reflux of bile into the duct system of the

pancreas would clearly be anatomically possible should the duodenal orifice become blocked, but Dawson and Langman (1961) concluded that a common channel as short as 3 mm would make biliary reflux possible. A common channel of 3 mm, or more, in length was found in about half their cases.

It has already been mentioned that variations in the course of the main pancreatic duct through the head of the pancreas are by no means uncommon. One striking variant of the course of the main duct through the head of the pancreas is when the duct forms a complete loop (Figs 1.4–1.5). The looped type of duct was recognised by Baldwin (1911) and Rienhoff and Pickrell (1945) and was demonstrated radiographically in autopsy material by Newman et al. (1958), who also showed that the duct of Wirsung may occasionally form a loop around the common bile duct before entering it. Marked looping of the bile duct is sometimes referred to as the formation of an ansa pancreatica (Dawson and Langman 1961). Some of the numerous variations in the course of the duct are illustrated in Figs 1.6–1.14.

The Accessory Pancreatic Duct

An accessory pancreatic duct (duct of Santorini) that usually drains the anterior and superior parts of the head of the pancreas is present in between 50% (Millbourn 1950) and over 70% of subjects (Birnstingl 1959–1960). This duct lies more ventrally than the main duct and in most cases there is a communication between the two ducts in the head of the pancreas. The accessory duct may have a duodenal

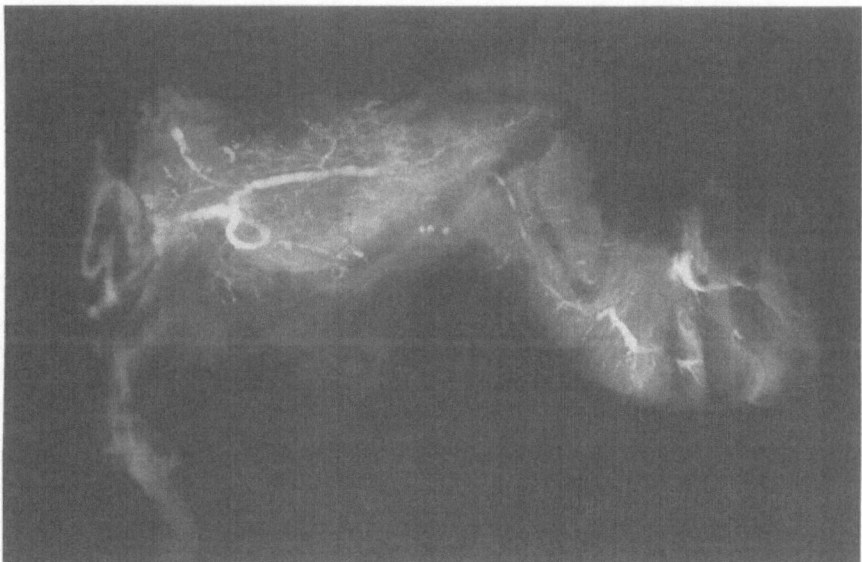

Fig. 1.5. Another example of the formation of a complete loop by the main pancreatic duct. The pancreas was obtained from a woman aged 84, who had died of carcinoma of the colon.

orifice of its own at the minor duodenal papilla (Figs 1.2–1.4), but, in some of the accessory ducts that reach the minor duodenal papilla, the orifice at the duodenal end may not be patent. The accessory duct then acts entirely as a tributary to the main pancreatic duct. In other cases a large tributary to the main duct (Fig. 1.7), may represent an accessory duct that has failed to establish independent drainage into the duodenum. If an accessory duct has both a patent duodenal orifice and a communication with the main pancreatic duct then there are at least the anatomical arrangements for an alternative route by which pancreatic secretion might reach the duodenum should the orifice of the main duct be blocked. In a small number of cases the main pancreatic duct has undergone atrophy by post-foetal life and the secretion from the whole gland reaches the duodenum at the minor papilla. The minor papilla is

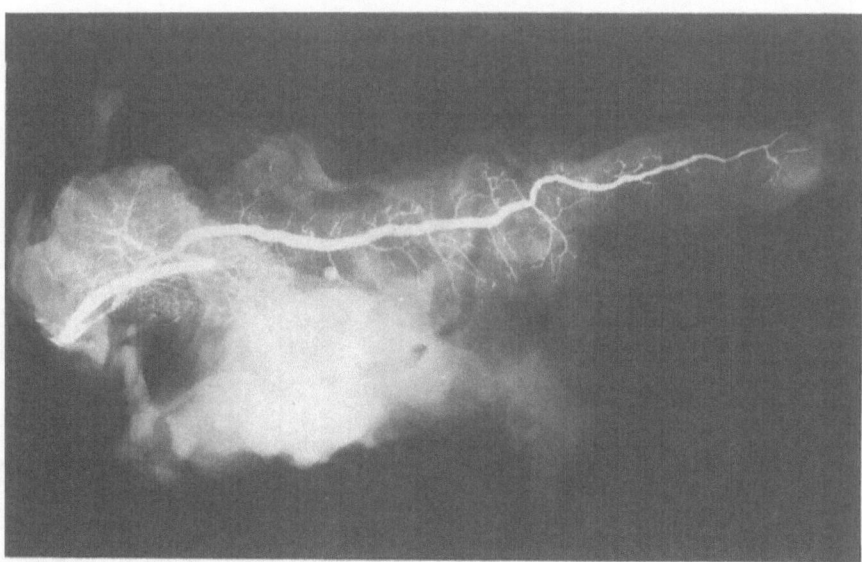

Fig. 1.6. Radiograph after the injection of the pancreatic ducts with barium sulphate. An accessory duct communicates with the main duct and appears to have discharged close to the orifice of the main duct at the duodenal papilla.

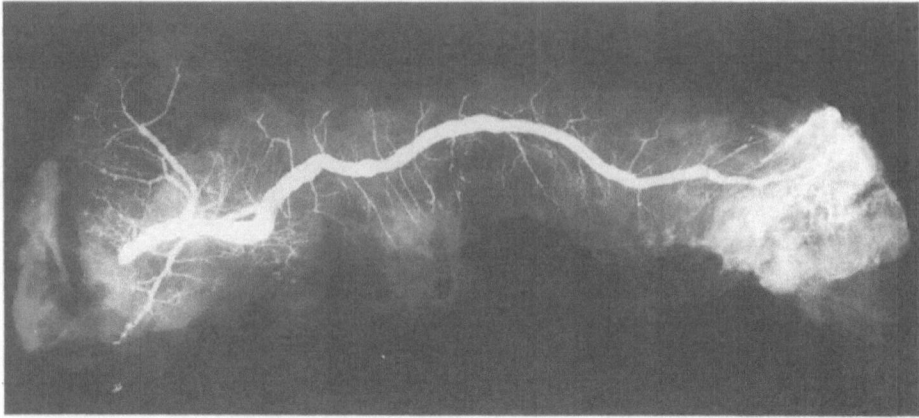

Fig. 1.7. Radiograph of the ducts after the injection of barium sulphate. In this case a duct that probably represents an embryonic duct that might have formed an accessory duct has become instead a tributary of the main duct.

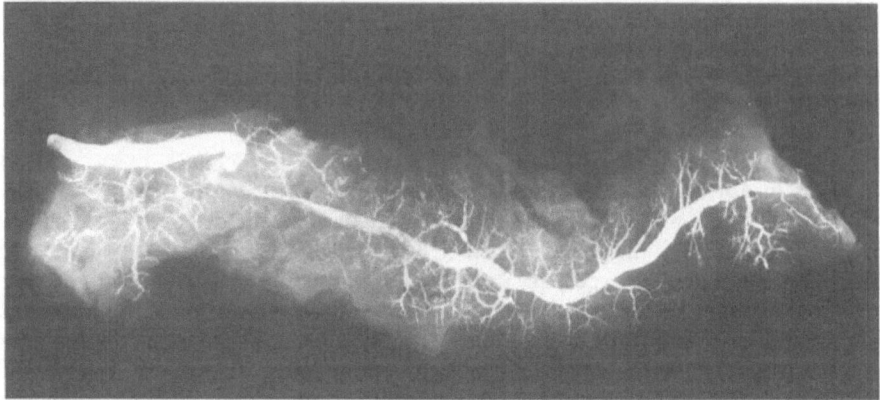

Fig. 1.8. Radiograph after injection of the pancreatic ducts with barium sulphate. Although lymph nodes that contained metastatic carcinoma from a carcinoma of the colon were present at the upper border of the pancreas the only recognisable filling defect is more likely to be associated with the superior mesenteric vessels than with the enlarged lymph nodes.

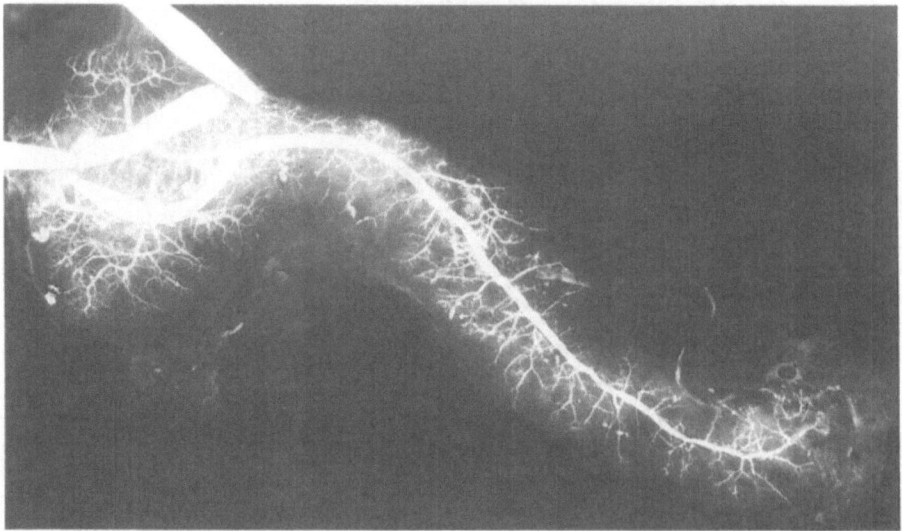

Fig. 1.9. Radiograph after the common bile duct and pancreatic ducts had been injected with barium sulphate. There is no accessory duct and a large tributary joins the main duct near the site where an accessory duct sometimes communicates. Calcification is present in the walls of the superior mesenteric and splenic arteries.

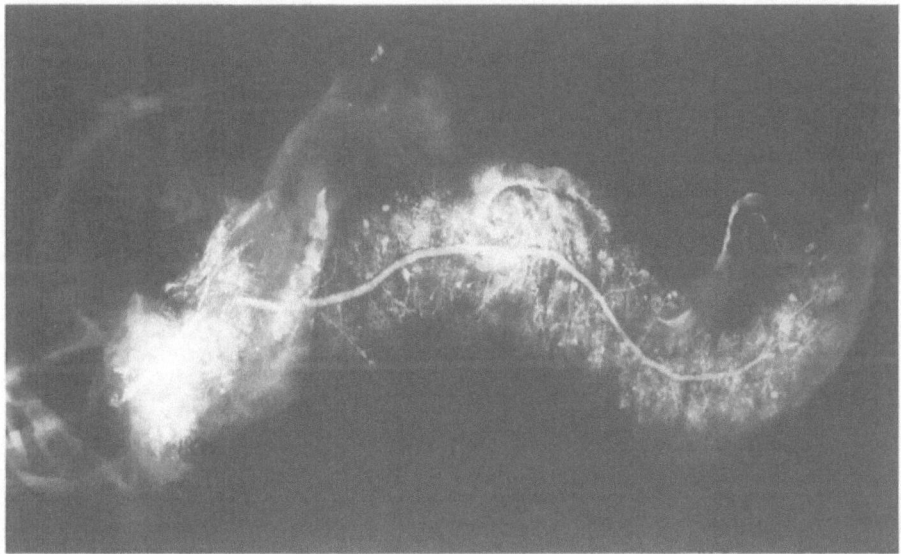

Fig. 1.10. In this radiograph, taken after injection of the pancreatic ducts with barium sulphate, there is an obvious filling defect in the duct system near the markedly calcified superior mesenteric artery. Calcification is also present in the wall of the splenic artery.

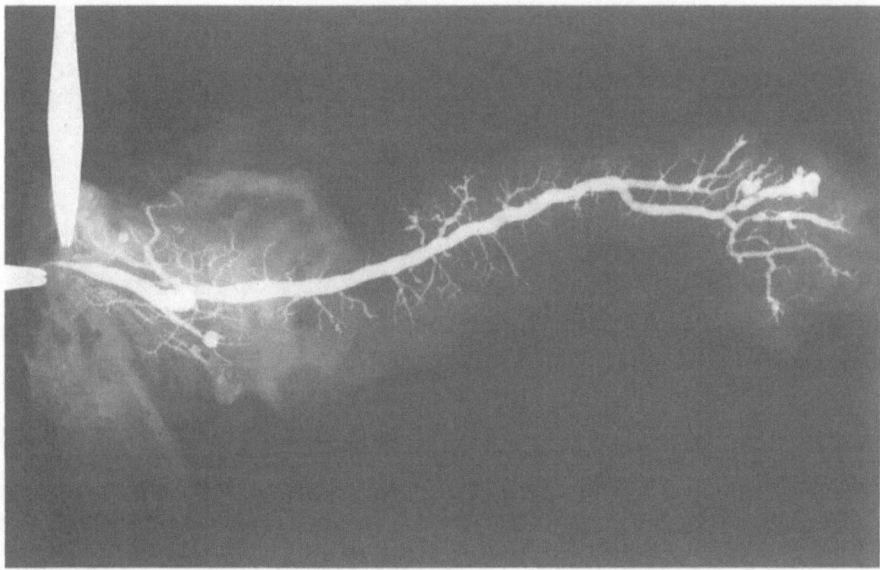

Fig. 1.11. In this radiograph of the pancreas after injection of the ducts with barium sulphate there is filling of only the main ducts and their major tributaries. Some of the "cysts" noted by Kreel and Sandin (1973) are present near the head and in the tail.

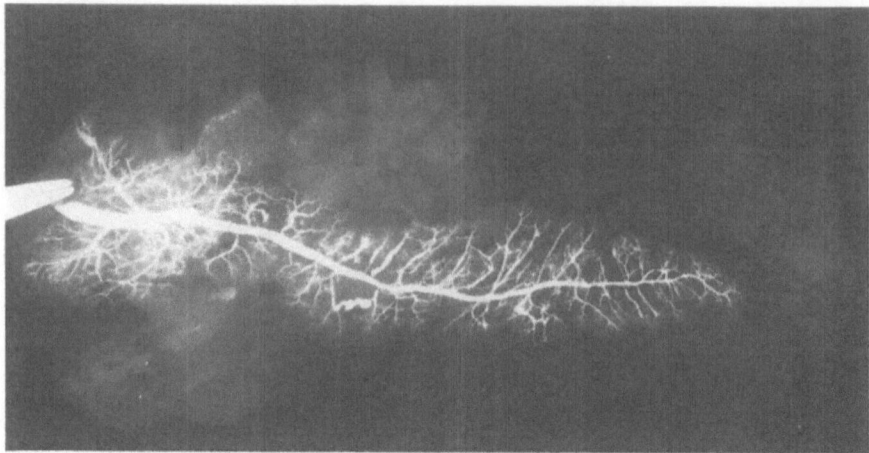

Fig. 1.12. Radiograph of the injected duct system in a woman aged 62, who died of a myocardial infarction. There is no accessory duct and there is an apparent absence of ducts near the partially calcified superior mesenteric artery.

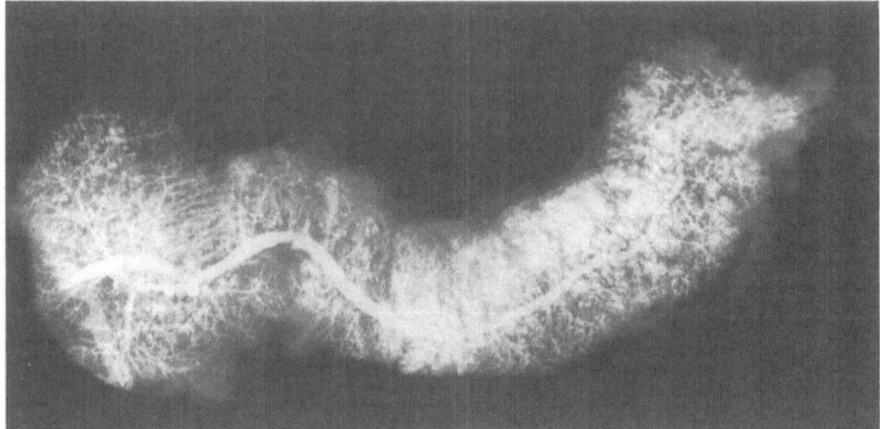

Fig. 1.13. Radiograph of a pancreas after the ducts had been injected with barium sulphate. In this case the injection has entered the glandular acini, perhaps as a result of autolysis of the gland.

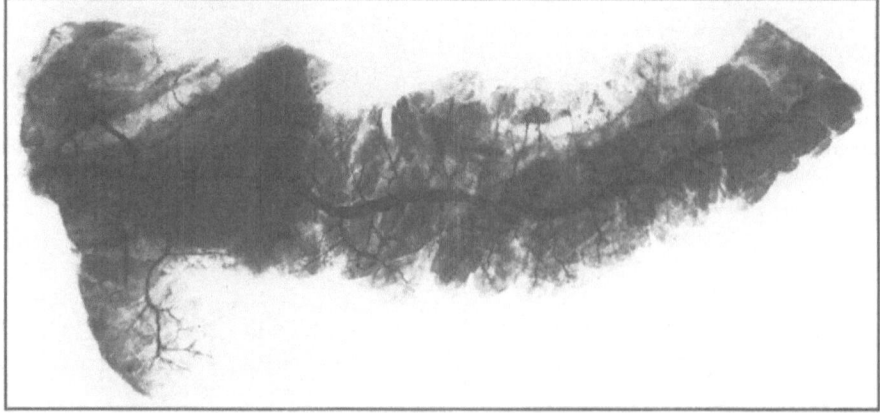

Fig. 1.14. The duct system of the pancreas demonstrated by the injection of vinyl acetate into the ducts from the tail of the gland, which has now been removed, followed by clearing of the gland in methyl salicylate. The clearing process took about a year.

usually situated about 2 cm (Baldwin 1911) proximal (cephalad) to the major papilla on the duodenal mucosa and on a plane ventral to the major papilla. It is easy to recognise the major papilla, but the minor papilla, though sometimes easily found, may be very inconspicuous. It could be identified, however, in each of the 100 specimens studied by Baldwin.

It is not surprising that there is some variation in the incidence of the various types of ductal arrangement found by different authors. The duct that drains the tail and body of the pancreas can easily be recognised and followed by dissection during its relatively straight course towards the head of the pancreas but it becomes much more difficult to follow the duct and to identify its tributaries and communications once it has entered the head of the gland. Injections of dye, latex or radio-opaque material may also give results that are difficult to interpret while unphysiologically high injection pressures, or the injection of a heavy liquid such as mercury, may force open orifices that may not, in fact, be patent.

There seems to be at least some agreement that, in about 90% of pancreases, the sole or main excretory channel is the duct (of Wirsung) that opens at the major duodenal papilla. In about 50%–70% of pancreases, an accessory duct (of Santorini) is present, which may transmit various amounts of secretion, from none up to all the gland's output, into the duodenum at the minor duodenal papilla. All the results seem to show that in most cases the main pancreatic duct joins the common bile duct and discharges through a common orifice. There is agreement also that, in a proportion of cases, the main pancreatic duct and the common bile duct have separate, though adjacent, orifices into the duodenum upon the major papilla. The frequency of such cases varies from an incidence of 20%–30% down to about 5% in the results of various observers. It is agreed also that a Santorini system and a Wirsung system may coexist with separate duodenal orifices and without communications within the gland. In such cases the Santorini system may be larger and more important. When the duct of Santorini is well developed, its course through the head of the gland is in a straight line without the angles or loops that are usual in the course of the duct of Wirsung. Two ducts of Santorini with two minor papillae in the duodenum and with a communication with the major duct system were found in a single case by Berman et al. (1960) in their series of 130 specimens. There is no significant difference between male and female duct patterns.

The presence of multiple minute accessory pancreatic ducts is said by Cross (1956) to be common-place. After examining 400 specimens he concluded that in most specimens the common bile duct in its intrapancreatic and intraduodenal portions is joined by many small ducts of pancreatic origin and that many small pancreatic ducts also enter the lumen of the bowel directly, particularly at the ampulla and in the second portion of the duodenum. It is true that when heterotopic pancreatic tissue, unconnected with the main pancreas, is present in the wall of the duodenum, the small ducts of the heterotopic glandular tissue discharge directly into the duodenum but ducts of the type described by Cross have not been recognised by most workers.

Pancreas Divisum

Rokitansky (1849) referred to the rare occurrence of a double pancreas, but in more recent times the term pancreas divisum has been given to the type of pancreas in which the two ductal systems do not unite or communicate. In this situation, the duct of Wirsung, normally the main duct, may be very small (no more than 1–2 cm in length), while the duct of Santorini, draining into the duodenum at the minor papilla, provides the main ductal system. The clinical significance of pancreas divisum will be discussed more fully in the chapter on malformations of the pancreas (pp. 30–31).

Interpretation of Pancreatograms

The development of pancreatography as a clinical procedure following cannulation of the biliary and pancreatic ducts endoscopically prompted various workers to obtain pancreatograms at routine postmortem examinations in subjects without known pancreatic disease, to establish the appearances of normal pancreatograms.

Birnstingl (1959–1960) undertook a combined radiographic and histological study to assess the anatomical variations that might influence the interpretation of pancreatograms obtained during operations upon patients with pancreatic disease. He found that the main pancreatic duct showed variations in calibre that ranged between 1.8 and 9.2 mm; he recommended caution in the interpretation of apparent dilatation of the ducts in pancreatograms. Birnstingl found that, in 10% of his 150 specimens, the main duct had a diameter of more than 6 mm. He found also that fusiform dilatation of the terminal part of the main pancreatic duct was a common normal variant with no associated histological abnormality, as was apparent stenosis of the duct at the level of the neck of the pancreas. In the secondary pancreatic ducts, dilatation and irregularity were common and closely reflected hyperplastic and metaplastic changes in the ductal epithelium.

With the advent of fibre-optic equipment that made it possible to cannulate the ampulla of Vater endoscopically, Kreel et al. (1973) were prompted to undertake a radiographic study of the pancreas at autopsy to ascertain its anatomical variations and to familiarise themselves with the normal ductular pattern. While the organs were still in place in the body, the duodenum was opened and the pancreatic duct was cannulated and injected with barium sulphate: radiographs were then obtained. In the 77 cases in which the procedure was carried out successfully there was great variation in size, shape and position of the pancreas and its ducts. Thus, although the head of the pancreas lay to the right of the spinal column in most cases, it lay directly on the spine in a significant number, and in a few (5%) it lay to the left of the spine. The level of the papilla of Vater also varied considerably from the usual levels between the second to the fourth lumbar vertebrae. In one case it was at the level of the body of the first lumbar vertebra, while in another it was as low as the level of the second sacral vertebra. It is, of course, well known that levels ascertained in a supine cadaver may not represent the levels that exist during life with the subject in the erect position, and the involvement of the pancreas in general enteroptosis (Glénard's disease) was recognised as long ago as 1903 by Keith.

Using their radiographs, the authors described the shape of the pancreas as being either oblique or L-shaped in the majority of their cases. Less often it was sigmoid horseshoe-shaped, or, occasionally transverse, and in a single case, an inverted V. Some of these shapes are illustrated in Figs 1.1–1.14.

Variations in the duct size and shape were common. In nine cases there was a distinct loop near the proximal end of the major duct (see Fig. 1.4). The width of the proximal part of the duct, as measured on the radiograph taken with the pancreas in situ, was less than 3 mm in 26%, 3–6 mm in 50% and 6–9 mm in 19% of the cases. In one normal pancreas it was slightly over 9 mm and in two pancreases, in which carcinoma of the head had caused almost complete obstruction of the duct, the width was also slightly over 9 mm.

Filling of an accessory duct was found in 24%. The accessory duct lay above the main duct in all but two cases. Although the accessory duct in one of these cases lay below the main duct, it ran across it to open into the duodenum at the minor papilla.

A filling defect in the duct system in the parts of the pancreas that lay close to the superior mesenteric vessels was common and was present in 44% of the cases. This filling defect has been found also by the authors and is illustrated in Figs 1.1–1.5. Deficient filling of the ducts near the splenic artery was noted by Kreel et al. (1973) in 5% of their cases. Primary or secondary carcinoma in the pancreas itself or in adjacent lymph nodes also caused filling defects. In one case separation of the peripheral lobules in the radiograph was found to be due to fatty infiltration.

The Effects of Age in Relation to Pancreatography

The effects of ageing upon the width of the pancreatic ducts was studied by Kreel and Sandin (1973) by retrograde pancreatography at necropsy in 120 cases. They found that the main pancreatic duct increased in width along its whole length at about 8% per decade and that in the elderly, widths of 1 cm can occur in the main duct in the head of the pancreas in the complete absence of obstruction. Ductular ectasia also tends to occur in the interlobular ductules and intralobular ductules, with the formation of cysts 1–2 cm in diameter. Narrowing of segments of the ducts with no recognisable stricture was also found. The length of the main duct was not found to be affected by ageing. Amongst findings that the authors considered to be unrelated to age was the presence of a loop on the main duct; this was present in 18% of cases. An accessory duct was present in 28% of cases, and a completely separate opening of the pancreatic duct from that of the common bile duct in 6% of cases. The presence of a filling defect in the duct system of the pancreas in the vicinity of the superior mesenteric vessels was unrelated to age.

The effects of age were found to complicate the interpretation of retrograde pancreatograms in the autopsy room preparations studied by Schmitz-Moormann et al. (1985). Their material consisted of 69 pancreases from cases without clinical or histological evidence of chronic pancreatitis that had their ducts injected through the duodenal papilla with contrast medium in the post-mortem room, and five pancreases from cases of chronic pancreatitis that had been injected similarly. A panel of six clinicians, all experienced in the interpretation of endoscopic retrograde pancreatograms, recognised all the cases of chronic pancreatitis but also made a false-positive diagnosis of chronic pancreatitis in 81% of the cases without pancreatitis because of pancreatitis-like lesions in the main duct and its side tributaries. On histological examination, a significant positive correlation was found between such appearances and perilobular fibrosis, which was suspected to be a result of age-dependent intraductal epithelial hyperplasia.

The Weight of the Normal Pancreas and Pancreatic Fat

Like the salivary glands, the pancreas in the well nourished has fat between the glandular lobules; the amount of fat seems to influence the size and shape of the gland, and, as in the salivary glands, replacement by fat may mask atrophy of the secretory tissue. In his study of the normal weight of the pancreas in the adult human being, Schaefer (1926) found in a study of 216 personally collected cases, whose pancreatic weights he analysed statistically, that the mean weight in women was 84.88 g (±14.95 g) and in men 90.31 g (±15.08 g).

Comparison of his findings in American subjects with those found in studies in England led him to suggest that there might be a racial difference between English and American people. He found there was a positive correlation between the normal weight of the adult pancreas and the normal body weight in both sexes, the correlation being higher in the female than in the male. A fairly high negative correlation was established between normal weights for the pancreas and age in the female, but no similar correlation could be established with certainty in the male. There was no correlation between the normal weight of the pancreas and stature in either sex.

Schaefer pointed out that he had carried out the work personally and that the pancreas had been carefully dissected away from all extraneous fatty tissue and large vessels in every case. It is often difficult to weigh the pancreas accurately unless special care is taken. Careful separation from the duodenum is tedious, the superior mesenteric vessels may seem to be embedded in the gland and mesenteric fat and lymph nodes may be intimately attached, while the removal of these structures may be complicated by upper abdominal disease or by obesity; thus the weights recorded for the pancreas

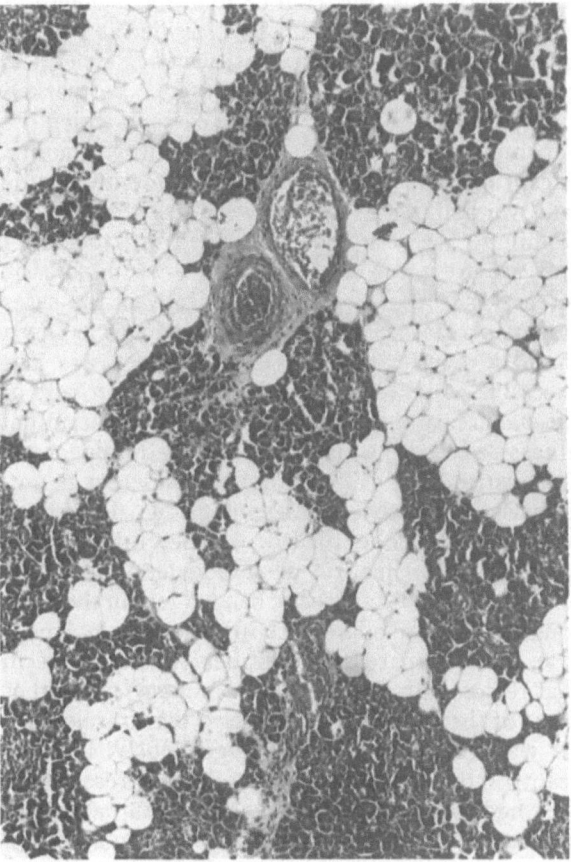

Fig. 1.15. Interlobular fat in a pancreas. Adiposity of such a degree is within the range of normality. H&E, × 60

at routine autopsies tend to be unreliable. Moreover, normal pancreases contain varying amounts of fat (Fig. 1.15). Ogilvie (1933) devised a method for the measurement of the islets of Langerhans that involved the incidental measurement of the percentage of adipose tissue that was present. He found that in a group of 19 non-obese subjects, eight male and 11 female, the average adipose component of the pancreas was 9.3%, while in a group of 19 obese subjects, all but two of which were female, the average adipose component was 17.1% with a scatter from 0 to 48.5%. More recently, the amount of fat in pancreases obtained at routine autopsies has been studied by Olsen (1978) in relation to the age and obesity of the subjects. One section of a block of tissue from the body of the pancreas in each of 394 cases was assessed microscopically and graded, according to the number of fat cells that were seen, into four grades. Sections in which only a few scattered fat cells were present in the exocrine parenchyma were classified as grade 1, while sections with partial or total replacement of the exocrine lobules by fat were classified as grade 4; intermediate degrees of adiposity were classified as grades 2 or 3. Cases in which there was marked autolysis were excluded, as were cases in which the pancreas contained primary or secondary tumours. Except for one, all the pancreases contained some fat. Over half the cases (51%) were assigned to grade 1, while 26% were assigned to grade 2, 15% to grade 3 and 8% to grade 4. No evidence of pancreatic disease had been recognised clinically in the cases with pancreases classified as grades 3 and 4. Olsen found a significant correlation between age and excessive body weight and the grade of fattiness of the pancreas, and also that a prolonged terminal illness reduced the amount of fat in the pancreas. The distribution of fat within the pancreas is not, however, entirely homogeneous as has been observed by Orci et al. (1979). They undertook a quantitative evaluation of adipocytes in the posterior part of the pancreatic head, a region they had found to be particularly rich in pancreatic polypeptide, and compared the number of adipocytes in that region with the number of adipocytes in other parts of the pancreas. They found that intralobular fat was not distributed homogeneously, it being scanty in the area of the head of the pancreas, where they had found the lobules to be rich in pancreatic polypeptide when compared with the remainder of the pancreas, but that extralobular fat was distributed homogeneously throughout the pancreas.

The studies that have been quoted above should make it clear that the variable amount of fat that is normally present in the pancreas makes it very difficult to recognise either hypertrophy or atrophy of the pancreatic parenchyma by simple weighing of the organ. The masking of atrophy of the glandular tissue by fatty replacement will be referred to later when pancreatic atrophy is discussed.

The weight of the pancreas in the final months of pre-natal life, at birth and in the first year following birth has been studied by Schulz et al. (1962), along with the weights of the other main organs of the foetus and infant. They found that in five male foetuses at the 5th month of gestation, the mean weight of the pancreas was 2.1 g, and in four female foetuses at the same gestational age, the mean weight was 1.4 g. In 91 male infants that were born alive at term but who lived for less than 1 week, the mean weight of the pancreas was 5.3 g (standard deviation 3.2, standard error of the mean 0.4) and in 55 liveborn female infants of the same age the mean weight was 5.6 g (standard deviation (SD) 2.8, standard error of the mean (SEM) 0.4). At the end of the first year after birth the mean weight of the pancreas in 19 male infants was 14 g (SD 6.0, SEM 1.6), and in 15 female infants 15 g (SD 8.0, SEM 2.7).

References

Baldwin WM (1911) The pancreatic ducts in man, together with a study of the microscopical structure of the minor duodenal papilla. Anat Rec 5:197–228

Berman LG, Prior JT, Abramow SM, Ziegler DD (1960) A study of the pancreatic duct system in man by the use of vinyl acetate casts of post mortem preparations. Surg Gynecol Obstet 110:391–403

Birnstingl M (1959–1960) A study of pancreatography. Br J Surg 47:128–139

Cross KR (1956) Accessory pancreatic ducts. Arch Pathol 61:434–440

Dawson W, Langman J (1961) An anatomical-radiological study of the pancreatic duct pattern in man. Anat Rec 139:59–64

Keith A (1903) On the nature and anatomy of enteroptosis (Glénard's disease). Lancet i:629–640

Kreel L, Sandin B (1973) Changes in pancreatic morphology associated with aging. Gut 14:962–970

Kreel L, Sandin B, Slavin G (1973) Pancreatic morphology, a combined radiological and pathological study. Clin Radiol 24:154–161

Lytle WJ (1959–1960) The common bile-duct groove in the pancreas. Br J Surg 47:209–212

Millbourn E (1950) On the excretory ducts of the pancreas in man, with special reference to their relations to each other, to the common bile duct and to the duodenum. Acta Anat 9:1–34

Newman HF, Weinberg SB, Newman EB, Northup JD (1958) The papilla of Vater and distal portions of the common bile duct and duct of Wirsung. Surg Gynecol Obstet 106:687–694

Ogilvie RF (1933) The islands of Langerhans in 19 cases of obesity. J Pathol Bacteriol 37:473–481

Olsen TS (1978) Lipomatosis of the pancreas in autopsy material and its relation to age and overweight. Acta Microbiol Scand Sect A 86:367–373

Orci L, Stefan Y, Malaisse-Lagae F, Perrelet A, Patel Y (1979) Pancreatic fat. N Engl J Med 301:1292

Rienhoff WF, Pickrell KL (1945) Pancreatitis: an anatomic study of the pancreatic and extrapancreatic biliary systems. Arch Surg 51:205–219

Rokitansky C (1849) A manual of pathological anatomy, vol. 2. Translated by Sieveking E. The Sydenham Society, London, p 177

Schaefer JH (1926) The normal weight of the pancreas in the adult human being: a biometric study. Anat Rec 32:119–132

Schmitz-Moormann P, Himmelmann GW, Brandes J-W et al. (1985) Comparative radiological and morphological study of human pancreas. Pancreatitis like changes in postmortem ductograms and their morphological pattern. Possible implications for ERCP. Gut 26:406–414

Schulz DM, Giordano DA, Schulz DH (1962) Weights of organs of fetuses and infants. Arch Pathol 74:244–250

Singh I (1956) Observation on the mode of termination of the bile and pancreatic ducts: anatomical factors in pancreatitis. J Anat Soc India 5:54–60

Stern CD (1986) A historical perspective of the accessory duct of the pancreas, the ampulla of Vater and pancreas divisum. Gut 27:203–212

2 Normal Microscopic Structure

The exocrine pancreas is a compound acinar gland, that is, it is formed by the branching of its main duct into subdivisions into which secretory units discharge their product. The secretory unit is the acinus and groups of acini form lobules that are surrounded by, and separated from neighbouring lobules by, delicate connective tissue septa (Fig. 2.1). Each acinus consists of a single layer of pyramidal broad-based cells that rest upon a basal lamina. The nucleus of the acinar cells lies towards the base of the cell and the basophilic cytoplasm towards the lumen of the acinus contains zymogen granules that are acidophilic and refractile (Fig. 2.2). The secretion of the acinus enters its lumen and is drained into the duct system by ductules that begin within the acinus as the centro-acinar cells. These are inconspicuous in routinely stained sections but they can be demonstrated by various techniques by which their staining reaction can be made to contrast with that of the acinar cells (Fig. 2.2).

The centro-acinar cells form part of the lining of the lumen of the acinus, which is lined in part by acinar cells only, and in part by acinar and centro-acinar cells mixed. While still within the acinus, the centro-acinar cells form an intra-acinar ductule by which the secretion of the acinar cells is conveyed to intercalated ducts, which, in turn, deliver the secretion to intralobular ducts that lead to interlobular ducts and, eventually, to the main duct or ducts. The three-dimensional reconstruction of the normal human pancreas carried out by Akao et al. (1986) has, however, shown that the above description is an over-simplification. They found that acini may be

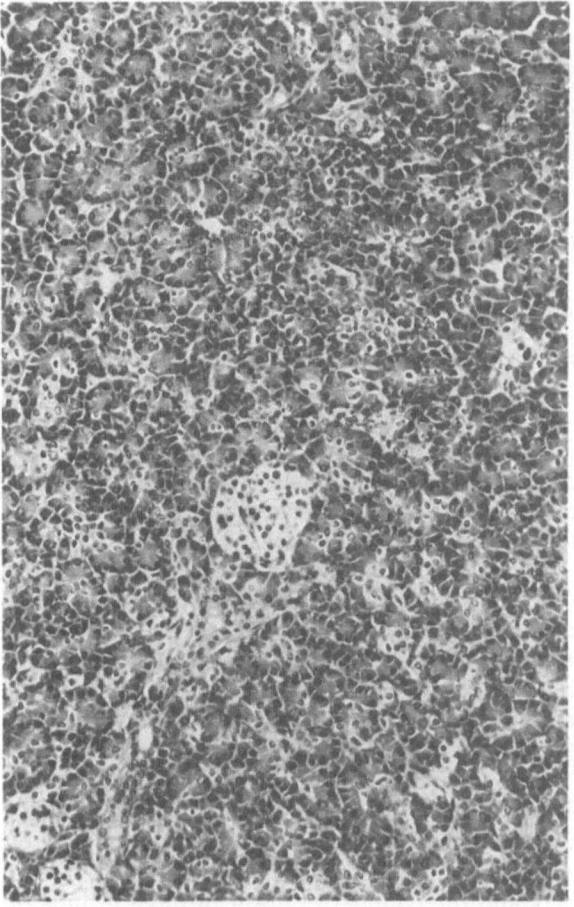

Fig. 2.1. Normal pancreas. Acini occupy most of the field but an islet of Langerhans is present near the centre. H&E, × 200

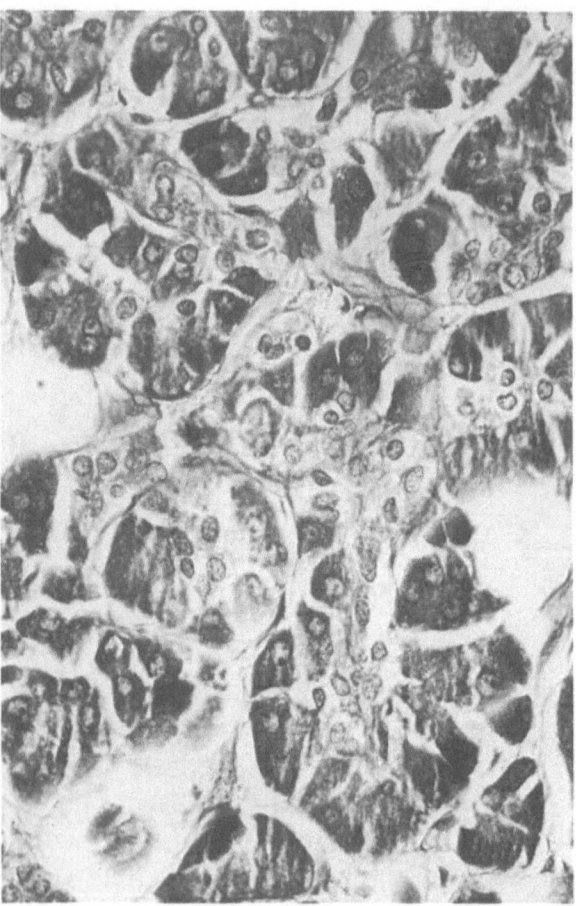

Fig. 2.2. Normal pancreas with dark-staining acinar cells and paler centro-acinar cells, some of which are in continuity with the cells of the intercalated ducts. Schiff–Unna–Pappenheim, ×600

interpolated between ducts and that lumina may form anastomotic loops surrounded by combinations of acinar and ductal cells.

It is stated by Hollender et al. (1983) that a certain proportion of the secretion of the acinar cells escapes from the acinus where the centro-acinar cells have not yet formed a complete ductule. It then enters the interstitial tissue of the pancreas to be removed by the lymphatics. The latter begin as periacinar and perilobular capillary networks that drain to the lymphatic vessels that lie alongside the blood vessels in the interlobular septa to reach the surface of the gland on which there is an anastomotic network of lymphatics. Beyond the surface of the gland the lymphatics drain through groups of lymph nodes of increasing size to join the intestinal lymph trunks that lead to the receptaculum chyli.

Ultrastructurally, the acinar cells contain an abundance of organelles, whereas the centro-acinar cells have an electron-lucent cytoplasm with few organelles. It has been suggested by Walters (1965) that the centro-acinar cells may act as reserve cells that can proliferate and mature to replace damaged or effete acinar, ductular or islet cells. Centro-acinar cells have been suggested also to be the cells that line the loculi of cystadenomas of the pancreas (Becker et al. 1965), while the experiments of Pour (1980) suggest their possible importance in the genesis of other, more common, types of pancreatic tumours.

On examination with the electron microscope the acinar cells are seen to have abundant endoplasmic reticulum in their basal parts and zymogen granules towards their apices. Ribosomes in groups are attached to the endoplasmic reticulum and there are also free ribosomes (Fig. 2.3). Mitochondria are found peripherally near the cell membranes. Some microvilli project from the apical cell border, and adjacent acinar cells are attached by junctional complexes that have been described in detail by Dixon (1979). The zymogen granules are electron dense and vary in size, the larger ones being 1.5 μm in diameter; they are limited by a smooth membrane and no internal structure can be distinguished (Fig. 2.3). Material, thought to represent earlier stages in the formation of zymogen granules, can sometimes be seen in the Golgi complexes that usually lie in a supranuclear position. The nuclei of the acinar cells are single, spherical and have a double nuclear membrane, inside which the chromatin, which is dispersed in the more central parts of the nucleus, becomes condensed.

Ultrastructurally the centro-acinar cells (Fig. 2.4) have nuclei that resemble those of the acinar cells but their cytoplasm contains little identifiable endoplasmic reticulum, only a few scattered ribosomes and some mitochondria. They have a few microvilli on their free borders. They closely resemble the cells of the intercalated ducts.

The main pancreatic duct is lined by tall columnar epithelial cells. Less tall columnar cells and cubical cells line the interlobular and intralobular ducts respectively, while the intercalated ducts are lined by low cuboidal cells. Argentaffin cells are found occasionally among the columnar cells of the larger ducts and their presence may explain the origin of the carcinoid tumours that have been reported as a rare type of pancreatic neoplasm (Peart et al. 1963).

The epithelial cells that line the pancreatic ducts secrete mucinous material and they have been classified by Roberts and Burns (1972) into four different types according to the histochemical reactions of their mucins. The cells that line the intralobular ducts are classified as type I; they

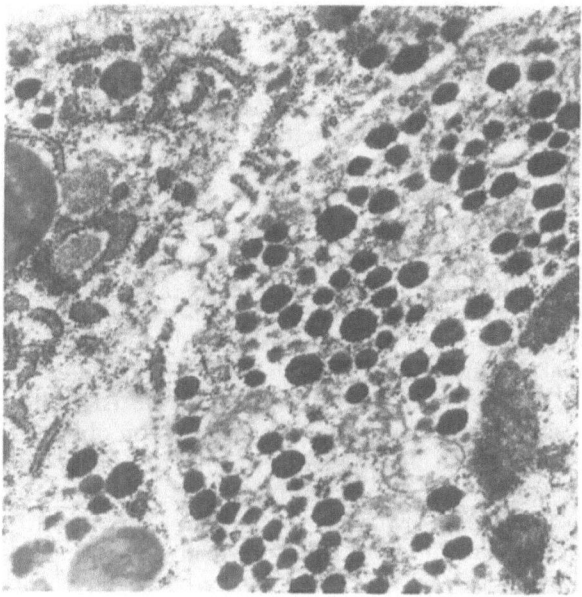

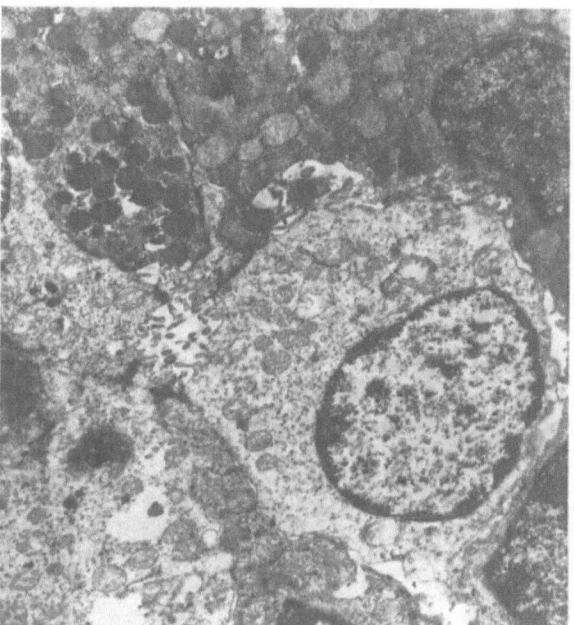

Fig. 2.3. Electron micrograph of a pancreatic acinar cell. Part of the nuclear membrane is visible. The cytoplasm contains zymogen granules and rough endoplasmic reticulum. × 28 000

Fig. 2.4. Electron micrograph of a centro-acinar cell. The cytoplasm contains mitochondria but zymogen granules are absent. A few microvilli can be seen. × 7000

secrete a sulphonated, periodate-reactive glycoprotein. The interlobular ducts are lined by type II and type III cells. The type II cells are low columnar cells and their secretion differs from that of the type I cells in that it contains either fewer sulphonate groups or more neutral glycoprotein. Type III cells are tall columnar cells that secrete a neutral periodate-reactive glycoprotein, while type IV cells are goblet cells and are present in small groups in the larger interlobular ducts. The latter cells were found in only four out of ten biopsies and, although the pancreases were believed to be normal, their presence may have been due to metaplasia. Their mucin is thought to be a weakly sulphonated periodate-reactive sialomucin and was histochemically similar to the mucin found in four mucus-secreting carcinomas of the pancreas. In general, the mucin secreted by the cells of the smaller ducts is sulphonated glycoprotein, but, as the size of the ducts increases, there is less sulphonated mucin in their lining cells, which then tend to secrete more neutral glycoprotein and sialomucin.

The material studied by Roberts and Burns consisted of surgical specimens from ten normal pancreases and of three normal pancreases obtained during autopsies in which the preservation was good. This relatively small collection may not have included all the possible normal variants but the findings are of interest in relation to the studies of

metaplasia and dysplasia of the ductal epithelium that will be discussed later.

The ultrastructure of the cells that form the intercalated ducts is similar to that of the centro-acinar cells, and the interlobular ducts are also lined by cells that are poor in cytoplasmic organelles other than mitochondria. They have interdigitating lateral cell membranes and occasional cilia that project into the lumen of the duct.

The Islets of Langerhans

The endocrine cells of the pancreas are scattered in clumps throughout the exocrine tissue, and are known as the pancreatic islets, or, in honour of their discoverer, as the islets of Langerhans. They have long been known to secrete insulin and, because of the importance of abnormalities of the secretion of insulin in diabetes mellitus, a great deal of information about the structure and function of the normal islets, and about the abnormalities of their structure and function, has been obtained. The book entitled *The Islets of Langerhans*, edited by Cooperstein and Watkins is a comprehensive review of the information that was available, up to 1981, about the structure, biochemistry, physiology and pathology of the islets.

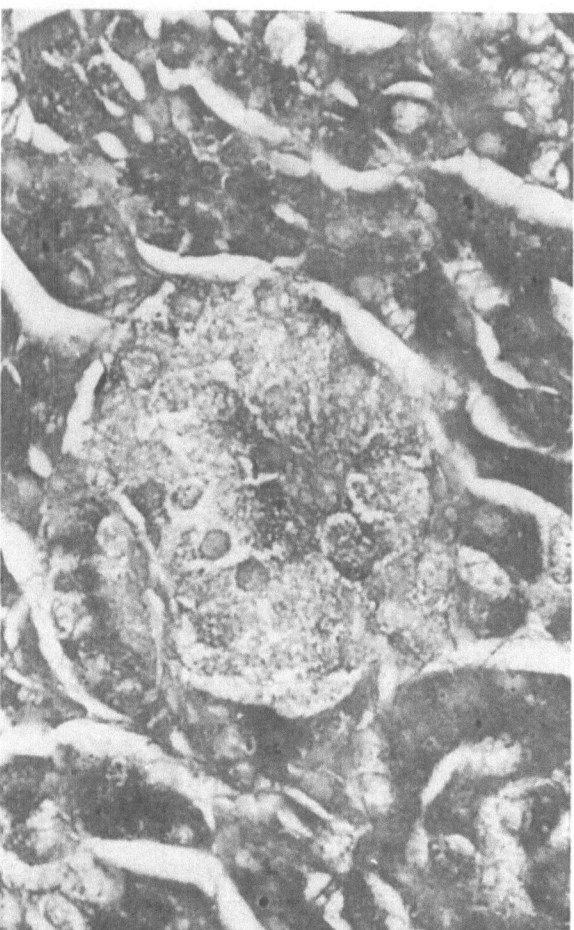

Fig. 2.5. A normal islet of Langerhans stained by Gomori's aldehyde fuchsin method for beta granules. Granules are present in
the cytoplasm of many of the islet cells. × 1000

The islets are highly vascular, with capillaries that
are usually wider than those in the exocrine tissue.
Connections between the vessels of the islets and the
adjacent exocrine tissue allow blood that has passed
through capillaries in contact with the islet cells to
flow next to exocrine glandular tissue where the
effects of the islet hormones are thought to
influence the metabolic activity of the exocrine pancreas (Henderson et al. 1981).

The islet cells are smaller and stain less densely
than the acinar cells and their nuclei are more
closely packed. Until the introduction of immunocytochemical methods, the recognition of the
various cells that make up the islets depended upon
staining methods, of which Gomori's aldehyde
fuchsin was one of the most commonly used. By this
method the granules of the beta cells (B cells) that
secrete insulin, stain a purple colour that may vary
in intensity from very dark to light purple or blue

(Fig. 2.5). The granules of the alpha (A) cells stain
with phosphotungstic acid haematoxylin, or with
the Grimelius silver stain; the alpha cells secrete
glucagon. Another type of islet cell that was first
identified by staining methods and has since been
shown to secrete somatostatin is the delta (D or A_1)
cell, while the PP, or F, cells, which cannot be
demonstrated by ordinary staining methods, have
been identified by their ultrastructure and have
been shown by immunocytochemical staining to
secrete pancreatic polypeptide. It is almost certain
that other types of islet cells exist, but their exact
structure and function has yet to be established.

The ultrastructure of the pancreatic islets has
received much study and the information obtained
up to 1981 has been reviewed by Munger (1981), and
by Klöppel and Lenzen (1984). The latter also
discuss the information obtained by immunocytochemical techniques. In electron micrographs the
most characteristic feature of the beta cells is the
heterogeneous shape of their secretory granules.
The granules have electron-dense cores of variable
shapes within large clear halos inside the smooth
limiting membrane of the granules (Fig. 2.6). At
high magnifications the dense cores have a crystal-
like structure. Beta cells usually have Golgi complexes and rough endoplasmic reticulum; they are
attached to each other and to alpha cells by tight-
and gap-junctions. Ultrastructurally the alpha cells
are more conspicuous than the beta cells because of
the density of the cores of their secretory granules
which are more uniform than those of the beta cells.
The cores lie eccentrically within the secretory granules and are surrounded by a halo that is much less
lucent than the halo that surrounds the cores of the
granules in the beta cells. The granules are usually
concentrated at the secretory pole of the cell. In
delta cells, the somatostatin that these cells have
been shown to secrete is stored in large granules
throughout the cytoplasm of the cells. The granules
have cores of variable electron density and are
closely surrounded by a membrane from which they
are not separated by a halo. PP cells are somewhat
similar ultrastructurally to alpha cells but the granules are said to differ in minor ways. The precise
identification of PP cells, however, depends upon
immunocytochemistry.

Immunocytochemical techniques depend upon
the treatment of sections that may contain peptide-
secreting cells with an antiserum that will become
attached specifically to whatever peptide has been
used as an antigen in the preparation of the antiserum. Cells in which the antiserum has become
attached to the product within the cell can then be
made visible when the sections are examined with
the light microscope. Antisera against insulin,

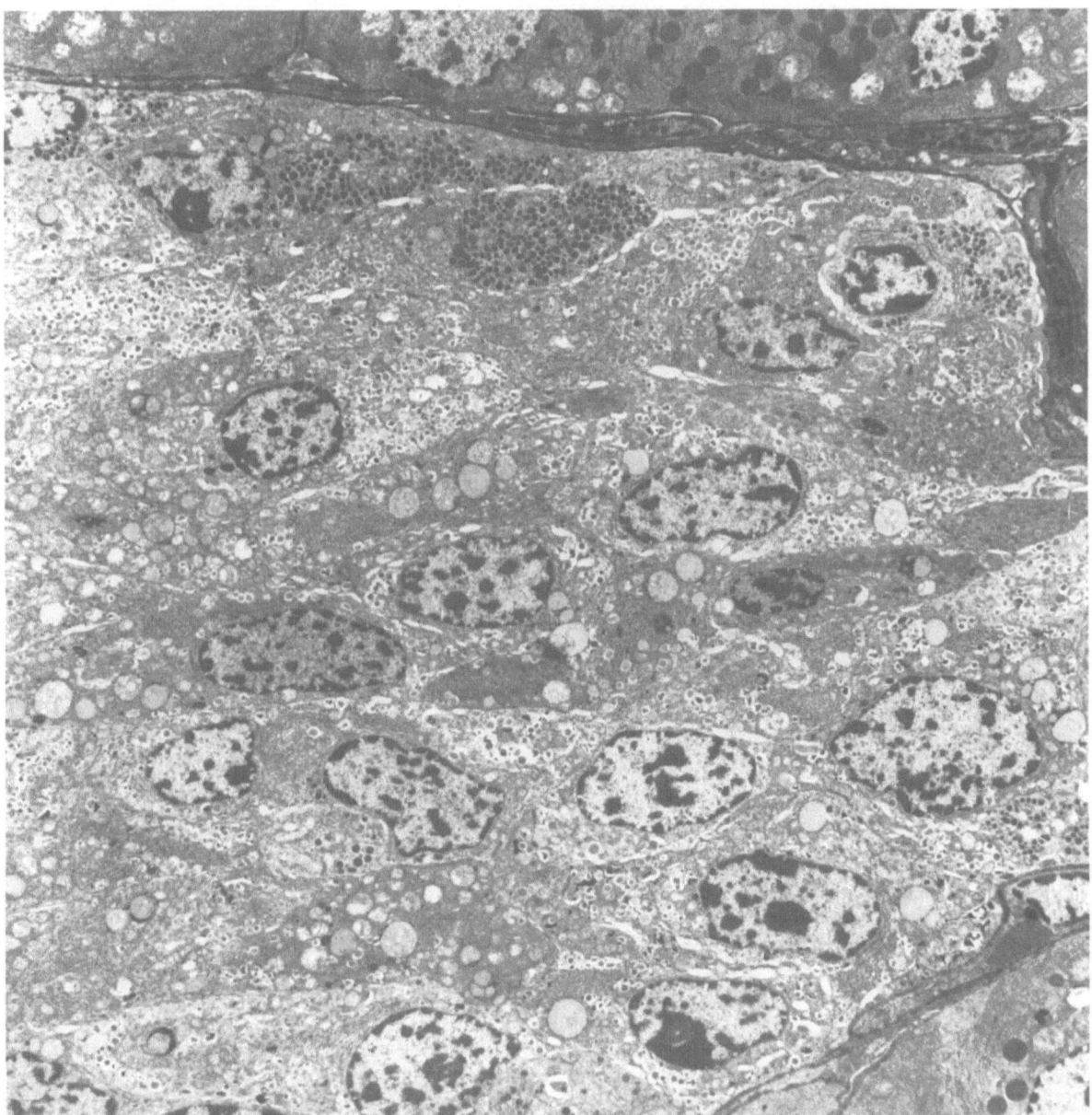

Fig. 2.6. An electron micrograph of a normal pancreatic islet. A single cell contains alpha granules, the cytoplasm of most of the other cells contains the characteristically irregular secretory granules of beta cells. × 3300

glucagon, somatostatin and pancreatic polypeptide have been prepared. When such an antiserum, an anti-insulin serum for example, is applied to a section that contains pancreatic islets then antibody will become attached to intracellular insulin in any beta cells that may be present. If the antibody has been labelled by having had the stable enzyme horseradish peroxidase attached to it, the site of the immune reaction can then be made visible by applying diaminobenzidine, which, in the presence of peroxidase and hydrogen peroxide, will form an insoluble brown polymer that can be seen microscopically. The brown colour will indicate the cells in which the anti-insulin antibody has reacted with insulin. The method can be made more sensitive by various indirect methods that make the site of the immune reaction visible (Heyderman 1979).

The application of such methods has shown that the beta cells tend to be situated in the centre of the islets (Fig. 2.7), alpha cells around the periphery

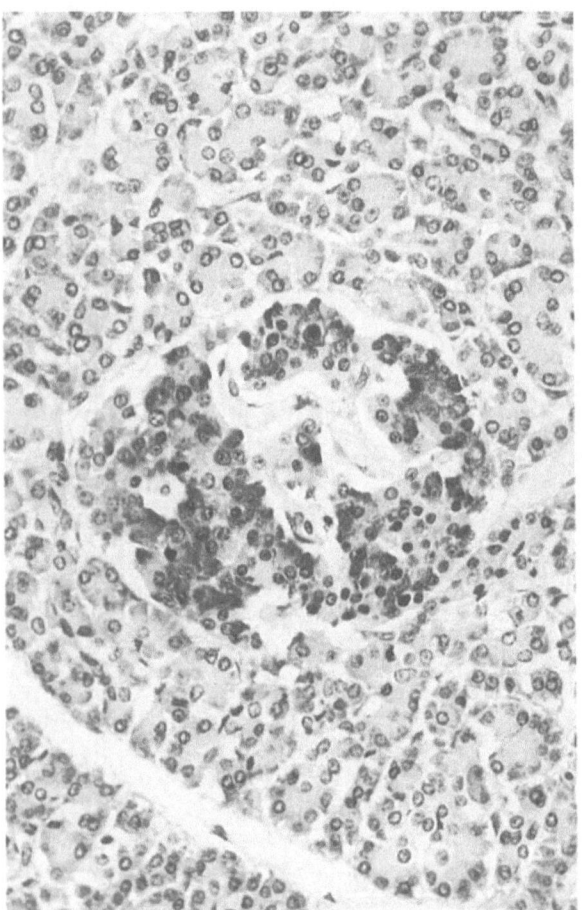

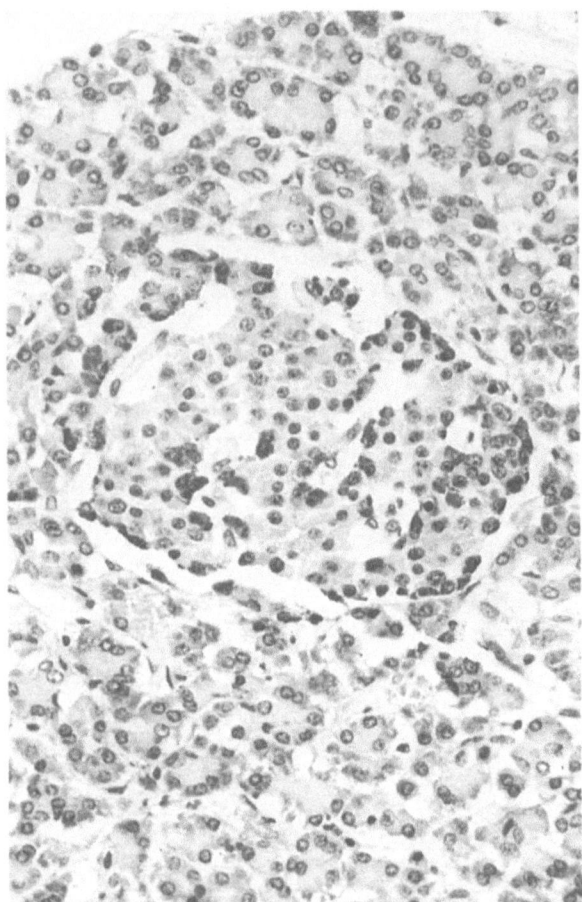

Fig. 2.7. The centre of the field is occupied by an islet that has been treated by an immunoperoxidase method for insulin. The cytoplasm of insulin-secreting cells has stained darkly by the method; such cells are mainly towards the centre of the islet. × 375

Fig. 2.8. The islet in this field has been stained by an immunoperoxidase method for glucagon. The glucagon-positive cells tend to be in the peripheral region of the islet. × 375

(Fig. 2.8) and along capillaries, and delta cells in a paracentral position (Fig. 2.9) where they mingle with alpha cells, while PP cells are found at the periphery (Klöppel and Lenzen 1984). The relative proportions of the types of endocrine cells that make up the islets vary in different parts of the pancreas. For example, the islets in the inferior and posterior parts of the head, areas derived from the ventral primordium, contain a high proportion of PP cells, although such cells are scanty in the islets throughout the rest of the gland. The proportions of the various types also differ somewhat at different ages between birth and maturity (Rahier 1988).

Occasional endocrine cells, other than those organised into islets, have been found in close contact with epithelial cells, both of the centro-acinar type and those lining the ducts (Bendayan 1987).

When islet cells have become neoplastic, the application of immunocytochemical methods allows the normal, or abnormal, peptide hormones that tumours may secrete, to be identified. Neoplastic islet cells have often been shown to secrete peptide hormones that are not produced by normal islet cells.

The Development of the Pancreas

Many descriptions of the embryological development of the pancreas are available. Such descriptions include that by Liu and Potter in 1962, and, more recently, that by McLean (1979), while Like and Orci (1972) and Clark and Grant (1983) have reported the

duct system, the duct of Wirsung, are contributed by the ventral component. The original duct of the dorsal pancreas usually persists as the accessory pancreatic duct, the duct of Santorini. The common variants of the duct system that may be found in adult life were described in the previous chapter, as were the variants of the relationship of the main pancreatic duct to the common bile duct where these two canals open into the duodenum. Although the progress of the development of the pancreas from its dorsal and ventral rudiments has been studied for the most part by reconstructions from serial sections, the progress of the developing pancreas has been demonstrated by dissections carried out by England (1983) in which, under low magnifications, the tiny buds in the embryonic duodenum can be seen, as can the various intermediate positions that they occupy before their eventual incorporation into the pancreas in its final form.

Microscopically, the pancreatic buds consist of epithelial tubules that lengthen and branch as they grow into the adjacent mesenchyme, which differentiates into the fibroblasts that provide the primitive pancreatic stroma. The side branches of the ducts form solid cellular buds that are the first stages in the development of the pancreatic lobules (Figs 2.10, 2.11), but acini cannot be recognised until the foetus has been developing for about 12 weeks, by which time endocrine cells that can be identified by immunocytochemical methods have already been present for 1 or 2 weeks (Heitz et al. 1984). In 1972, Like and Orci carried out their light and electron microscopic study of the development of the pancreatic islets in 20 human embryos and foetuses between 8 and 23 weeks' gestational age. They found that no epithelial structures, other than primitive pancreatic tubules, were present at 8 and 8.5 weeks, but that by 9 weeks alpha cells were identified, followed by delta cells and, somewhat later, at 10.5 weeks, by beta cells. Their impression was that alpha and delta cells were the predominant endocrine cells during early human pancreatic development. It is of interest that other endocrine cells that Like and Orci tentatively identified in the developing human pancreas included serotonin-, gastrin-, epinephrine- and norepinephrine-producing cells. Clark and Grant (1983), using the immunoperoxidase method to identify the endocrine cells in human foetal pancreases, also found that endocrine cells were present at 9 weeks; they found that alpha, beta, PP and delta cells were all present by that time.

Because they were not concerned with foetuses of more than 23 weeks' gestational age, studies of the type that have just been referred to do not confirm an interesting observation made by Liu and Potter in 1962. These workers, in their study of 130 human

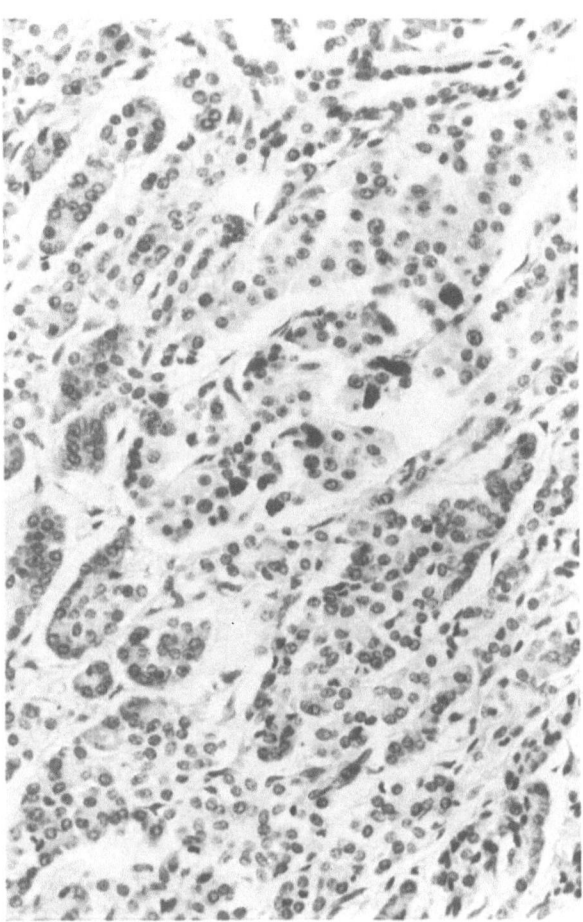

Fig. 2.9. An islet stained by the immunoperoxidase method for somatostatin. × 375

results of their studies of the embryogenesis of the endocrine cells of the human pancreas. In 1984, Pearse also discussed the development of the pancreatic islet cells, and offered evidence that they formed part of a diffuse neuroendocrine system.

There seems to be general agreement that the rudiments of the pancreas are one dorsal and one ventral outgrowth from the abdominal foregut. These appear early in the fifth week of intrauterine life. At first the buds are separate, but the clockwise rotation of the gut that begins during the fifth week of embryonic life leads to the fusion of the smaller ventral bud (part of which atrophies) with the larger dorsal one during the seventh embryonic week; by the eighth week, the ducts of the two structures have anastomosed, the neck, body and tail of the now single organ having been formed from the dorsal component. The head and the widest channel of the

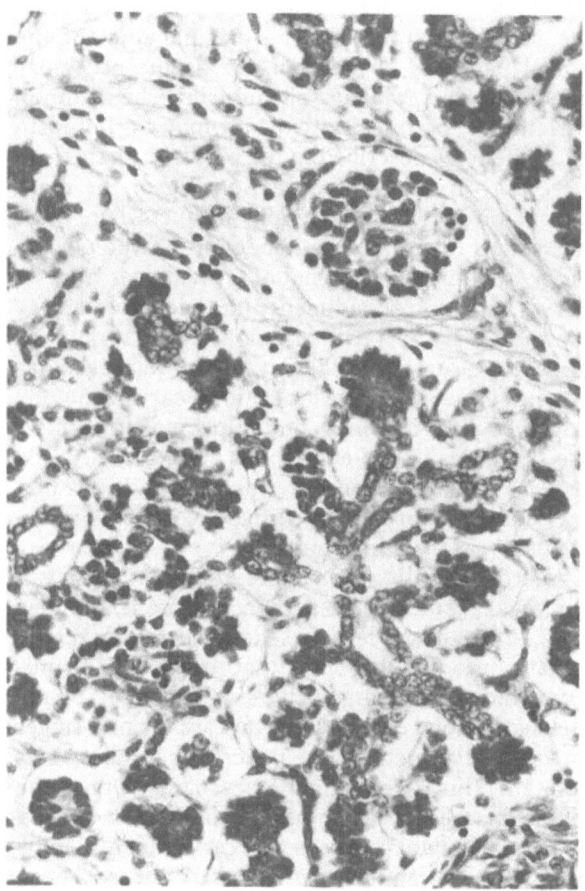

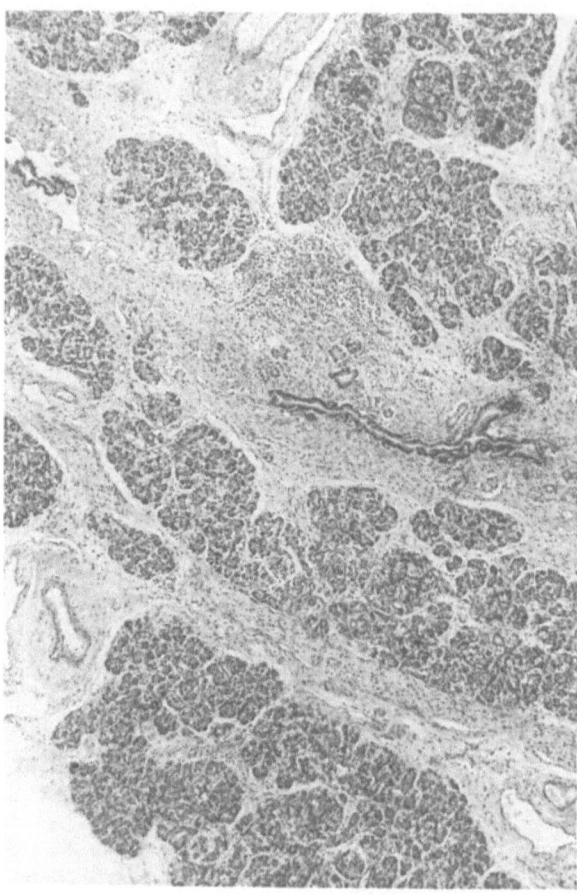

Fig. 2.10. Immature pancreas in a 22-week-old foetus. Tubules and acinar buds are present in a background of loose fibrous tissue. H&E, × 375

Fig. 2.11. Immature pancreas in a 29-week-old foetus. The ducts and lobules of acini lie in abundant interstitial fibrous tissue, parts of which are infiltrated by round cells. H&E, × 60

embryos and foetuses aged between 4 weeks' gestational age and full-term, found that two generations of pancreatic islets appeared during foetal development. They identified primary islets that originated from the primitive pancreatic ducts during the eighth week of gestation and reached maturity during the fifth month, after which they underwent a degeneration that was associated with lymphocytic infiltration of the interlobular connective tissue. The degenerate primary islets were replaced by secondary islets that began to form from the terminal ducts during the third month of gestation and then increased in size and number throughout foetal life to provide the permanent islets.

The abundant literature that deals with the functional development of the pancreatic islets has been reviewed by Baxter-Grillo et al. (1981).

There are many morphological observations to the effect that the pancreatic islets develop from the

pancreatic ductules, and are thus of entodermal origin, but Pearse (1984), who has demonstrated the presence of the neuron-specific gamma-isomer of enolase in islet cells, argues that they must have a neuroectodermal origin and that, with the endocrine cells of the gastrointestinal tract, they form a diffuse neuroendocrine system.

The publications on the development of function in the exocrine component of the foetal and neonatal pancreas have been reviewed by Lebenthal et al. (1986). In the pre-natal stages, homogenates from the pancreas of human foetuses have been studied for the presence of exocrine pancreatic enzymes. The results indicate that very small amounts of lipase and amylase may be present at about 16 weeks of gestation with trypsin appearing at approximately 20 weeks. There is a marked increase in the activity of the exocrine enzymes between 32 weeks of gestation and birth. After birth the digestive enzymes of the pancreas have been investigated in samples of fluid aspirated from the duodenum and the results indicate that it takes about a year for the full complement of pancreatic enzymes to appear, while adult levels are not reached until between 18 months and 2 years of age.

Epithelial Metaplasia and Dysplasia in the Pancreas

The many minor lesions that may be found incidentally in pancreases collected at autopsies upon patients without known pancreatic disease have been recorded by Stamm (1984). The incidence of such lesions increases with increasing age of the patients. Metaplasia of the pancreatic epithelium has attracted the attention of pathologists in relation to the aetiology of both pancreatitis and cancer of the pancreas; it is not uncommon. Rich and Duff (1936), for example, in their study of the pathogenesis of acute haemorrhagic pancreatitis, found metaplasia of the epithelium of the branches of the pancreatic duct in routine sections in 18.6% of 150 consecutive autopsies on individuals over 25 years of age. They believed that the metaplasia led to partial obstruction followed by dilatation of the acini and ductules behind the obstruction. They found metaplasia of the duct epithelium in 13 of 24 cases of haemorrhagic pancreatitis and formed the impression that obstruction caused by metaplasia of the epithelium of the ducts might lead to acinar rupture with escape of secretion. Their opinion was that, although the effect of such rupture was often trivial, it might, in many cases of acute haemorrhagic pancreatitis, have played an important part in the pathogenesis of the disease.

In the pancreatic ducts, the epithelial metaplasia may be a change from the normal columnar epithelial lining of the ducts to one of the mucin-producing goblet cells, or the normal columnar epithelium may be transformed into stratified squamous epithelium (Figs 2.12–2.14). Conversion to the mucin-secreting type of epithelium is the commoner type of metaplasia (Fig. 2.15); this change may occur, not only in the epithelium of the large ducts, but also in that of ductules and acini (Walters 1965). Multilayered squamous metaplasia occurs mainly in the ductules, but, according to Walters, the mechanism of both types of transformation is probably similar. Walters suggested that the pancreatic exocrine parenchyma contains cells capable of proliferation and differentiation in certain direc-

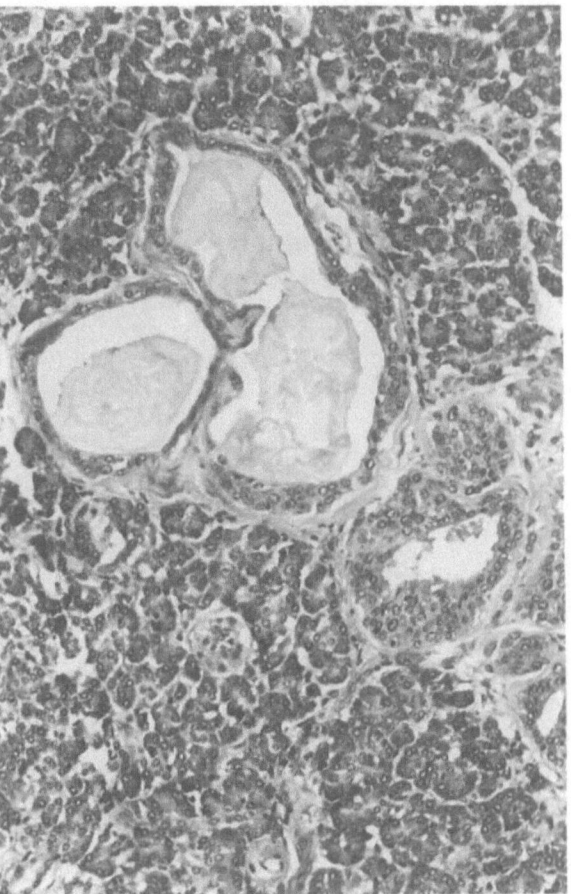

Fig. 2.12. Squamous metaplasia of the lining cells of small ducts, some of which are distended by hyaline secretion found incidentally during an autopsy. H&E, × 150

tions under normal or abnormal conditions. Normally such cells contribute to the replenishment of the lining epithelium of the intercalary ductules, but, under certain conditions such as ductal obstruction, they may also contribute zymogen-producing or even islet cells, while, in the presence of interstitial fibrosis, these proliferating cells may take on goblet cell or, less frequently, squamous cell characteristics. The appearance of goblet cells within the acini was, he believed, due to proliferation and maturation of centro-acinar ductular cells that acted as reserve cells. In the pancreases from 200 almost consecutive necropsies Walters found goblet cell metaplasia of the ductular, and sometimes of the acinar, epithelium in 55 instances, whereas squamous metaplasia occurred only ten times.

The mucin produced by metaplastic pyloric gland-like cells in the pancreatic ducts has been

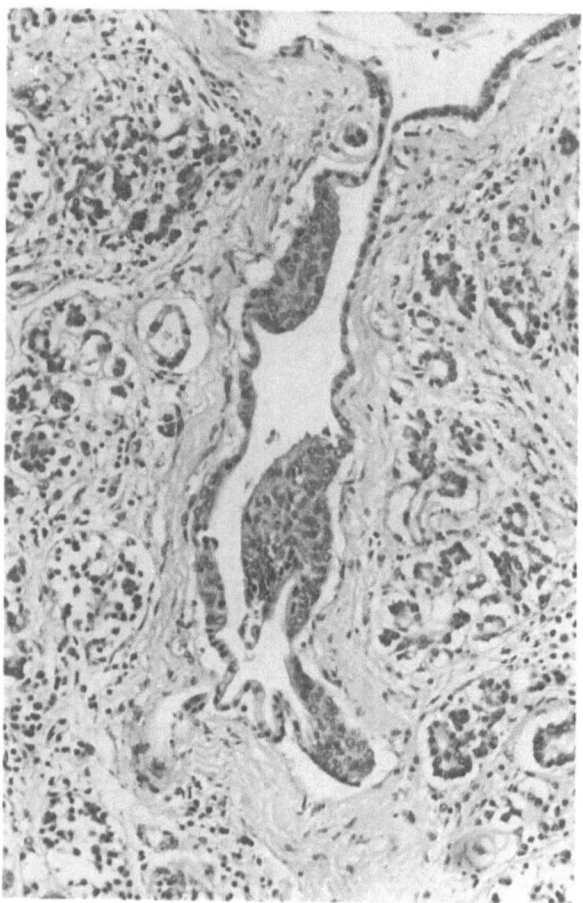

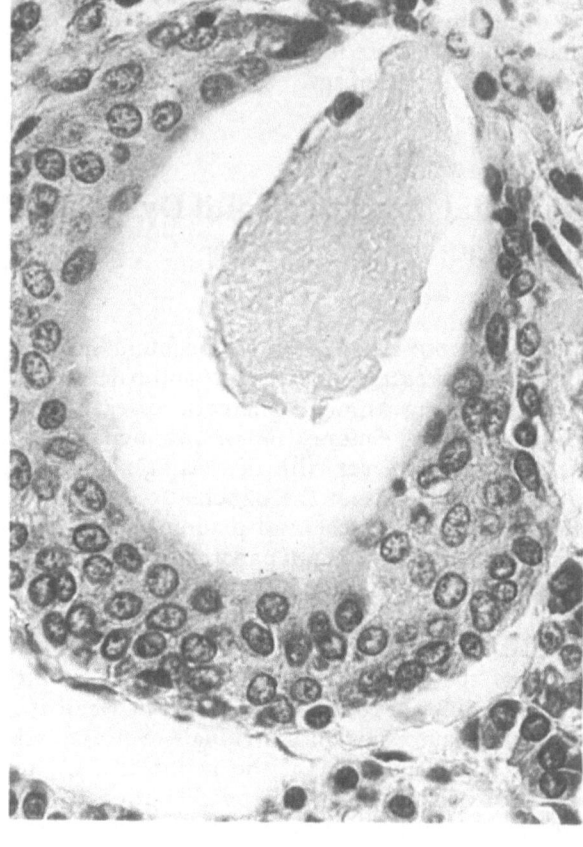

Fig. 2.13. Patchy squamous cell metaplasia in a small duct; an incidental finding. H&E, × 150

Fig. 2.14. Another small duct lined by cells that have undergone squamous cell metaplasia. H&E, × 600

studied histochemically by Roberts (1974) and compared with the mucins found in normal and neoplastic pancreases by Roberts and Burns (1972). Roberts found that the mucin produced by the metaplastic epithelium was of the neutral type and that it was similar, both morphologically and histochemically, to the secretion produced by normal juxtapyloric glands, and was similar also to the secretion of the metaplastic mucous glands found in the small intestine in certain cases of Crohn's disease, as well as in the mucosa of the gall bladder in some cases of chronic cholecystitis.

Neither Walters nor Roberts concerned themselves with dysplastic changes in the metaplastic epithelial cells that they studied, but Longnecker et al. (1980), in their study of the 108 pancreases that they scanned for acinar cell and ductal lesions, noted that some of the acinar cell abnormalities were similar to the atypical acinar cell nodules found in carcinogen-treated experimental animals. The inci-

dence of nodules was higher among patients with a history of heavy cigarette smoking or with a history of alcohol abuse. The principal cytological changes that they observed in the acini were a reduction of the basophilia of the cytoplasm of the cells, with reduction also of the cytoplasmic mass and zymogen content, or, occasionally the presence of cytoplasmic vacuoles. Reduced cytoplasmic basophilia was the most common of these changes and was present in 29 of the 108 pancreases. Ductal epithelial abnormalities were more common than focal dysplasia of the acinar cells. Mucous cell hypertrophy was noted in 65 cases and squamous metaplasia in 31, with papillary epithelial hyperplasia in 23. Some glands contained more than one type of epithelial abnormality. In one case there was marked atypical hyperplasia of the ductal epithelium.

The association of epithelial dysplasia with chronic pancreatitis has been studied by Volkholz et al. (1982); they found that in 280 operative speci-

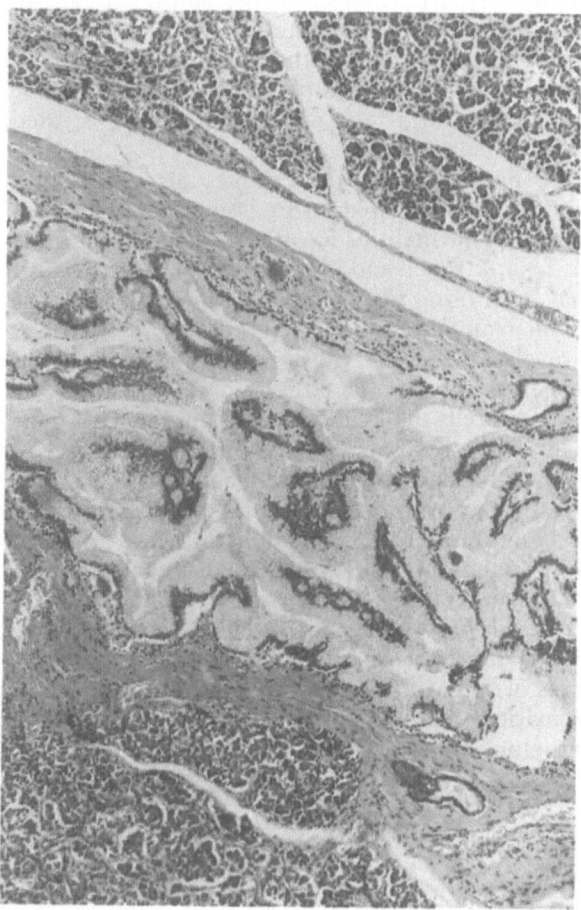

Fig. 2.15. A duct lined by cells that have undergone goblet cell metaplasia. H&E, × 60

mens of chronic pancreatitis there were 112 (40%) with dysplasias of the ductal epithelium. Because pancreatic carcinoma usually has its origin in the epithelium of the ducts, these workers limited themselves to epithelial proliferations in the ducts, but they noted also a lesion that they called tubular accumulation. The latter consisted of foci of very small dilated ducts, closely packed in groups and surrounded by fibrosis. The authors graded the epithelial lesions according to the three grades of dysplasia that have been recognised in the epithelia of other organs, but they assigned none of their cases to grade III, a grade that signifies borderline malignancy. The changes that they included in grade I were: extra tallness of the cylindrical epithelium, double rows of cylindrical epithelium, mucoid transformation of the epithelium, pseudopapillary hyperplasia, papillary hyperplasia with connective tissue stroma within the epithelial projections, and multilayered epithelial metapla-

sia. To be placed in grade I these epithelial changes had to be free from atypical cells, that is cells with enlarged slightly polymorphous or hyperchromatic nuclei, and free from disturbances of stratification within multilayered epithelium. Of the 112 cases of chronic pancreatitis with changes in the ductal epithelium, 92 (32.9%) were placed in grade I. The changes that were an indication for assigning cases to grade II were: pseudopapillary hyperplasia with atypia of the cells, papillary hyperplasia with atypia, and multilayered epithelial metaplasia with atypia (Fig. 2.16). The criteria for atypia were enlargement and hyperchromatism of nuclei with visible nucleoli, occasional mitotic figures and increased basophilia of the cytoplasm of the cells. Of the 112 cases with dysplasia of the ductal epithelium, 20 cases (7.1%) were classified as grade II. Ductular accumulation was found 18 times.

Dysplasia tended to be most marked in areas in which there was marked scarring of the gland with obstruction to the outflow of secretion. Thus the frequency of epithelial dysplasias was greatest in uniformly scarred glands. Such results neither prove nor dispel the suspicion, felt by various workers, that chronic pancreatitis predisposes to carcinoma of the pancreas.

The prevalence, distribution and clinical associations of ductal mucinous hyperplasia were also studied by Allen-Mersh (1985) in 102 non-malignant pancreases. He found the condition in over 60% of specimens, frequently associated with fibrosis. The most significant clinical association was with corticosteroid treatment. In later work (1988) his findings led him to suggest that the hyperplasia might be a proliferative response to exogenous agents liable to injure the pancreas, and that an association between ductal mucinous hyperplasia and occlusion of the accessory papilla might explain the susceptibility of pancreas divisum to pancreatitis.

Volkholz and his colleagues (1982) stated that the dysplasias with which they were concerned were unrelated to the presence, or otherwise, of tumours in organs other than the pancreas, but Burry (1974) has described the case of a young woman whose death was caused by a hepatocarcinoma. The hepatocarcinoma was superimposed upon cirrhosis of the liver, and, when the other organs were examined microscopically, extreme dysplasia was found in the renal epithelium, along with dysplasia of the cells of the endocrine and exocrine pancreas. The woman had not been an alcoholic and no history of the ingestion of a toxin that might have injured the hepatocytes or other cells could be established. Virological investigations that might have shown an association with

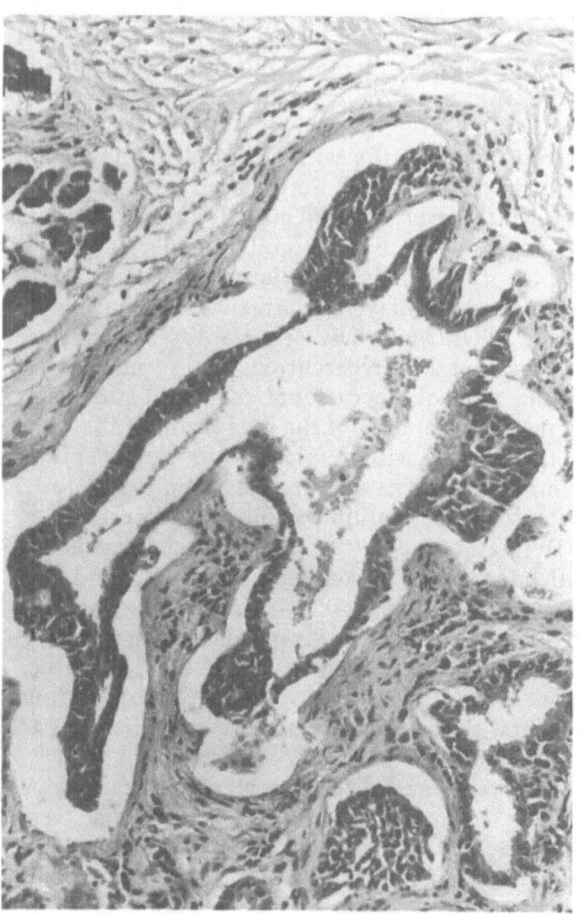

Fig. 2.16. Hyperchromatic dysplastic epithelium lining a pancreatic duct. There was no associated neoplasia. H&E, × 150

nuclear hyperchromasia in the epithelial cells of organs such as the lung, uterine cervix and urinary tract (Koss et al. 1965). One of the present authors has seen a marked example of these changes in the pancreas from a fatal case of busulphan-treated myeloid leukaemia.

Dysplasia of the pancreas may also occur as a congenital malformation in association with congenital abnormalities in other organs (Ivemark et al. 1959; Strayer and Kissane 1979). Such lesions may, according to Ivemark and his colleagues, be familial, and, in a photomicrograph in the paper by Strayer and Kissane, the pancreatic abnormality is one in which the pancreatic acini are lined by flattened cells that leave a central lumen within the acini, while each acinus is seen to have branched from a duct and to be surrounded by loose connective tissue. The authors found that, although a certain number of normal acini were present, abnormal tissue made up the bulk of the pancreas.

Experimental work of the type carried out by Rao et al. (1989) has shown that, in rodents, pancreatic ductular and interstitial cells are capable of transforming into hepatocytes but no such transformation has yet been recognised in human pathology.

Pancreatic Injury, Repair and Regeneration

Injury

Injury of the pancreas without associated injuries to neighbouring organs is uncommon, but multiple injuries that include damage to the pancreas are relatively common in motor car and motor cycle accidents, in any type of crushing injury of the lower thorax or upper abdomen, and in child abuse. The organs that may be damaged in association with pancreatic injury are the liver, spleen, transverse colon and duodenum. Penetrating injuries such as gunshot or stab wounds may involve the pancreas, and the pancreas may be damaged during procedures such as splenectomy or gastrectomy. In blunt injuries to the upper abdomen a severe blow in the mid-line can rupture the body of the pancreas by driving the gland against the vertebral column behind it. An injury of this type may split the pancreas into two pieces, with division of the duct and the formation of a large retroperitoneal haematoma. Laceration of the tail of the pancreas tends to be associated with

hepatitis B were not carried out. The dysplastic changes in the pancreas consisted of occasional acinar cells with enlarged, irregular and hyperchromatic nuclei, while many islet cells showed similar nuclear atypia.

Two other examples of atypia in the pancreas in association with neoplasms have been reported by Shinozuka et al. (1980). In one of their cases the neoplasm was an insulin-secreting adenoma of islet cells, while in the other it was a carcinoma of the bronchus. The pancreatic lesions resembled those found in rats that had been given carcinogenic chemicals and consisted of multiple nodules that were well demarcated from the surrounding acinar tissues and were composed of zymogen-containing acinar cells with a pale pink cytoplasm. The authors discussed the possibility that such nodules might be presursors of acinar cell carcinoma of the pancreas. Prolonged therapy with busulphan may cause cellular enlargement and rupture of the spleen, while injury to the head of the pancreas tends to be associated with damage to the duodenum. It has been emphasised by Torrance (1979) that, from his own experience and from his study of the publications on pancreatic injury, a considerable number of pancreatic injuries have followed apparently minor trauma, especially in children. The effects of such injuries may not be recognised until a pseudocyst has developed. The danger of pancreatic injuries depends upon the effects of leakage from ruptured ducts and upon the severe haemorrhage that may occur retroperitoneally or into the lesser sac of the peritoneum. Such haemorrhage may mask a rupture of the pancreatic duct.

Acute pancreatitis may also follow injury to the pancreas and such injuries may be the result of operative procedures, such as gastrectomy (Warren 1951; Pendower and Tanner 1959–1960) or the diagnostic procedure of translumbar aortography (Imrie et al. 1977). In the cases of pancreatitis that followed subtotal gastrectomy, Warren found no consistent aetiological pattern.

The possibility that retroperitoneal fibrosis with ureteric obstruction might be a late sequel of injury to the pancreas was considered by Pollock (1974) who carried out a long-term follow-up of four patients who had had non-penetrating injuries of the pancreas, but no late ureteric obstruction attributable to retroperitoneal fibrosis was found.

Healing and Regeneration

The healing of wounds in the pancreas appears to depend upon the extent to which the wound injures the ducts; if leakage from injured ducts can be prevented, healing will occur without complications, but if leakage from either the main or accessory duct or one of their larger tributaries occurs, the development of a pseudocyst is likely. In such a cyst, a wall of granulation tissue develops but, as in a peptic ulcer, a conflict between the healing process and the effects of digestive enzymes becomes established and, as a rule, it is not until surgical drainage has reduced the damaging effects of the pancreatic juice that a pseudocyst will heal, leaving some residual scar tissue.

In humans, as in experimental animals, the healthy pancreas seems to have sufficient reserves of functional capacity to allow substantial resection of the organ to be carried out, following injury for example, without subsequent diabetes or impairment of digestive function; but it is not known to what extent the human pancreas can regenerate after

partial pancreatectomy. Functionally, however, Pap et al. (1987) were able to demonstrate a significant degree of recovery of the exocrine function in 25 patients in whom about 60% of pancreatic mass had been removed by distal pancreatectomy for the relief of chronic pancreatitis. They attributed the improvement in function to regeneration of acinar cells, an opinion in keeping with conclusions reached by Elsässer et al. (1986). Glucose tolerance was frequently depressed.

In 1969 McMinn summarised the earlier experimental work on regeneration of the pancreas after partial pancreatectomy in several types of animal. In dogs there was marked proliferation of the ducts but less formation of new acini than in the guinea pig and rabbit, while in work done later than that reviewed by McMinn, it was found by Pearson et al. (1975) that there was significant regeneration of the pancreas in rats subjected to partial pancreatectomy. In baboons, however, it was found by the Russian workers Raitzina et al. (1965) that, after partial pancreatectomy, the remaining glandular tissue became enlarged by hypertrophy that eventually restored the normal weight of the pancreas. The acini and the islets in the hypertrophied glandular tissue increased in size, but there was no regrowth of glandular tissue on the wounded surface of the organ.

Experimental studies have also been undertaken to determine whether the disappearance of acini that follows ligation of the pancreatic duct can be reversed. In dogs in which ductal ligation has caused a complete absence of acinar tissue, successful restoration of the continuity of the duct is followed, in about 4 months, by the return of acinar secretion. After reviewing the experimental publications, and the results of surgical procedures designed to relieve obstruction of the pancreatic ducts in humans, Tiscornia and Dreiling (1966) felt convinced that the pancreas has a remarkable ability to regenerate its parenchyma and to recover its exocrine secretory capacity. To obtain such regeneration and recovery it is essential to restore duct-to-intestinal continuity, or to relieve ductal obstruction. The degree of regeneration that can occur in humans after the relief of ductal obstruction by sphincterotomy has been illustrated by Doubilet and Mulholland (1956). These authors also stated that the regeneration that follows the restoration of ductal drainage is derived from the ductular system, from which both acinar tissue and islets can be formed.

Regeneration of acinar tissue that has been destroyed by the toxic necrosis that can be induced in rats by the administration of ethionine has also been noted by various workers, and such work has been reviewed by McMinn. This type of regeneration may also be derived from the intra-acinar ductular cells (centro-acinar cells), but surviving, though damaged, acinar cells seemed to Herman and Fitzgerald (1962) to be more likely to be responsible for the regeneration. It was noted by Lehv and Fitzgerald (1968) that the regeneration that followed ethionine-induced necrosis was more rapid than the regeneration that followed surgical resection. They suggested that different mechanisms might be responsible for the stimulation of DNA synthesis.

In experiments on the carcinogenic effects of various nitroso compounds upon the pancreas of the Syrian golden hamster, Pour (1980) found that toxic necrosis of certain groups of acinar cells, especially around the islets, was associated with enlargement of centro-acinar and intercalary ductular cells that led to the formation of pseudoductules or tubules, with the formation of new islets that contained beta cells.

There seems to be general agreement that, in animal experiments, regenerating pancreatic tissue can form islets of Langerhans that include beta cells. Such work has been reviewed by Gepts (1981), but it is clear that the ability to regenerate, though it varies from species to species, is not unlimited. In juvenile diabetics that have died soon after the onset of the disease there are usually signs of regeneration in the pancreatic islets and this is thought to explain the temporary remissions that may follow the first clinical signs of the disease. Such remissions are, however, only temporary and, in patients that die after a longer interval, beta cells can no longer be recognised, probably because attempts at regeneration have been frustrated by the abnormal conditions of immunity that have been demonstrated to be present in type I diabetics. Some optimism has, however, been created by the discovery that nicotinamide, a derivative of the B_3 vitamin nicotinic acid, will prevent both chemically-induced diabetes mellitus in animal models and the spontaneous development of insulin-dependent diabetes in animals genetically destined to become diabetic. The substance is non-toxic and it preserves residual beta cell function and enhances beta cell regeneration in partially pancreatectomised rats. Furthermore, nicotinamide promotes the growth of cultured human foetal islet cells (Picot et al. 1993; Eizirik et al. 1993).

References

Akao S, Bockman DE, Lechene de la Porte P, Sarles H (1986) Three-dimensional pattern of ductuloacinar associations in normal and pathological human pancreas. Gastroenterology 90:661–668

Allen-Mersh TC (1985) What is the significance of pancreatic ductal mucinous hyperplasia? Gut 26:825–833

Allen-Mersh TC (1988) Pancreatic ductal mucinous hyperplasia: distribution within the pancreas, and effects of variation in ampullary and pancreatic duct anatomy. Gut 29:1392–1396

Baxter-Grillo D, Blázques E, Grillo TAI, Sodoyez J-G, Sodoyez-Goffaux F, Foà PP (1981) Functional development of the pancreatic islets. In: Cooperstein SJ, Watkins D (eds) The islets of Langerhans. Academic Press, New York, pp 35–49

Becker WF, Welsh RA, Pratt HS (1965) Cystadenoma and cystadenocarcinoma of the pancreas. Ann Surg 161:845–863

Bendayan M (1987) Presence of endocrine cells in pancreatic ducts. Pancreas 2:393–397

Burry AF (1974) Extreme dysplasia in the renal epithelium, and dysplasia of endocrine and exocrine pancreas in a young woman dying from hepatocarcinoma. J Pathol 113:147–150

Clark A, Grant AM (1983) Quantitative morphology of endocrine cells in human fetal pancreas. Diabetologica 25:31–35

Cooperstein SJ, Watkins D (eds) (1981) The islets of Langerhans. Biochemistry, physiology, and pathology. Academic Press, New York

Dixon JS (1979) Histology: ultrastructure. In: Howat HT, Sarles H (eds) The exocrine pancreas. Saunders, London, pp 31–49

Doubilet H, Mulholland JH (1956) Eight-year study of pancreatitis and sphincterotomy. JAMA 160:521–528

Eizirik DL, Sandler S, Palmer JP (1993) Repair of pancreatic beta cells. A relevant phenomenon in early IDDM. Diabetes 42:1383–1391

Elsässer H-P, Lütcke H, Kern HF (1986) Acinar and duct cell replication and regeneration. In: Go VLW, Gardner JD, Brooks FP, Lebenthal E, Di Magno EP, Scheele GA (eds) The exocrine pancreas: biology, pathobiology, and diseases. Raven Press, New York, pp 45–53

England MA (1983) A colour atlas of life before birth. Normal fetal development. Wolfe Medical Publications, London, p 127

Gepts W (1981) Islet changes in human diabetes. In: Cooperstein SJ, Watkins D (eds) The islets of Langerhans. Academic Press, New York, pp 339–341

Heitz PU, Beglinger C, Gyr K (1984) Anatomy and physiology of the exocrine pancreas. In: Klöppel G, Heitz HU (eds) Pancreatic pathology. Churchill Livingstone, London, pp 3–21

Henderson JR, Daniel PM, Fraser PA (1981) The pancreas as a single organ: the influence of the endocrine upon the exocrine part of the gland. Gut 22:158–167

Herman L, Fitzgerald PJ (1962) Restitution of pancreatic acinar cells following ethionine. J Cell Biol 12:297–312

Heyderman E (1979) Immunoperoxidase technique in histopathology: application, methods and controls. J Clin Pathol 32:971–978

Hollender LF, Lehnert P, Wanke M (1983) Acute pancreatitis. An interdisciplinary synopsis. Urban and Schwarzenberg, Munich, p 34

Imrie CW, Goldring J, Pollock JG, Wall JK (1977) Acute pancreatitis after translumbar aortography. Br Med J iii:681

Ivemark B, Oldfelt B, Zetterström R (1959) Familial dysplasia of kidneys, liver and pancreas: a probably genetically determined syndrome. Acta Pediatr 48:1–11

Klöppel G, Lenzen S (1984) Anatomy and physiology of the endocrine pancreas. In: Klöppel G, Heitz PU (eds) Pancreatic pathology. Churchill Livingstone, London, pp 133–153

Koss LG, Melamed MR, Mayer K (1965) The effect of busulphan on human epithelia. Am J Clin Pathol 44:385–397

Lebenthal E, Lev R, Lee PC (1986) Prenatal and postnatal development of the human exocrine pancreas. In: Go VLW, Gardner JD, Brooks FP, Lebenthal E, Di Magno EP, Scheele GA (eds) The exocrine pancreas: biology, pathobiology, and diseases. Raven Press, New York, pp 33–43

Lehv MD, Fitzgerald PJ (1968) Pancreatic acinar cell regeneration IV. Regeneration after surgical excision. Am J Pathol 53:513–535

Like AL, Orci L (1972) Embryogenesis of the human pancreatic islets: a light and electron microscopic study. Diabetes 21 (Suppl 2):511–534

Liu HM, Potter EL (1962) Development of the human pancreas. Arch Pathol 74:439–452

Longnecker DS, Shinozuka H, Dekker A (1980) Focal acinar cell dysplasia in human pancreas. Cancer 45:534–540

McLean JM (1979) Embryology of the pancreas. In: Howat HT, Sarles H (eds) The exocrine pancreas. Saunders, London, pp 3–14

McMinn RMH (1969) Tissue repair. Academic Press, London, pp 356–359

Munger BL (1981) Morphological characterisation of islet cell diversity. In: Cooperstein SJ, Watkins D (eds) The islets of Langerhans. Academic Press, New York, pp 3–34

Pap A, Flautner L, Karacsonyi S, Szecseny A, Varro V (1987) Recovery of pancreatic function after distal resection for chronic pancreatitis: regeneration or merely functional amelioration. M Sinai J Med 54:409–412

Pearse AGE (1984) Islet development and the APUD concept. In: Klöppel G, Heitz PU (eds) Pancreatic pathology. Churchill Livingstone, London, pp 125–132

Pearson KW, Scott D, Torrance HB (1975) Pancreatic regeneration following pancreatic resection. Gut 16:404–405

Peart WS, Porter KA, Robertson JIS, Sandler M, Baldock E (1963) Carcinoid syndrome due to pancreatic duct neoplasm secreting 5-hydroxytryptophan and 5-hydroxytryptamine. Lancet i:239–243

Pendower JEH, Tanner NC (1959–1960) Pancreatitis following gastrectomy. Br J Surg 47:145–147

Picot F, Reimers JI, Anderson HU (1993) Nicotinamide: biological actions and therapeutic potential in diabetes prevention. Diabetologia 36:574–576

Pollock AV (1974) Pancreatic trauma and idiopathic retroperitoneal fibrosis: a long-term follow-up study of 4 patients. Br J Surg 61:112

Pour P (1980) Experimental pancreatic ductal (ductular) tumors. In: Fitzgerald PJ, Morrison AB (eds) The pancreas. Williams and Wilkins, Baltimore, pp 111–139

Rahier J (1988) The diabetic pancreas: a pathologist's view. In: Lefèbvre PJ, Pipeleers DG (eds) The pathology of the endocrine pancreas. Springer-Verlag, Berlin, pp 19–21

Raitzina SS, Farutina LM, Kashintzeva VN (1965) Regenerative hypertrophy of pancreas in monkey. (In Russian, English summary) Arkh Anat Gistol Embriol 49:43–48

Rao MS, Dwivedi RS, Yeldandi AV et al. (1989) Role of periductal epithelial cells of adult rat pancreas in hepatocyte lineage. A change in the differentiation commitment. Am J Pathol 134:1069–1086

Rich AR, Duff GL (1936) Experimental and pathological studies on the pathogenesis of acute haemorrhagic pancreatitis. Bull Johns Hopkins Hosp 58:212–260

Roberts PF (1974) Pyloric gland metaplasia of the human pancreas. A comparative histochemical study. Arch Pathol 97:92–95

Roberts PF, Burns J (1972) A histochemical study of mucins in normal and neoplastic human pancreatic tissue. J Pathol 107:87–94

Shinozuka H, Lee RE, Dunn JL, Longnecker DS (1980) Multiple atypical acinar cell nodules of the pancreas. Hum Pathol 11:389–391

Stamm BH (1984) Incidence and diagnostic significance of minor pathologic changes in the adult pancreas at autopsy: a systematic study of 112 autopsies in patients without known pancreatic disease. Hum Pathol 15:677–683

Strayer DS, Kissane JM (1979) Dysplasia of the kidneys, liver, and pancreas: report of a variant of Ivemark's syndrome. Hum Pathol 10:228–234

Tiscornia OM, Dreiling DA (1966) Does the pancreatic gland regenerate? Gastroenterology 51:267–271

Torrance B (1979) Traumatic lesions of the pancreas. In: Howat HT, Sarles H (eds) The exocrine pancreas. Saunders, London, pp 340–351

Volkholz H, Stolte M, Becker V (1982) Epithelial dysplasias in chronic pancreatitis. Virchows Arch A 396:331–349

Walters MN-I (1965) Goblet-cell metaplasia in ductules and acini of the exocrine pancreas. J Pathol Bacteriol 89:569–572

Warren KW (1951) Acute pancreatitis and pancreatic injuries following subtotal gastrectomy. Surgery 29:643–657

3   Congenital Pancreatic Abnormalities

Congenital Absence of the Pancreas

Because the pancreas develops, like the liver and biliary system, by outgrowths from the mid-gut, absence of the pancreas and of the liver occurs in monstrous foetuses that lack the intestinal tract; survival is impossible. Less severe failures in the development of the pancreas have been associated sufficiently often with retardation of foetal growth to suggest that insulin, and perhaps glucagon also, may be necessary growth factors for the foetus. The suggestion seems to have been made first by Sherwood et al. (1974) who reported a defect in both somatic and cell growth in two siblings in whom agenesis of the pancreas was confirmed at autopsy. In 1977, Van Assche et al. found that there was a reduction of foetal endocrine pancreatic tissue and of the insulin-producing beta cells in a small series of pregnancies complicated by severe foetal growth retardation. They believed themselves to be the first to have noted the association.

Complete absence of pancreatic tissue has been described in a live-born infant by Lemons et al. (1979). They reported the case of a female child with a gestational age of 41 weeks by dates, but with clinical and radiological features more in keeping with 36 weeks, findings they interpreted as indications of intrauterine growth retardation. A left diaphragmatic hernia was recognised and was repaired soon after birth, but the child died at the age of 24 h. At autopsy there was no recognisable pancreatic tissue at the usual site nor was any exocrine or endocrine pancreatic tissue found on microscopic examination of all the organs. In addition to the repaired diaphragmatic hernia there was bilateral pulmonary hypoplasia, a ventricular septal defect, malrotation of the intestine, absence of the gall bladder, uterus didelphus and bilateral hydronephrosis with hydro-ureter. The authors suggested that the absence of the secretion of insulin had caused retardation of foetal growth. They were able to refer to other cases of growth retardation associated with congenital absence of the pancreas as well as reports of retardation of growth associated with extreme hypoplasia of the pancreas or absence of the islets of Langerhans.

Congenital Absence of the Islets of Langerhans

Absence of any recognised islets of Langerhans has been reported by Dodge and Laurence (1977). Their case was a small-for-dates male infant that developed acute metabolic acidosis and diabetes mellitus soon after birth and died at the age of 40 h. The baby was the fourth child of healthy unrelated parents whose first child, also a male, had died at 48 h under similar circumstances.

Congenital Absence of Insulin-Secreting Cells

An example of this type of congenital deficiency has been reported by Wong et al. (1988). Their patient was a male child who was recognised as having diabetes mellitus on the day after birth and died at the age of three days. On histological examination of the pancreas there were small inconspicuous islets of Langerhans in which no insulin-secreting cells could be demonstrated by immunocytochemistry. Because there was no insulitis the authors attributed the absence of insulin-secreting cells to a failure of development.

Congenital Short Pancreas

Two adult cases of partial agenesis of the pancreas have been reported by Glinsky et al. (1985). The diagnosis was made by endoscopic retrograde pancreatography. Growth and development of the other organs seemed normal but one of the two patients was an insulin-dependent diabetic. Diabetes mellitus was said by the authors to be commonly associated with this type of pancreatic abnormality.

Agenesis of the Dorsal Pancreatic Bud

An example of this type of agenesis, with asplenia, cardiac abnormalities and visceral isomerism, was described by Leese et al. (1989). They referred to 20 cases reported in the literature. This abnormality predisposes to recurrent attacks of pancreatitis with eventual exocrine and endocrine pancreatic failure. They stated that agenesis of the ventral pancreas is very rare.

Pancreas Divisum

This term is misleading, for a truly divided pancreas is so rare that morbid anatomists who have spent a working lifetime in the autopsy room may never have recognised the condition. Pancreas divisum, however, as understood by endoscopists, is relatively common. It is a superficially normal pancreas in which no communication has developed between the duct of the dorsally derived pancreas and the duct of the embryonic ventral pancreas, which normally forms most of the main pancreatic duct. The lack of communication between the two ducts makes the accessory duct (of Santorini), which enters the duodenum at the minor papilla, responsible for the drainage of the tail, body, neck and some of the upper part of the head of the gland. Under such circumstances, a very short duct of Wirsung drains only the lower part of the head and discharges into the duodenum at the major duodenal papilla in association with the orifice of the common bile duct. In over 1850 successful cannulations of Vater's papilla, Rösch et al. (1976) identified such an arrangement of the ducts in 63 patients, an incidence of 3.4%, and Gregg (1977) recognised the condition in 33 patients of 1100 on whom he had carried out endoscopic retrograde cholangiopancreatography, an incidence of 3%. Most of the patients on whom endoscopy had been carried out had symptoms that suggested episodes of pancreatitis and, because the orifice of the accessory duct is small and difficult to cannulate, it has been suggested that inadequate drainage predisposes to attacks of pancreatitis in the regions of the gland that secrete into the accessory duct (Cotton and Kizu 1977; Cotton 1980). Cotton's experience was that only 3.6% of 169 patients with primary biliary tract disease, who underwent pancreatography incidentally to cholangiography, had pancreas divisum but that 25.6% of 78 patients with unexplained recurrent pancreatitis had the anomaly. Such findings, combined with results obtained in Hungary by Tulassy and Papp (1980) seemed to indicate that pancreas divisum predisposes to pancreatitis. Mitchell et al. (1979), however, did not agree. They found an incidence of 4.7% of pancreas divisum in a series of 449 successful pancreatograms and, although their 21 cases of pancreas divisum included four patients with clinical evidence of pancreatitis and two with possible pancreatic disease, they did not consider the anomaly to be clinically relevant. They found, moreover, that an abnormal pancreatogram suggestive of pancreatitis was present in 116 of 428 patients (27.1%) with a normally fused duct system, and they interpreted their findings as suggesting that failure of the embryonic ducts to fuse did not predispose to pancreatitis. Scepticism about the significance of pancreas divisum as a cause of pancreatitis was also expressed by workers such as Delhaye et al. (1985) and Sugawa et al. (1987), who produced results that failed to confirm that pancreas divisum predisposed to pancreatic disease.

The suggestion that a combination of unfused ducts along with relative stenosis of the duodenal orifice of the dorsal duct predisposed to pancreatitis led to attempts to improve the drainage of the gland by operative enlargement of the ductal orifices, but in the hands of surgeons such as Richter et al. (1981), Gregg et al. (1983, 1984) and Britt et al. (1983), such procedures had only limited success. A reason why they were not always successful has been put forward by Warshaw et al. (1983), who suggested that recurrent attacks of acute pancreatitis led to the establishment of irreversible chronic pancreatitis. Chronic pancreatitis with marked periductal fibrosis was, however, found unexpectedly in two out of three patients with pancreas divisum in whom Thompson et al. (1981) removed the tail of the pancreas and had it examined microscopically.

In patients in whom chronic pancreatitis has become established, pancreatectomy is often necessary and the results of pancreatectomy in 14 such patients were published by Blair et al. (1984). Good relief of pain was obtained in 11 of these patients at the expense of steatorrhoea in two and diabetes in one. The presence of chronic pancreatitis of varying severity was confirmed pathologically in all the excised specimens. Moreover, in two cases it was possible to fix and mount the pancreaticoduodenectomy specimens in a way that allowed a comparison of the dorsal and ventral portions of the pancreas. In both there was chronic pancreatitis that was limited to the dorsal part of the gland, the ventral part being normal. Such evidence has a strong appeal to the histopathologist as support for the view that pancreas divisum predisposes to pancreatitis in the dorsally derived regions of the gland. The need for the additional factor of stenosis of the minor papilla is emphasised by the results of Rusnak et al. (1988). They operated upon 11 patients in whom intractable symptoms were associated with pancreas divisum, combined with delayed ductal drainage. In one of these, pancreaticoduodenectomy was necessary and examination of the excised specimen confirmed that there was obstruction of the outlet of the dorsal duct, while pancreatitis was limited to the parts of the gland drained by that duct.

Although the significance of pancreas divisum remains controversial, the histopathological evidence seems to support the view that when papillary stenosis is combined with the ductal anomaly, recurrent attacks of pancreatitis will occur and will lead eventually to chronic disease. The attacks may begin in childhood (Adzick et al. 1989), but are more likely to begin in early adult life. The radiological

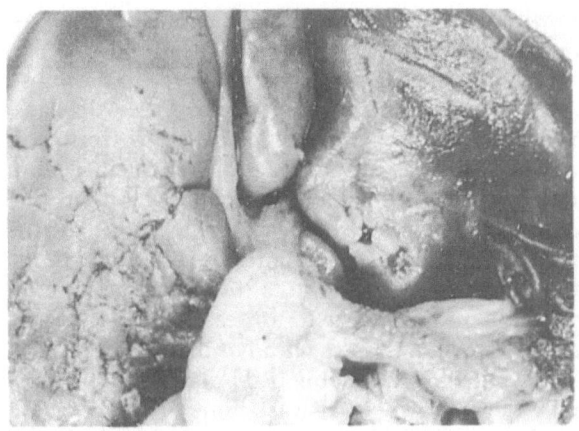

Fig. 3.1. Annular pancreas in an infant. Dissection has displayed the abnormality of the head of the pancreas, which is still attached by the bile duct and blood vessels to the liver. (Courtesy of Irene M. Irving)

appearances are said to be characteristic, provided cancer or previous injury can be excluded (Warshaw and Cambria 1984; Agha and Williams 1987).

Annular Pancreas

This is a well known anomaly (Fig. 3.1); it is quite rare but its recognition is said to have increased in recent years, even though Ravitch (1973) was able to refer to reports of over 350 cases published up to 1967. The increase is likely to be the result of better identification, rather than a change in prevalence, for, as has been pointed out by Lloyd-Jones et al. (1972), asymptomatic cases are easily missed.

The condition is one in which glandular pancreatic tissue, in continuity with the head of the pancreas, extends to encircle the duodenum. In 85% of cases (Ravitch 1973) it is the second part of the duodenum that is encircled, usually proximal to the papilla of Vater; in the remaining cases it is either the first or the third part of the duodenum that is surrounded. The annulus forms a thin flat ring and is usually drained by a duct that enters the duct of Wirsung. In most cases the abnormally situated pancreatic tissue extends between the muscle bundles of the duodenum, as has been demonstrated by Hyden (1963). This is not invariable, however, as is illustrated by Ravitch (1973) in a specimen from a neonate who died in the first week of life with congenital heart disease as well as the pancreatic abnormally.

It seems that the abnormal embryonic mechanisms that result in annular pancreas are not always the same. The normal pancreas develops from two buds from the primitive duodenum: one ventral and one dorsal. The dorsal lobe remains dorsal, but the ventral anlage, which appears on the root of the liver diverticulum, accompanies the bile duct on its migration to the left towards the dorsal surface of the duodenum, where it unites with the dorsal anlage to form part of the head of the pancreas. The ventral anlage is at first bilobed but its left lobe normally degenerates. In at least some of the cases of annular pancreas that have been studied, it seems that the left lobe not only persists but grows, first round the right side of the duodenum, then in front of it to join the rest of the pancreas, thus forming a ring around the duodenum. When the abnormality has been caused by this mechanism, the duct from the encircling pancreas passes behind the duodenum to join the duct of Wirsung. This has been demonstrated, for example, by Ikeda and Irving (1984), who made a three-dimensional reconstruction of an annular pancreas from a foetus with an estimated gestational age of 18 weeks.

In other cases, however, the duct from the annulus courses from right to left, anterior to the duodenum, or, in yet others, there may be multiple small ducts, each of which drains separately into the duodenum. The presence of a duct that passes from right to left in front of the duodenum suggests that overgrowth of the dorsal anlage may have been responsible for, or may have contributed to, the development of the annulus. Mechanisms to explain the variants of the anatomy of different cases of annular pancreas are discussed by authors such as Ikeda and Irving (1984) and again by Irving (1990).

Evidence that the annulus originated from the ventral primordium in an adult case of annular pancreas has been presented by Rode et al. (1988). These workers carried out immunostaining of horizontal sections through the entire specimen and found that the annulus contained islets with characteristics that they maintained were those of islets derived from the ventral primordium. In addition to such immuno-histochemical features, the islets in the annulus had the jagged outline of the islets seen in the ventrally derived part of the anatomically normal pancreas. Moreover, on morphometry, the nuclei of the acinar cells had a significantly smaller diameter, as seen in cells with a ventral origin. The two embryonic parts of the pancreas were also affected by pancreatitis of differing grades of severity. Endoscopically, the annular duct was shown to empty at the major papilla, with the other draining to the minor papilla.

In the excised specimen a communication between the two ducts was demonstrated.

Symptoms attributable to annular pancreas are usually those of duodenal obstruction, but such symptoms are not necessarily immediate. In about half the reported cases, however, trouble developed during the first year of life and over half of these had symptoms during the first week of life. Regarding such neonatal cases, Lister (1978) has raised the question of whether it is the pancreatic annulus or lack of duodenal development that causes the obstruction. The duodenum is usually markedly narrowed, or has its lumen completely obliterated, but the abnormally sited pancreatic tissue may surround only a part of the atretic or stenotic duodenum. Lister believes that the duodenal abnormality is the primary lesion and that the pancreatic annulus develops as a secondary effect.

In the reported cases of duodenal obstruction by annular pancreas in adults, with ages ranging from 21 to 70 years, inflammation in the pancreatic tissue usually accounted for the obstruction. Patients reported by Glinsky et al. (1987) and Rode et al. (1988) illustrate this.

As has already been mentioned, annular pancreas may not be an isolated abnormality: imperforate anus, oesophageal atresia with tracheo-oesophageal fistula, congenital heart disease and other congenital lesions have all been associated (Ravitch 1973). More recently, Adeyemi (1988) has reported a combination of annular pancreas and partial situs inversus in three babies in whom duodenal obstruction developed within a few days of birth. In all three patients the partial situs inversus was attributed to malrotation of the duodenum, pancreas, liver, stomach and, indirectly, the spleen. All the babies recovered after the duodenal obstruction had been relieved surgically.

There have been at least two reports that suggest that annular pancreas may be a familial malformation: Montgomery et al. (1971) reported the occurrence of the lesion in a brother and a sister, and Jackson and Apostolides (1978) found four cases in two generations of one family.

Pancreatic Fibrosis, Bilateral Renal Dysplasia, Intrahepatic Biliary Dysgenesis and Situs Inversus Totalis

A report by Hiraoka et al. (1988) records the case of a Japanese newborn infant in whom severe pancreatic fibrosis was associated with renal dysplasia, intrahepatic biliary dysgenesis and total situs inversus. The chromosomal analysis was normal, but the authors found that another child, with no known blood relationship to their patient, had been born in the same town in a remote area. They offered no explanation for this coincidence.

Aberrant Pancreatic Ducts

An aberrant pancreatic duct, communicating with a gastric duplication cyst and with the main pancreatic duct, was found by Hoffman et al. (1987) by endoscopic retrograde pancreatography to be the cause of recurrent attacks of acute pancreatitis in a young woman. When the patient was operated upon, the cyst, later shown to be lined by mucosa similar to that of the gastric antrum, was found to communicate with the aberrant duct, which lay in an abnormal lobe of the pancreas. The cyst did not communicate with the stomach and was removed without entering the stomach. The aberrant pancreas and its duct were separated from the normal pancreas and were removed with the cyst. Areas of pancreatitis were noted in the aberrant pancreatic tissue. Following the operation, the patient had no further attacks of pancreatitis throughout the year during which she was followed up. The authors could find only five published reports in which there were similar abnormalities.

Another report of an abnormal connecting duct, in this case between the main pancreatic duct and the common bile duct, is that by Rosseland et al. (1988). Their patient was a young woman who had attacks of upper abdominal pain accompanied by hyperamylasaemia; when the connecting duct was ligated and divided the patient was relieved of her symptoms.

Heterotopia of Pancreatic Tissue

Aberrant pancreas, in which glandular acini, ducts and well differentiated islets can be recognised microscopically, is by no means uncommon in organs derived, like the normally situated pancreas, from entoderm. In such organs its presence is the result, according to Willis (1962), of heteroplastic differentiation of parts of embryonic entoderm that do not normally produce pancreas. Such areas of heterotopia occur in the stomach, small intestine,

mesentery, Meckel's diverticulum (and other vitellointestinal remains), large intestine, gall bladder, liver, abdominal and mediastinal cysts, and lung. Pancreatic tissue in the spleen, again according to Willis, is an incorporated aberrant extension of the pancreas proper, while the pancreatic pseudocyst reported in the left kidney by Stept et al. (1971) is thought to have been the result of pancreatitis with erosion of the left kidney, which progressed to form a pseudocyst.

Frequency in Various Organs

The most frequent sites for accessory pancreatic tissue are the walls of the stomach or duodenum, followed by the jejunum. In a table of cases recorded up to 1944, combined with 41 surgical cases of their own, Barbosa et al. (1946a) showed that the duodenum was the site in 27.7% of cases, the stomach in 25% and the jejunum in 15.9%; a Meckel's diverticulum was the site in 5.3%. In all other sites the incidence was much lower.

The same authors stated that aberrant pancreatic tissue was found somewhere in the abdomen about once in every 500 laparotomies at the Mayo Clinic. They also stated (Barbosa et al. 1946b) that pancreatic tissue occurring away from the main gland had been found in 1.7% of routine autopsies at the Mayo Clinic between 1939 and 1943. In a later series of 212 cases from the Mayo Clinic, all of which were clinical cases and not cases in which the aberrant tissue had been found incidentally at autopsy, Dolan et al. (1974) reported that the stomach was the site in 81 cases, the duodenum in 77 and the upper jejunum in 33, followed by Meckel's diverticulum in 11 and the ileum in three. There were single cases in which the sites were: the common bile duct, the umbilicus, the gall bladder, the hilus of the spleen, the papilla of an accessory pancreatic duct, outside the stomach near the left gastric artery, and anterior to the duodenal end of the main pancreas. In the latter two cases, and in the case where the aberrant tissue lay at the hilus of the spleen, the aberrant pancreatic tissue is likely to have been due to abnormal extension from the pancreas rather than to heteroplasia. In some sites, especially in the jejunum, heterotopic pancreatic tissue may be entirely without symptoms, but, even in the jejunum, intussusception may be initiated by the area of thickening of the wall caused by the pancreatic tissue. In the stomach, heterotopic pancreatic tissue seems very often to be associated with symptoms. In a case reported by Tanemura et al. (1987), ectopic pancreas in the bulb of the duodenum was associated with completely developed heterotopic fundic glands.

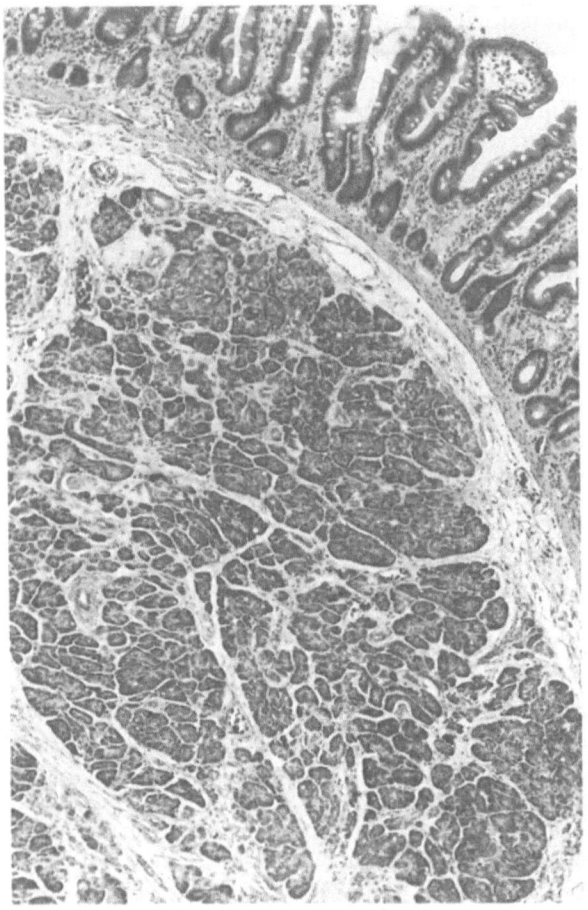

Fig. 3.2. Heterotopic pancreas in the submucosa of the jejunum. H&E, × 60

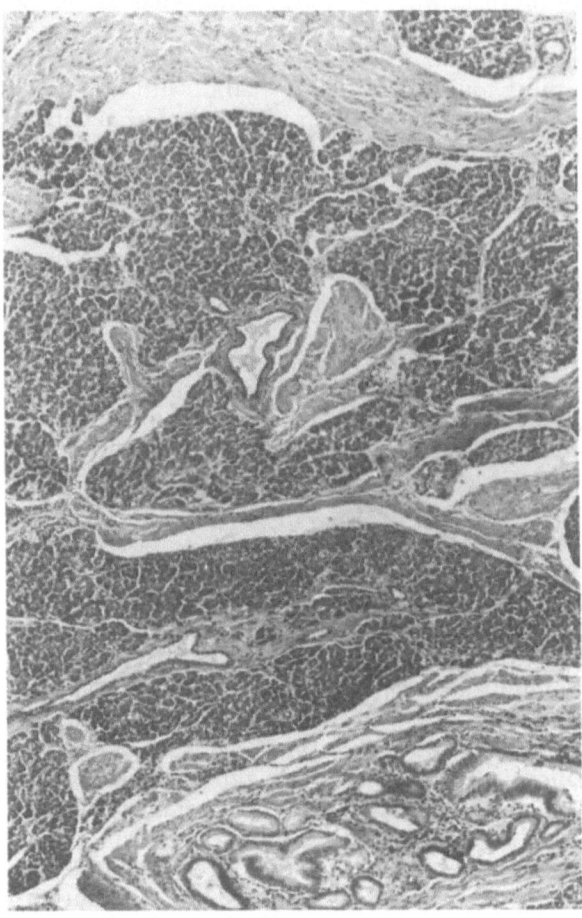

Fig. 3.3. Heterotopic pancreas mixed with the fibres of the duodenal muscularis. H&E, × 66

Appearances

In the bowel wall, the heterotopic tissue forms rounded or lobulated, white or yellowish nodularities that are usually between 1 cm and 4 cm in diameter. Most commonly, the glandular tissue lies in the submucosa, but it may lie between the fibres of the muscularis, subserosally or on the serosal surface (Figs 3.2–3.5). In certain cases the pancreatic tissue may extend through more than one, or all, of the layers of the bowel wall. The resemblance to normally situated pancreas is most easily recognised with the naked eye when the heterotopic tissue is on the serosal surface (Fig. 3.6). The submucosal and intermuscular types usually require microscopic examination for their identification. Microscopically the heterotopic tissue resembles normal pancreas with acini arranged in lobules, ducts and islets of Langerhans, though all of these components may

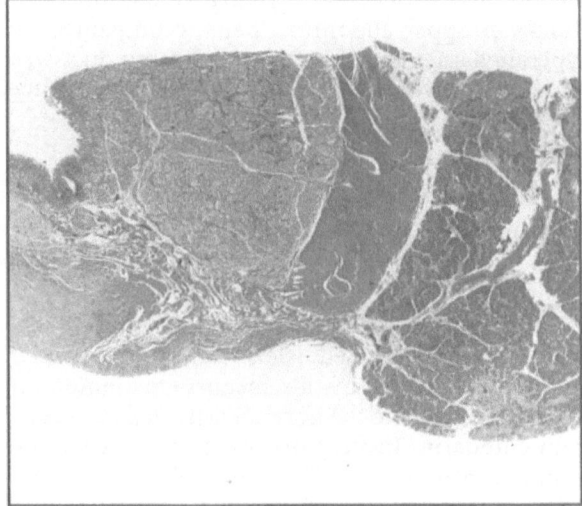

Fig. 3.4. Heterotopic pancreas in the duodenal subserosa. H&E, × 4

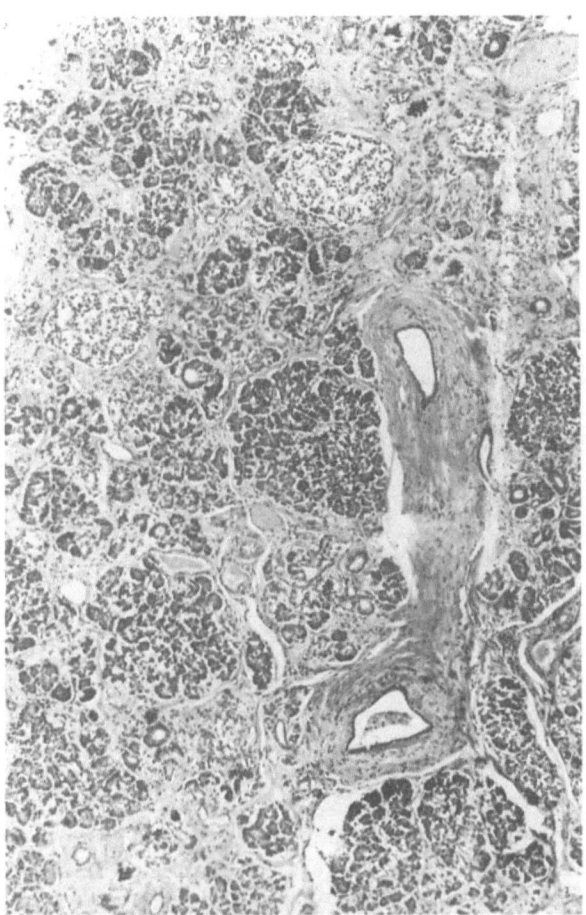

Fig. 3.5. Heterotopic pancreas, with islets of Langerhans, in the duodenum. H&E, × 60

not be present. In particular, islets often cannot be detected with routine stains, and although immunological stains may reveal some positive cells in such cases, this is by no means invariable. The small ducts do not usually form a common duct but instead drain independently into the intestine. It is said (Barbosa et al. 1946a) that heterotopic pancreatic tissue is vulnerable to the same afflictions that may affect the normally situated pancreas; namely cyst formation, haemorrhagic necrosis, inflammation and simple and malignant neoplasia.

Symptoms

In pancreatic heterotopia in the duodenum, symptoms may be absent but there are reports, for example that of Branch and Gross (1935), of mucosal ulceration with haemorrhage over ectopic pancreas in the duodenum, although Dolan et al. (1974) found

that necrosis and ulceration were rare when excised heterotopic pancreas was examined microscopically. Heterotopic pancreas may be mistaken for neoplasm on macroscopic examination, and even microscopically, when there is infiltration of muscle. Many of the reported examples of pancreatic heterotopia in the duodenum were found incidentally during operations for peptic ulcers of the duodenum, but in other cases obstruction of the duodenum itself, or of the common bile duct at the duodenal papilla, seems to have occurred. Carcinoma at the duodenal papilla was suspected by Barbosa et al. (1946a) to have arisen in heterotopic pancreas, and obstruction of both the common bile duct and the pancreatic duct has been reported (Pearson 1951). More recently, Coupland et al. (1987) have described a case of obstructive jaundice due to ectopic pancreas in the submucosa and muscularis around the ampulla of Vater. A traction effect, with the formation of a duodenal diverticulum was noted by Baldwin as long ago as 1911.

Particularly in the stomach, aberrant pancreas may be a component of tumour-like lesions that cause symptoms, and in 1951 Palmer was able to find reports of 215 cases of histologically proven aberrant pancreatic tissue in the stomach. Most of the examples occurred in patients between 25 and 55 years old and epigastric pain was the usual complaint, with, in about one-quarter of the patients, symptoms suggesting pyloric obstruction. It was, in fact, the pyloric region of the stomach that was involved in about one-quarter of the 174 subjects in which a gastric location of the pancreatic tumour was stated. The incidence seems to be low in the fundus and cardia. Occasionally there may be more than one "polyp" with a component of pancreatic tissue (Wheelock et al. 1949). Unlike the completely differentiated aberrant pancreatic tissue found in the small intestine, the gastric lesions form organoid adenomyomatous structures that are seen with the naked eye as small masses on the mucosal surface. These may be hemispherical, conical, cylindrical or nipple-like, and their size may be between a few millimetres and 4–5 cm in diameter; most are 1–3 cm in diameter. The most characteristic macroscopic feature is the orifice of a duct that can sometimes be found on the surface of the "polyp" by the use of a fine probe. Occasionally there is more than one duct. According to Stewart and Taylor (1925) the tumour-like lesions of the stomach differ from simple heterotopias in having a varied structure that suggests that, while they probably originate from epithelial buds similar to those that form simple pancreatic heterotopias, they have differentiated in two directions: pancreatic and gastrointestinal. Each of their four cases had a combination of pancreatic

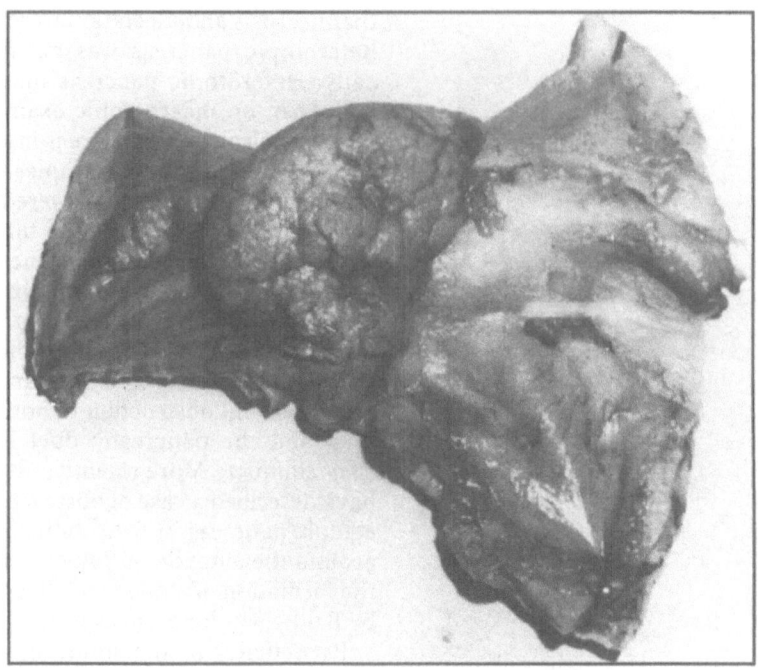

Fig. 3.6. Macroscopic appearance of heterotopic pancreas in the subserosa of the pylorus. The pancreatic tissue measured 2.5 cm in diameter: it was an incidental autopsy finding in a man aged 78 who died of bronchopneumonia associated with chronic bronchitis and emphysema.

tissue with secretory glandular tissue of gastro-intestinal type, along with undifferentiated, duct-like tissue that seemed to be neoplastic. All four contained muscle that appeared to be an integral part of the lesion (Fig. 3.7). A more recent example of a gastric lesion of this type has been described by Zarling (1981).

In addition to the tumour-like lesions of the stomach that have just been discussed, heterotopic pancreatic tissue with an uncomplicated structure may occur in the wall of the stomach (Mitchell and Angrist 1943); this occurred surrounding the pyloric canal and caused fatal pyloric obstruction in the 5-year-old girl reported by MacKinnon and Nash (1957).

The formation of cysts, 0.5–3 cm in diameter, is an uncommon feature of heterotopic pancreatic tissue. It has been reported in the duodenum and in the stomach (Claudon et al. 1988) where it may cause unusual endoscopic and radiographic appearances.

Malignancy

As has been mentioned, malignant tumours may arise in heterotopic pancreatic tissue. A brief note of carcinoma in aberrant pancreas in the jejunum was published by Seidelin in 1912–1913, and in 1923 Nicholson described a case of carcinoma of accessory pancreas in the stomach. He referred to two other reported cases, while, more recently, Goldfarb et al. (1963) gave an account of a possible case. The patient was a woman aged 55, whose gastric adeno-carcinoma contained an area of heterotopic pancreatic tissue in which the ducts resembled the ducts of the well differentiated carcinoma and, as there was no line of demarcation between the heterotopic and neoplastic tissues, it was concluded that the carcinoma had arisen from the pancreatic tissue. In earlier reports, for example that by Duff et al. (1943), who reported a carcinoma of the duodenum and that of Zak (1956), who reported a carcinoma in a jejunal diverticulum, the suggestion that the cancers might have originated from heterotopic pancreas depended entirely upon the histological resemblance of these carcinomas to carcinoma in the normally situated pancreas.

Other Complications

Heterotopic pancreas may cause problems in other ways. In Meckel's diverticula (Figs 3.8–3.10) its presence is normally of no significance, but Willis (1962) noted acute haemorrhagic necrosis in an "inflamed"

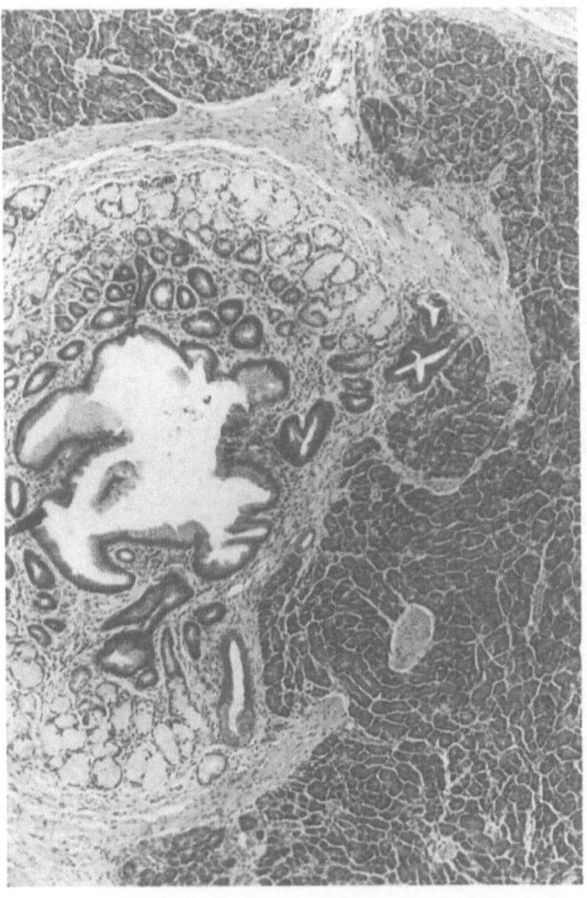

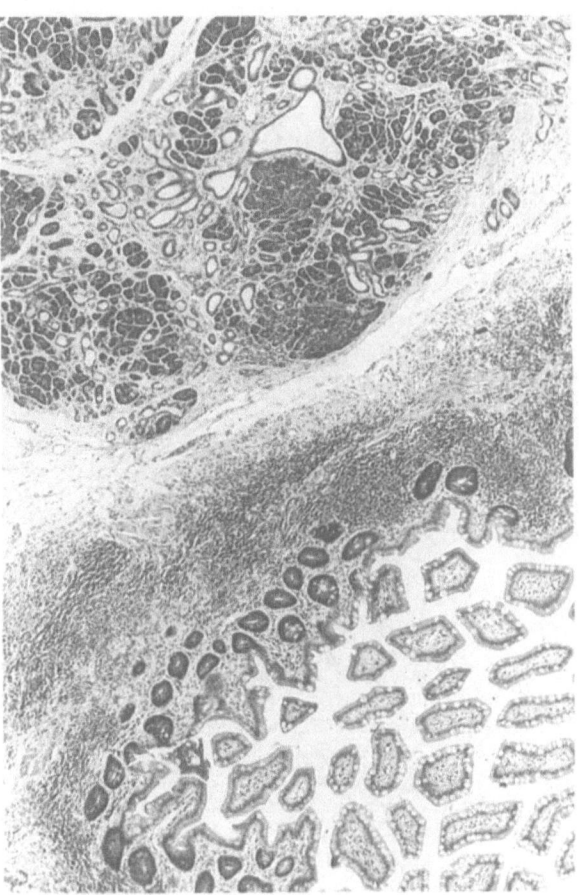

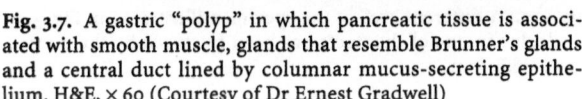

Fig. 3.7. A gastric "polyp" in which pancreatic tissue is associated with smooth muscle, glands that resemble Brunner's glands and a central duct lined by columnar mucus-secreting epithelium. H&E, × 60 (Courtesy of Dr Ernest Gradwell)

Fig. 3.8. Pancreatic tissue, with acini and ducts, but without islets, in the wall of a Meckel's diverticulum. H&E, × 41

Meckel's diverticulum removed from a boy aged 17. Inflammation of heterotopic pancreas may also be an unexpected finding at autopsy (Benbow 1988). At the umbilical region of the abdominal wall, vitelline remnants may form cystic lesions that contain heterotopic pancreas (Barbosa et al. 1946a), while in the large intestine Burne (1958) found pancreatic tissue that caused intussusception in a diverticulum of the transverse colon. In the oesophagus, heterotopic pancreatic tissue that caused symptoms was found by Razi (1966). His case was a man aged 43 who vomited blood and was found at operation to have a soft lobulated mass, 4 cm in diameter, on the right border of the oesophagus, well above the gastro-oesophageal junction but below the diaphragm. By frozen sections the mass was recognised to be pancreatic tissue. It was embedded in the outer wall of the oesophagus and did not extend to its inner muscular layer or mucosa. The tissue was enucleated

without interrupting the continuity of the oesophagus. It contained acini, ducts and islets of Langerhans.

In the biliary tract, pancreatic heterotopia may be mistaken for a true neoplasm in the vicinity of the common bile duct or ampulla of Vater (Weber et al. 1968; Coupland et al. 1987) or, as in one of the patients reported by Pearson (1951), aberrant pancreas in the ampulla of Vater may obstruct both the common bile duct and the duct of Wirsung. In Pearson's patient, although the pancreatic tissue measured only 25 × 20 × 20 mm after it had been excised, and although the orifices of the common bile duct and of the duct of Wirsung were separated by a distance of 4 mm, the abnormal tissue had blocked both ducts. Microscopically, the aberrant pancreatic tissue contained pancreatic acini and ducts but no islets. The appearance of the photomicrograph suggests that calcification had occurred

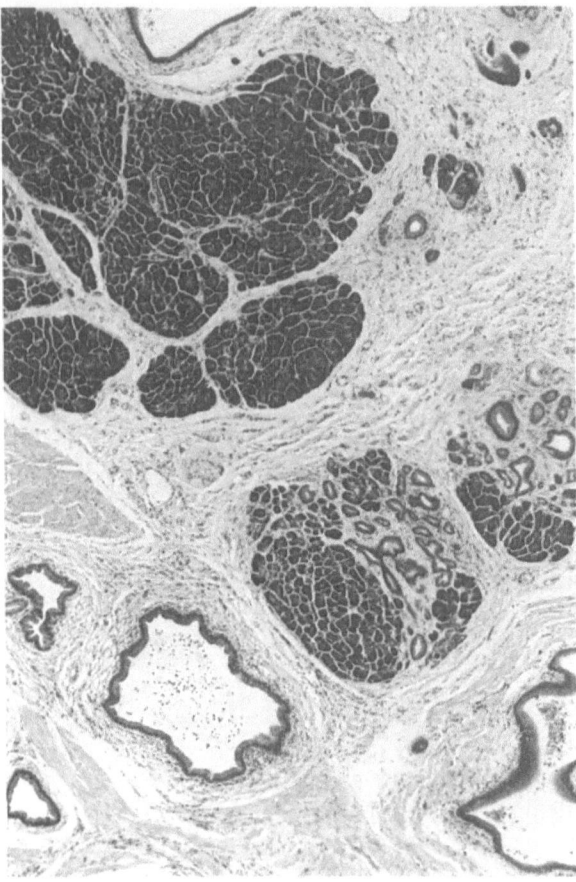

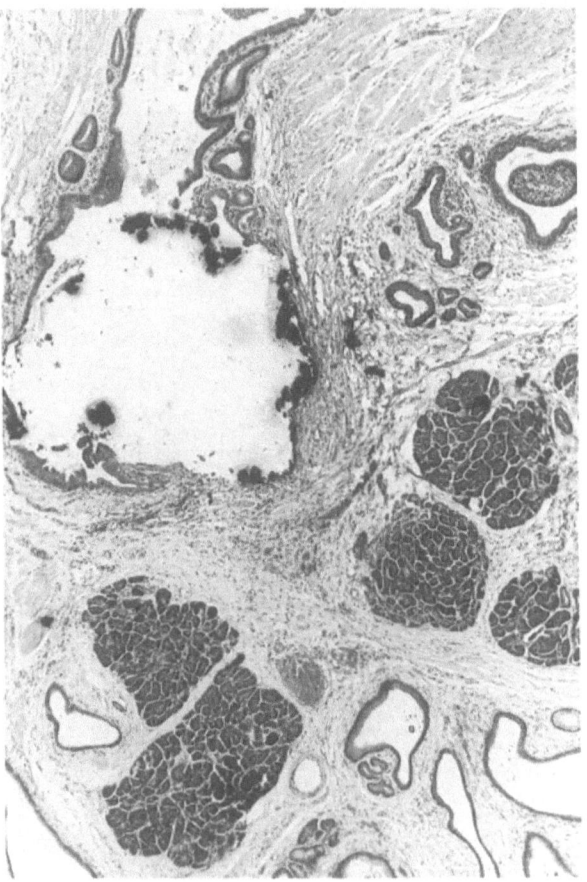

Fig. 3.9. Pancreatic tissue with ducts and smooth muscle in the wall of a Meckel's diverticulum. H&E, × 41

Fig. 3.10. A different area of the specimen illustrated in Fig. 3.9. A calculus in one of the ducts has been fractured by the microtome. H&E, × 41

in the pancreatic tissue, but Pearson does not comment on this, and there is nothing else in the photomicrograph to suggest that the obstructive effects of the aberrant tissue might have been precipitated by inflammation.

An apparently symptomless nodule on the neck of a human gall bladder with multiple projections was reported by Thorsness (1940), who could find records of only three other examples of the condition in man, although there are reports of the condition in the dog (Mann 1922; Higgins 1926). Ectopic pancreatic tissue and ectopic duodenal mucosa were incidental findings in the wall of a cyst removed from the perineum of a 9-year-old girl and reported by Narasimharao et al. (1987); the cyst was due to duplication of the rectum and had caused a chronic perianal fistula.

In the liver, pancreatic heterotopia may be of clinical importance, although its recognition in this site

is very rare. In the patient reported by Mobini et al. (1974), a mass of 7 cm in diameter and weighing 109 g, and attached to the left lobe of the liver by a pedicle, was palpable clinically. The greater part of the excised specimen was a cyst lined by tall columnar cells and interpreted by the authors as a retention cyst, but aberrant pancreatic tissue was found in the liver tissue that formed the pedicle of the lesion. Islet tissue was not found in the pancreatic tissue in that case, but in 1941 Ballinger reported a patient in which hypoglycaemia was attributed to a supposed islet cell carcinoma, whose origin was attributed to aberrant pancreatic tissue within the liver. At that time, however, it had not been recognised that hypoglycaemia is sometimes caused by a primary liver cell carcinoma.

A case of heterotopic pancreas in lymph nodes has been reported by Murayama et al. (1978). The authors could find no previous report of authentic pancreatic heterotopia in lymph nodes. The ectopic tissue was in nodes around the common hepatic artery and exocrine, endocrine and pancreatic ductal structures were present.

General Aspects

In general, it is in tissues derived from entoderm that heteroplasia may give rise to pancreatic tissue, but aberrant extensions of an otherwise normal pancreas may become incorporated in the spleen or its capsule (Weidman 1913); when accessory splenic tissue is embedded in the pancreas it may have strands of pancreatic tissue in its trabeculae (Willis 1962). A cystadenoma, indistinguishable from the mucin-secreting type of cystadenoma of the pancreas, was found by Satake et al. (1979) at the hilum of the spleen of a 48-year-old woman. The cystic tumour (which measured 16 × 26 × 17 cm) had been palpable as a left subcostal mass and was completely separated from the normal pancreatic tail; its origin was attributed to detached and heterotopic pancreatic tissue within the spleen.

In the thorax, heterotopic pancreatic tissue has been found in abundance in a large mediastinal cyst in a woman aged 19 (Shillitoe and Wilson 1957), and in a pulmonary malformation supplied with blood by two anomalous arterial branches from the lower thoracic aorta, as described by Kellett et al. (1962). In the latter case, the authors suggested that the developing lung tissue supplied by the abnormal blood vessels had undergone intralobar sequestration and had failed to develop into lung tissue, the bronchial entoderm having instead undergone heteroplastic differentiation into mature pancreatic tissue containing curved bars of cartilage, reminiscent of bronchial cartilage, around the ducts of the pancreatic tissue. The authors felt that the stimulus to the abnormal development might be related to the anomalous arterial blood supply of the sequestered pulmonary tissue.

Finally, there is a possible association between the chromosomal aberration of trisomy 18 and heterotopic pancreas; ectopic pancreas was present in four of the 84 necropsy cases of this condition tabulated by Warkany et al. (1966).

Pancreatic Tissue in Teratomas

Willis (1960) states that pancreatic tissue, including islets of Langerhans, may be present as one of the components of well differentiated teratomas. He does not, though, make any comments about frequency and sites; indeed his comments may be based on a single, personally observed example of an intrapericardial teratoma in a boy who died at about 9 months of age (Willis 1946). A more recent case report (Honicky and de Papp 1973) describes a 5-year-old boy with a mediastinal mass associated with asymptomatic hypoglycaemia and hyperinsulinaemia. After surgical excision of the mass, in which an abundance of islet cell tissue was found, glucose and insulin levels in the blood returned to normal.

Others have described systematic studies of collections of teratomas: Schlumberger (1946) studied 16 teratomas of the anterior mediastinum in adults of military age, and found pancreas in eight of them, including islets of Langerhans in seven. In one of these cases, pancreatic elements were so closely associated with a focus of adenocarcinoma that it was suggested that the former had given rise to the latter. Berry et al. (1969) studied 58 sacrococcygeal teratomas, 17 gonodal teratomas and 16 from other sites; pancreas was present in only three specimens, all from the sacrococcygeal area.

A more recent study, carried out in Japan (Suda et al. 1984) included 469 teratomas from various sites. There were 353 ovarian and 80 testicular lesions, none of which contained pancreatic tissue. In contrast, 34 teratomas from the anterior mediastinum, retroperitoneal space and sacrococcygeal region included 17 specimens that contained pancreatic tissue, with islets of Langerhans in 14 of them. There was no pancreatic tissue in two intracranial teratomas. Although there have been some recent advances in our understanding of the biology of teratomas, a recent review of the topic (Fox 1987) contains no explanation for the contrasting results of the study by Suda and his colleagues.

Accessory Spleens Within the Pancreas

Accessory spleens are common: they were found in almost 10% of a large series of consecutive autopsies upon adult male patients (Halpert and Györkey 1959; Halpert and Alden 1964). Of the accessory spleens found by these workers, at least one in six was embedded in the tail of the pancreas. Such intrapancreatic inclusions of splenic tissue are easily recognised with the naked eye by their red colour and general resemblance to normally situated splenic tissue. They are commonly about 1 cm in

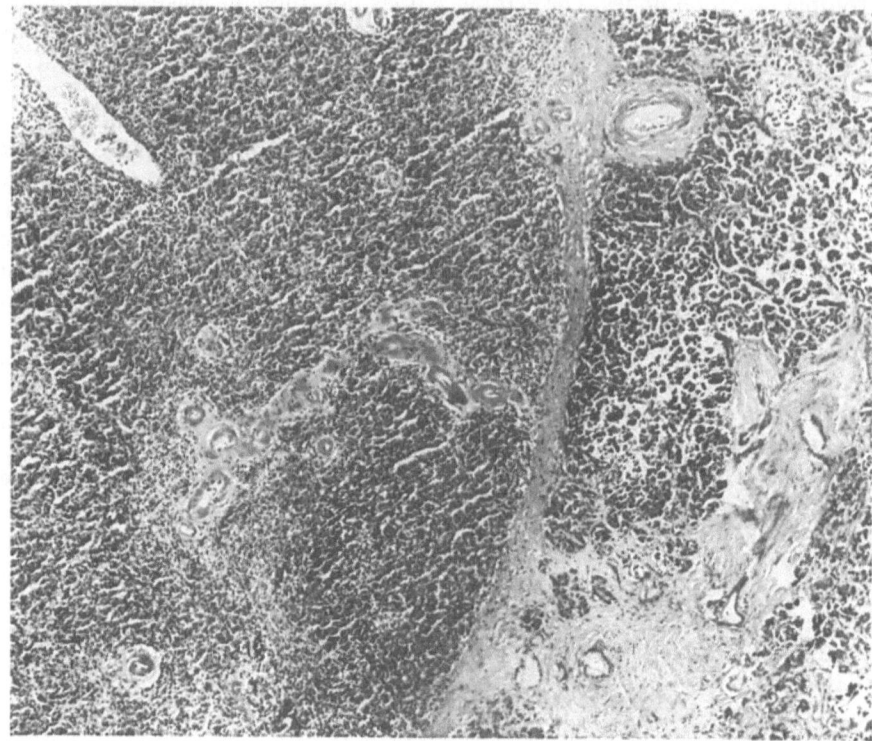

Fig. 3.11. Splenic tissue within the pancreas. In this case a partial capsule separated the splenic tissue, left, from the pancreatic tissue, right. H&E, × 60

diameter; the largest found by Halpert and Alden was 3.5 cm in diameter and the smallest 0.3 cm. Microscopically, the splenic inclusions may have a complete capsule, or the capsule may be incomplete, becoming thin and eventually disappearing in places, or, as in the case noted by Willis (1962), there may be no capsule. When a capsule is present it may contain lumina, lined by cuboidal cells that resemble pancreatic ducts and structures that resemble islets of Langerhans (Halpert and Györkey 1957), while the trabeculae within the splenic tissue may contain pancreatic tissue and ducts (Willis 1962). The pancreatic tissue near the splenic inclusion, especially if the capsule is incomplete, may contain small clumps of lymphocytes, and the glandular tissue may seem either rudimentary or atrophic, sometimes with conspicuous groups of islet cells.

Splenic inclusions within the pancreas are of practically no clinical importance, although they are said by Halpert and Györkey (1959) to participate with the main spleen in diseases that cause splenic changes, although granulomatous and metastatic neoplastic lesions are not always duplicated in the accessory tissue. In one of their cases, splenic tissue within the pancreas contained a deposit of columnar cell carcinoma that had originated in the pan-

creas; the main spleen contained no secondary carcinoma. Splenic inclusions within the pancreas are illustrated in Figs 3.11 and 3.12.

Congenital Cysts of the Pancreas

Congenital cystic lesions of the pancreas that are quite unrelated to cystic fibrosis of the pancreas (mucoviscidosis) are not very uncommon if the small single or multiple cysts of the pancreas that may be found incidentally, post-mortem, are truly congenital. Such cysts cause no symptoms; they have a thin fibrous wall and are lined by a columnar or cubical type of epithelium (Fig. 3.13). Two cystic lesions are illustrated in Figs 3.14 and 3.15 – they were unassociated with cysts in any other organ.

Cystic lesions of the pancreas large enough to be recognised at birth or in early infancy are most unusual. Miles (1959) could find reports of only eight examples in infants under 2 years of age: of these, only two were demonstrable at birth. The patient reported by Miles was that of a female black baby, whose abdomen was distended at birth and

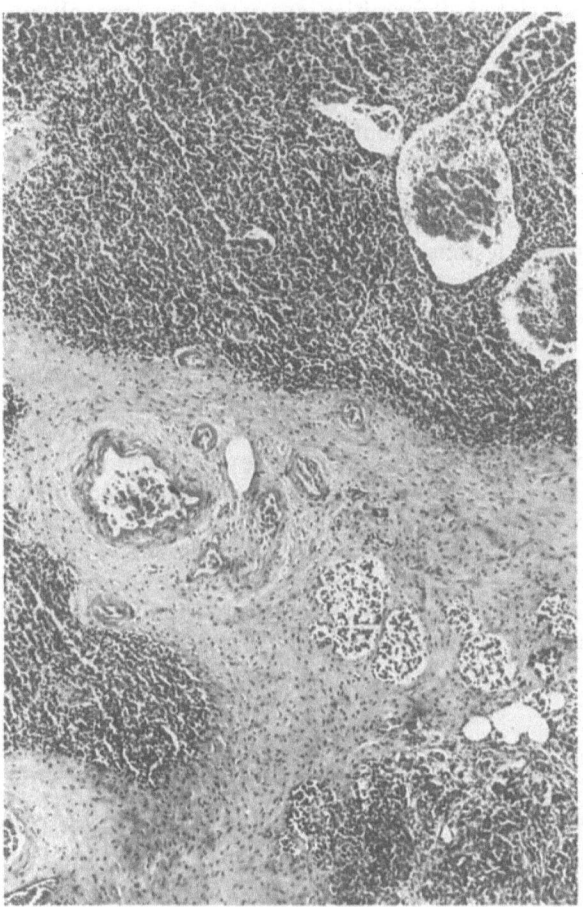

Fig. 3.12. Splenic tissue within the pancreas. Islets of Langerhans are present in the splenic trabeculae. H&E, × 60

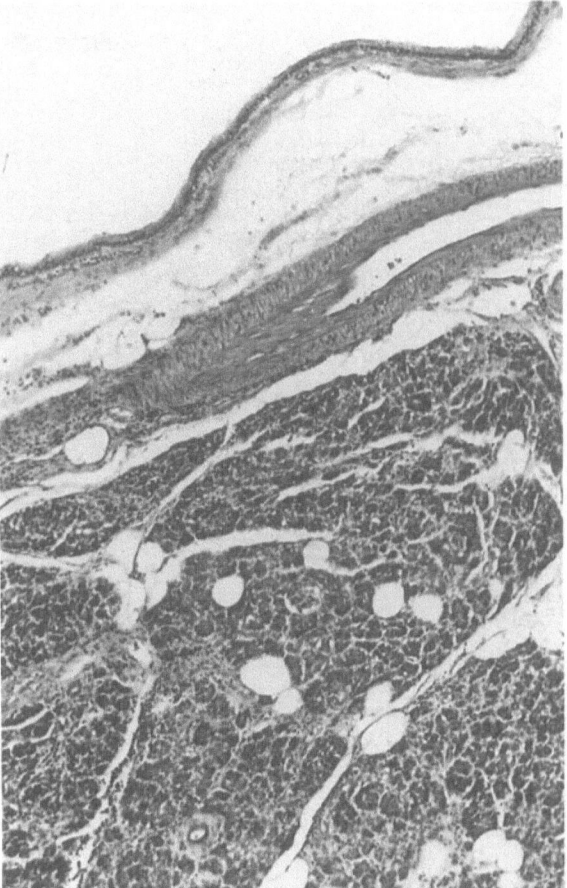

Fig. 3.13. The wall of one of several small cysts found incidentally at autopsy in a patient who had died of myeloproliferative disease. Such cysts are believed to be congenital. No neurological or other components of Lindau's disease were present in this patient. H&E, × 60

from whose pancreas a thin-walled multilocular cyst, 23 × 13 × 6 cm, was removed when the child was 8 days old. The cyst arose from the lower margin of the head and body of the pancreas and bulged forwards, separating the layers of the transverse mesocolon, to present between the stomach, which was displaced upwards, and the transverse colon. Lobular extensions of the cyst partially surrounded and partially obstructed the transverse colon. The cyst was excised with a margin of normal pancreatic tissue and could be dissected away from the other structures with which it was in contact. The cyst was made up of many thin-walled spaces filled with clear serous fluid. Microscopically the loculi were of various sizes. Some were lined by well differentiated, stratified squamous epithelium, others by cuboidal epithelium or by a single layer of flattened or columnar epithelium. Many duct-like spaces,

lined by stratified squamous epithelium, traversed the sections and the cystic spaces were separated by a fibrous stroma in which there were blood vessels and scattered clumps of well differentiated pancreatic acinar cells with a few islets of Langerhans. There was no significant enzymatic activity in the cystic fluid. The child recovered from the operation rather slowly, with some varus deformity of the feet, but, helped by built-up shoes, she was almost normal by about the age of 3 years.

The lack of important associated congenital deformities in the above patient contrasts with the severe associated deformities in the patient reported by de Lange and Janssen (1948). In a prematurely born female baby there was a pancreatic cyst, big enough to cause abdominal distension, along with developmental anomalies of the brain, polydactyly, and anterior displacement of the anus. Such

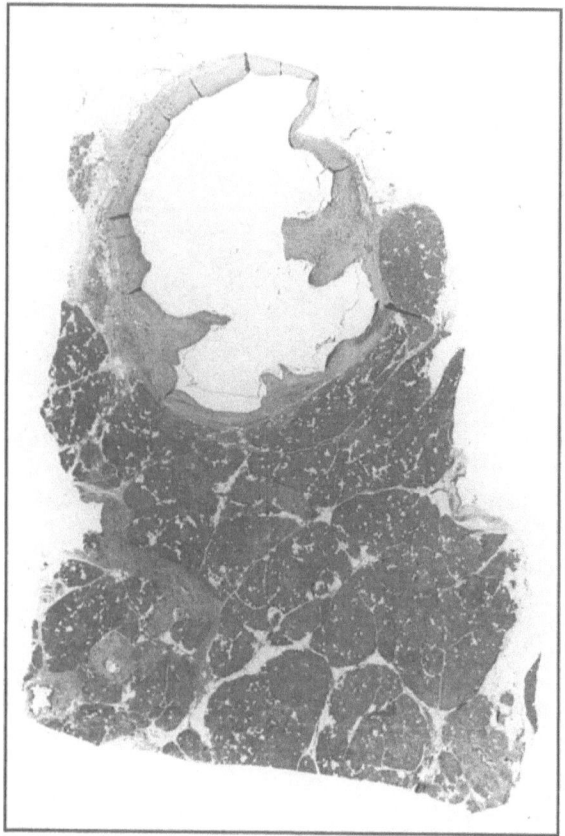

associated deformities are not, however, always present. Power (1961), for example, partially removed a pancreatic cyst with a fibrous wall and a lining of flattened epithelium from a 23-day-old boy. The child's development was normal once the fistula, caused by marsupialisation of the remnants of the cyst, had healed. Nevertheless, the presence of a pancreatic cyst is a cause for anxiety that other congenital lesions may be present, and Warkany (1971) quotes Seifert (1956) to the effect that isolated pancreatic cysts have been seen repeatedly in association with situs inversus and cystic kidneys. A developmental pancreatic cyst may also cause episodes of pancreatitis associated with osteolytic lesions and subcutaneous fat necrosis, as in the case of a 7-year-old girl described by Hollingworth et al. (1979). The child's symptoms were relieved by the removal of a developmental cyst that lay between the pancreas and the colon. The cyst had a fibrous wall and contained pancreatic acini and islets of Langerhans as well as intestinal glandular tissue. The pancreas itself seemed normal.

Fig. 3.14. A very low-power view of one of the cysts present in the pancreas in the case illustrated in Fig. 3.13. H&E, × 4

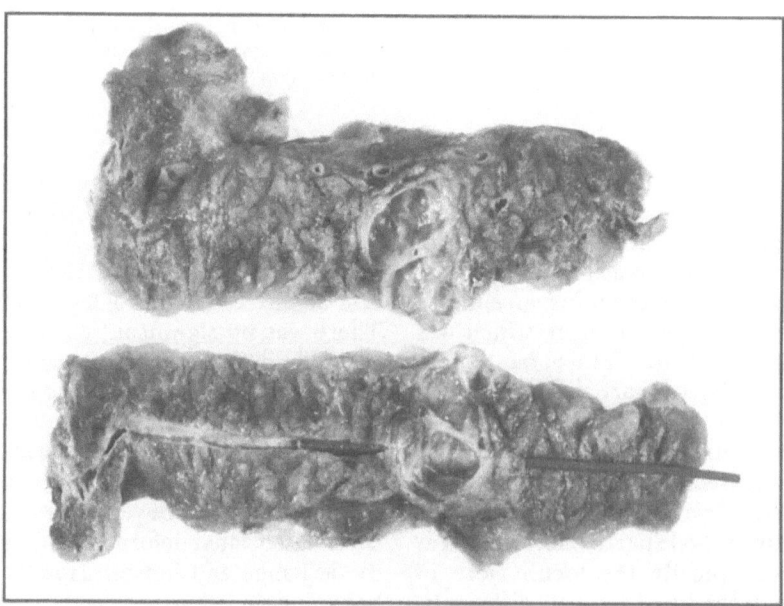

Fig. 3.15. A thin-walled loculated cyst, believed to be congenital, found incidentally in a pancreas. The pancreas has now been bisected. The probe in the pancreatic duct does not enter the cyst but, when barium sulphate was injected into the duct, the cyst was radiologically visualised.

Pancreatic Cysts Associated with Renal Cystic Disease

Congenital cystic disease of the kidneys is now recognised as being of several types. In the adult type of polycystic renal disease, cysts are commonly found post-mortem in the liver; they were found in 75 of the 184 cases of bilateral polycystic disease of the kidneys examined by Dalgaard (1957), but he found no cysts in the pancreas. According to Heptinstall (1966), however, pancreatic cysts may be found in about 10% of patients with polycystic disease of the kidneys, but the presence of such cysts may not be recognised without microscopic examination (Bigelow 1953).

In the infantile type of polycystic renal disease, a condition that is not compatible with prolonged survival, pancreatic cysts may be found as well as the cystic bile ducts that are invariably present within the liver, and the experiments of McGeoch and Darmady (1976) suggested that deficiency of the ouabain-sensitive enzyme sodium-potassium-activated adenosine triphosphatase, inherited as an autosomal recessive trait, may be responsible for the anomalies. The pancreatic cysts, which are formed by dilated ducts lined by flattened cells, seem, unlike the renal lesions, to be of no clinical importance. Similarly, the pancreatic cysts occasionally associated with congenital hepatic fibrosis, as noted by Kerr et al. (1961), have no clinical effects. Pancreatic cysts, of no apparent clinical significance, have also been noted (Kennedy et al. 1991) in the oral–facial–digital syndrome type 1, along with renal cysts and cystadenomatous bile ducts.

Von Hippel–Lindau Disease

In 1884 Pye-Smith noted the presence of cysts in the pancreas associated with cysts in the kidney and a cyst in the cerebellum, in the body of a man aged 27. Although "there was no trace of new growth or of blood crystals or pigment" in the cerebellar cyst it seems likely that Pye-Smith's case was an example of the condition that was later studied by Lindau (1926), and is now known as Lindau's syndrome, or von Hippel–Lindau disease. Although the pancreatic cysts in this inherited disease may be striking, as was illustrated in Lindau's communication to the Royal Society of Medicine in November 1930, they seldom cause ill effects; other components of the syndrome are usually of more importance in the

clinical management of the disease. In fact, pancreatic cysts are by no means invariably present; they were present in only two of Lindau's own 16 patients. When cysts are present they vary considerably in size and number. In Pye-Smith's case much of the pancreas seemed normal but about eight or nine cysts were scattered in the gland, mostly in the tail. Their sizes varied from that of a hemp seed to that of a hazel nut and they contained clear fluid; some projected from the surface.

In 1947, Kinney and Fitzgerald reported on the lesions in two cases of the syndrome. In one there were only a few small cystic spaces in the pancreas; they were lined by a low columnar epithelium and the adjacent pancreas was microscopically normal. In the other case, however, the pancreas weighed 370 g and measured 29 cm in length, 9 cm in width and 4–6 cm in thickness. It appeared macroscopically to be made up mainly of cysts that measured from 0.1 cm to 3 cm in diameter, but occasional areas of normal pancreas could be seen between the cysts. The walls of the cysts were paper thin, grey and translucent, and the spaces were filled with straw-coloured fluid. Microscopically, the cysts had fibrous walls and a lining of low columnar epithelium. In the areas where the cysts were most numerous there was fibrous replacement of some of the adjacent pancreatic acini, with compression of the remaining acini. In the regions in which cyst formation was less marked, the pancreatic tissue between the cysts was normal. The islets of Langerhans were unaffected. In the case reported by Davison et al. (1936) a cystadenoma that had been attached by a pedicle was removed six years before the patient's death, after which a few small cysts that contained clear fluid were found in the region of the head of the pancreas, and at the hilum of the spleen.

As has been mentioned already, the pancreatic component of von Hippel–Lindau disease is usually of minor clinical importance. The many components of the syndrome, including the vascular neoplasms of the retina and central nervous system, associated with the name of von Hippel, and the hereditary nature of the condition, have been described in detail by Lamiell et al. (1989). These authors have reviewed the contributions that led to the recognition that, in addition to haemangioblastomas of the retina and central nervous system, with or without cysts in the pancreas, victims of the disease are liable to develop simple or malignant tumours in many organs. The authors' conclusions were based on their own study of 43 members of a single kindred, and the lesions reported in 511 other cases in the medical literature. From this experience, they include the following lesions in the syndrome:

1. Cerebellar, spinal, medullary or cerebral haemangioblastoma;
2. Retinal haemangioblastoma;
3. Multiple renal cysts, with or without, renal adenocarcinoma;
4. Pancreatic cysts, cystadenocarcinoma or islet cell tumour;
5. Phaeochromocytoma;
6. Epididymal cystadenoma.

Their advice is that the syndrome should be suspected if at least one of the above conditions should occur in a member of a family in which at least one relative has, or has had, a lesion of the central nervous system or of an eye, or renal cysts or renal adenocarcinoma. Genetic studies have shown that the inheritance is of the autosomal dominant type and that the gene is located on the short arm of chromosome 3; and, by screening other members of the vulnerable kindred for presymptomatic conditions in already diagnosed or in undiagnosed relatives, the authors found and treated many early lesions associated with this syndrome.

The pancreatic lesions they found in the kindred were cysts in five of the males and in eight of the females. In ten of these 13 cases the cysts were multiple. Two of the males and two (or possibly three) of the females had pancreatic malignancy. In one of these the malignancy was pancreatic adenocarcinoma, while in another it was islet cell carcinoma. The possible third case had cystic lesions that were suspected of being malignant. Such lesions, as the authors point out, are definite, though uncommon, manifestations of von Hippel–Lindau disease. Other rare manifestations include pancreatic exocrine insufficiency (Fishman and Bartholomew 1979) and pancreatic endocrine insufficiency (Thompson et al. 1989)

Dermoid Cysts

There are a few reports of dermoid cysts in the pancreas and such cysts can be explained only as being due to a congenital abnormality in which a totipotential cell in an embryonic rest in the pancreas develops into a cystic tumour.

In 1977 Assawamatiyanont and King were able to refer to about ten recognised cases when they reported one of their own. In the case reported by De Courcy in 1943 the cyst was removed surgically from a 2-year-old female infant. A hard nodular mass, about the size of a small orange, was palpable clinically and, when laparotomy was undertaken, the tumour was found to be embedded in the middle portion of the pancreas. It was removed and, when opened, was found to be cystic and to contain "all the elements comprising a dermoid cyst." The patient reported by Assawamatiyanont and King was that of an 11-year-old girl who had a mass 9 × 8 × 6 cm removed from the body of the pancreas. The mass was found to be a benign dermoid cyst filled with hair and pasty sebaceous material. Dermoid cysts of the pancreas have also been found in adults. The case described by Dennis in 1923 was a man aged 40 whose pancreatic cyst had calcareous material in its lining and contained grumous, greasy material, as well as a few short hairs, while Judd's patient (Judd 1921; Masson and Caylor 1929) was a woman of 33 whose cyst, which had been enlarging gradually for 9 years, was in the body and tail of the pancreas. After its removal the cyst measured 15 cm in diameter, and its contents were hair, creamy sebaceous material and thin grey fluid. The wall of the cyst contained a tooth, said to be an incisor, together with squamous epithelium, sebaceous glands, hair follicles, sweat glands and connective tissue.

Pancreatic Lymphoepithelial Cysts

In 1985 Lüchtrath and Schriefers reported a multilocular cyst of the pancreas with walls that had the microscopic appearances of a branchial cyst, a type of pancreatic cyst that they believed had not been recognised previously. The cyst was removed from a 36-year-old man who had lost weight and who had leucocytosis. The cyst was recognised by computed tomography and ultrasonography; it was removed with the distal 10 cm of the pancreas, and the patient made a good recovery. After it had been cut, the cyst measured 9 × 5 × 2 cm and consisted of multiple loculi separated by thin septa. Microscopically, the walls were lined by mature, stratified squamous epithelium attached to lymphoreticular tissue with small germinal centres, and the authors felt that the structure of the wall was exactly similar to that of the so-called branchiogenic cyst that may occur in the sides of the neck.

A cyst with microscopically similar walls has also been found in the pancreas by Truong et al. (1987). This cyst differed from that reported by Lüchtrath and Schriefers (1985) only in that it consisted of a single loculus and lacked the fibrous septa that divided the cyst illustrated by Lüchtrath and Schriefers into multiple loculi. The cyst described by

Truong et al. was removed from a 35-year-old man who had had persistent diarrhoea and upper abdominal pain for 3 months. Endoscopic retrograde cholangiopancreatography showed a patent pancreatic duct that seemed to be compressed by a mass in the pancreas; the presence of a mass was confirmed by computed tomography and ultrasonography. At laparotomy, a smooth well circumscribed mass compressed, but did not invade, the pancreas, from which it was dissected easily, although the cyst ruptured during its removal. It consisted of a single loculus filled with semisolid tan-grey material that had a slightly laminated appearance on its cut surface. The cyst formed a mass $4 \times 6 \times 6$ cm and the wall, from which the contents could be separated without difficulty, was 0.3 cm thick and had a smooth shiny inner surface and a thin outer fibrous layer. Microscopically, the contents consisted of keratinous material, while the lining was of keratinising squamous epithelium that was almost completely surrounded by lymphoid tissue in which there were occasional lymphoid follicles. The outer parts of the lymphoid layer contained foci of pancreatic tissue in which there were ducts, acini and islets. After the removal of the cyst, the patient's symptoms disappeared and he was well 5 months later.

Both groups of authors speculate about the histogenesis of these lymphoepithelial cysts of the pancreas without reaching a definite conclusion. In an attempt to check the suggestion that the cysts may have arisen from benign epithelial inclusions within peripancreatic lymph nodes, Truong et al. (1987) examined 435 nodes from the region of the pancreas, obtained during autopsies and operations, but found neither squamous epithelial inclusions nor heterotopic pancreatic tissue in the nodes. Their failure does not, however, exclude an origin from at least the latter source, for heterotopic pancreatic tissue has been reported in lymph nodes by Murayama et al. (1978).

Pancreatic Atrophy

The presence of a certain amount of fat in most pancreases has already been mentioned in relation to the weight of the normal pancreas, but marked atrophy of the glandular tissue, especially of the acinar cells, regardless of the cause of the atrophy, usually leads to adipose replacement of the secretory tissue (Walters 1966). Thus, quite substantial degrees of atrophy of the pancreas may escape notice during routine autopsies. Increasing age alone tends to be associated with an increase in the diameter of the ducts (Kreel and Sandin 1973). Andrew (1944) described the development of locules and cavities as ageing progressed in the pancreases of Wistar rats and of man, along with a tendency for the epithelium of the interlobular ducts to undergo squamous metaplasia. An example of very marked dilatation of the pancreatic ducts with glandular atrophy in the absence of obstruction of the ducts, and without fatty replacement, is illustrated in Figs 3.16 and 3.17. In that patient, the abnormality of the pancreas was an incidental finding in a man aged 81 who died from a perforated duodenal ulcer; he was not known to have had any symptoms of pancreatic disease.

A rare but well-recognised type of primary atrophy of the pancreas, in which there is almost complete disappearance of the acinar cells and a loss to a lesser extent of the islets of Langerhans, with varying degrees of fatty replacement, has been described by Bartholomew et al. (1959). No cause for the atrophy has been determined and the infiltration of the organ by fat may be so great that it produces a condition of lipomatous pseudohypertrophy. This may occur in adults who are neither obese nor diabetic and who may, or may not, have clinical evidence of exocrine pancreatic insufficiency. An example of lipomatous pseudohypertrophy of the pancreas is illustrated in Fig. 3.18. In that case the pancreas weighed 740 g, about eight times the average weight of the pancreas in a woman. The patient, who died of heart disease, was aged 82; she was not obese. Shortly before her death she was found to be diabetic with a blood sugar of 350 mg/100 ml.

Bartholomew et al. (1959) were able to refer to published reports of six patients, to which they added an account of their own two patients. The youngest two patients in the eight tabulated by Bartholomew et al. were both 47 years old; the ages of the others were between 61 and 80 years. Only two had diabetes and the patient reported by Robson and Scott (1953) had steatorrhoea. In such mature or elderly patients it seems much more likely that the deficiency of pancreatic tissue, and its replacement by fat, is the result of atrophy of a previously normal pancreas, rather than a lifelong pancreatic deficiency. The development of a lipoma within the pancreas had been suggested as a cause, but a primary lipoma with subsequent pressure atrophy of the gland is unlikely to cause diffuse enlargement without distortion of the original shape; the shape of the gland was retained in all the reported cases. Two patients with pseudohypertrophic lipomatous atrophy of the pancreas that developed adenocarcinoma in the fatty gland have

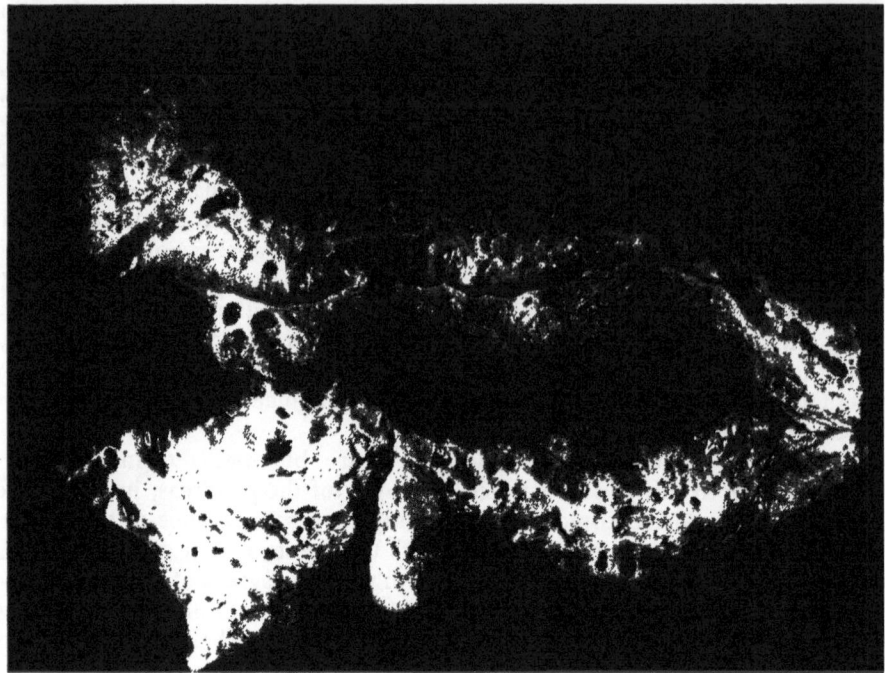

Fig. 3.16. Atrophy of the pancreas with dilatation of the ducts. No explanation for the condition of the pancreas was found. The specimen was obtained from the body of a man aged 81, who died because of a perforated duodenal ulcer. He also had atheromatous narrowing of the circumflex branch of the left coronary artery and fibrosis of the left ventricle. There was no history of disease of the pancreas. (Courtesy of Dr Peter Laidler)

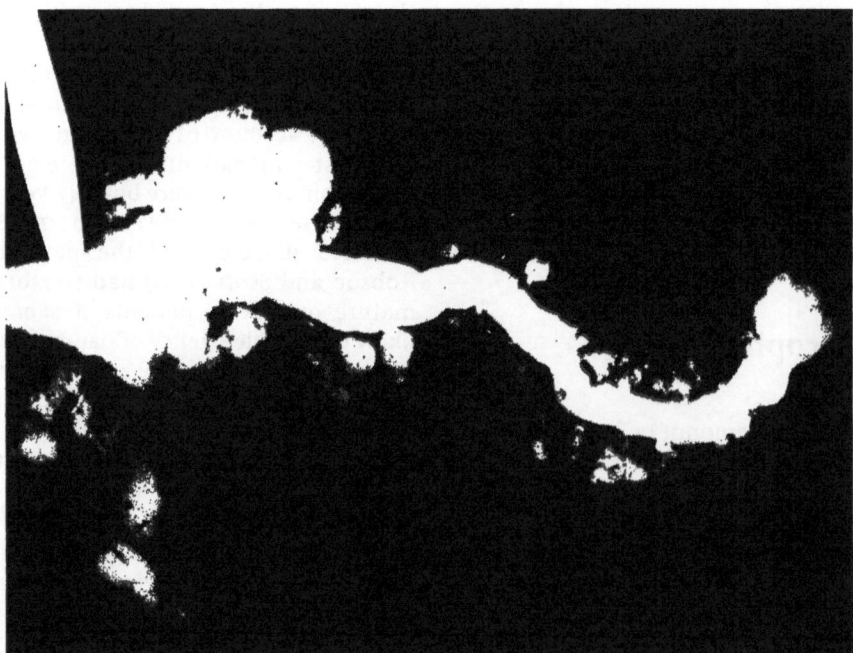

Fig. 3.17. Radiograph of the pancreas illustrated in Fig. 3.16, after the ducts had been injected with barium sulphate.

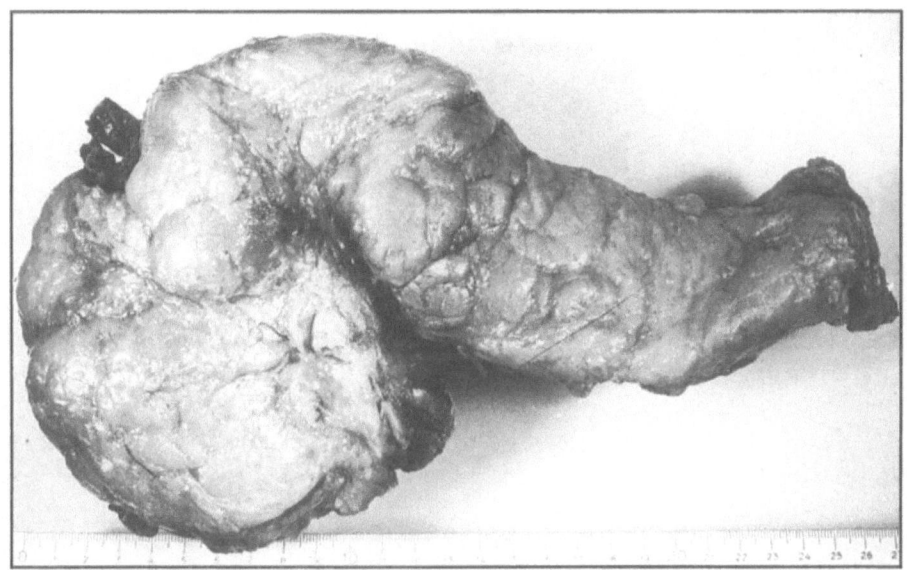

Fig. 3.18. Extreme liposis of a pancreas weighing 740 g. The loss of pancreatic parenchyma associated with the liposis is illustrated in Figs 3.19–3.22. (Courtesy of Dr William Taylor)

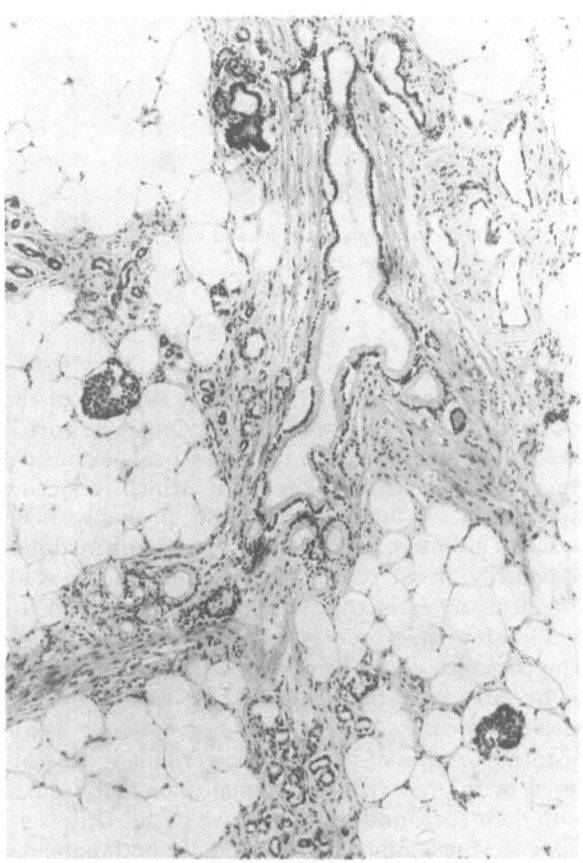

Fig. 3.19. One of the few scattered areas of pancreatic parenchyma that remained in the fat that replaced most of the pancreas illustrated in Fig. 3.18. H&E, × 60

been reported by Salm (1960, 1968). In that reported by Salm in 1960 the ducts of the enlarged (weight 175 g), fatty pancreas were dilated and filled with calcareous casts. Microscopically, partial squamous metaplasia was found in the dilated ducts. The exocrine parenchyma was missing except in the immediate vicinity of the ducts, and had been replaced by fat. The islets of Langerhans were quite numerous.

In most of the reported cases the microscopic appearances have resembled those in that illustrated in Figs 3.19–3.22. The metaplasia of the epithelium of the ducts noted by Salm (1960) is unusual and, although the carcinoma in the head of the gland was small, the effects of obstruction of the ducts cannot be excluded. In more typical cases the exocrine tissue disappears and is replaced by fat, except for the ducts and a few remnants of acinar tissue near the ducts, while the islets of Langerhans are prominent and often arranged in clusters. Their cells, however, may be small, and, even in patients without diabetes, it is difficult to recognise alpha and beta cells, while the nuclei are deeply staining and possibly pyknotic in many of the islet cells. Some fibrous septa traverse the fatty tissue and the ducts and ductules are surrounded by a sheath of loose fibrous tissue. Sometimes there are some clumps of lymphocytes in the fatty tissue. The ducts are lined by cuboidal or columnar mucus-secreting epithelium. Fatty change in other organs is variable; some degree of fatty change, such as is common in autopsy material, may be present in the liver. In the

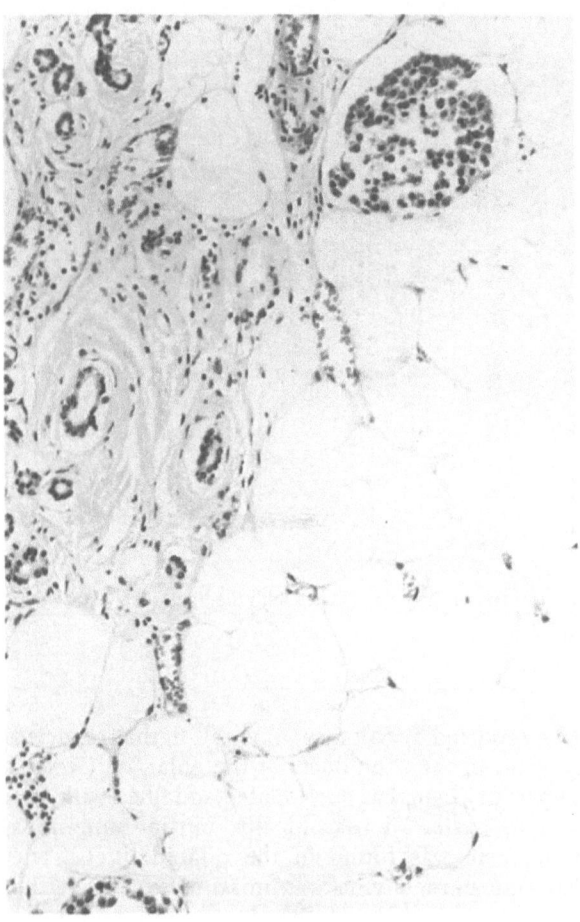

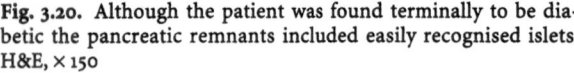

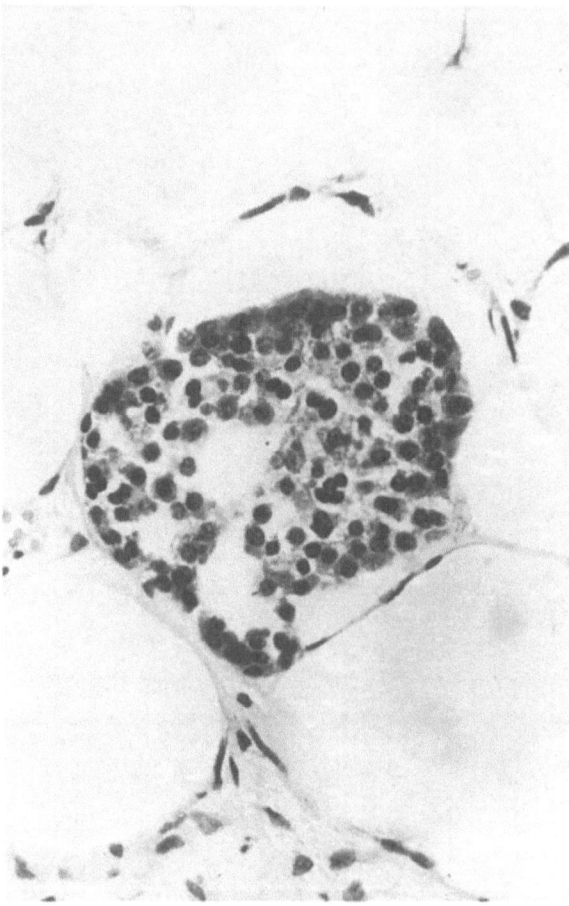

Fig. 3.20. Although the patient was found terminally to be diabetic the pancreatic remnants included easily recognised islets. H&E, × 150

Fig. 3.21. An islet surrounded by fat and without other types of pancreatic tissue. H&E, × 375

patient reported by Robson and Scott there was a possible increase of fat in the parathyroid glands, the body being emaciated elsewhere, except for the pancreas, and, in the patient whose pancreas is illustrated in Figs 3.19–3.22, there was quite marked fatty replacement of the one submandibular gland that was examined microscopically.

Congenital Pancreatic Hypoplasia with Haematological Abnormalities (Shwachman–Diamond Syndrome)

In 1964 Bodian et al. reported two patients with congenital hypoplasia of the pancreas, pointing out that

this condition differed from cystic fibrosis of the pancreas. They reviewed 18 previously reported cases in which the pancreas had been examined microscopically, and three in which exocrine hypoplasia of the pancreas had probably been present, although this had not been confirmed histologically. In the patients reported by Bodian et al. the electrolytes in the sweat were normal and the condition of the pancreas was ascertained by biopsy. The pancreas could be recognised macroscopically to be fatty in both cases and this was confirmed microscopically. There were no signs of cystic fibrosis. Groups of islets of Langerhans were scattered in the fat with some small pancreatic ducts with their surrounding connective tissue. Only very few exocrine acini could be found. In both patients, repeated haematological investigations were carried

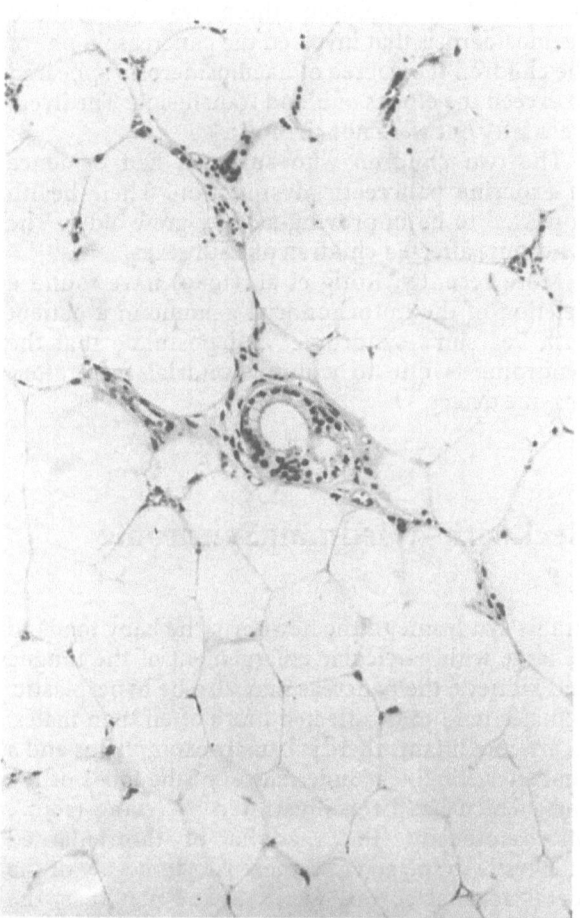

Fig. 3.22. A small duct surrounded by fat and without other types of pancreatic tissue. H&E, × 150

tory granules; there was some vacuolation of the cytoplasm. The nuclei were enlarged and irregular, had prominent nuclear membranes, pale or empty nucleoplasm, and contained striking central intra-nuclear inclusions. Intracytoplasmic inclusions were also present. The islets of Langerhans were relatively prominent and were composed of large cells with distinct cell borders, clear cytoplasm and large pyknotic nuclei. The excretory ducts were decreased in number and the remaining ducts were surrounded by fibrous tissue. They were empty and undilated.

Since the publications of Bodian et al. and Shwachman et al. in 1964, various other reports from different parts of the world have appeared. The syndrome is usually referred to as the Shwachman–Diamond syndrome and a variety of findings in addition to the pancreatic and haematological abnormalities have been reported. These reports have been reviewed by Anderson (1979); she mentions dwarfism, metaphyseal abnormalities, small chest and dyspnoea, immune deficiency, recurrent infections, abnormal liver function, mild cirrhotic changes in the liver, nonspecific mild enteropathy and other congenital abnormalities, which include Hirschsprung's disease. The abnormalities may be multiple.

The syndrome has a familial incidence, with several reports of siblings having been affected, but no pattern of inheritance has yet been recognised. The sexes are affected equally. Illustrations of the macroscopic and microscopic appearances of the pancreas were reproduced by Anderson (1979).

The two patients described as examples of lipomatous pseudohypertrophy of the pancreas by Beresford and Owen (1957) may have been cases of congenital hypoplasia of the pancreas that survived until early adult life. The first was that of a woman who was aged 27 at the time of her death. She was of dwarf stature and had generalised scleroderma, rheumatic heart disease and chronic pulmonary tuberculosis. During her terminal illness she developed a haemorrhagic tendency. The second patient was a man aged 23, who suffered from coeliac disease in childhood. He died of bronchopneumonia; a lipomatous pseudohypertrophic pancreas weighing 330 g was found post-mortem.

Neurological complications of the Shwachman–Diamond syndrome have been reported by Steinspir and Vinters (1985), who found central pontine myelinolysis in a child, and by Mah et al. (1987), who found focal pontine leucoencephalopathy in an adult woman who died of infective complications of the syndrome.

out. In their conclusions the authors stated that there was sometimes a curious association between haemotological disturbances of varying severity and congenital hypoplasia of the exocrine pancreas. The disturbances might include anaemia, thrombocytopenia or neutropenia, and were sometimes associated with hypoplasia of the corresponding cellular elements in the bone marrow. Their studies suggested a familial incidence.

The haematological features of the syndrome received more attention in the paper, published also in 1964, by Shwachman et al. Pancreatic biopsy was carried out in one of their patients, and representative sections from the tail and body of the pancreas were examined. There was marked displacement of the exocrine pancreatic glandular tissue by fat. The remaining acinar cells were large and lacked secre-

Juvenile Nephronophthisis with Calcification of Basal Ganglia and Pancreatic Insufficiency

The association of clinically unimportant congenital cysts of the pancreas with congenital cystic disease of the kidneys has been mentioned earlier in this chapter, but important functional failure of the pancreas with anatomical atrophy and fat replacement in association with this type of chronic juvenile renal failure, now considered to be synonymous with medullary cystic disease of the kidneys, has been described by Raafat et al. (1988). Their patient was a girl who died when she was 4 years old. She had had the various clinical manifestations of progressive renal failure due to juvenile nephronophthisis, with diarrhoea and reduced faecal chymotrypsin, followed later by hyperglycaemia and neurological abnormalities. At autopsy, in addition to the renal lesions, some hepatic fibrosis, and microscopic areas of calcification in the basal ganglia, the pancreas was seen to be much shrunken and fatty. Microscopically, the entire exocrine pancreas was replaced by fat. The islets of Langerhans also appeared to be reduced, but contained some beta cells when staining with an anti-insulin peroxidase antiperoxidase stain was carried out.

Refractory Sideroblastic Anaemia with Vacuolisation of Marrow Precursors and Exocrine Pancreatic Dysfunction

What is claimed by the authors to be a new syndrome of anaemia and exocrine pancreatic dysfunction was described in 1979 by Pearson et al. The syndrome, in which bone marrow and exocrine pancreatic dysfunction were associated in four unrelated children, differed in several respects from the syndrome described by Shwachman et al. (1964) and by Bodian et al. (1964). The anaemia was of the refractory sideroblastic type and very marked vacuoles were present in the precursors of the red and white cells in the bone marrow, with ringed sideroblasts and haemosiderosis. Two of the children died and were found at autopsy to have extensive pancreatic fibrosis, with acinar atrophy but normal islets. The ducts were not obstructed or dilated. The pancreases were not enlarged by fat and were of normal size. In both children there was generalised haemosiderosis that involved the pancreas; in one of the children the degree of haemosiderosis appeared to exceed the effects of blood transfusion. The livers were fatty but were not cirrhotic.

The two children who survived had evidence of exocrine pancreatic dysfunction. Their health appeared to be improving as they grew older. The syndrome affected children of both sexes.

More recently, Rotig et al. (1989) have found a deletion of the mitochondrial genome in a patient with Pearson's syndrome, and postulate that the syndrome is due to a mitochondrial respiratory enzyme defect.

Beckwith–Wiedman Syndrome

In this syndrome of the newborn, the baby tends to be large with particular enlargement of the tongue and kidneys; the pancreas may also be hyperplastic. Females tend to be affected more often than males. In affected infants there is usually exomphalos and a characteristic linear indentation of the lobes of the ears, which has been illustrated by Irving (1967). Microscopically, the medulla of the enlarged kidneys is dysplastic and there is cytomegaly of the foetal adrenal cortex, while, in the pancreas, the islets may be enlarged and form confluent masses, although this is not invariably present. The enlargement of the tongue may interfere with respiration and, if there is hyperplasia of the pancreatic islets, there may be hypoglycaemia, which can be fatal. By 1986 there had been reports of 388 cases of this syndrome (Koh et al. 1986) and a number of these had been complicated by malignant tumours such as nephroblastoma, adrenal carcinoma or hepatoblastoma. Koh and his colleagues reported the successful removal of a pancreatoblastoma from a West Indian baby with the syndrome.

References

Adeyemi SD (1988) Combination of annular pancreas and partial situs inversus: a multiple organ malrotation syndrome and duodenal obstruction. J Pediatr Surg 23 : 88–191

Adzick NS, Shamberger RC, Winter HS, Hendren WH (1989) Surgical treatment of pancreas divisum causing pancreatitis in children. J Pediatr Surg 24 : 54–58

Agha FP, Williams KD (1987) Pancreas divisum: incidence, detection and clinical significance. Am J Gastroenterol 82 : 315–320

Anderson M (1979) Pancreatic disease in childhood. In: Howat HT, Sarles H (eds) The exocrine pancreas. Saunders, London, pp 313–339

Andrew W (1944) Senile changes in the pancreas of Wistar Institute rats and of man with special regard to the similarity of locule and cavity formation. Am J Anat 74:79–144

Assawamatiyanont S, King AD (1977) Dermoid cysts of the pancreas. Am Surg 43:503–504

Baldwin WM (1911) The pancreatic ducts in man, together with a study of the microscopical structure of the minor duodenal papilla. Anat Rec 5:197–228

Ballinger J (1941) Hypoglycemia from metastasizing insular carcinoma of aberrant pancreatic tissue in the liver. Arch Pathol 32:277–285

Barbosa JJ DeC, Dockerty MB, Waugh JM (1946a) Pancreatic heterotopia: a review of the literature and report of 41 authentic cases of which 25 were clinically significant. Surg Gynecol Obstet 82:527–542

Barbosa JJ DeC, Dockerty MB, Waugh JM (1946b) Pancreatic heterotopia: surgical cases. Proc Staff Meet Mayo Clin 21:246–255

Bartholomew LG, Baggenstoss AH, Morlock CG, Comfort MW (1959) Primary atrophy and lipomatosis of the pancreas. Gastroenterology 36:563–572

Benbow EW (1988) Simultaneous inflammation in entopic and ectopic pancreas. J Clin Pathol 41:430–434

Beresford OD, Owen TK (1957) Lipomatous pseudohypertrophy of the pancreas. J Clin Pathol 10:63–66

Berry CL, Keeling J, Hilton C (1969) Teratoma in infancy and childhood: a review of 91 cases. J Pathol 98:241–252

Bigelow NH (1953) The association of polycystic kidneys with intracranial aneurysms and other related disorders. Am J Med Sci 225:485–494

Blair AJ, Russell CG, Cotton PB (1984) Resection for pancreatitis in patients with pancreas divisum. Ann Surg 200:590–594

Bodian M, Sheldon W, Lightwood R (1964) Congenital hypoplasia of the exocrine pancreas. Acta Paediatr Scand 53:282–293

Branch CD, Gross RE (1935) Aberrant pancreatic tissue in the gastrointestinal tract. Arch Surg 31:200–224

Britt LG, Samuels AD, Johnson JW (1983) Pancreas divisum: is it a surgical disease? Ann Surg 197:654–661

Burne JC (1958) Pancreatic and gastric heterotopia in a diverticulum of the transverse colon. J Pathol Bacteriol 75:470–471

Claudon M, Verain AL, Bigard MA et al. (1988) Cyst formation in gastric heterotopic pancreas: report of two cases. Radiology 169:659–660

Cotton PB (1980) Congenital anomaly of pancreas divisum as cause of obstructive pain and pancreatitis. Gut 21:105–114

Cotton PB, Kizu M (1977) Malfusion of dorsal and ventral pancreas: a cause of pancreatitis [abstract]. Gut 18:A400

Coupland RM, Aukland P, Harrison DA (1987) Heterotopic pancreas: a rare cause of obstructive jaundice. J R Coll Surg Edinb 32:168–169

Dalgaard OZ (1957) Bilateral polycystic disease of the kidney. Acta Medica Scand Suppl 328:1–255

Davison C, Brock S, Dyke CG (1936) Retinal and central nervous hemangiomatosis with visceral changes (Von Hippel–Lindau's disease). Bull Neurol Inst N Y 5:72–93

De Courcy JL (1943) Dermoid cyst of pancreas. Ann Surg 118:394–395

de Lange C, Janssen TAE (1948) Large solitary pancreatic cyst and other development errors in a premature infant. Am J Dis Child 75:587–594

Delhaye M, Engelholm L, Cremer M (1985) Pancreas divisum: congenital anatomic variant or anomaly? Gastroenterology 89:951–958

Dennis WA (1923) Dermoid cyst of the pancreas. Surg Clin North Am 3:1319–1322

Dodge JA, Laurence KM (1977) Congenital absence of islets of Langerhans. Arch Dis Child 52:411–413

Dolan RV, ReMine WH, Dockerty MB (1974) The fate of heterotopic pancreatic tissue. A study of 212 cases. Arch Surg 109:762–765

Duff GL, Foster HL, Bryan WW (1943) Primary carcinoma of the infra-ampullary portion of the duodenum. Arch Surg 46:494–503

Fishman RS, Bartholomew LG (1979) Severe pancreatic involvement in three generations of von Hippel–Lindau disease. Mayo Clin Proc 54:329–331

Fox H (1987) Biology of teratomas. Recent Adv Histopathol 13:33–43

Glinsky NH, Del Favero G, Cotton PB, Lees WR (1985) Congenital short pancreas: a report of two cases. Gut 26:304–310

Glinsky NH, Lewis JW, Flueck JA, Fried AM (1987) Annular pancreas associated with diffuse chronic pancreatitis. Am J Gastroenterol 82:100–106

Goldfarb WB, Bennett D, Monafo W (1963) Carcinoma in heterotopic pancreas. Ann Surg 158:56–58

Gregg JA (1977) Pancreas divisum: its association with pancreatitis. Am J Surg 134:539–543

Gregg JA, Monaco AP, McDermott WV (1983) Pancreas divisum: results of surgical intervention. Am J Surg 145:488–492

Gregg J, Solomon J, Clark G (1984) Pancreas divisum and its association with choledochol sphincter stenosis. Am J Surg 147:367–371

Halpert B, Alden ZA (1964) Accessory spleens in or at the tail of the pancreas. Arch Pathol 77:652–654

Halpert B, Györkey F (1957) Accessory spleen in the tail of the pancreas. Arch Pathol 64:266–269

Halpert B, Györkey F (1959) Lesions observed in accessory spleens of 311 patients. Am J Clin Pathol 32:165–168

Heptinstall RH (1966) Pathology of the kidney, 1st edn. Churchill, London, p 85

Higgins GM (1926) An aberrant pancreas in the wall of the gall bladder of the dog. Anat Rec 33:149–161

Hiraoka K, Horatake J, Horie A, Miyagawa T (1988) Bilateral renal dysplasia, pancreatic fibrosis, intrahepatic biliary dysgenesis and situs inversus totalis in a boy. Hum Pathol 19:871–873

Hoffman M, Sugerman HJ, Heuman D, Turner MA, Kisloff B (1987) Gastric duplication cyst communicating with aberrant pancreatic duct: a rare cause of recurrent acute pancreatitis. Surgery 101:369–372

Hollingsworth P, Isaacs D, Bydder G (1979) Recurrent osteolytic lesions and subcutaneous fat necrosis in association with a developmental pancreatic cyst. Arch Dis Child 54:790–792

Honicky RE, de Papp EW (1973) Mediastinal teratoma with endocrine function. Am J Dis Child 126:650–653

Hyden WH (1963) The true nature of annular pancreas. Ann Surg 157:71–77

Ikeda Y, Irving IM (1984) Annular pancreas in a fetus: three-dimensional reconstruction. J Pediatr Surg 19:160–164

Irving IM (1967) Exomphalos with macroglossia: a study of eleven cases. J Pediatr Surg 2:499–507

Irving IM (1990) Duodenal atresia and stenosis: annular pancreas. In: Lister J, Irving IM (eds) Neonatal surgery. 3rd edn. Butterworth, London, pp 427–430

Jackson LG, Apostolides P (1978) Autosomal dominant inheritance of annular pancreas. Am J Med Genet 1:319–321

Judd ES (1921) Cysts of the pancreas. Minn Med 4:75–82

Kellet HS, Lippard D, Willis RA (1962) Two unusual examples of heteroplasia in the lung. J Pathol Bacteriol 84:421–425

Kennedy SM, Hashida Y, Malatack JJ (1991) Polycystic kidneys, pancreatic cysts and cystadenomatous bile ducts in the oral-facial-digital syndrome type 1. Arch Pathol Lab Med 115:519–523

Kerr DNS, Harrison CV, Sherlock D, Milnes Walker R (1961)

Congenital hepatic fibrosis. Q J Med 30:91–117

Kinney TD, Fitzgerald PJ (1947) Lindau–von Hippel disease with hemangioblastoma of the spinal cord and syringomyelia. Arch Pathol 43:439–455

Koh THH, Cooper JE, Newman CL, Walker TM, Kiely EM, Hoffman EB (1986) Pancreatoblastoma in a neonate with Wiedemann-Beckwith syndrome. Eur J Pediatr 145:435–438

Kreel L, Sandin B (1973) Changes in pancreatic morphology associated with aging. Gut 14:962–970

Lamiell JM, Salazar FG, Hsia YE (1989) Von Hippel-Lindau disease affecting 43 members of a single kindred. Medicine 68:1–29

Leese T, Chiche L, Bismuth H (1989) Pancreatitis caused by congenital anomalies of the pancreatic ducts. Surgery 105:125–130

Lemons JA, Ridenour R, Orsini EN (1979) Congenital absence of the pancreas and intrauterine growth retardation. Pediatrics 64:255–257

Lindau A (1926) Studien über Kleinhirncysten. Acta Pathol Microbiol Scand Suppl 1:1–129

Lindau A (1930–1931) Discussion on vascular tumours of the brain and spinal cord. Proc R Soc Med 24:363–370

Lister J (1978) Duodenal atresia and stenosis: annular pancreas. In: Rickham PP, Lister J, Irving IM (eds) Neonatal surgery, 2nd edn. Butterworth, London, pp 357–358

Lloyd-Jones W, Mountain JE, Warred KW (1972) Annular pancreas in the adult. Ann Surg 176:163–170

Lüchtrath H, Schriefers KH (1985) Pankreaszyste unter den Bild einer sogenannten Branchiogenenzyote. Pathologe 6:217–219

McGeoch JEM, Darmady EM (1976) Polycystic disease of the kidney, liver and pancreas: a possible pathogenesis. J Pathol 119:221–228

MacKinnon D, Nash FW (1957) Pyloric obstruction due to pancreatic heterotopia in a child. Br Med J i:87–88

Mah V, Nelson L, Vintero HV (1987) Focal pontine leukoencephalopathy in a patient with the Shwachman-Diamond syndrome. Can J Neurol Sci 14:608–610

Mann FC (1922) Accessory pancreas in the dog. Anat Rec 19:263–268

Masson JC, Caylor HD (1929) Dermoid cyst of the pancreas. Surg Clin North Am 9:837–839

Miles RM (1959) Pancreatic cyst in the newborn. Ann Surg 149:576–581

Mitchell CJ, Lintott DJ, Ruddell WAJ, Losowsky MS, Axon ATR (1979) Clinical relevance of an unfused pancreatic duct system. Gut 20:1066–1071

Mitchell N, Angrist A (1943) Myo-epithelial hamartoma of the gastrointestinal tract (Clarke). Ann Intern Med 19:952–964

Mobini J, Krouse TB, Cooper DR (1974) Idiopathic pancreatic heterotopia: review and report of a case presenting as an abdominal mass. Am J Dig Dis 19:64–70

Montgomery RC, Poindexter MH, Hall GH, Leigh JE (1971) Report of a case of annular pancreas of the newborn in two consecutive siblings. Pediatrics 48:148–149

Murayama H, Kikuchi M, Imai T, Yamamoto Y, Iwata Y (1978) A case of heterotopic pancreas in lymph node. Vichows Arch [A] 377:175–179

Narasimharao KL, Patel RV, Malik AK, Mitra SK (1987) Chronic perianal fistula: beware of rectal duplication. Postgrad Med J 63:213–214

Nicholson GW (1923) The importance of congenital malformation in tumour formation. Guy's Hosp Rep 73:37–64

Palmer ED (1951) Benign intramural tumors of the stomach. Medicine 30:81–96

Pearson HA, Lobel JS, Kocoshis SA et al. (1979) A new syndrome of refractory sideroblastic anemia with vacuolization of marrow precursors and exocrine pancreatic dysfunction. J Pediatr 95:976–984

Pearson S (1951) Aberrant pancreas: review of literature and

report of 3 cases, one of which produced common and pancreatic duct obstruction. Arch Surg 63:168–184

Power WH (1961) Pancreatic cyst in infancy: recovery after marsupialization. Br Med J ii:625–626

Pye-Smith PH (1884) Cyst of the cerebellum with numerous small cysts in the pancreas and kidneys. Trans Pathol Soc Lond 36:17–21

Raafat F, Morita M, Lau M, Taylor C-M, White RHR (1988) Juvenile nephronophthisis with calcification of basal ganglia and pancreatic insufficiency. Arch Pathol Lab Med 112:630–633

Ravitch MM (1973) Anomalies of the pancreas. In: Carey LC (ed) The pancreas. Mosby, St Louis, MO, pp 404–427

Razi M (1966) Ectopic pancreatic tissue of esophagus with massive upper gastrointestinal bleeding. Arch Surg 92:101–104

Richter JM, Schapiro RH, Mulley AG, Warshaw AL (1981) Association of pancreas divisum and pancreatitis, and its treatment by sphincteroplasty of the accessory ampulla. Gastroenterology 81:1104–1110

Robson HN, Scott GBD (1953) Lipomatous pseudohypertrophy of the pancreas. Gastroenterology 32:74–81

Rode J, Dowsett J, Russell RCG (1988) The annular pancreas derives from the ventral primordium [abstract]. J Pathol 155:351A

Rösch W, Koch H, Schnaffner O, Demling L (1976) The clinical significance of pancreas divisum. Gastrointest Endosc 22:206–207

Rosseland AR, Ettvik LP, Gundersen B, Baakka A (1988) Abnormal connecting duct between the common bile duct and the pancreatic duct. Br J Surg 75:385

Rotig A, Colonna M, Bonnefont JP et al. (1989) Mitochondrial DNA deletion in Pearson's marrow/pancreas syndrome. Lancet i:902–903

Rusnak CH, Hosie RT, Kuechler PM, McHattie JD, Piercey JR, Cameron RD (1988) Pancreatitis associated with pancreas divisum: results of surgical intervention. Am J Surg 155:641–643

Salm R (1960) Scirrhous adenocarcinoma arising in a lipomatous pseudohypertrophic pancreas. J Pathol Bacteriol 79:47–52

Salm R (1968) Carcinoma arising in a lipomatous pseudohypertrophic pancreas, Br Med J iii:293

Satake, K, Uchima K, Yamashita K, Yashimota T, Umeyayama K (1979) Pancreatic cystadenoma of the spleen. Am J Surg 137:670–672

Schlumberger HG (1946) Teratoma of the anterior mediastinum in a group of sixteen men of military age: a study of sixteen cases and a review of theories of genesis. Arch Pathol Lab Med 41:398–444

Seidelin H (1912–1913) Carcinoma of the jejunum from aberrant pancreas germ [abstract]. J Pathol Bacteriol 17:428

Seifert G (1956) Die Pathologie des kindlichen Pankreas. Thieme, Leipzig. Quoted in Warkany J (1971) Congenital malformations. Year Book, Chicago, pp 729–735

Sherwood WC, Chance GW, Hill DE (1974) A new syndrome of familial pancreatic agenesis: the role of insulin and glucagon in somatic and cell growth [abstract]. Pediatr Res 8:360

Shillitoe AJ, Wilson JE (1957) Enterogenous cyst of thorax with pancreatic tissue as a constituent. J. Thorac Surg 34:810–814

Shwachman H, Diamond LK, Oski FA, Khaw K-T (1964) The syndrome of pancreatic insufficiency and bone marrow dysfunction. J Pediatr 65:645–663

Steinspir KD, Vinters HV (1985) Central pontine myelinosis in a child with the Shwachman-Diamond syndrome. Hum Pathol 16:741–743

Stept LA, Johnson SH, Marshall M, Price SE (1971) Intrarenal pancreatic disease. J Urol 106:15–18

Stewart MJ, Taylor AL (1925) Adenomyoma of the stomach. J Pathol Bacteriol 28:195–202

Suda K, Mizuguchi K, Hebisawa A, Wakabayashi T, Saito S (1984) Pancreatic tissue in teratoma. Arch Pathol Lab Med 108:

835–837

Sugawa C, Walt AJ, Nunez DC, Masuyama H (1987) Pancreas divisum: is it a normal anatomic variant. Am J Surg 153 : 62–66

Tanemura H, Uno S, Suzuki M et al. (1987) Heterotopic gastric mucosa accompanied by aberrant pancreas in the duodenum. Am J Gastroenterol 82 : 685–688

Thompson MH, Williamson RCN, Salmon PR (1981) The clinical relevance of isolated ventral pancreas. Br J Surg 68 : 101–104

Thompson RK, Peters JI, Sirinek KR, Levine BA (1989) Von Hippel–Lindau syndrome presenting as pancreatic endocrine insufficiency: a case report. Surgery 105 : 598–604

Thorsness ET (1940) An aberrant pancreatic nodule arising on the neck of a human gall bladder from multiple outgrowths of the mucosa. Anat Rec 77 : 319–329

Truong LD, Rangdaeng S, Jordan PH (1987) Lymphoepithelial cyst of the pancreas. Am J Surg Pathol 11 : 899–903

Tulassy Z, Papp J (1980) New clinical aspects of pancreas divisum. Gastrointest Endosc 26 : 143–146

Van Assche FA, De Prins F, Aerts L, Verjans M (1977) The endocrine pancreas in small-for-dates infants. Brit J Obstet Gynaecol 84 : 751–753

Walters MN-I (1966) Adipose tissue of the exocrine pancreas. J Pathol Bacteriol 92 : 547–557

Warkany J (1971) Congenital malformations. Year Book, Chicago, pp 729–735

Warkany J, Passarge E, Smith LB (1966) Congenital malformations in autosomal trisomy syndromes. Am J Dis Child 112 : 502–517

Warshaw AL, Cambria RP (1984) False pancreas divisum: acquired pancreatic duct obstruction simulating the congenital anomaly. Ann Surg 200 : 595–599

Warshaw AL, Richter JM, Schapiro RH (1983) The cause and treatment of pancreatitis associated with pancreas divisum. Ann Surg 198 : 443–450

Weber CM, Zito PF, Becker SM (1968) Heterotopic pancreas: an unusual cause of obstruction of the common bile duct. Am J Gastroenterol 49 : 153–159

Weidman FD (1913) Aberrant pancreas in the splenic capsule. Anat Rec 7 : 133–139

Wheelock MC, Atkinson AJ, Teloh HA (1949) Case report: aberrant pancreatic tissue in the stomach wall. Gastroenterology 13 : 594–596

Willis RA (1946) An intrapericardial teratoma in an infant. J Pathol Bacteriol 58 : 284–286

Willis RA (1960) Pathology of tumours, 3rd edn. Butterworth, London, pp 960–961

Willis RA (1962) The borderland of embryology and pathology, 2nd edn. Butterworth, London, pp 295, 327–329

Wong KC, Tsek K, Chan JKC (1988) Congenital absence of insulin-secreting cells. Histopathology 12 : 451–455

Zak FJ (1956) Aberrant pancreatic carcinoma in jejunal diverticulum. Gastroenterology 30 : 529–534

Zarling EJ (1981) Gastric adenomyoma with coincidental pancreatic rest: a case report. Gastrointest Endosc 27 : 175–177

4 Effects upon the Pancreas of Disease in Various Organs and Systems

It seems likely that a certain amount of functional disturbance of the pancreas will occur during almost any severe illness, especially when there is fever, bacteraemia or toxaemia, but studies of pancreatic function are usually irrelevant and unjustified in the diagnosis and treatment of such diseases. During scarlet fever, for example, Veghelyi (1949) demonstrated an increased concentration of pancreatic enzymes in the pancreatic juice and a rise in the pancreatic enzymes in the blood during the first days of the illness. This was followed, after the first week, by a fall in the activity of the pancreatic enzymes in the duodenal juice and a marked increase in the blood levels of these enzymes, with a return to normality during the fourth week. In illnesses in which shock has occurred, or if there has been hypothermia, the effects upon the pancreas may be very marked. These effects are discussed in the chapter on pancreatitis. In arterial disease, especially if hypertension of the malignant type is present, or if there is periarteritis nodosa, there may be infarcts or other marked lesions in the pancreas; these lesions are discussed in a separate chapter. In cirrhosis of the liver and in ulcerative colitis it is common for a variety of lesions, which have usually had no recognisable effect upon the patient's illness, to be found at autopsy. In renal failure, and some other conditions associated with dehydration, a characteristic type of acinar ectasia may be found in the pancreas, although there is seldom any clinical or biochemical evidence of pancreatic damage.

When multiple blood transfusions or haemolytic anaemic have caused haemosiderosis, the pancreas is usually conspicuously involved along with other organs, although, if the deposition of haemosiderin has taken place during the terminal stages of a fatal illness, only a trivial reaction to the presence of the pigment may occur, and there are no clinical effects. The deposition of haemosiderin that occurs in haemochromatosis will be discussed in the chapter on the pancreatic lesions associated with diabetes mellitus.

In systemic amyloidosis, the pancreas may be involved along with other organs, though the involvement is scarcely ever sufficient to cause clinical effects, but in senile amyloidosis, in which deposition of amyloid is restricted to the islets, the process may cause diabetes mellitus.

In congestive cardiac failure and in portal hypertension, pancreatic changes have been described but such lesions seem to be unimportant and indefinite. Inconstant changes have also been reported following death from burning and being struck by lightning. In Reye's syndrome the pancreas may be affected to some extent by fatty change, but much less so than the liver, and it has been suggested, because there are marked vacuoles in the exocrine cells of the pancreas in bovine mannosidosis (Jolly and Thompson 1977), that similar vacuoles may be present in the pancreatic cells in human mannosidosis. The few reports of the study of autopsy material from human cases of this rare disease have been mainly concerned, however, with the nervous and reticuloendothelial systems, and do not include any description of the microscopic appearances of the pancreas.

The commonest inherited disease, at least in Europe, that involves many systems, is, of course, cystic fibrosis and in this condition lesions of the pancreas are usually, but not invariably, severe and important.

Cystic Fibrosis (Fibrocystic Disease of the Pancreas, Pancreatic Fibrosis, Mucoviscidosis)

Incidence

In European countries the incidence is at least one in 2000 live births; it is suspected by many that the incidence may be much higher. Bodian for example, in London in 1952, estimated the incidence to be one in 1300, while in America in 1956, di Sant' Agnese thought the incidence might be as high as one in 600. A more recent estimate of the incidence in the British population is that about 500 children are born each year with cystic fibrosis (Williams et al. 1991). The incidence is much lower in non-Caucasian races.

Systemic Nature

Early reports of patients with the disease and the analysis of 49 examples by Andersen in 1938 tended to focus attention upon the anatomical and functional abnormalities of the pancreas as the cause of the disease, while alimentary disturbances, such as the malabsorption and fatty diarrhoea of young children, or the meconium ileus that was commonly fatal in the newborn, were attributed entirely to the failure of pancreatic enzymes to reach the intestine. The early publications have been reviewed by authors such as Andersen (1938), Baar (1953) and May (1954). The work of Farber (1944), however, led him to suggest that what had been called cystic fibrosis of the pancreas, or pancreatic fibrosis, was in fact a systemic disease that involved mucous glands throughout the body, the pancreatic achylia being only a part, albeit a characteristic part, of the syndrome. Farber's conclusion was based upon the findings in 87 post-mortem examinations at the Boston Children's Hospital, and confirmation of the systemic nature of the disease was provided by published work, edited by Bodian (1952), from the Hospital for Sick Children in London. The London workers suggested the name mucosis for the disease, but, when it was shown by di Sant' Agnese and his colleagues (1953) that the sodium and chloride content of the sweat was three or four times greater than normal in children with the condition, it was realised that glands other than mucous glands

behaved abnormally, as did the pancreas itself, which is, of course by no means a true mucous gland. No anatomical abnormality has yet been demonstrated in the sweat glands (Munger et al. 1961; Bartman and Landing 1966), but examination of the sweat for its sodium and chloride content has become an important diagnostic test.

If a child with cystic fibrosis does not die from meconium ileus in the neonatal period, the effects of pancreatic insufficiency become much less of a threat to the child's life than the very marked vulnerability to respiratory infection. Other systems too may be affected to a greater or lesser extent; for example, biliary cirrhosis may develop and cause portal hypertension and eventual liver failure. Males that reach maturity are usually sterile, and, in tropical conditions, salt loss in the sweat may cause heat prostration. Those in whom the pancreatic component of the syndrome has been absent, although other components have been present, have now been reported (Oppenheimer and Esterly 1973), and the condition is now usually referred to simply as cystic fibrosis or mucoviscidosis.

Inheritance

The inheritance is of the autosomal recessive type and in Britain the carrier rate is about 1 in 25, that is about 4% of the population. Thus there are 2.5 million carriers and this means that one in every 600 pregnancies will have a high risk (25%) of producing a child with cystic fibrosis (Brock 1990). The genetic cause of cystic fibrosis has been found to be on chromosome 7 (Rommens et al. 1989; Riordan et al. 1989; Kerem et al. 1989). There are many mutations within the gene, but, in the British population, there are only four of significance. Of these 76% are of the type that have been given the title of delta F508, usually written using the Greek capital delta, as ΔF508. Two other mutations can be detected, which increases the percentage of identifiable carriers to 85%.

A method by which the community can be scanned for the identifiable cystic fibrosis genes has been pioneered by Williams et al. (1991). The method requires samples of DNA from the people to be tested; sufficient DNA can be obtained painlessly from the cells of the buccal mucosa by rinsing the mouth with 5–10 ml of sterine saline. After the cells have been lysed to liberate their DNA, the polymerase chain reaction can be applied to amplify specific regions of the DNA for three of the four cystic fibrosis mutations found in the British population to be identified. One mutation, however, remains unidentifiable at present, thus, while positive tests are significant in the detection of carriers, negative results may be false negatives. In the meantime, the work of identifying the remaining mutations continues optimistically.

Prenatal recognition of the identified abnormal genes is possible in DNA obtained from the foetal cells in the chorionic villi of the placenta or in the amniotic fluid. Prenatal diagnosis, at least at present, is usually reserved for pregnancies in which both parents are known to be carriers. In families in which a child with cystic fibrosis has been born, and from whom nucleated cells are available, indirect methods involving the use of DNA markers known to be situated in the vicinity of the cystic fibrosis gene, whether its structure is known or not, may indicate the presence of the gene. The genetics, the carrier tests and tests used during pregnancy for the recognition of the cystic fibrosis genes have been described, without technical details, by Brock (1990).

Pathophysiology

The abnormal genes that cause cystic fibrosis are believed to do so by failing to synthesise the protein that normally regulates the transport of chloride ions into and out of certain types of cell (a transmembrane regulator). The absence of this regulator is responsible for the high concentration of salt in the sweat and probably also for the pancreatic and gastrointestinal abnormalities of function. In the pancreas, the defective secretory function leads to progressive anatomical changes, while in the lungs the abnormally viscid secretions, combined probably with defective ciliary function in the tracheobronchial epithelial cells, favour bacterial infections.

In addition to the genetic studies already mentioned, there has been much research into physicochemical abnormalities of the secretions, especially in relation to the transport of ions and into the glycosaminoglycans secreted. Cells from patients and their parents have been grown in culture and the enzymes associated with their lysosomes and other subcellular compartments have been studied. The vulnerability of these patients to infection has led to much work on their capacity for inflammatory and immune responses. Special attention has been devoted to the study of cystic "fibrosis factors" in the serum and other biological fluids from patients, and from their close relations. Such factors include a substance that impairs the action of the cilia of cultured ciliated cells. The serum from such patients has also been found by some to have an abnormally great capacity to bind calcium; this seems to have some relationship to IgG. It is thus suspected that

there is some link between circulating factors, calcium, IgG, the abnormalities of the secretions, and a defect in transport of ions. Other research has involved the autonomic nervous control of the exocrine gland. Some of the results of such experimental work are conflicting.

Much of the research into the basic defect in cystic fibrosis has been reviewed in publications such as those of di Sant' Agnese and Davis (1976), di Sant' Agnese (1979), Park and Grand (1981), and Lebenthal et al. (1986), whose bibliography contains 310 references.

Pancreatic Lesions

The pancreatic lesions in cystic fibrosis vary from apparent normality (Oppenheimer and Esterly 1973) to marked macroscopic and microscopic abnormalities.

Macroscopic Features

One of the early descriptions of the pancreas (Clarke and Hadfield 1924) states that, "Lying in the position of the pancreas was a shrunken-looking mass of fat running through which was a strand of gland-tissue containing many cell-islets." That patient, a girl who had suffered from fatty diarrhoea, probably from birth, with much retardation of development, had survived for 4 years and 4 months, and, as the abnormalities of the pancreas depend to a great extent upon the time that the patient has survived, such appearances in the pancreas were those of a fairly advanced stage of the disease.

In the 49 patients analysed by Andersen (1938), it was found that cystic fibrosis of the pancreas was described in 45 and fatty replacement of the acinar tissue in four. In many of Andersen's own cases she could detect no macroscopic abnormalities in the pancreas but, as her experience of the disease increased, she felt she could recognise certain features with the naked eye. The shape, colour and size of the gland were often normal, but sometimes it seemed abnormally small. On section, it tended to be unusually firm and occasionally there was a grating sound as the knife passed through calcified concretions. The lobules seemed rounded rather than having the normal diamond shape and many were fused together by fibrous tissue. In four out of five of her own cases, attempts to dissect out the pancreatic duct were unsuccessful because the lumen seemed to end in fibrous tissue between 5 mm and 15 mm from the ampulla of Vater but, because it is difficult to dissect out the pancreatic ducts in small children, she did not regard this as proof that the ducts were atretic. In some of the previously published cases she referred to, the duct was described as normal, or patent, or dilated.

In a later (1944) study of 87 infants and children with pancreatic insufficiency, Farber confirmed almost all of these observations. He found that in the majority of his cases there was no congenital atresia or stenosis, the ducts, especially in the head of the gland, tending to be dilated and to contain yellow or white plugs that could sometimes be recognised with the naked eye when a cross section was made. Farber was able to provide photographs of three specimens that illustrated the appearance of the surface of the pancreas: the first was from a child who had survived for 5 years and 7 months; the second had died at 3 years and 10 months; and the third child had died at 3 weeks of age because of meconium ileus. Irregularity and distortion of the surface of the gland can be recognised in his illustrations.

The question of patency or otherwise of the terminal pancreatic duct system received special study by Allen and Baggenstoss (1955). They made serial sections of the head of the pancreas and papilla of Vater in eight cases of fibrocystic disease of the pancreas, and found that in six the main duct was patent; in two, the main duct was abnormal; in one, the duct became atretic in the duodenal musculature; while in the other the duct was narrowed in the papilla of Vater. In all cases there was atresia of many of the interlobular and intralobular ducts.

Microscopic Features

There have been many descriptions of the microscopic appearances of the pancreas in cystic fibrosis, and there is general agreement that the most marked changes tend to be found in patients that have survived longest. Thus, in the very young, or in the premature baby, changes, though sometimes recognisable, may not be found. Oppenheimer and Esterly (1973), for example, in their study of 37 infants who had died from meconium ileus, could recognise no pancreatic lesions in ten of their cases, nine of whom were less than 1 month old. When the tissues throughout the body were studied, however, lesions compatible with a diagnosis of cystic fibrosis were found in 34 of the 37 cases, while changes that suggested cystic fibrosis were found in the remaining three. These authors concluded that the occurrence of meconium ileus was always a manifestation of cystic fibrosis.

The difficulty in interpreting the significance of the microscopic appearances of the pancreas in the very young have been pointed out by Emery (1951)

and by May (1954), who drew attention to the relatively large fibrous component of the pancreas in early infancy. However, Menten and Kinsey (1949) found a retention of acinous secretion that was not related to cystic disease of the pancreas, or to clinical symptoms, in 35 (13.7%) of the 256 autopsies carried out in the University of Pittsburg's Children's Hospital between 1944 and 1947. In the immature pancreas, too, lymphocytic infiltration associated with the degeneration of the primary type of islets is marked at about the sixth month of gestation, although, by birth, lymphocytes are inconspicuous (Liu and Potter 1962). Nevertheless, Imrie et al. (1979), by the application of quantitative methods to the study of the development of the exocrine pancreas, were able, by an assessment of the acinar volume in infants of 42 weeks of post-conceptional age, to discriminate between cases of cystic fibrosis and normal controls.

Moderately severe lesions of the pancreas have been found in children who have died of meconium ileus soon after birth. May (1954), for example, describes his experience of the presence of definite mild dilatation of the acini by homogeneous secretion in a biopsy of the pancreas of an infant who was operated upon for meconium ileus during the first day after birth. The dilatation had increased considerably by the fourth day after birth, when the child died and was examined post-mortem. Such appearances are illlustrated in Fig. 4.1.

The appearances described by Dorothy Andersen (1938) as cystic fibrosis of the pancreas, comprise acini that contain concretions of various sizes around which the acinar cells are flattened to form a thin epithelial wall. The smaller concretions are surrounded by relatively normal cells, which may, occasionally, contain eosinophilic granules. The degree of flattening of the epithelium depends, as a rule, upon the size of the concretions. The small ducts contain material similar to that in the acini and tend to be difficult to distinguish from the acini. The concretions are more or less deeply eosinophilic, the smaller being homogeneous, while the larger are often laminated with eosinophilic central material surrounded by a paler substance; occasionally they may be calcified. Sometimes, in the cysts that contain the paler material, there may be desquamated epithelial cells, a few phagocytes, or a rare polymorphonuclear leucocyte. The size of the cysts varies from case to case, but large ones are not often seen in the youngest infants. Surrounding the acini, and also the lobules, there are moderate to large amounts of fibrous tissue (Fig. 4.2), the quantity corresponding roughly to the age of the child.

The fibrous tissue includes fibroblasts or young fibrocytes and is always infiltrated by lymphocytes,

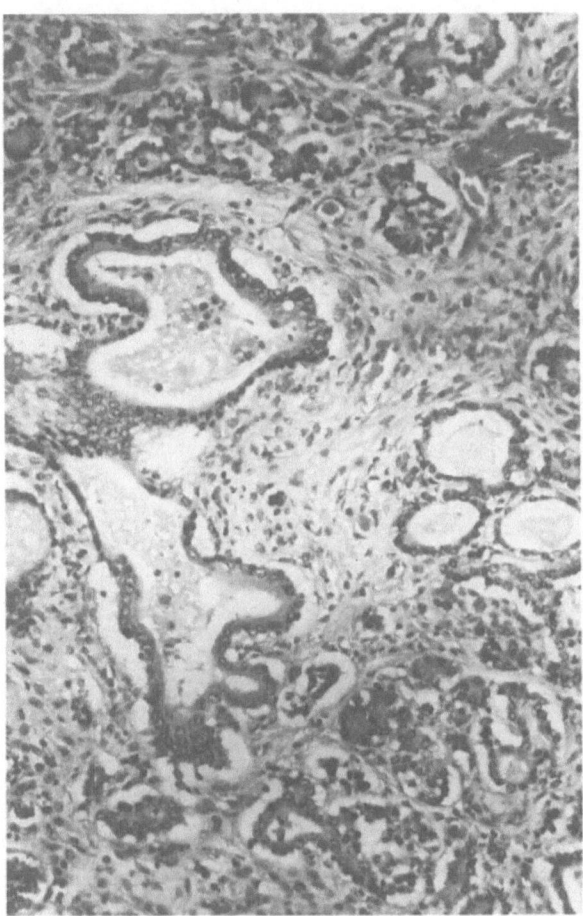

Fig. 4.1. A group of dilated ducts with adjacent ectatic acini in the pancreas of a child that died of purulent bronchitis at the age of 2 months, having been operated upon at the age of 1 month for meconium ileus. H&E, × 150

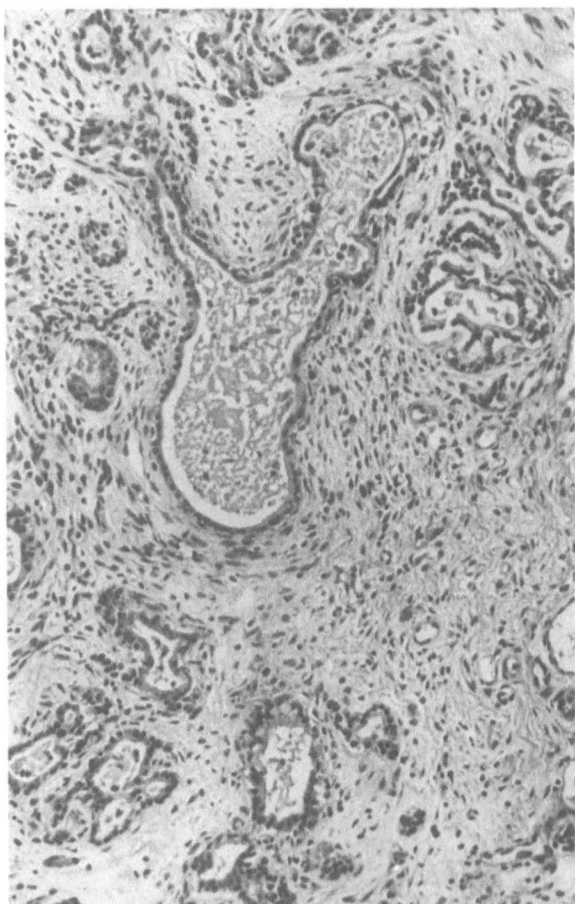

Fig. 4.2. Another focal area of dilated ducts in the pancreas illustrated in Fig. 4.1. Acini have almost disappeared from the vicinity of the secretion-filled dilated ducts and the few acini that remain in the background of fibrous tissue resemble small ducts. H&E, × 150

plasma cells and phagocytes. Sometimes the infiltration is sufficient to warrant a diagnosis of subacute or chronic pancreatitis, and may include occasional polymorphonuclear leucocytes. The islets of Langerhans are usually normal in number and appearance. Farber (1943, 1944) considered the islets to be unaffected by the process in the exocrine pancreas. His interpretation of the microscopic appearances was that the obstruction began in the acini with inspissation of the secretion, and that dilatation of the ducts occurred later, to be followed by atrophy of the acini and fibrous replacement of the organ; the final picture resembled that caused by experimental obstruction of the pancreatic ducts in animals. Later work, for example that of Bodian (1952), supported the suggestion that the obstructive effects were due to abnormal secretion that adhered excessively to the walls of the spaces in which it lay

to cause widespread, but patchy, obstruction within the acini and small ducts.

Stages in this progressive pancreatic damage are shown in Figs 4.3–4.15.

Nature and Effects of Retained Secretion

Histochemical studies of the nature of the retained secretion, for example those of Baar (1953) and of Walters and Gibb (1965), have shown that, although the material in the ectatic acini is a mucoprotein, it does not react with stains for mucopolysaccharides. Acid mucopolysaccharides are present, however, in the larger ducts. As the cysts enlarge and the acinar cells atrophy, as occurs in patients who survive for a number of years, acid mucopolysaccharides accumulate, while goblet cells become conspicuous and

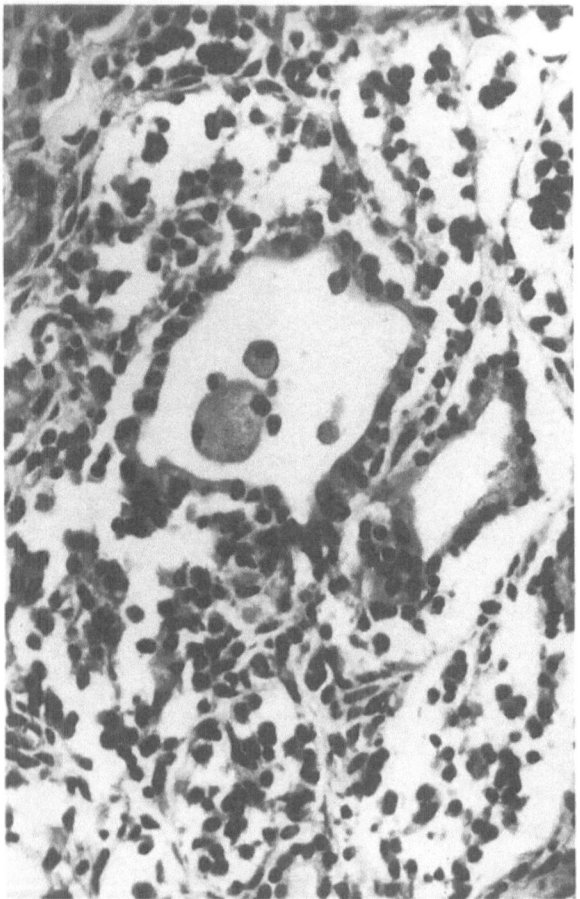

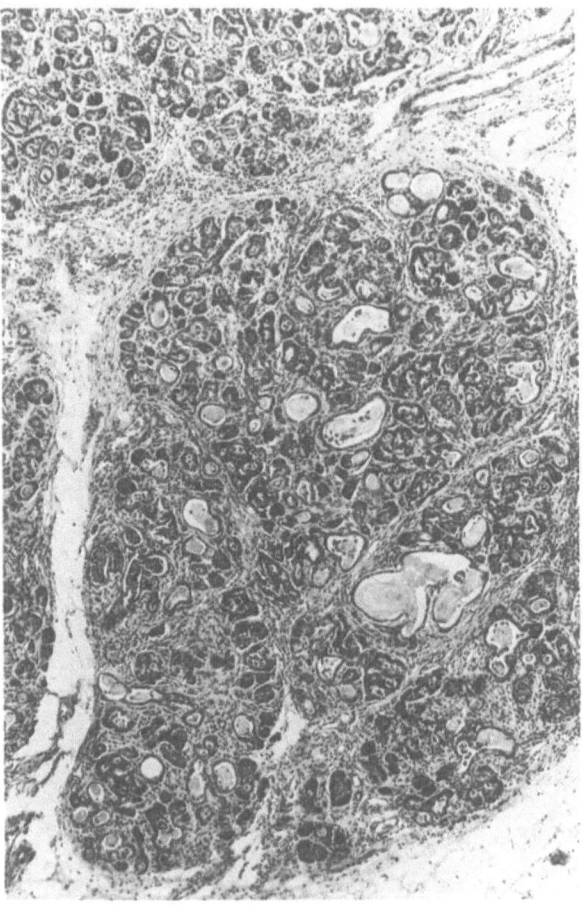

Fig. 4.3. Mononuclear and binuclear phagocytes filled with ingested secretion in a dilated acinus lined by atrophic epithelium in the pancreas illustrated in Figs 4.1. and 4.2. Many of the surrounding acini are disorganised and collapsed. H&E, × 375

Fig. 4.4. A pancreatic lobule that has become isolated by interstitial fibrosis in a child who died at the age of 1 year with cystic fibrosis. Within the lobule, dilated ducts are associated with ectatic and partially atrophic acini. H&E, × 50

may undergo papillary hyperplasia. In such cases, fat as well as fibrous tissue may replace the glandular tissue that has undergone atrophy. Walters (1965), from his study of the pancreases of 15 children with cystic fibrosis, has suggested that the basic abnormality is proliferation of the centro-acinar and intercalary ductular cells, followed by necrosis that leaves detritus, whose effect is to cause inspissation of the secretion within the ducts and acini. He considered ductular occlusion to be more important than intra-acinar obstruction in causing pressure atrophy of the acinar epithelium.

It has already been said that the pancreatic lesions become more marked as the child gets older, and, when no pancreatic lesions can be recognised at autopsy on a baby who has died soon after birth, it is suspected that pancreatic damage would have developed postnatally if the child had survived. The stage of the development of the pancreatic damage does not, however, correlate with the severity, or otherwise, of the symptoms of the associated malabsorption, as was found by Bostick and Rinehart (1950) in a series of 20 children between the ages of 20 days and 12 years.

It is usual to attribute the damaging effects of the retained secretion to its mechanical pressure upon the acinar cells and, in general, this seems to be true. However, here and there in certain pancreases the intra-acinar secretion may provoke an inflammatory reaction in which polymorphonuclear leucocytes are much more conspicuous than was suggested by Andersen (1938) (Fig. 4.6) while in the more advanced stages of pancreatic damage, there is a pseudomyxomatous appearance in the fibrous tissue within obliterated ducts (Figs 4.14, 4.15). Such obliteration of ducts within the pancreas resembles, at least partially, the organic obliteration of the intestine that may be provoked in utero by inspis-

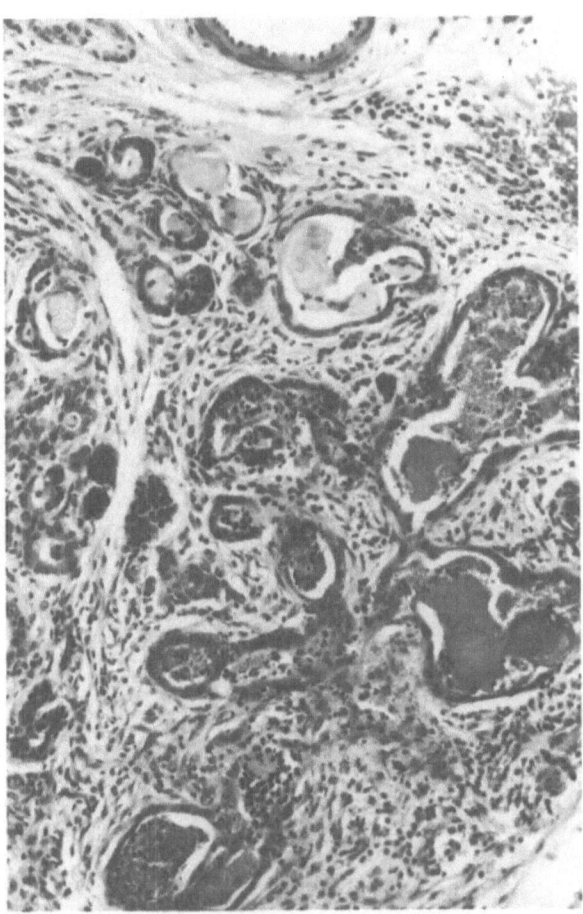

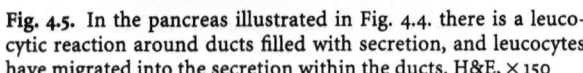

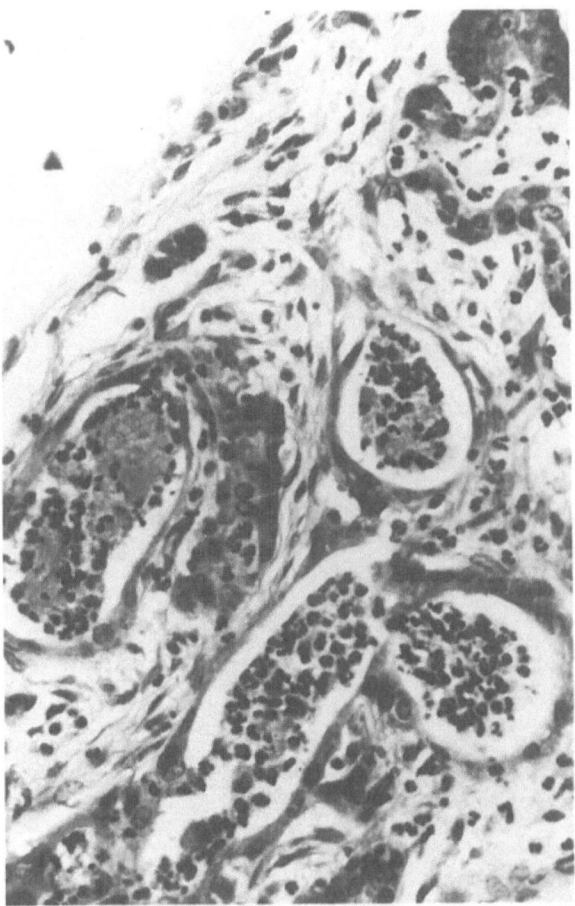

Fig. 4.5. In the pancreas illustrated in Fig. 4.4. there is a leuco-cytic reaction around ducts filled with secretion, and leucocytes have migrated into the secretion within the ducts. H&E, × 150

Fig. 4.6. The cells that have reacted to secretion within the ducts include many polymorphonuclear leucocytes. H&E, × 375

sated meconium in cystic fibrosis, as described by Zuelzer and Newton (1949), who also described similar obliteration of the cystic duct in older infants. Such obliterative effects may account for the apparent atresia of the pancreatic duct that was found by Andersen in four of the five cases in which she attempted to dissect out the ducts, and by Allen and Baggenstoss in two of the eight cases they studied.

Ultrastructure

The ultrastructural changes in the atrophic acinar cells in the pancreas in cystic fibrosis have been described by Porta et al. (1964), who found that there was dilatation of the ergastoplasm, reduction in the number of zymogen granules, spherulation of the mitochondria, and atrophy of the microvilli. The

changes illustrated in the review by Lebenthal et al. (1986) are very similar and show distension of the lumen of an acinus by fibrillar and granular mater-ial, which extends into interacinar vacuoles, while the surrounding acinar cells contain few dense gran-ules and distended endoplasmic reticulum contain-ing granular material. Zymogen granules are reduced and fibrous tissue and fibroblasts are present beneath the acinar basement membrane; these later progressively replace the exocrine acini. An interlocular duct is shown to be filled by dense fibrillar material.

Changes in the Islets of Langerhans

In the earlier studies of the pancreas in cystic fibrosis the islets of Langerhans were found to be normal, but, in later observations, for example those

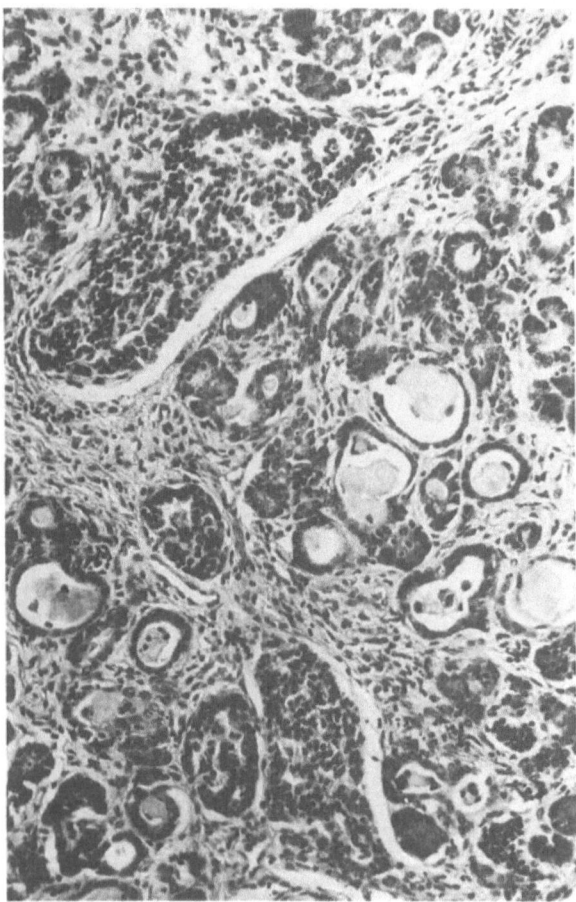

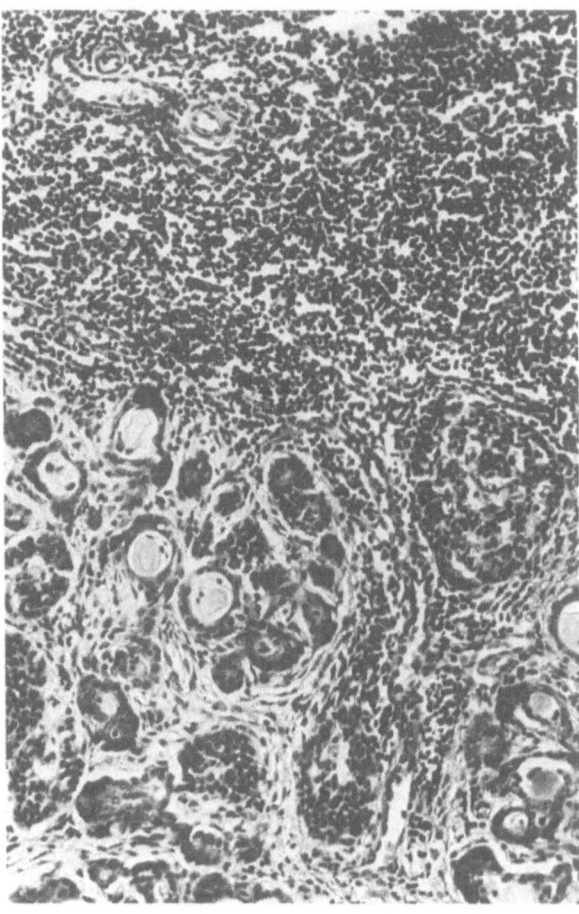

Fig. 4.7. Numerous islets of Langerhans, some of which appear to be enlarged, associated with interstitial fibrosis and ectatic acini in another part of the pancreas illustrated in Fig. 4.6. H&E, × 150

Fig. 4.8. An area of interstitial lymphocytic infiltration in the pancreas illustrated in Fig. 4.7. H&E, × 150

of Brown and Madge (1971), a genuine increase of islets (rather than an apparent increase due to atrophy of the exocrine pancreas), has been found, with the formation of new beta cells and argyrophilic cells. Such neo-formation of islets (nesidioblastosis) (Fig. 4.7) might be expected to prevent the development of diabetes mellitus, but it has become well recognised that diabetes occurs in about 10% of the older children with cystic fibrosis (Anderson and Goodchild 1976), while it has been shown that plasma insulin and glucose-dependent insulinotrophic peptide responses are significantly lower in patients with cystic fibrosis. Fasting levels of pancreatic polypeptide, too, are significantly lower as shown by Adrian et al. (1980); these authors suggest that the pancreatic polypeptide-producing cells of the islets may be particularly vulnerable to the effects of this disease.

An immunohistochemical study of the endocrine component of the pancreas in cystic fibrosis was carried out by Iannucci et al. (1984). Their material consisted of the pancreases of 17 patients who had suffered from cystic fibrosis, some also with diabetes mellitus. They found that, at the end of the first decade of life in the patients without diabetes, nesidioblastosis was marked and the islets were normal. Some exocrine glandular tissue was still present and had the usual lesions of cystic fibrosis. In the pancreases of the young adults who had had diabetes as well as cystic fibrosis there appeared to be a decrease in the number of islets with reduction of the number of insulin-containing cells in each islet, as well as reduction in the size of the islet cells, and fibrosis and amyloid deposition in the islets. The exocrine glandular tissue was completely replaced by fat.

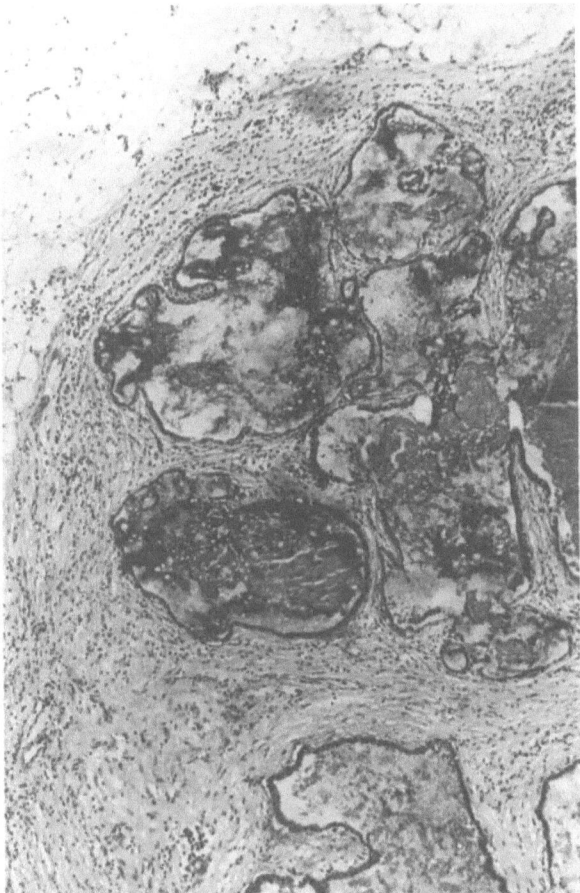

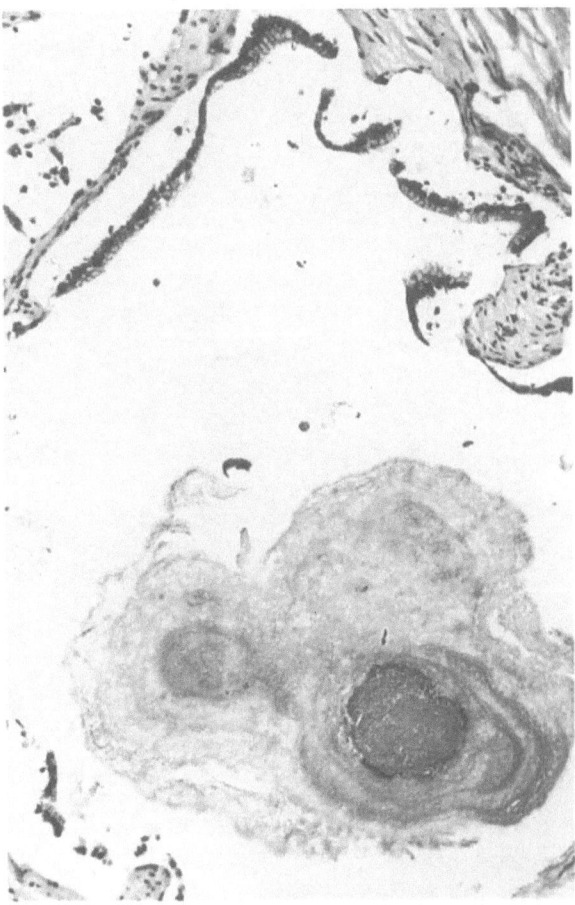

Fig. 4.9. Spaces filled with strongly PAS-positive secretion. The spaces have a lining of atrophic epithelium. Acini are unrecognisable and it is not obvious whether the secretion-filled spaces represent the remains of ducts or acini. The spaces are surrounded by fat. This pancreas was obtained from a boy with cystic fibrosis who survived until the age of 12 years before he died of respiratory infection. Periodic acid–Schiff, × 60

Fig. 4.10. Early calcification in secretion within a duct in the pancreas illustrated in Fig. 4.9. The epithelium that lines the duct has undergone goblet cell metaplasia. H&E, × 135

The Pancreas in Patients who have Survived to Become Adults

The early descriptions of the pancreatic changes in cystic fibrosis were of material from infants or from young children, but it is now commonplace for patients with cystic fibrosis to grow to adulthood, and in 1976 it was possible for di Sant' Agnese and Davis to write a review based upon 75 of their own adult patients and 232 cases from the literature. If adult patients with cystic fibrosis die and are examined post-mortem the most characteristic abnormalities are non-pancreatic and consist of focal biliary cirrhosis, obstructive lesions of the male genital tract and obstructive bronchopulmonary disease with colonisation of the respiratory secretions by

Staphylococcus aureus or *Pseudomonas aeruginosa* (Vawter and Shwachman 1979).

Some form of pancreatic atrophy is, however, usually present, and Vawter and Shwachman described four patterns of abnormality. In the pattern that they classify as type i, the changes are intralobular and consist of loss of zymogen granules, the acinar cells having undergone de-differentiation to resemble canalicular cells, while the lumina contain eosinophilic deposits that extend to the smallest radicals. In type ii there is exocrine atrophy with intralobular and perilobular fibrosis, and segmental ectasia of ducts or microcysts that contain amorphous and laminated eosinophilic masses. Type iii is more severe, with complete acinar atrophy, occasional ruptured mucoceles and

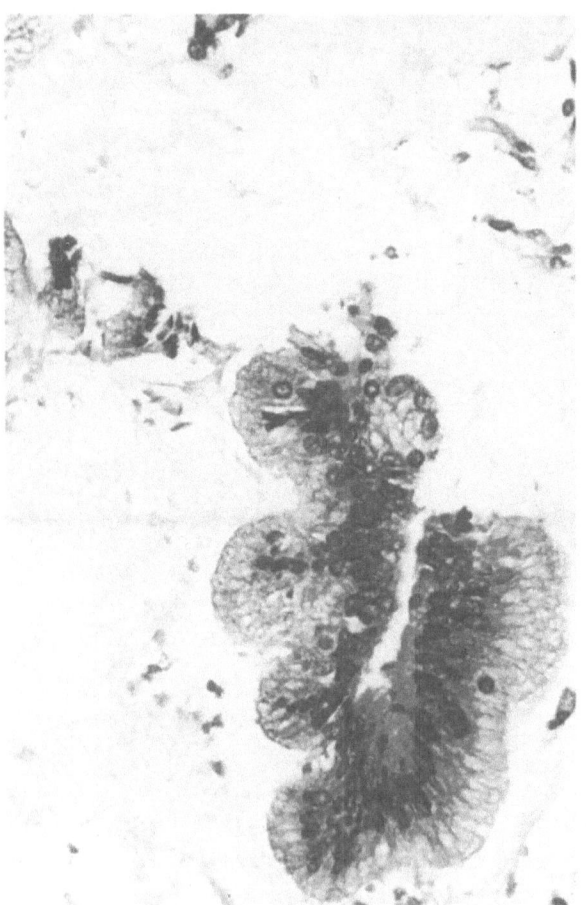

Fig. 4.11. Papillary hyperplasia of epithelium that has undergone goblet cell metaplasia in a duct in the pancreas illustrated in Fig. 4.10. H&E, × 375

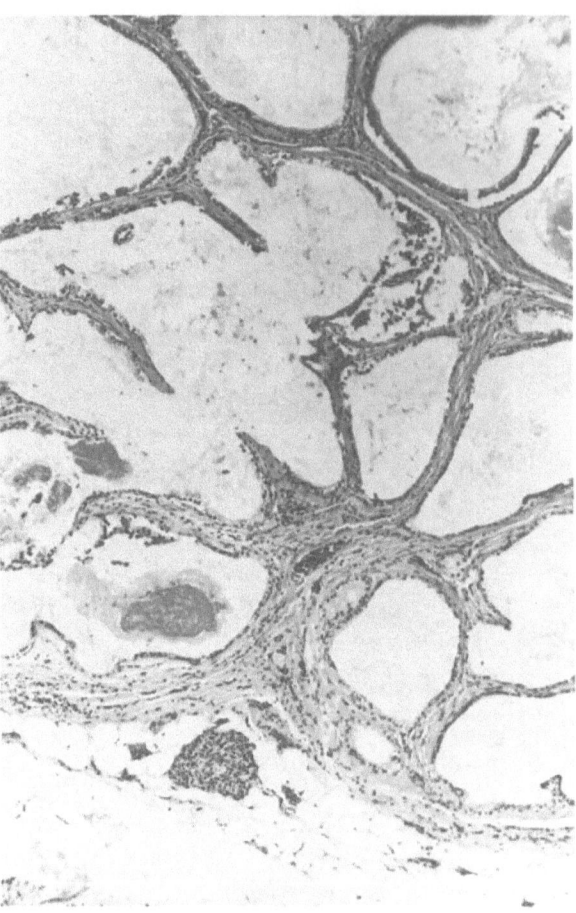

Fig. 4.12. Glandular atrophy that has left spaces, some of which contain partially calcified concretions, with an atrophic islet in the surrounding fat and what appears to be the remnant of an islet among the glandular spaces. The photomicrograph is of another part of the pancreas shown in Fig. 4.11. H&E, × 66

liposclerosis, while in type iv there is total acinar loss with obliteration of some of the ducts. This causes areas of scarring in which central fibrosis is surrounded by liposclerotic tissue that contains scattered islets (Fig. 4.13), while unobliterated ducts contain mucus and are lined by epithelium that has undergone goblet cell metaplasia (Fig. 4.11). Various regions of the pancreas may contain different types of lesion, type iv lesions being found typically in the tail with less advanced lesions in the body and head.

In young adults, cystic fibrosis may be complicated by recurrent attacks of acute pancreatitis (Shwachman et al. 1975). Jaundice due to compression of the intrapancreatic portion of the common bile duct in an adult with cystic fibrosis has been reported by Lambert et al. (1981).

Haemosiderosis of the Pancreas

Causes of Accumulation of Iron

The three main ways in which abnormally large amounts of iron can accumulate in the body have been described by Bothwell and Charlton (1972) as: first, excessive absorption from a normal diet; secondly, excessive dietary iron; and, thirdly, parenteral iron overload.

Excessive absorption from a normal diet occurs in the genetic disorder idiopathic haemochromatosis. The pancreatic lesions in idiopathic haemochromatosis are described in Chap. 6, along with the pancreatic lesions of diabetes mellitus. Accumulation of iron also occurs in the "iron-

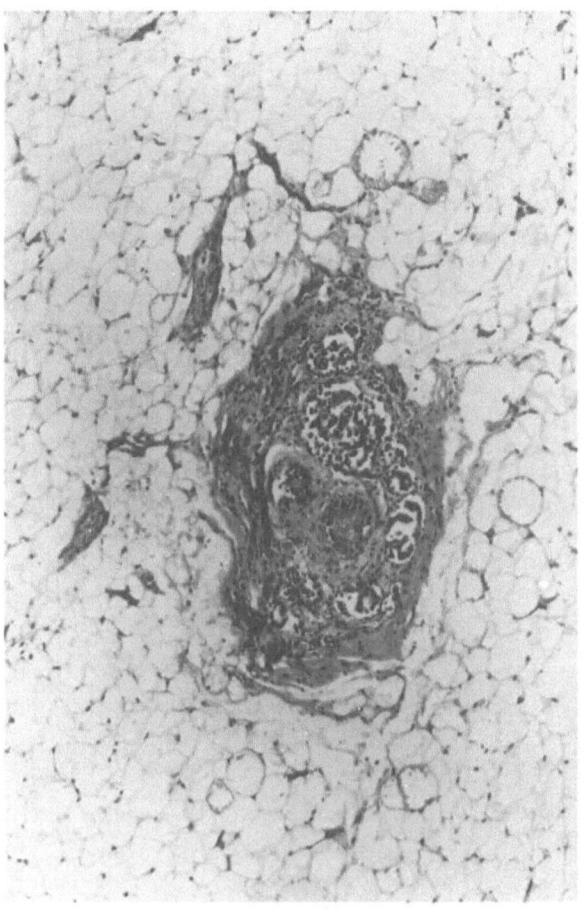

Fig. 4.13. Atrophic duct and glandular remnants in an area of replacement by fat in the pancreas shown in Fig. 4.12. H&E, × 70

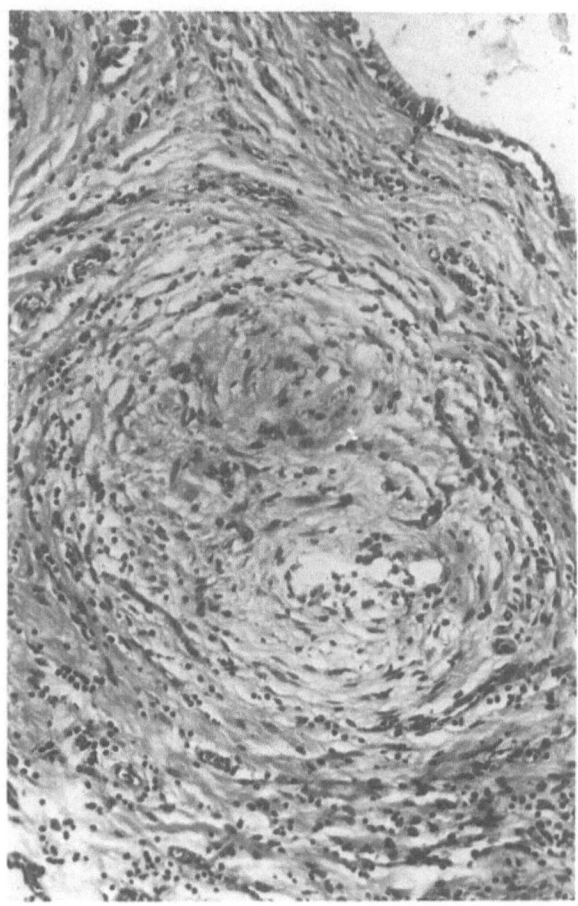

Fig. 4.14. Obliteration of a duct by cellular fibrous tissue in the pancreas shown in Fig. 4.13. H&E, × 150

loading" types of anaemia because, although erythropoiesis is increased, it is ineffective, and iron absorbed from a normal diet lies unused in depots throughout the body, while the rapid destruction of abnormal red cells, with liberation of iron, aggravates the accumulation. An excess of iron in the diet is thought to account for the overloading with iron that is common in men of the Bantu race of southern Africa and is attributed to large amounts of ionic iron derived from iron vessels used in the making of fermented drinks. So much iron reaches the mucosa of the upper small intestine that it overwhelms the normal mechanism that excludes unwanted iron. Parenteral iron overload is the result of multiple blood transfusions such as are necessary in the management of hypoplastic and other forms of refractory anaemia; this is the commonest type of iron overload met in routine pathology in the autopsy room.

The accumulated iron is in the form of the yellowish-brown pigment haemosiderin. This can be detected with the naked eye in the pancreas, as well as in many other organs, if the amount is large. The Prussian blue reaction will confirm that the pigmentation is due to haemosiderosis, and may indicate that haemosiderin is also present in sites that are not obviously pigmented. Microscopically, the presence of haemosiderin can be demonstrated by the method of Perls. Haemosiderin is generally believed to consist of aggregates of ferritin, and, although ferritin is water soluble and thus disappears during ordinary fixation, the aggregates that form haemosiderin are insoluble. Ferritin is a macromolecular complex of protein and colloidal ferric hydroxide-phosphate within a protein shell arranged in micelles; these contain between 17% and 23% by weight of iron (Crichton 1971). Although ferritin cannot be seen with the light microscope, it has a characteristic appearance under the electron microscope.

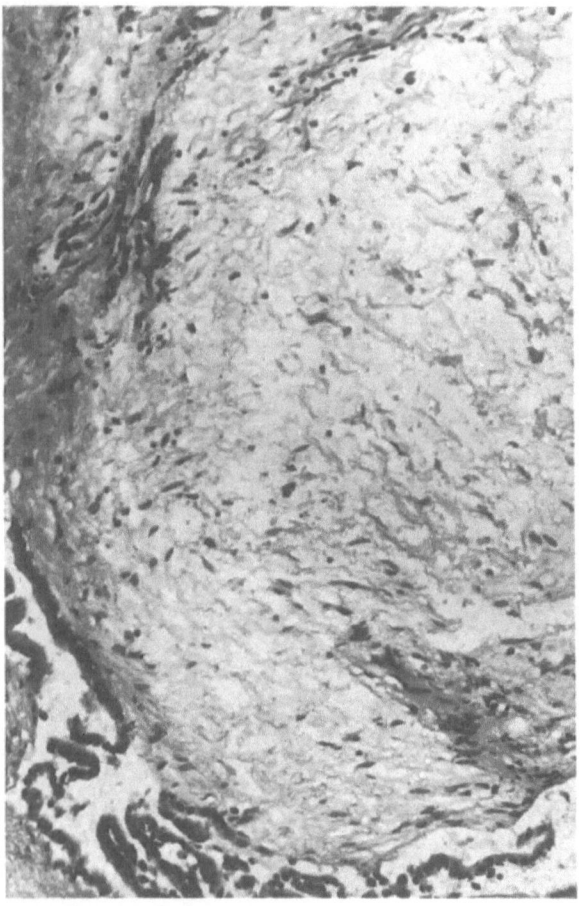

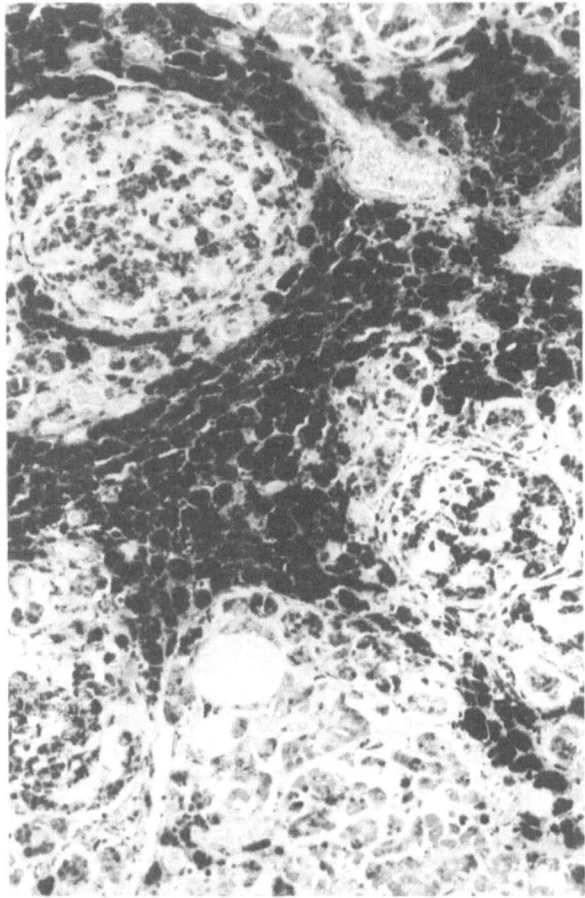

Fig. 4.15. An area of pseudomyxomatous reaction in the pancreas shown in Fig. 4.14. H&E, × 150

Fig. 4.16. Haemosiderosis of the pancreas due to multiple blood transfusions given to treat aplastic anaemia. The pigment is most abundant within cells in the interlobular areas but smaller granules of haemosiderin are present in the cells of the islets. The patient was not diabetic but tests of glucose tolerance were not carried out. (Courtesy of Dr T. Helliwell) Perls' stain, × 150

Similarity of Haemosiderosis and Haemochromatosis

As far as the pancreas is concerned, the distinction between haemosiderosis and haemochromatosis by microscopic examination, without clinical and biochemical information, is almost impossible (MacDonald and Mallory 1960). It has been said (Bothwell and Charlton 1972) that in idiopathic haemochromatosis the haemosiderin is found predominantly in the parenchymal cells of the affected organs, while in haemosiderosis the haemosiderin is mainly in the reticuloendothelial cells, but, in the pancreas, the appearances in these two conditions can be indistinguishable, especially if the haemosiderosis is of the very marked type that follows multiple blood transfusions (Fig. 4.16). In

haemosiderosis the pigment is most abundant in the stroma where it is associated with an increase of interlobular fibrous tissue in which lie coarse granules of haemosiderin, apparently extracellularly. Rather smaller granules of haemosiderin are present in the cytoplasm of the acinar cells and in the ductal epithelial cells, while much smaller granules may stipple the cells of the islets. The islets usually contain much less stainable iron than the exocrine cells and in some cases the islets may have none. Diabetes mellitus is not usually associated with the haemosiderosis caused by refractory anaemias or by multiple blood transfusions, but it is said (Isaacson et al. 1961) that diabetes is frequent in the small proportion of Bantu subjects whose pancreatic parenchyma contains significant amounts of iron. It is now recognised that if marked haemosiderosis is

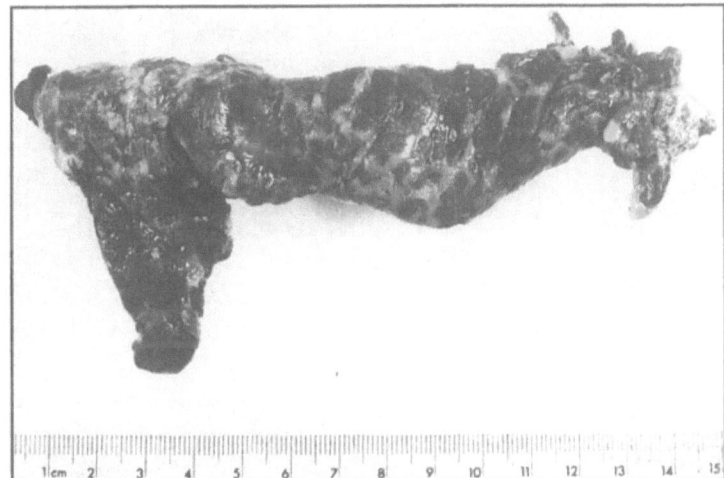

Fig. 4.17. The macroscopic appearance of the pancreas of the woman referred to in the text, whose haemosiderosis developed after portacaval anastomosis had been carried out because of cirrhosis of the liver.

present for long enough a type of haemochromatosis indistinguishable from hereditary haemochromatosis will develop.

Haemosiderosis Associated with Hepatic Cirrhosis

An accumulation of haemosiderin in the pancreas, as well as in many other organs, is occasionally associated with cirrhosis of the liver. The mechanism by which this occurs is not clear, but it has been suggested by Tisdale (1961) that portacaval anastomosis may favour its deposition. Marked deposition of iron can, however, sometimes be found in many organs, including the pancreas, in patients who have died from hepatic failure due to portal cirrhosis for which no portacaval anastomosis has been carried out, as has been reported by Sabesin and Thomas (1964).

The following case history contains evidence that the haemosiderosis in this situation can develop during 1 year. A woman, who was 47 at the time of her death, had been found during a cholecystectomy 5 years previously, to have cirrhosis of the liver. One year before her death, portacaval anastomosis was carried out to relieve portal hypertension with splenomegaly. A biopsy of the liver at that time confirmed that cirrhosis was present; no iron was present in sections stained by Perls' method. A year later, hepatic coma developed and an attempt was made to relieve this by extracorporeal pig liver perfusion, but improvement was only temporary and the patient died. At the post-mortem examination there was macronodular cirrhosis of the liver with a patent portacaval anastomosis and absence of the gall bladder. The liver, pancreas, salivary glands, myocardium, gastric mucosa, skin, thyroid, pituitary

and adrenal glands, as well as the choroid plexus, all contained much haemosiderin on microscopic examination, and, in the case of the liver, pancreas (Figs 4.17 and 4.18) and gastric mucosa, the haemosiderosis could be seen macroscopically as a rusty brown colour. The spleen, which weighed 598 g, contained no haemosiderin. There were multiple acute duodenal ulcers.

Also in infants with subacute or chronic liver disease, iron is liable to accumulate, distributed in the organs as in haemochromatosis. In 13 of the 15 infants studied by Witzleben and Uri (1989) the pancreas contained iron. These infants did not have portacaval anastomoses.

Other Pancreatic Lesions Associated with Hepatic Disease

Haemosiderosis is by no means the only lesion of the pancreas that has been reported in association with cirrhosis of the liver; it seems to be much less common in cirrhosis of the liver, including alcoholic cirrhosis, than an interstitial fibrosis without haemosiderosis.

The earlier reports of fibrosis of the pancreas in association with portal cirrhosis were reviewed by Stinson et al. in 1952. These workers compared the findings in the pancreases of 75 patients who had died of cirrhosis of the liver with the pancreatic abnormalities in 75 subjects in whom there was no hepatic disease. A wide variety of pancreatic lesions was found in both groups, but, in patients with cirrhosis of the liver, there was a significantly higher

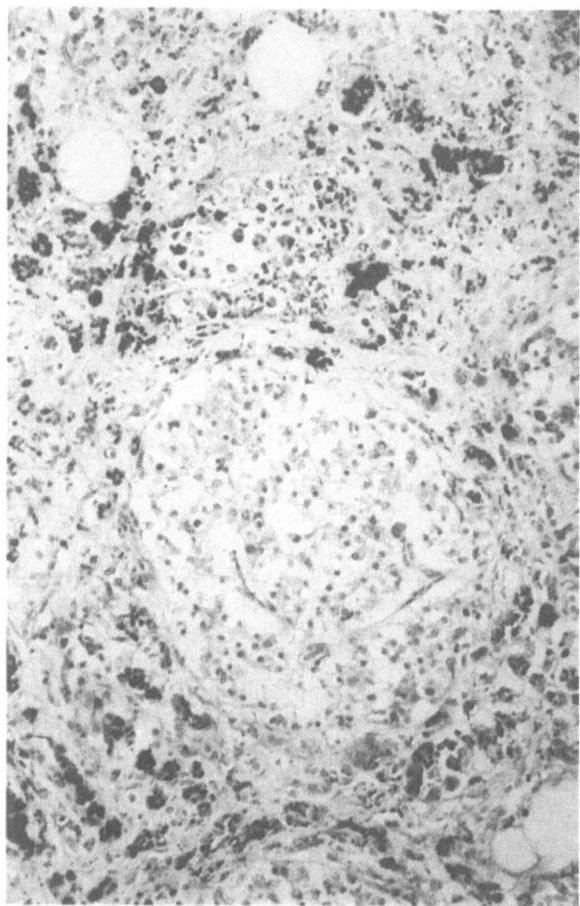

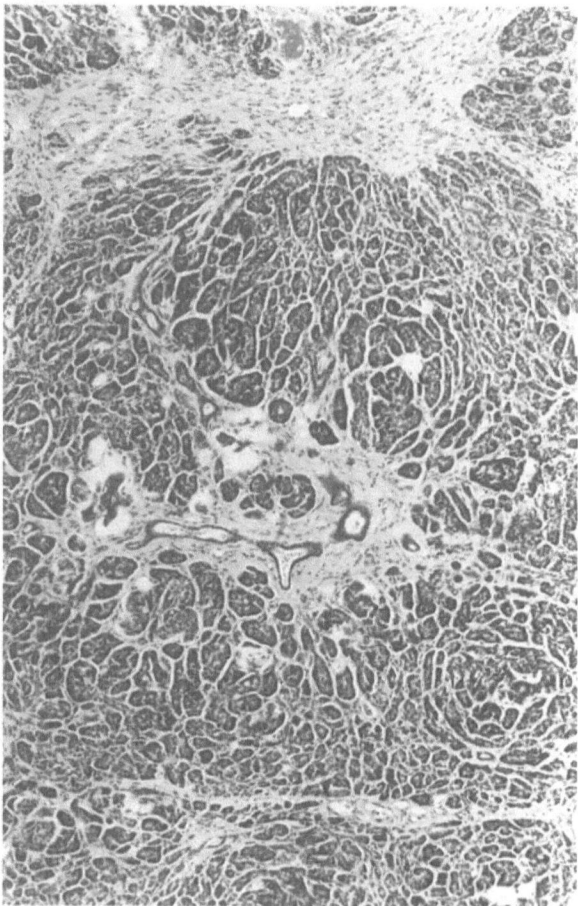

Fig. 4.18. The microscopic appearance of the pancreas illustrated in Fig. 4.17. Haemosiderin pigment is abundant in the exocrine tissues but the islet, like the other islets throughout the specimen, contains no pigment. Perls' stain, × 300

Fig. 4.19. Interstitial fibrosis of the pancreas found incidentally in a man aged 59, who died of bronchopneumonia associated with carcinoma of the caecum that was locally infiltrative but had not metastasised. There was also cirrhosis of the liver, believed to be alcoholic, and an old cerebral infarct. The pancreatic changes were not recognised with the naked eye. (Courtesy of Dr William Taylor) H&E, × 60

incidence of interstitial inflammation, moderate and severe interlobular fibrosis, and acinar and ductal dilatation. Deposits of pigment were present in the pancreas of only one of the cirrhosis patients; one of the patients in the control group also had deposits of pigment. The authors concluded that the factors causing the liver disease in the cirrhotic patients might have caused the pancreatic pathologies also. In their survey of the autopsy data of 530 patients, of whom 148 had alcoholic cirrhosis of the liver, Martin and Bedossa (1989) recognised a type of diffuse fibrosing pancreatitis that was significantly more common in the patient group with alcoholic cirrhosis compared with other groups, including a group of alcoholics without cirrhosis of the liver. The fibrosis was intralobular and was without

inflammatory infiltration or abnormalities of the intralobular ducts. It did not appear to have caused clinical effects and was always an unexpected incidental finding at autopsy. An example of pancreatic fibrosis in association with alcoholic cirrhosis of the liver is illustrated in Fig. 4.19.

In primary biliary cirrhosis of the liver, although anatomical evidence of pancreatic involvement is lacking, tests of pancreatic function show that the pancreas may be involved. Klass et al. (1979), for example, found that, in six of 11 patients with primary biliary cirrhosis, there was functional evidence of asymptomatic pancreatic disease that did not correlate with the depth of the jaundice or with the presence of the sicca syndrome. Epstein et al. (1980, 1982), however, interpreted the pancreatic

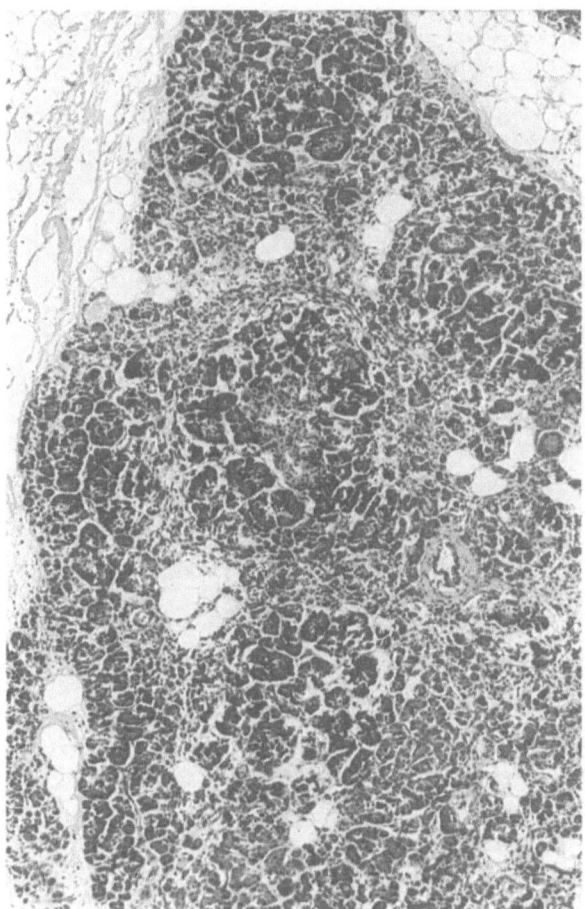

Fig. 4.20. The effect of chronic passive congestion upon the pancreas. The central parts of the lobules, where the islets are usually situated, are well preserved, but the exocrine cells at the periphery of the lobules are atrophic. The patient, a woman aged 37, died with extreme chronic passive congestion of the organs because of stenosis of the mitral and aortic valves of the heart. H&E, × 60

hyposecretion that they demonstrated in primary biliary cirrhosis as evidence that this condition was a "dry gland" disease.

Chronic Venous Congestion

The effects of chronic venous congestion upon the pancreas are not usually considered to be of any importance, but, in the 7th edition of MacCallum's *Textbook of Pathology*, published in 1940, it is stated that in chronic venous congestion of the pancreas the acini near the islets are well preserved, while those at a distance from the islets are atrophic or

necrotic; this is illustrated in Fig. 256 of that edition. Such damage is in keeping with the distribution of the arterial branches within the pancreatic lobules by which the islets are supplied by glomerular-like structures formed by the termination of the, usually, single artery that enters each lobule, the other parts of the lobule receiving oxygenated blood only after the vicinity of the islet has been supplied (Opie 1910; Wharton 1932), an arrangement that makes the parts of the lobule at a distance from the islets particularly vulnerable to the effects of anoxia.

Although the histopathological effects of chronic venous congestion upon the pancreas have received little recent study, evidence has been produced by Webb et al. (1980) that impaired pancreatic function in extrahepatic portal venous obstruction may be the result of pancreatic damage due to the local chronic venous congestion, caused in turn by the portal venous obstruction. Since that time Shibayama et al. (1992) have shown that pancreatic perilobular necrosis is found relatively commonly at autopsy in liver disease; it was present in 41% of their cases with liver disease compared with 13% of autopsies in which no liver disease was found. Chronic passive congestion of the pancreas is illustrated in Figs 4.20 and 4.21.

Pancreatic Lesions Associated with Chronic Ulcerative Colitis

Although clinical signs of pancreatic disease are not usually recognisable in ulcerative colitis, Ball et al. (1950) found interstitial pancreatitis at necropsy in 46 of 86 consecutive cases of active chronic ulcerative colitis, with 11 additional cases in which interstitial fibrosis and acinar atrophy were present. The incidence was far in excess of similar lesions found in a control group, but the authors could not identify the factors responsible for the pancreatic lesions. In 46 cases in the series, dilatation of the pancreatic acini was also present.

Pancreatic Lesions Associated with Uraemia and Dehydration

In 1947, Baggenstoss reported that he had noted dilatation of the pancreatic acini (Fig. 4.22) in 39% of 85 cases of chronic glomerulonephritis that ended in uraemia, in 42% of 85 cases of systemic hyper-

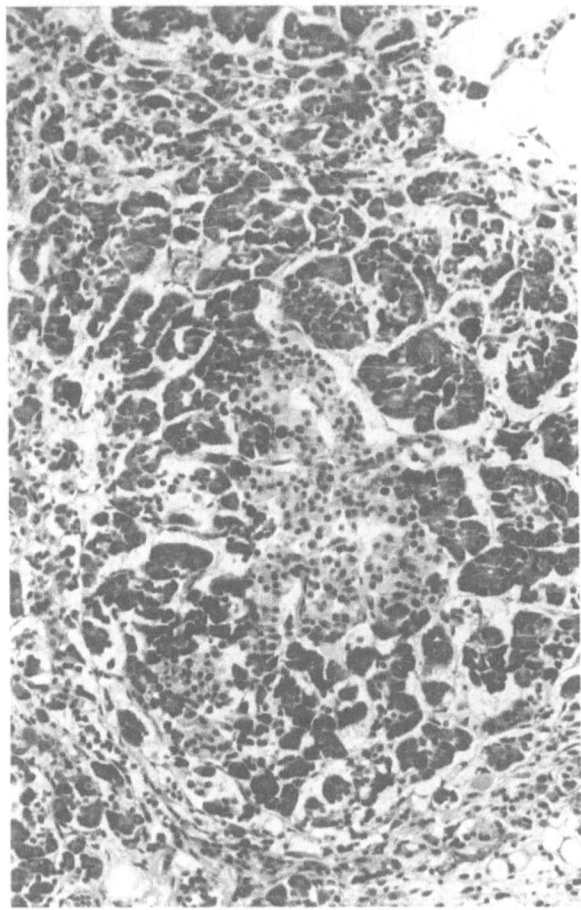

Fig. 4.21. A higher power view of the pancreas illustrated in Fig. 4.20. H&E, × 150

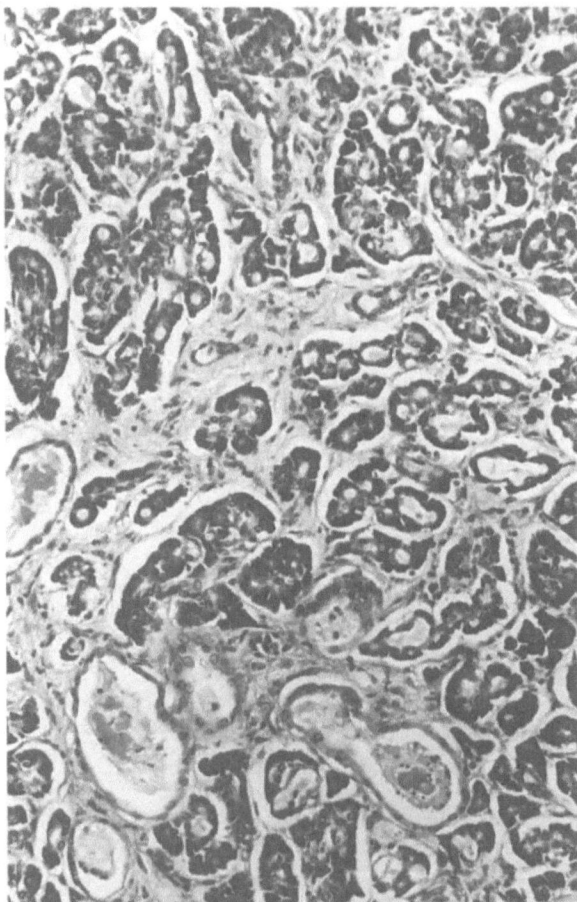

Fig. 4.22. Ectasia of the acini and ductules of the pancreas from a woman who died in uraemia because of congenital cystic disease of the kidneys. H&E, × 150

tension that had ended in uraemia and in 52 of 100 cases in which uraemia had been the result of various other causes. He also noted that uraemic pericarditis and the pancreatic lesion tended to be associated. In a later communication (1948a), he reported that he had found the pancreatic lesion in 20% of 200 control cases in which uraemia had been absent. In the controls, the lesion tended to be associated with vomiting and dehydration. In a further study (1948b), Baggenstoss, having found the lesion in association with carcinoma of the stomach, severe infections and chronic ulcerative colitis, speculated that, in addition to inspissation of the pancreatic secretion due to dehydration, neural alteration of the nature of the secretion or failure of the pancreatic cells to repair themselves because of protein deficiency due to malnutrition might contribute to the development of the lesion. The later stages of the lesion, as well as its development, were studied by Stein and Powers (1956).

These authors, having found either the focal or the diffuse type of lesion in 21% of 358 consecutive necropsies in adults, then traced the progress of the focal type of lesion, from an accumulation of inspissated secretion within the lumen of an acinus, to atrophy, and eventual disappearance of the acinar cells with surrounding inflammation, collapse of the lobules and fibrosis. The ductules were not involved in the process and the end-result was a focus of parenchymal scarring, with the loss of acini, an increase of fibrous stroma, infiltration by chronic inflammatory cells, and an apparent increase in the number of normal-appearing ductules. The resemblance of pancreatic acinar ectasia to the early stages of cystic fibrosis of the pancreas was pointed out by Walters and Gibb (1965), who studied the intraluminal material histochemically and identified it as a mucoprotein.

In the later stages of uraemia due to chronic renal failure there may of course be widespread

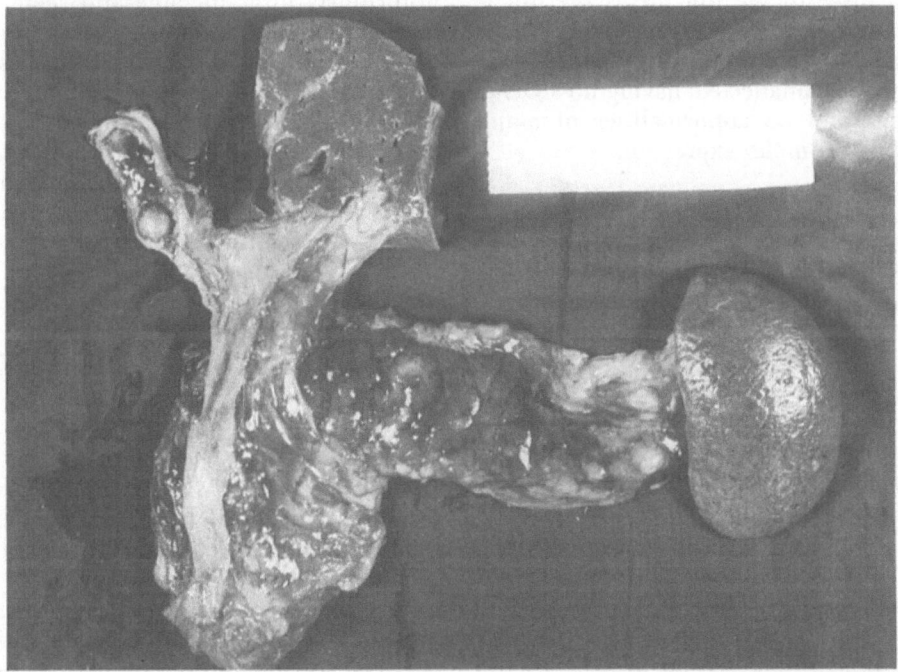

Fig. 4.23. Purpuric haemorrhage into the pancreas in a woman who died of renal failure due to chronic glomerulonephritis. The whole pancreas was haemorrhagic and acute haemorrhagic pancreatitis was suspected, especially as the gall bladder contained a calculus, but neither necrosis nor inflammation was found microscopically in the pancreas. Much purpuric haemorrhage was also present in the walls of the oesophagus, stomach, small intestine and colon. The haemorrhage had caused no clinical effects and was thought to have occurred terminally.

purpuric haemorrhage, which may involve the pancreas; such a case is illustrated in Fig. 4.23. The appearance of the pancreas in this case suggested the diagnosis of acute haemorrhagic pancreatitis but neither necrosis nor inflammation was found microscopically.

The pancreatic abnormalities found postmortem in patients whose end-stage renal disease had been treated by chronic haemodialysis have been studied by Vaziri et al. (1987, 1988). Their 78 cases included 22 with pancreatitis (16 chronic, two haemorrhagic, one acute and three acute superimposed on chronic). In one of the cases of pancreatitis there was a history of heavy alcohol consumption and in six there were signs of biliary disease. Other lesions found quite frequently included fibrosis, haemosiderin deposits, calcification, cystic changes, amyloidosis and abscesses. In addition, hyalinisation, atrophy or absence of islets of Langerhans, and necrosis of peripancreatic fat were present in several cases. Inspissated secretions, focal ductular epithelial metaplasia and dilatation were noted in some patients. A number of the latter lesions were of course related to the causes of the renal failure, which included diabetic nephropathy, polycystic kidney disease, systemic

sclerosis and amyloid disease. The authors concluded that these findings, when compared with those of Baggenstoss, for example, in the days before the use of long-term dialysis, indicated a considerable increase of pancreatic lesions in patients who had been sustained by long-term haemodialysis.

The Pancreas in Acute Graft Versus Host Disease

This condition has been described in the main by Foulis et al. (1989). In four cases in a series of 26 bone marrow transplant recipients, 14 of whom had evidence of acute graft versus host disease at autopsy, the pancreas, as well as other organs, was involved. The pancreatic lesions, believed by the authors to be pathognomonic, were in the ducts of the exocrine tissue and consisted of marked atypia of the epithelium accompanied by a mild lymphocytic infiltrate. In the more severe cases this was associated with ulceration and haemorrhage into the lumen. In three of the four cases the ductal epithelium showed clear hyperexpression of class I and class II major histocompatability complex antigens. The islets were unaffected, having no signs of cellular damage and no abnormalities of major histocompatability complex expression.

Pancreatic Lesions in Toxaemia of Pregnancy

Eclampsia is now a rare complication of pregnancy and there are few recent reports of the condition of the pancreas in fatal cases, but Haukland et al. (1987) found that, in 13 patients with pre-eclampsia, there were statistically significant rises in the serum concentrations of cationic trypsinogen and amylase, which suggested a concomitant injury of the pancreas. This suggestion was supported by Goodlin (1987).

In their study of the pathology of toxaemia of pregnancy, Sheehan and Lynch (1973) used material from 677 fatal cases, from 377 of which they undertook detailed histological re-examination. These included five in whom acute interstitial pancreatitis was found. There were multiple patches of fat necrosis in the lobules of fat at the surface of the pancreas, with extension along the larger septa in the gland, associated with oedema and infiltration by monocytes and other inflammatory cells. Where the fat necrosis was in contact with pancreatic acini there was a superficial band of necrosis of the pancreatic cells. In one of the cases there were signs of healing; in two others there were several minute infarcts each 0.2–0.3 mm in diameter, with complete central coagulative necrosis and nuclear pyknosis and cytoplasmic eosinophilia of the peripheral cells. These lesions were not associated with fat necrosis. A single patient, who had died in toxaemic coma, had haemorrhagic pancreatitis with massive necrosis of the pancreatic tissue. Sheehan and Lynch followed the description of their own cases by a review of earlier reports of pancreatic necrosis or pancreatitis in eclampsia and during pregnancy. They found that well over 100 cases had been published.

Pancreatic Lesions Associated with Death from Lightning Stroke

The lesions found in the bodies of people that have died because they have been struck by lightning are notoriously unpredictable and seem to be determined by chance combined with the conditions that determine the conductivity of the tissues. Lesions that have been described include the two examples reported by Lynch and Shorthouse (1949) of haemorrhage and necrosis in the tail of the pancreas, with arborescent marks on the skin. These authors could find no previous reports of pancreatic damage in fatal cases of lightning stroke.

Pancreatic Lesions in Fatal Cases of Burning

In 1963, Sochor and Mallory published a study of the lesions found in the lungs of 41 patients who had died from burns. Although their main interest was in the pulmonary lesions, they noted incidentally that in five cases there was haemorrhage into the pancreatic islets, interstitial pancreatitis in four, an islet cell adenoma in one, acinar changes that suggested uraemia in one, and fibrosis of the pancreatic islets in one. The significance of haemorrhage into the islets has been rejected by Warren et al. (1966), who consider the lesion to be an artefact, or at least an agonal change. The finding of clinically unsuspected interstitial pancreatitis is, as has been pointed out in the chapter on acute pancreatitis, commonplace in material from routine autopsies.

Amyloidosis

The pancreas may be involved, along with other organs, in systemic amyloidosis, either when it is associated with chronic inflammatory disease or when it is of the primary type (Figs 4.24, 4.25). In addition, localised amyloidosis may occur in the islets of Langerhans in old age, and, as this may be important in relation to the development of maturity-onset diabetes mellitus, that lesion is discussed in the chapter on the pancreas in diabetes mellitus.

In systemic amyloidosis, other than the senile type, the pancreatic involvement is seldom of clinical importance and is found only when a complete autopsy with microscopic examination of all the main organs is carried out. True involvement of the exocrine pancreas should also be distinguished from the mere involvement of blood vessels or of nerves within the pancreas.

The numerous publications on the distribution of amyloid amongst the various organs in different

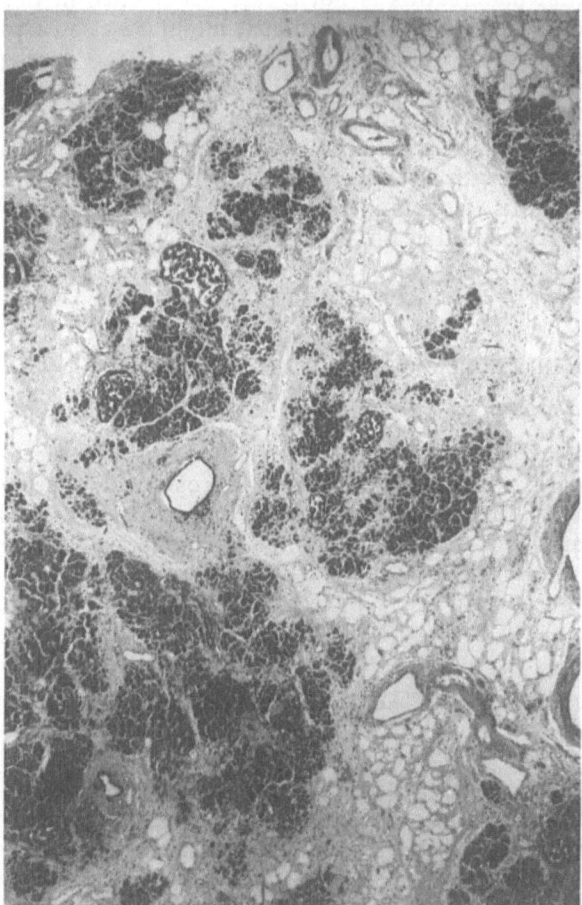

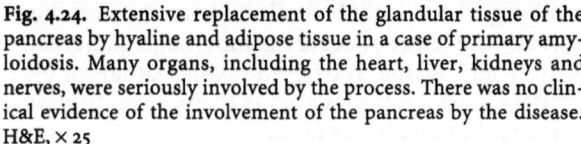

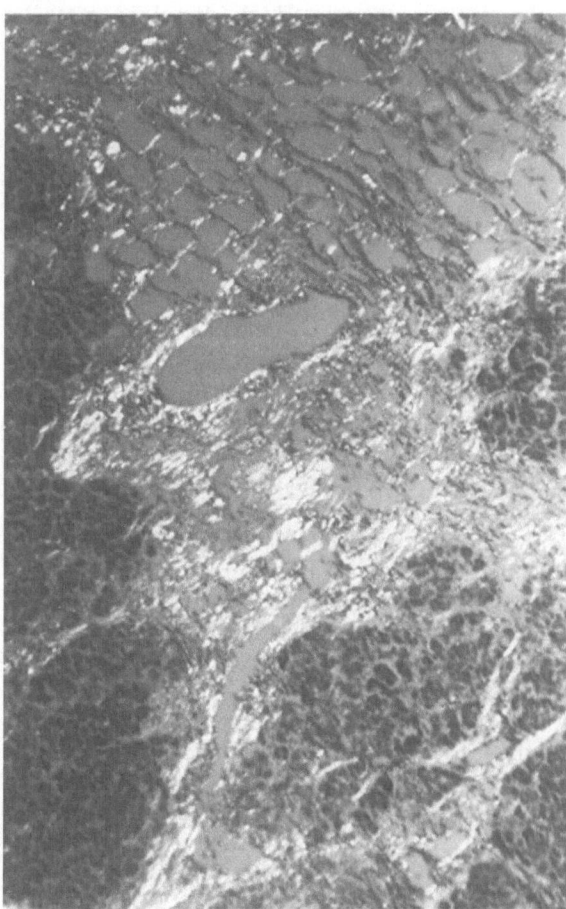

Fig. 4.24. Extensive replacement of the glandular tissue of the pancreas by hyaline and adipose tissue in a case of primary amyloidosis. Many organs, including the heart, liver, kidneys and nerves, were seriously involved by the process. There was no clinical evidence of the involvement of the pancreas by the disease. H&E, × 25

Fig. 4.25. The dichroic reaction given by the hyaline material in the pancreas shown in Fig. 4.24. when examined with crossed prisms after staining with Congo red. × 60

types of amyloidosis have been reviewed by Pirani (1976). He found that, in 413 cases of amyloidosis associated with chronic inflammatory diseases, some of which were cases of his own and some of which were from publications by others, the pancreas was involved in 23%, although, in a series of 252 cases collected by Battaglia and quoted by Pirani, amyloidosis associated with chronic inflammatory diseases involved the pancreas in only 6%. In what these authors classified as primary amyloidosis, of which Pirani had 165 cases and Battaglia 66, involvement of the pancreas was found in 22% of Pirani's cases and 30% of Battaglia's, while, in amyloidosis associated with plasma cell dyscrasias, Pirani found pancreatic involvement in two out of 12 cases in which the plasma cell lesions were osteolytic (plasma cell myelomatosis) and in

three of 22 cases in which the plasma cell lesions were not osteolytic.

In concluding his review, Pirani made the comment that, in spite of the progress that has been made in ascertaining the chemical composition of amyloid and the pathogenesis of amyloidosis, little is known that explains its distribution in different tissues.

Another study of the organs affected by amyloid disease was that carried out by Looi (1989), whose material consisted of 25 cases of systemic AA amyloidosis (i.e. amyloidosis associated with chronic inflammatory disease). Material from the pancreas was available in only 13, but the secretions from 12 were positive for amyloid. Looi noted that, in the earlier stages of the deposition of amyloid, only the small arteries of the pancreas were affected, but that, as the disease progressed, the amyloid material infiltrated beyond the arteries into the stroma and along the basement membrane of the acini, causing parenchymal atrophy.

Wilson's Disease (Hepatolenticular Degeneration)

Ultrasonic evidence for pancreatic enlargement in Wilson's disease has been reported by Minns et al. (1982). They suggested that the enlargement might represent a congestive pancreatitis due to portal hypertension. Dixon and Walshe (1983), however, after examining the pancreas by computed tomography in 23 patients with Wilson's disease, came to the conclusion that an apparent prominence of the pancreas was likely to be due to enlargement of the spleen, which compressed the pancreas in its long axis and caused it to buckle. Their letter to *The Lancet* contains an illustration of such distortion of the pancreas in Wilson's disease. They commented that the presence or absence of pancreatitis could be resolved by histological studies. No abnormalities of the pancreas were observed with the naked eye by Wilson (1912), and the overloading with copper that occurs is almost exclusively in the liver, brain, kidney and cornea (Sass-Kortsak and Bearn 1978). It may even be that the inadequate transport of copper that is an essential feature of Wilson's disease could deprive the pancreas of the copper that is necessary for its normal function. Experimental work (Smith et al. 1982) has shown that copper deficiency will cause atrophy of the pancreatic acinar tissue, at least in rats. Studies of pancreatic function do not seem to have been carried out in cases of Wilson's disease, but the results might be interesting (Pitchumoni et al. 1986). Steatorrhoea, due to pancreatic insufficiency, was present in one of the patients described by Danks et al. (1990).

Systemic Lupus Erythematosus

A clinical diagnosis of pancreatitis was made by Reynolds et al. (1982) in 20 patients with systemic lupus erythematosus, in four of whom no contributing factors other than systemic lupus erythematosus could be ascertained. No serious complication of the pancreatitis occurred in any of the patients, despite continued steroid therapy. The authors concluded

that pancreatitis is not a rare occurrence in this disease, and suggested that it might be related in part to the vasculitis that has been found during periods when the disease is active. More recently, Wolman et al. (1988) have also reported a case of acute pancreatitis, unrelated to drug therapy, in a patient with systemic lupus erythematosus; the pancreatitis was fulminant and its complications eventually caused death.

Progressive Systemic Sclerosis

Pancreatic lesions in the generalised form of scleroderma (progressive systemic sclerosis) do not seem to be of clinical significance, but areas of fibrosis and sclerosis have sometimes been observed (Piper and Helwig 1935).

Alpha₁ Antitrypsin Deficiency

There are conflicting opinions about whether inherited deficiency of this protease inhibitor, normally formed in the pancreas, makes the pancreas unduly susceptible to agents, such as alcohol, that may cause it injury (Novis et al. 1975; Braxel et al. 1982). Svenberg et al. (1988) attributed, in two of their patients, the onset of acute haemorrhagic pancreatitis after endoscopic retrograde pancreatography to this deficiency. In both patients the pancreatitis was severe and in one it was fatal.

Nephropathic Cystinosis

Nephropathic cystinosis is an inherited abnormality of metabolism in which cystine accumulates within many cell types, including cells of the kidney, bone marrow, liver, spleen, lymph nodes, cornea, conjunctiva, thyroid and pancreas. Renal glomerular failure has usually developed by about the age of 10 years, but in patients in whom life is prolonged by dialysis or renal transplantation, the accumulation of cystine crystals in other organs may create problems. One such patient, in whom malabsorption due to pancreatic exocrine insufficiency developed at the age of 17 years, has been reported by Fivush et al. (1988).

References

Adrian TE, Mckiernan J, Johnston DI et al. (1980) Pancreatic gut hormone abnormalities in cystic fibrosis [abstract]. Gut 21: A448

Allen RA, Baggenstoss AH (1955) The pathogenesis of fibrocystic disease of the pancreas. Am J Pathol 31: 337-351

Andersen DH (1938) Cystic fibrosis of the pancreas and its relation to celiac disease. Am J Dis Child 56: 344-399

Anderson CM, Goodchild MC (1976) Cystic fibrosis. Blackwell, Oxford, pp 1-23

Baar HS (1953) Fibrocystic disease of the pancreas. Lancet ii: 80-83

Baggenstoss AH (1947) The pancreas in uremia [abstract]. Am J Pathol 23: 908

Baggenstoss AH (1948a) The pancreas in uremia: a histopathologic study. Am J Pathol 24: 1003-1017

Baggenstoss AH (1948b) Dilatation of the acini of the pancreas. Arch Pathol 45: 463-473

Ball WP, Baggenstoss AH, Bargen JA (1950) Pancreatic lesions associated with chronic ulcerative colitis. Arch Pathol 50: 347-358

Bartman J, Landing BH (1966) Morphology of the sweat apparatus in cystic fibrosis. Am J Clin Pathol 45: 455-459

Bodian M (1952) Fibrocystic disease of the pancreas. Heinemann, London, pp 67-104

Bostick WL, Rinehart JF (1950) Pathologic lesions in cystic fibrosis of the pancreas. J Pediatr 37: 469-477

Bothwell TH, Charlton RW (1972) Haemosiderosis. Br J Hosp Med 8: 437-444

Braxel C, Versieck J, Lemey G, Vanballenberge L, Barbier F (1982) Alpha-1-antitrypsin in pancreatitis. Digestion 23: 93-96

Brock D (1990) Genetic carrier tests and tests during pregnancy. Cystic Fibrosis Research Trust, Bromley, Kent, pp 1-10

Brown RE, Madge GE (1971) Cystic fibrosis and nesidioblastosis. Arch Pathol 92: 53-57

Clarke C, Hadfield G (1924) Congenital pancreatic disease with infantilism. Q J Med 17: 358-364

Crichton RR (1971) Ferritin: structure, synthesis and function. N Engl J Med 284: 1413-1422

Danks DM, Metz G, Sewell R, Prewett EJ (1990) Wilson's disease in adults with cirrhosis but no neurological abnormalities. Br Med J iii: 331-332

di Sant' Agnese PA (1956) Fibrocystic disease of the pancreas, a generalised disease of exocrine glands. JAMA 160: 846-853

di Sant' Agnese PA (1979) Cystic fibrosis (fibrocystic disease of the pancreas; pancreatic fibrosis; mucoviscidosis). In: Nelson WE, Vaughn VC, McKay RJ, Behrman RE (eds) Nelson textbook of pediatrics, 11th edn. Saunders, Philadelphia, pp 1988-2001

di Sant' Agnese PA, Davis PB (1976) Medical progress - research in cystic fibrosis. N Engl J Med 295: 481-485, 534-541, 597-602

di Sant' Agnese PA, Darling RC, Perera GA, Shea E (1953) Abnormal electrolyte composition of sweat in cystic fibrosis of the pancreas. Pediatrics 12: 549-563

Dixon AK, Walshe JM (1983) Pancreatic distortion due to splenomegaly in Wilson's disease [letter]. Lancet ii: 47

Emery JL (1951) Postnatal changes in the lobulation and connective tissue of the pancreas. J Anat 85: 159-162

Epstein O, Lake-Bakaar G, McKavanagh S, Sherlock S (1980) Pancreatic hyposecretion in primary biliary cirrhosis (PBC)-a "dry gland" disease. Gut 21: A448-449

Epstein O, Chapman RWG, Lake-Bakaar G, Foo AY, Rosalki SB, Sherlock S (1982) The pancreas in primary biliary cirrhosis and primary sclerosing cholangitis. Gastroenterology 83: 1177-1182

Farber S (1943) Pancreatic insufficiency and the celiac syndrome. N Engl J Med 229: 653-657

Farber S (1944) Pathologic changes associated with pancreatic insufficiency in early life. Arch Pathol 37: 238-250

Fivush B, Flick JA, Gahl WA (1988) Pancreatic exocrine insufficiency in a patient with nephropathic cystinosis. J Pediatr 112: 49-51

Foulis AK, Farquharson MA, Sale GE (1989) The pancreas in acute graft versus host disease in man. Histopathology 14: 121-128

Goodlin RC (1987) The effect of severe pre-eclampsia on the pancreas: changes in the serum cationic trypsinogen and pancreatic amylase [letter]. Br J Obstet Gynaecol 94: 1228

Haukland HH, Florholmen J, Øian P, Maltau JM, Burhol PG (1987) The effect of severe pre-eclampsia on the pancreas: changes in the serum cationic trypsinogen and pancreatic amylase. Br J Obstet Gynaecol 94: 765-767

Iannucci A, Mukai K, Johnson D, Burke B (1984) Endocrine pancreas in cystic fibrosis: an immunohistochemical study. Hum Pathol 15: 278-284

Imrie J, Fagan D, Sturgess J (1979) Quantitative evaluation of the development of the exocrine pancreas in cystic fibrosis and control infants. Am J Pathol 95: 697-708

Isaacson C, Seftel HC, Keeley KJ, Bothwell TH (1961) Siderosis in the Bantu: the relationship between iron overload and cirrhosis. J Lab Clin Med 58: 845-853

Jolly RD, Thompson KG (1977) Mannosidosis - pathogenesis of lesions in exocrine cells. J Pathol 121: 59-62

Kerem B-S, Rommens JM, Buchanan JA et al. (1989) Identification of the cystic fibrosis gene: genetic analysis. Science 245: 1073-1080

Klass HJ, Braganza JM, Warnes TW (1979) Pancreas in primary biliary cirrhosis (PBC) [abstract]. Gut 20: A443

Lambert JR, Cole M, Crozier DN, Connon JJ (1981) Intrapancreatic common bile duct compression causing jaundice in an adult with cystic fibrosis. Gastroenterology 80: 169-172

Lebenthal E, Lerner A, Heitlinger L (1986) The pancreas in cystic fibrosis. In: Go VLW, Gardner JD, Brooks FP, Lebenthal E, Di Magno FP, Scheele GA (eds) The exocrine pancreas: biology, pathobiology and diseases. Raven Press, New York, pp 753-817

Liu HM, Potter EL (1962) Development of the human pancreas. Arch Pathol 74: 439-452

Looi LM (1989) Histomorphological variations in systemic AA amyloidosis: clues of AA protein polymorphism. Histopathology 14: 111-120

Lynch MJG, Shorthouse PH (1949) Injuries and death from lightning. Lancet i: 473-478

MacCallum WG (1940) Textbook of pathology, 7th edn. Saunders, Philadelphia, pp 483-484; Fig. 256

MacDonald RA, Mallory GK (1960) Hemochromatosis and hemosiderosis; study of 211 autopsied cases. Arch Intern Med 105: 686-700

Martin E, Bedossa P (1989) Diffuse fibrosis of the pancreas: a peculiar pattern of pancreatitis in alcoholic cirrhosis. Gastroenterol Clin Biol 13: 579-584

May CD (1954) Cystic fibrosis of the pancreas in infants and children. Thomas, Springfield, pp 10-17

Menten ML, Kinsey WC (1949) Asymptomatic retention of pancreatic secretion. Arch Pathol 47: 90-96

Minns RA, Eden OB, Hendry GMA (1982) Pancreatic enlargement and Wilson's disease. Lancet ii: 337-338

Munger GL, Brusilow SW, Cooke RE (1961) An electron microscopic study of exocrine sweat glands in patients with cystic fibrosis of the pancreas. J Pediat 59: 497-511

Novis BH, Bank S, Young GO, Marks IN (1975) Chronic pancreatitis and Alpha-1-antitrypsin. Lancet ii: 748-749

Opie EL (1910) Disease of the pancreas, 2nd edn. Lippincott, Philadelphia, Fig. 18

Oppenheimer E, Esterly J (1973) Cystic fibrosis of the pancreas:

morphologic findings in infants with and without pancreatic lesions. Arch Pathol 96 : 149–154

Park RW, Grand RJ (1981) Gastrointestinal manifestations of cystic fibrosis: a review. Gastroenterology 81 : 1143–1161

Piper WN, Helwig EB (1935) Progressive systemic sclerosis: visceral manifestations in generalised scleroderma. Arch Dermatol 72 : 535–546

Pirani CL (1976) Tissue distribution of amyloid. In: Wegelius O, Pasternack A (eds) Amyloidosis. Academic Press, London, pp 33–49

Pitchumoni CS, Scheele G, Lee PC, Lebenthal E (1986) Effects of nutrition on the exocrine pancreas. In: Go VLW, Gardner JD, Brooks FP, Lebenthal E, Di Magno FP, Scheele GA (eds) The exocrine pancreas: biology, pathobiology and diseases. Raven Press, New York, p 394

Porta E, Stein A, Patterson P (1964) Ultrastructural changes of the pancreas and liver in cystic fibrosis. Am J Clin Pathol 42 : 451–465

Reynolds JC, Inman RD, Kimberley RP, Chuong JH, Kovacs JE, Walsh MB (1982) Acute pancreatitis in systemic lupus erythematosus: report of twenty cases and a review of the literature. Medicine 61 : 25–32

Riordan JR, Rommens JM, Kerem B-S et al. (1989) Identification of the cystic fibrosis gene: cloning and characterisation of complementary DNA. Science 245 : 1066–1072

Rommens JM, Iannuzi MC, Kerem B-S et al. (1989) Identification of the cystic fibrosis gene: chromosome walking and jumping. Science 245 : 1059–1065

Sabesin SM, Thomas LB (1964) Parenchymal siderosis in patients with preexisting portal cirrhosis. Gastroenterology 46 : 477–485

Sass-Kortsak A, Bearn AG (1978) Hereditary disorders of copper metabolism. In: Stanbury JB, Wyngaarden JB, Fredrickson DS (eds) The metabolic basis of inherited disease, 4th edn. McGraw-Hill, New York, p 1108

Sheehan HL, Lynch JB (1973) Pathology of toxaemia of pregnancy. Churchill Livingstone, Edinburgh, pp 682–683

Shibayama Y, Hashimoto K, Makata K (1992) Pathogenesis of pancreatic perilobular necrosis in patients with liver disease. J Pathol 167 : 421–424

Shwachman H, Lebenthal E, Khaw KT (1975) Recurrent attacks of acute pancreatitis in patients with cystic fibrosis with normal pancreatic enzymes. Pediatrics 55 : 86–95

Smith PA, Sunter JP, Case RM (1982) Progressive atrophy of pancreatic acinar tissue in rats fed a copper-deficient diet supplemented with D-penicillamine or triethylene tetramine: morphological and physiological studies. Digestion 23 : 16–30

Sochor FM, Mallory GK (1963) Lung lesions in patients dying of burns. Arch Pathol 75 : 303–308

Stein AA, Powers SR (1956) Pancreatic acinar ectasia. Arch Pathol 62 : 494–496

Stinson JC, Baggenstoss AH, Morlock CG (1952) Pancreatic lesions associated with cirrhosis of the liver. Am J Clin Pathol 22 : 117–126

Svenberg T, Haggmark T, Strandovik B, Slezak P (1988) Haemorrhagic pancreatitis after ERCP in patients with alpha-1-antitrypsin deficiency [letter]. Lancet i : 772

Tisdale WA (1961) Parenchymal siderosis in patients with cirrhosis after porta-caval shunt surgery. N Engl J Med 265 : 928–932

Vawter GF, Shwachman H (1979) Cystic fibrosis in adults: an autopsy study. Pathol Annu 14 (Part 2) : 357–382

Vaziri ND, Dure-Smith B, Miller R, Mirahmadi M (1987) Pancreatic pathology in chronic dialysis patients – an autopsy study of 78 cases. Nephron 46 : 347–349

Vaziri ND, Chang D, Malekpour A, Radahat S (1988) Pancreatic enzymes in patients with end-stage renal disease maintained on hemodialysis. Am J Gastroenterol 83 : 410–412

Veghelyi PV (1949) Pancreatic function in scarlet fever. Pediatrics 4 : 94–101

Walters N-I (1965) The ductular cell in pancreatic cystic fibrosis. J Pathol Bacteriol 90 : 45–52

Walters N-I, Gibb DGA (1965) Cystic fibrosis and acinar ectasia of the pancreas: histochemical comparison of the intraluminal secretions. J Pathol Bacteriol 89 : 89–93

Warren S, Le Compte PM, Legg MA (1966) The pathology of diabetes mellitus. Kimpton, London, pp 81, 121

Webb L, Smith-Laing G, Lake-Bakaar G, McKavanagh S, Sherlock S (1980) Pancreatic hypofunction in extraportal venous obstruction. Gut 21 : 227–231

Wharton GK (1932) The blood supply of the pancreas with special reference to that of the islands of Langerhans. Anat Rec 53 : 55–76

Williams C, Williamson B, Watson E (1991) Carrier screening for cystic fibrosis in the community. Bull R Coll Pathol 73 : 4–5

Wilson SAK (1912) Progressive lenticular degeneration: a familial nervous disease associated with cirrhosis of the liver. Brain 34 : 295–509

Witzleben CL, Uri A (1989) Perinatal hemochromatosis: entity or end result. Hum Pathol 20 : 335–340

Wolman R, de Gara C, Isenberg D (1988) Acute pancreatitis in systemic lupus erythematosus: report of a case unrelated to drug therapy. Ann Rheum Dis 47 : 77–79

Zuelzer WW, Newton WA (1949) The pathogenesis of fibrocystic disease of the pancreas: a study of 36 cases with special reference to the pulmonary lesions. Pediatrics 4 : 53–69

5 The Effects of Arterial Disease upon the Pancreas

The pancreas receives a generous supply of arterial blood, which is not surprising, because of the important exocrine and endocrine functions of the gland. The arteries that supply the pancreas can show a certain amount of anatomical variation and are liable to be affected by certain congenital or acquired defects that are rare, but which may have catastrophic effects. Both the arteries and arterioles of the pancreas are vulnerable to the effects of systemic hypertension and arteriosclerosis. The latter effects may be of importance in the aetiology of diabetes mellitus of the maturity-onset type, and of acute haemorrhagic pancreatitis, while true infarcts of the pancreas may occur in the malignant type of essential hypertension, certain cases of glomerulonephritis with hypertension, and some cases of periarteritis nodosa.

Anatomy of the Arteries of the Pancreas

The arterial supply of the pancreas has been studied by Woodburne and Olsen (1951) by dissection, and by Falconer and Griffiths (1949–1950) by dissection and the injection-corrosion technique.As far as the major arterial vessels are concerned, these workers found the descriptions in the standard anatomical textbooks to be correct in that deviations from the usual pattern are rare. The arteries concerned are branches of the coeliac axis and the superior mesenteric artery. The head of the pancreas, which shares its arterial supply with the adjacent parts of the duodenum, is supplied by arteries carrying blood from both the coeliac axis and from the superior mesenteric artery. The body and tail of the pancreas are usually supplied with arterial blood derived from the coeliac axis through the splenic artery and its branches. The dorsal pancreatic artery, however, a vessel present in 90% of cases, may receive its blood either through the coeliac axis or through the superior mesenteric artery. This vessel, which has a typical course and pattern of branches, may arise variously from the coeliac axis itself or from the splenic or hepatic branches of the coeliac axis, or, instead of receiving its blood through the coeliac axis, it may be a branch of the superior mesenteric artery.

The formation of arterial arcades is characteristic of the blood supply of the pancreas. Two arcades – one anterior, the other posterior – supply the head of the pancreas and the adjacent duodenum. The anterior arcade is formed by the almost constant anterior superior pancreaticoduodenal artery from the gastroduodenal artery. It forms an anastomosis with the less constant anterior inferior pancreaticoduodenal artery from the superior mesenteric system. The posterior arcade is contributed to from above by the posterior superior pancreaticoduodenal artery and is usually completed by a posterior inferior pancreaticoduodenal artery that arises in most cases from the superior mesenteric system.

The inferior pancreaticoduodenal vessels are much more variable in the details of their origin than the superior vessels. The many variations have been studied by Michels (1962) by dissection, and, as the vessels concerned are between 1 mm and 2 mm in diameter, his results compare surprisingly well with those obtained angiographically by Finlay and Herlinger (1977). Commonly, the anterior and posterior arcades are in communication with the splenic artery via the right and uncinate branch of the dorsal pancreatic artery. The dorsal pancreatic artery is usually a branch of the splenic artery, but it may arise from the superior mesenteric, middle colic or hepatic arteries, and even, very rarely, as an independent branch of the coeliac axis. It descends behind the pancreas and divides into right and left branches. The right branch communicates with the pancreaticoduodenal arcades, and the left branch, the transverse pancreatic artery, provides a communication with the blood supply of the body of the pancreas and with that of the spleen. The pancreatica magna artery is a fairly constant superior pancreatic branch of the splenic artery, which enters the body of the pancreas at the junction of its middle and left third; it is present in over 60% of cases. The tail of the pancreas receives its arterial supply from caudal branches of the splenic artery or its left gastroepiploic branch.

Aneurysms of the Pancreatic Arteries

Until angiography became available, aneurysms of the visceral arteries were seldom recognised during life. Such aneurysms of the pancreatic arteries are still rare, but reports are accumulating of their recognition and surgical cure after having been diagnosed and localised angiographically. Some of the reports do not include an opinion on the origin of the aneurysms, but the cases in which a cause has been recognised make it clear that there are several different aetiologies.

Congenital Aneurysms

Two different types of congenital aneurysm may occur within the pancreas or on its surface. The first of these is the arteriovenous aneurysm, which may be part of the Osler–Weber–Rendu type of hereditary telangiectasia, as has been described in the lungs by Hales (1956), and in the abdominal region by Halpern et al. (1968). In this lesion its congenital nature is undoubted. A case of this type in which there was a diffuse arteriovenous malformation in the body and tail of the pancreas, with involvement of the head to a lesser extent, has been described by Chuang et al. (1977). This lesion would by itself have caused portal hypertension, but the severe bleeding from oesophageal varices that led to the diagnosis and an attempt to cure the patient surgically was precipitated by the onset of alcoholic cirrhosis of the liver.

The authors' own experience of an arteriovenous aneurysm within the pancreas in the Osler–Weber–Rendu syndrome is as follows. A girl in whom a diagnosis of the Osler–Weber–Rendu syndrome had been established during her childhood after she had had a haemorrhage from oesphageal varices, and whose father had died of an upper abdominal intraperitoneal haemorrhage, married and became pregnant at the age of 20 years. Shortly before delivery was due she developed signs of an intra-abdominal haemorrhage. Rupture of an aneurysm of the splenic artery was suspected and emergency splenectomy was carried out after resuscitation, but she died as the operation was being completed. At post-mortem, a ruptured aneurysm 1 cm in diameter on the splenic artery at the hilum of the spleen was identified and multiple arteriovenous communications between the splenic artery and the splenic and pancreatic veins within the tail of the pancreas were found, along with marked intimal thickening in the portal venous system. The ruptured aneurysm on the splenic artery resembled the aneurysms of the splenic artery described in the Osler–Weber–Rendu syndrome by Schuster (1937). In this patient, as in that reported by Chuang et al. (1977), an additional factor had been added to the portal hypertension caused by the arteriovenous communication, for pregnancy has been recognised by Lennie and Sheehan (1942) to increase the tendency to rupture of aneurysms of visceral arteries, especially aneurysms of the splenic artery.

Another type of "congenital" aneurysm of an artery supplying the pancreas has been described by Shallow et al. (1946). In this type, the aneurysm is believed to be the counterpart of the aneurysmal lesions that are well recognised to occur on the intracranial arteries, especially the anterior half of the circle of Willis and its branches. The lesion described by Shallow et al. involved the inferior pancreaticoduodenal artery and was close to the first bifurcation of the artery. The aneurysm, which was saccular, was 4 cm in diameter and had an ostium 1 cm in length and 3 mm across. It had ruptured, and its contents of grey laminated ante-mortem thrombus were in direct communication

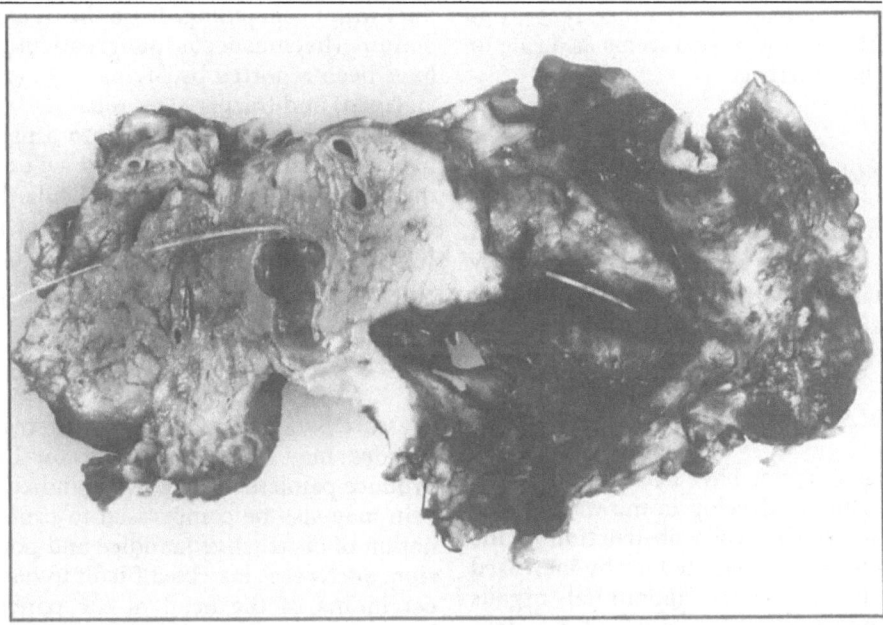

Fig. 5.1. A coronal section through a pancreas, the tail and distal body of which has become a pseudocyst following infarction. A marker in the main pancreatic duct demonstrates that the duct communicates with the cyst. The orifice of a ruptured artery, resembling a ruptured artery in the floor of a peptic ulcer, is present on the posterior wall of the pseudocyst. A smaller cyst near the neck of the pancreas is the remnant of another infarct that has become cystic. The patient was a man aged 33 in whom renal failure with hypertension due to chronic glomerulonephritis was treated by a renal transplant. Haemorrhage into the pseudocyst caused death. Atheromatous narrowing of the splenic artery was very marked and thrombi at various stages of organisation were present within the pancreatic arterial branches.

with a large haemorrhage into the pancreas, retroperitoneum and peritoneal cavity. There were three fusiform dilatations of the artery distal to the ruptured aneurysm. Defects similar to those demonstrated in aneurysms of arteries at the base of the brain by Forbus (1930) were found microscopically. In describing these lesions the authors wrote the word "congenital" within inverted commas because of the uncertainty that exists about the true congenital nature of such aneurysms and of the defects that lead to their development (Glynn 1940). In many of the reported cases of aneurysm of the visceral arteries the exact nature of the aneurysm has not been determined but, in general, when there are multiple arteriovenous communications, the lesions are assumed to be congenital or to be the result of congenital abnormalities for, as has been pointed out by van Way et al. (1971), arterial aneurysms of the congenital type may, by rupturing, cause arteriovenous communications.

Arteriosclerotic Aneurysms

Arteriosclerosis has been diagnosed as the cause of aneurysms of the pancreaticoduodenal artery in a number of the reported cases. In their review in 1968 West et al. found that, in eight (including one of their own) cases of the 14 recorded up to that time, the aneurysm was attributable to the effects of arteriosclerosis.

Inflammatory Aneurysms

Inflammation too may cause aneurysms of the arteries of the pancreas, usually as a result of damage to branches of the peripancreatic arteries by pancreatitis (White et al. 1976) or by a pseudocyst (Harris et al. 1975; Walter et al. 1977); the splenic artery may be eroded if it becomes involved in the wall of a pseudocyst (Kadell and Riley 1967). The small orifice of a ruptured aneurysm can be recognised in the wall of the pseudocyst illustrated in Fig. 5.1.

Mycotic aneurysms of the arteries within the pancreas have not been reported, although there are said to have been cases of mycotic aneurysm of the splenic artery (Spittel et al. 1961) and of a non-pancreatic branch of the superior mesenteric artery (Keehan et al. 1978). The generalised arteritis of periarteritis nodosa may cause microscopic aneurysms of arteries within the pancreas (Gruber 1929), but thrombosis within the aneurysms seems as a rule to prevent serious haemorrhage.

Traumatic Aneurysms

Traumatic aneurysms may develop in and around the pancreas following non-penetrating injury (West et al. 1968), or following penetrating injuries and operations.

Non-traumatic Aneurysms

Non-traumatic aneurysms have been found radiologically to be liable to develop in the walls of the small pancreatic arteries when obstruction of the coeliac axis has to be compensated for by increased blood supply to the upper abdominal organs through collateral vessels from the superior mesenteric artery. There are no reports of the rupture of such aneurysms. Proud and Chamberlain (1978), who recognised these aneurysms, suggest that they may regress if compression of the coeliac axis can be relieved.

Haemorrhage Due to Rupture of Aneurysms

The effects of aneurysms of the arteries of the pancreas are usually due to rupture with massive haemorrhage, to pressure by a haematoma (false aneurysm) around the aneurysm, or to pressure by the aneurysm itself. Rupture of an aneurysm may also occur with the formation of an arteriovenous fistula and the development of portal hypertension. The haemorrhage that follows catastrophic rupture of an aneurysm of a pancreatic artery is retroperitoneal at first, with the development of a haematoma within the pancreas, transverse mesocolon, upper periaortic region, around the adrenal glands and upper poles of one or both kidneys. By the time that laparotomy or autopsy is carried out, haemoperitoneum is usually present as well, the extravasated blood having ruptured into the lesser sac of the peritoneum and escaped through the aditus of the lesser sac into the main peritoneal cavity. Less severe, but life-threatening, haemorrhage may occur into the duodenum, with haematemesis or melaena if a haematoma in the head of the pancreas erodes the duodenal mucosa; bleeding into the duodenum may also occur following the rupture of an aneurysm into the pancreatic

duct with haemorrhage from the duct into the duodenum (haemosuccus pancreaticus). Such cases have been reported by Bivins et al. (1978), Lung et al. (1980) and Harper et al. 1984.

If an aneurysm ruptures into a pseudocyst that has been drained, haemorrhage will occur through the drain site or through any fistula that may have been created. The various types of haemorrhage that may complicate pancreatic disease have been discussed by Walter et al. (1977).

Effects of Pressure by Aneurysms

Pressure by aneurysms of the pancreaticoduodenal arcades may affect the common bile duct and produce painless obstructive jaundice, or the portal vein may also be compressed to produce a combination of obstructive jaundice and portal hypertension. Such cases may be difficult to distinguish from carcinoma of the head of the pancreas, even at laparotomy, because the true nature of the mass in the head of the pancreas may not be recognised.

In the case recorded by Catanzaro et al. (1957) however, a mass 4 cm in diameter could be felt to pulsate and there was a palpable bruit. An aneurysm no more than 1 cm or 2 cm in diameter may be surrounded by a much larger haematoma. The mass in the head of the pancreas in the case reported by Lambert and Hyde (1960) was 15 cm in diameter. Attacks of pancreatitis may also be precipitated by pressure upon the pancreatic duct, as in the patient reported by Hendrick (1956), in whom the removal of an aneurysm 4 cm in diameter and 6 cm long from the pancreaticoduodenal artery in the region of the neck of the pancreas effected a cure for recurrent attacks of pancreatitis. Pancreatitis, however, does not explain the upper abdominal pain experienced by some patients, for example in one of the cases reported by Harris et al. (1975). The patient, a woman aged 54, had complained of recurrent pain in the epigastrium and right upper abdominal quadrant for several months. Selective coeliac angiography demonstrated a calcified aneurysm, 2 cm in diameter, in the gastroduodenal artery and two calcified aneurysms, each 1 cm in diameter, in the pancreaticoduodenal artery. Removal of the aneurysm of the gastroduodenal artery, and ligation of the pancreaticoduodenal artery without removal of its aneurysms, cured the patient of her symptoms. The pancreas was examined during the operation and was found to be normal. The aneurysm that was removed was diagnosed pathologically as being due to arteriosclerosis.

Effects of Arteriosclerosis of the Pancreatic Arteries

With advancing age there is an increased incidence of arteriosclerotic and arteriolosclerotic lesions in the arteries of the pancreas. Several studies have been undertaken to correlate such changes with lesions of the pancreatic parenchyma. The earlier work in this field has been reviewed by Gruber (1929), while the more recent publications, especially those on the relationship between arterial and arteriolar lesions and maturity-onset diabetes mellitus, have been reviewed in publications such as those of Lazarus and Volk (1962), Warren et al. (1966) and Volk and Wellmann (1977). Moschcowitz (1951, 1956) interpreted his observations as indicating a relationship between arterial disease and adult diabetes in that he found that hyalinised islets in adult diabetes were nearly always associated with arteriosclerosis of the pancreatic vessels. He suggested that the lesion of the islets was a result either of an extension of the hyalinisation of the afferent arteriole into the capillaries of the islet, or of diminution of the blood supply to the islet. He went on to suggest that, in cases of diabetes in which the islets seemed normal, their functional failure to produce adequate amounts of insulin was due to an impairment of the grosser blood supply. While it seems likely that Moschcowitz's explanation for the hyaline lesion of the islets is correct, there remains a serious discrepancy in the association between the presence of hyaline islets and the presence of clinical diabetes mellitus.

Discrepancies also exist in the observations of different workers upon the association between arteriosclerosis of the pancreatic arteries and diabetes mellitus. Lazarus and Volk (1961) found that marked arteriosclerosis within the pancreas was almost twice as common (66%) and more occlusive in diabetes than in the pancreases of non-diabetic patients, in whom the incidence of sclerotic arterial lesions was only 34% and lesions were less severe. Warren et al. (1966), however, found that only 7.4% of the pancreases in their collection of material from patients with diabetes had marked arteriosclerosis. They concluded that, while they could not exclude arteriosclerosis as a factor in the production of diabetes, it was "hardly of outstanding importance". They stated also that, although the splenic artery may be extremely sclerosed and calcified, there is frequently very little change in its branches to the pancreas.

General atrophy of the pancreatic exocrine glandular tissue with fatty replacement has also been attributed to obliterative arterial disease (Lazarus and Volk 1962), but the arteriosclerotic lesions illustrated by these authors in this condition may be entirely coincidental. Marked examples of exocrine atrophy with lipomatous pseudohypertrophy, but without arteriosclerotic lesions, have been reported (Davie 1938; Høyer 1949; Bartholomew et al. 1959). Diffuse or focal interacinar fibrosis, without signs of chronic pancreatitis, is, however, usually attributed to the effects of arteriosclerosis.

It should be noted that arteriosclerosis in the pancreas does not always indicate generalised arteriosclerosis. Only five of the 18 cases with pancreatic arteriosclerosis studied by Stamm (1984) had general arteriosclerosis.

Arterial Lesions in Relation to Acute Haemorrhagic Pancreatitis

Because the appearances of the pancreas in acute haemorrhagic pancreatitis are those of haemorrhagic infarction, or are indistinguishable from those of haemorrhagic infarction, it is not surprising that the possible vascular factors in the aetiology of acute pancreatitis have received attention from various investigators. The results of experimental work suggest that disturbances of the microcirculation are the essential factors in the development of haemorrhagic pancreatitis, but there are reports of human examples of the disease that implicate arterial obstruction as an aetiological factor. In the case described by Gambill et al. (1948), a large artery within the pancreas was demonstrated to have been eroded by what was thought to have been less severe preceding pancreatitis and to have been occluded by thrombus to cause haemorrhagic infarction, giving the picture of acute haemorrhagic pancreatitis in the tail and in a portion of the body of the gland. In the case described by Guice et al. (1987), thrombosis of a pancreatic artery associated with invasive aspergillosis was thought to have caused haemorrhagic pancreatitis .

Embolisation of arterial branches within the pancreas by cholesterol and other atheromatous material from atheromatous ulcers in the intima of the aorta has also been suggested to be of importance in the aetiology of acute pancreatitis (Probstein et al. 1957; Pollak 1968).

Large emboli in the hepatic and pancreaticoduodenal arteries are referred to in the paper by Moberg et al. (1968) as having caused an infarct in the liver and what was described as acute pancreatitis. There was no clinical evidence of pancreatitis, and it seems likely that the pancreatic lesion was, in fact, an infarct.

Pancreatic Infarction

Clinical Significance

Although it is sometimes impossible to distinguish between haemorrhagic infarction of the pancreas and acute haemorrhagic pancreatitis, there are cases in which there are lesions in the pancreas that are obvious infarcts of the anaemic type, and the observations of McKay et al. (1958) have established that pancreatic infarction undoubtedly exists as a separate pathological entity. The status, however, of pancreatic infarcts as lesions of clinical significance is less clear, for in some cases the lesions found postmortem seem to have had no clinical effects, but, in at least some of the cases reported by McKay et al., the infarcts seem to have caused upper abdominal pain with nausea and vomiting. The serum enzymes were estimated in only a few of the patients, but no disturbances of the enzymes was demonstrated.

Incidence

Pancreatic infarcts are rare; they were found by McKay et al. in only 0.19% of 21 481 consecutive necropsies at the Mayo Clinic. Such rarity is in keeping with the rich arterial blood supply of the pancreas from the ramifications of two separate branches of the abdominal aorta, with numerous communications between the two systems. Infarcts thus tend to occur only in cases of generalised arterial disease in which thrombosis of a pancreatic artery is associated with occlusive disease of the collateral vessels. According to Pollak (1968) it is the more dramatic effects of the generalised arterial disease upon organs such as the heart, kidneys or brain that make the clinical recognition of pancreatic infarcts so rare; he reports his experience of myocardial infarction associated with clinically unsuspected pancreatic infarction.

The reports of patients with pancreatic infarcts published between 1900 and 1954 have been reviewed by McKay et al. (1958). They found 28, to which could be added the pancreatic infarcts noted by Baló (1926) in his account of fatal cases of periarteritis nodosa with polyneuritis. This account included the information that infarcts, or fresh nodules of vascular disease with necrosis, were present in the pancreas in two of the cases, while in the third the pancreas was atrophic and contained scarred nodules associated microscopically with arteries that were either completely occluded or narrowed by proliferating connective tissue.

Causes

McKay et al. searched the records of the Mayo Clinic and found 41 cases in which they decided that there were pancreatic lesions that were infarcts as distinct from other abnormalities of the pancreas that caused necrosis. They eliminated all the cases in which the presence of fat necrosis in the extrapancreatic tissue, or of marked peripancreatic or intrapancreatic haemorrhage, suggested a diagnosis of acute haemorrhage pancreatitis; they also eliminated cases in which there was diffuse inflammation that was not in the immediate vicinity of the infarcts. They did not include fibrous lesions that might have been healed infarcts, for such scars could not be distinguished from injuries due to other causes of pancreatic damage.

Although the infarcts were associated with various primary diseases, the two predominant primary conditions were periarteritis nodosa and malignant essential hypertension; one or other of these two arterial disorders was present in 66% of the cases in the series. Embolism was an unusual cause and was present in only three, two of which were cases of subacute bacterial endocarditis, while the third was infarction of the left ventricle with mural thrombosis. Thrombosis of the splenic or superior mesenteric arteries in the absence of periarteritis nodosa caused the infarcts in only two of the cases.

McKay et al. confirmed the importance of periarteritis nodosa as a cause of pancreatic infarcts, as previously noted by Baló (1926) and by Froboese (1949), and also of malignant hypertension, as noted by Klemperer and Otani (1931), Aufdermaur (1947) and Hranilovich and Baggenstoss (1953). The relative rarity, in the absence of periarteritis nodosa, of thrombosis of the major arteries to the pancreas as a cause of pancreatic infarction is probably because of the effective collateral circulation that exists in the splanchnic area and whose importance has been emphasised by Rob (1965). It seems that occlusion of the superior mesenteric artery by thrombosis or embolism does not cause infarction of the pancreas

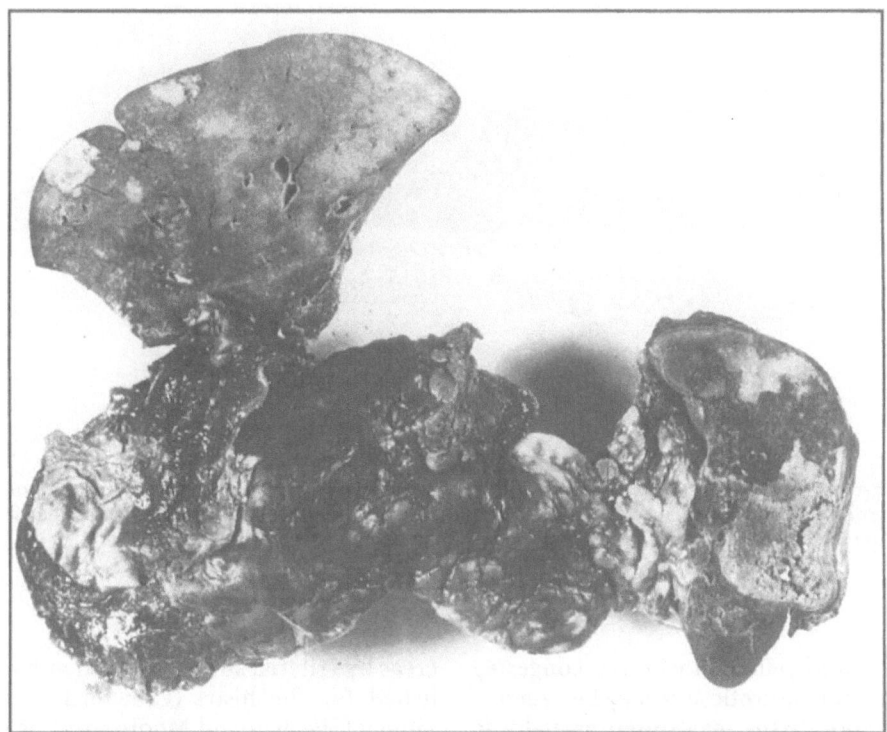

Fig. 5.2. Haemorrhagic infarction of the whole pancreas, with anaemic infarcts in the spleen and in the subcapsular region of the liver, caused by embolism of the coeliac axis by mural thrombus from the left ventricle of the heart.

(Droller 1972). In two cases in Droller's series, even occlusion of the coeliac axis causing hepatic necrosis and duodenal gangrene does not appear to have caused obvious pancreatic damage.

Sudden occlusion of the coeliac axis can, however, sometimes include infarction of the pancreas, along with the production of infarcts in the liver and spleen, as illustrated in Fig. 5.2. The patient was a woman, 67 years old, who was diagnosed clinically as having a myocardial infarct and atrial fibrillation. While in hospital she had sudden abdominal pain that suggested pancreatitis, but a definite diagnosis of pancreatitis was not made because there was no elevation of the serum amylase. Her general condition was considered to be too poor for laparotomy and she died within a few hours. Post-mortem the abdomen contained blood-stained fluid, large infarcts were present in the liver and spleen, and the pancreas was haemorrhagic throughout. The coeliac axis was completely blocked by thrombus from its orifice for a distance of about 1 cm, that is, for most of the length of the trunk of the vessel. The coeliac trunk was free from recognisable disease, both macroscopically and microscopically, and the thrombus was taken to be embolic from the heart, in which mural thrombus was attached to the endo-

cardium of the left ventricle in association with a large myocardial infarct of the left ventricle. There was no fat necrosis in the vicinity of the pancreas or elsewhere in the body.

In eight of the 41 cases with pancreatic infarcts collected by McKay et al. no marked occlusive lesions were found in the arteries, but, in seven of these, death had been preceded by shock or congestive cardiac failure with hypotension. Cardiac failure with hypotension is now recognised to be a cause of infarction of various parts of the alimentary canal and it seems likely that the pancreas, supplied as it is by some of the same arteries, is similary vulnerable to the effects of hypotension.

Macroscopic Features

The size of pancreatic infarcts varies from microscopic lesions that involve a single lobule, 2 mm or less in diameter, to macroscopically obvious areas of necrosis 3 cm or 4 cm in diameter (Fig. 5.3), or, as in the case illustrated in Fig. 5.2, the whole gland may be affected. Infarcts that involve three or more lobules can usually be recognised with the naked eye. As with infarcts in other organs, the necrotic

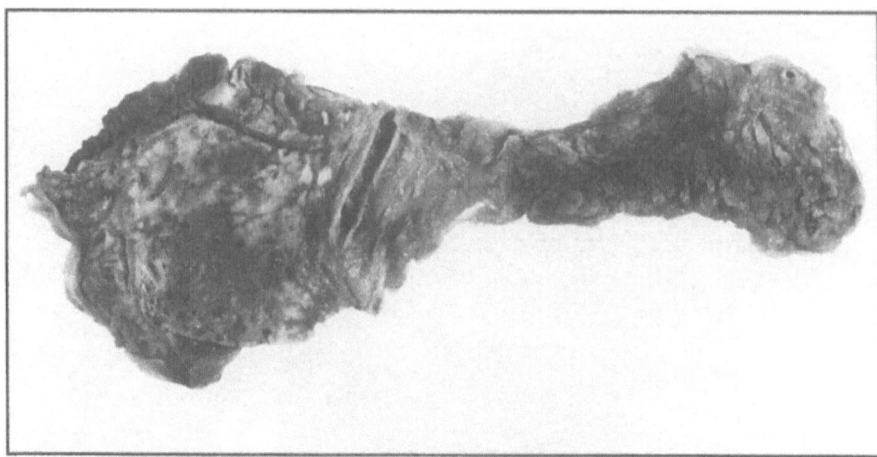

Fig. 5.3. A coronal section through the pancreas, second part of duodenum and superior mesenteric artery, showing an infarct that is partly haemorrhagic and partly anaemic. It occupies most of the head of the pancreas. The patient was a 52-year-old woman who died of renal failure due to malignant hypertension that complicated systemic sclerosis.

area may be pale and yellowish with red congested margins, or the whole necrotic area may be haemorrhagic. The necrotic tissue may soften partially to become caseous or it may liquefy, leaving a cavity filled with brown or almost black fluid. The large infarct illustrated in Fig. 5.1 became liquefied and formed a pseudocyst that communicated with the main pancreatic duct. A small aneurysm of an artery in the wall of the pseudocyst later ruptured and caused uncontrollable haemorrhage.

Large macroscopically obvious infarcts may occur in any part of the gland. Such infarcts are usually single and an occluded artery can sometimes be recognised with the naked eye in the adjacent glandular tissue. The smallest infarcts are usually multiple and scattered throughout the pancreas. The occluded vessels cannot be recognised macroscopically.

Microscopic Features

The dead area usually becomes more eosinophilic than the adjacent normal glandular tissue because the nuclei undergo karyolysis or fragment, while granules disappear leaving the acinar cells with pink-staining cytoplasm and absent or degenerate nuclei. In some lesions the outline of the cells is retained, but in others, probably older lesions, the glandular tissue breaks down to leave granular debris. The granules disappear from the islets in the necrotic area and, in lesions that are probably older, even the outline of the islets disappears. An assessment of the approximate age of infarcts of the pan-

creas by criteria, such as those that have been established for the heart (Crawford 1977) or for the kidney (Sheehan and Moore 1952), is not justifiable because so many pancreatic infarcts are clinically silent. A zone of congested vessels and extravasated red cells usually surrounds the necrotic glandular tissue but this is not invariable (Fig. 5.4). A reaction of polymorphonuclear leucocytes can usually be recognised beyond the margins of the infarcts. Migration of polymorphonuclear leucocytes into the dead area and a zone of dead polymorphs within the area of necrosis are not usually recognisable. Older lesions become encapsulated by proliferating fibroblasts (Fig. 5.5). However, as has been pointed out by McKay et al., the microscopic appearances may vary considerably (Figs 5.6–5.10), and in some infarcts there may be so much extravasation of blood into and around the infarct that the lesion resembles a haematoma. Fat in the interstitial tissues of the pancreas may be included in the area of necrosis but extensive necrosis of fat is unusual.

Relationship to Haemorrhagic Pancreatitis

The rarity of infarcts of the pancreas would suggest that they are pathological curiosities and of little real importance, but there is experimental work that suggests that, at least occasionally, infarction may initiate acute haemorrhagic pancreatitis. Thus Block et al. (1954) found that, in the rat, complete devascularisation of portions of the pancreas usually produced pancreatic infarcts, but occasionally acute pancreatitis developed in the ischaemic

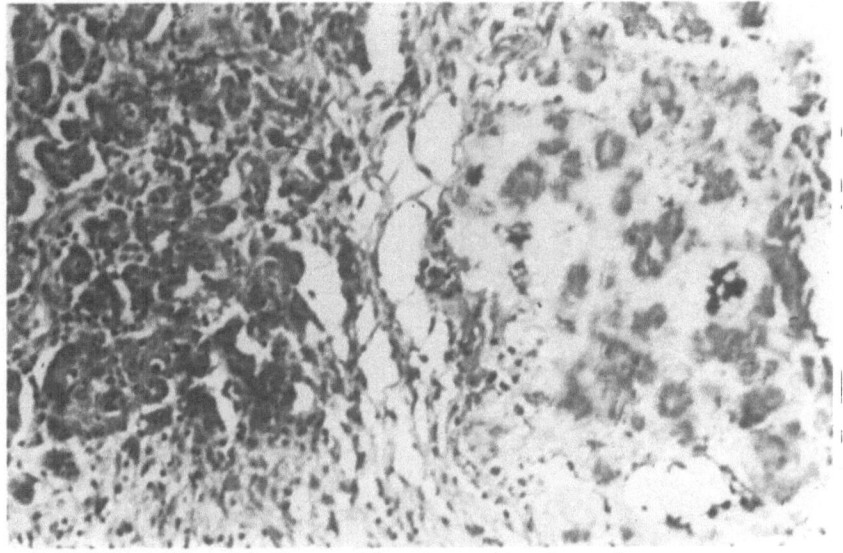

Fig. 5.4. The edge of a pancreatic infarct in which karyolysis is almost complete. There is very little adjacent inflammatory reaction. H&E, × 40

areas. As a rule, however, these workers found that procedures in addition to devascularisation were necessary to produce pancreatitis that resembled the human disease, a finding in keeping with the results of the earlier experiments of Popper et al. (1948). The experiments of Pfeffer et al. (1962), in which it was found that, when sterile polythene microspheres were injected into the pancreatic circulation, the severity of the pancreatitis produced was inversely proportional to the size of the microspheres injected, suggest that disturbance of the microcirculation is of more importance than gross arterial occlusion. However, Baggenstoss (1973), from his large experience of experimental pancreatic lesions, as well as of the histopathology of human pancreatic disease, has come to the conclusion that infarction of the pancreas is unlikely to initiate acute pancreatitis.

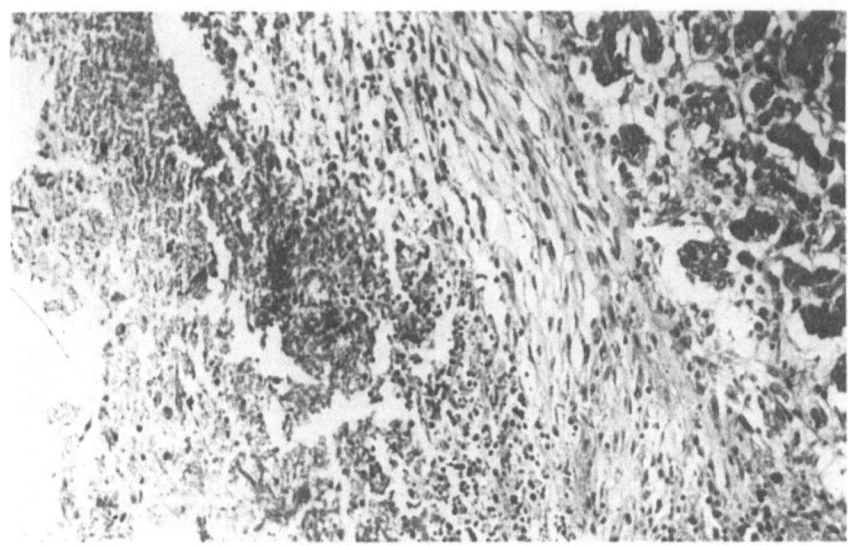

Fig. 5.5. Fibroblasts forming a capsule around a pancreatic infarct. H&E, × 40

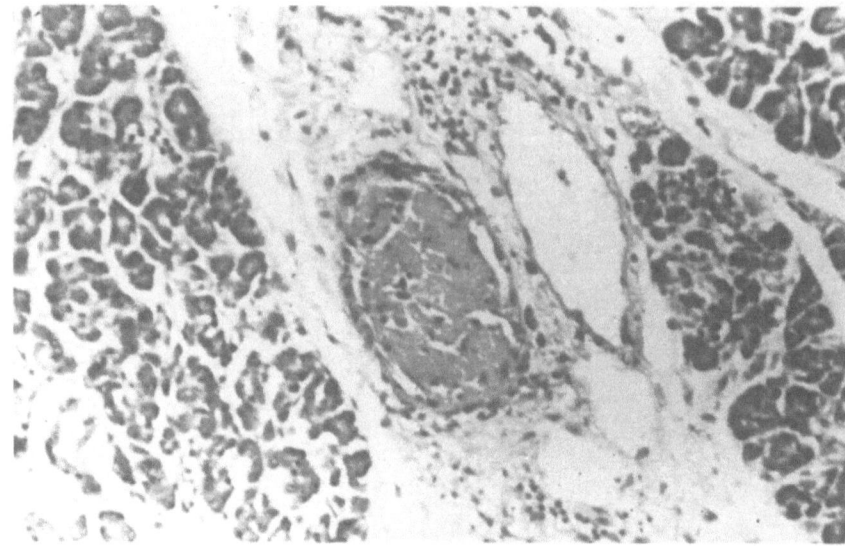

Fig. 5.6. Early organisation of thrombus in a small artery near the pseudocyst illustrated in Fig. 5.1. H&E, × 40

Injury to the Arteries of the Pancreas

Injuries to the pancreas are uncommon (Sturim 1966; Owens and Wolfman 1973) but operations in the vicinity are common, and accidental injury to the arteries may complicate operations upon the stomach or duodenum. Ischaemia of the pancreas, however, does not usually follow such operations, but, during splenectomy, a recurrent branch of the splenic artery that was found in about one-third of the specimens examined by Baronovsky et al. (1951), and which supplies branches to the tail of the pancreas, is liable, according to these authors, to be destroyed, with consequent damage to the tail of the pancreas, which may lead to the formation of a pancreatic fistula.

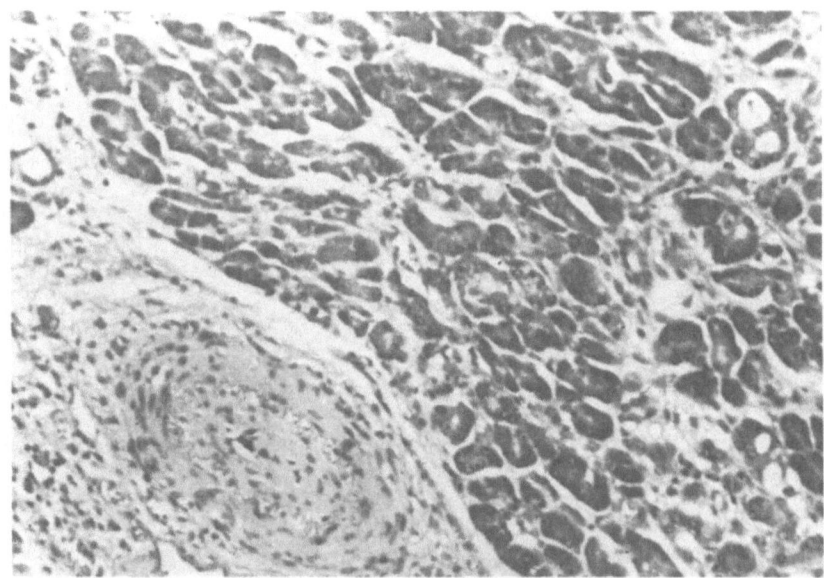

Fig. 5.7. Intimal fibrosis that has obliterated a small artery in the same pancreas as that illustrated in Fig. 5.6. H&E, × 40

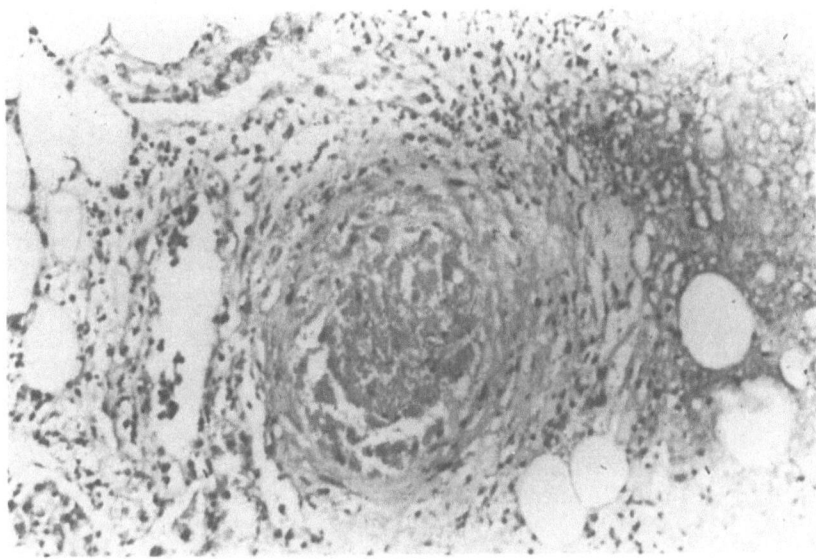

Fig. 5.8. Unorganised thrombus in a small artery near the margin of the infarct illustrated in Fig. 5.3. H&E, × 40

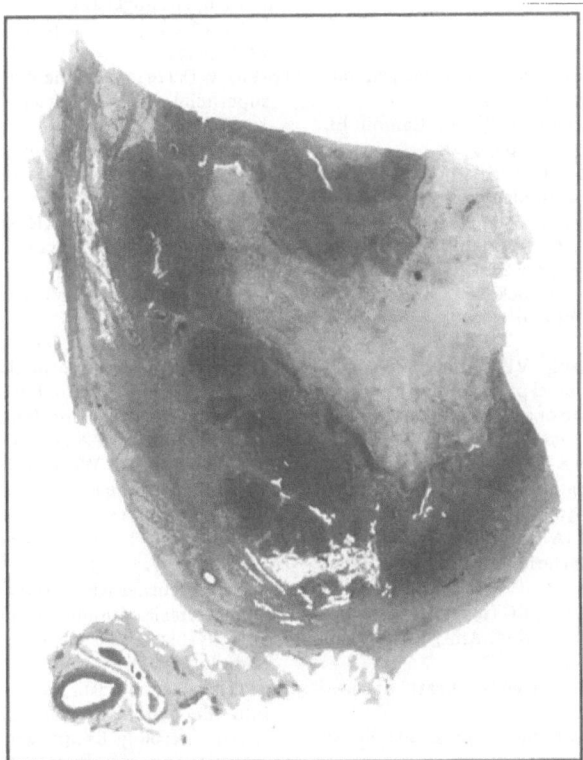

Fig. 5.9. A section of an anaemic infarct in the pancreas of a man aged 52, who suffered a cerebral haemorrhage due to hypertension that was entering the malignant phase. H&E, × 4

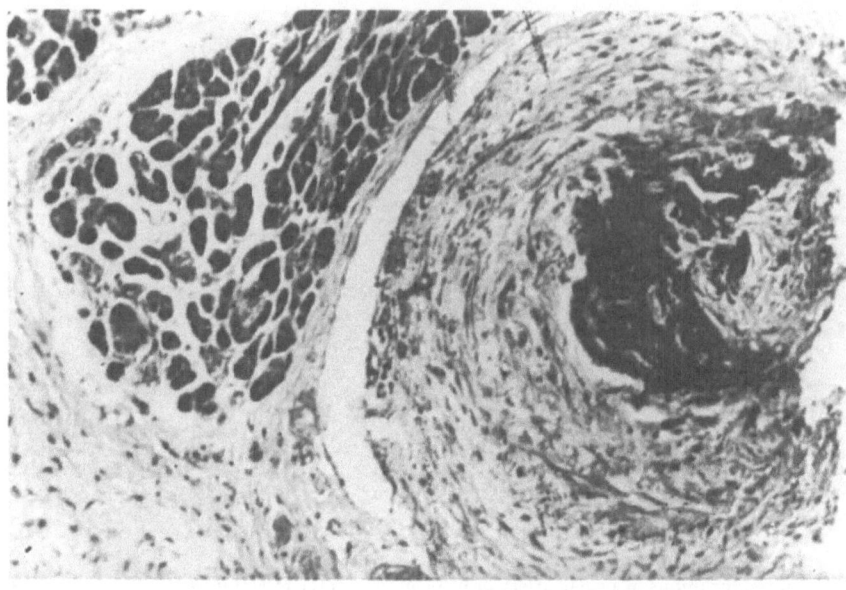

Fig. 5.10. Organised thrombus in an artery within the pancreas of a man aged 50, who died of congestive cardiac failure due to systemic hypertension, diagnosed clinically as being of the maglignant type but unassociated with fibrinoid necrosis of the arterioles postmortem. Anaemic infarcts that had not been suspected clinically were present in the pancreas at autopsy. H&E, × 20

References

Aufdermaur M (1947) Über Pankreasnekrosen als Folge generalisierter Arteritis. Gastroenterologia 72 : 81–95

Baggenstoss AH (1973) Pathology of pancreatitis. In: Gambill EE (ed) Pancreatitis. Mosby, St Louis, MO, pp 179–212

Baló J (1926) Über eine Häufung von Periarteritis-nodosa-Fallen, nebst Beiträgen zur Polyneuritis infolge von Periarteritis nodosa. Virchows Archiv 259 : 773–794

Baronovsky ID, Walton W, Noble JF (1951) Occult injury to the pancreas following splenectomy. Surgery 29 : 852–857

Bartholomew LG, Baggenstoss AH, Morlock CG, Comfort MW (1959) Primary atrophy and lipomatosis of the pancreas. Gastroenterology 36 : 563–572

Bivins BA, Sachatello CR, Chuang VP, Brady P (1978) Hemosuccus pancreaticus (hemoductal pancreatitis): gastrointestinal haemorrhage due to rupture of a splenic aneurysm into the pancreatic duct. Arch Surg 113 : 751–753

Block MA, Wakim KG, Baggenstoss AH (1954) Experimental studies concerning factors in the pathogenesis of acute pancreatitis. Surg Gynecol Obstet 99 : 83–90

Catanzaro FP, Merlino A, Palumbo JA (1957) Aneurysm occurring in the pancreaticoduodenal arteries treated by excision. N Engl J Med 256 : 847

Chuang VP, Pulmano CM, Walter JF, Cho KG (1977) Angiography of pancreatic arteriovenous malformation. Am J Roentgenol 129 : 1015–1018

Crawford T (1977) Pathology of ischaemic heart disease. Butterworth, London, p 97

Davie TB (1938) Massive replacement of the pancreas by adipose tissue. J Pathol Bacteriol 46 : 473–479

Droller H (1972) Atheromatous disease of the vessels supplying the gut. Age Ageing 1 : 162–167

Falconer CWA, Griffiths E (1949–1950) The anatomy of the blood vessels in the region of the pancreas. Br J Surg 37 : 334–344

Finlay DB, Herlinger H (1977) The intrapancreatic anatomy as an index of adequacy of pancreatic arteriography. Clin Radiol 28 : 595–599

Forbus WD (1930) On the origin of miliary aneurysms of the superficial cerebral arteries. Bull Johns Hopkins Hosp 47 : 239–284

Froboese C (1949) Beitrag zur Stütze der rheumatischen Äetiologie der Periarteritis nodosa und zum subtotalen Pankreasinfarkt. Virchows Archiv 317 : 430–448

Gambill EE, Baggenstoss AH, van Patter WG, Power MH (1948) Acute hemorrhagic pancreatitis; study of a patient having disseminate fat necrosis, hypocalcemia, hypopotassemia, uremia, diabetes mellitus and bilateral hydrothorax. Gastroenterology 11 : 371–381

Glynn LE (1940) Medial defects in the circle of Willis and their relation to aneurysm formation. J Pathol Bacteriol 51 : 213–222

Gruber GB (1929) Thrombosen und Infarkte im Gebiet der Bauchspeicheldrüse. In: Henke F, Lubarsch O (eds) Handbuch der pathologischen Anatomie 5 : 305–319

Guice KS, Lynch M, Weatherbee L (1987) Invasive aspergillosis: an unusual cause of hemorrhagic pancreatitis. Am J Gastroentrol 82 : 563–565

Hales MH (1956) Multiple arteriovenous fistulae of the lungs. Am J Pathol 32 : 927–943

Halpern M, Turner AF, Citron BP (1968) Hereditary hemorrhagic telangiectasia: an angiographic study of abdominal visceral angiodysplasias associated with gastrointestinal hemorrhage. Radiology 90 : 1143–1149

Harper PC, Gamelli RL, Kaye MD (1984) Recurrent hemorrhage into the pancreatic duct from a splenic artery aneurysm. Gastroenterology 87 : 417–420

Harris RD, Anderson JE, Coel MN (1975) Aneurysms of the small pancreatic arteries: a cause of upper abdominal pain and intestinal bleeding. Radiology 115 : 17–20

Hendrick JW (1956) Treatment of aneurysm of the pancreaticoduodenal artery by excision. Ann Surg 144:1051–1053

Høyer A (1949) Lipomatous pseudohypertrophy of the pancreas with complete absence of exocrine tissue. J Pathol Bacteriol 61:93–100

Hranilovich GT, Baggenstoss AH (1953) Lesions of the pancreas in malignant hypertension: review of one hundred cases at necropsy. Arch Pathol 55:443–456

Kadell BM, Riley JM (1967) Major arterial involvement by pancreatic pseudocysts. Am J Roentgenol 99:632–635

Keehan MF, Kistner RL, Banis J (1978) Angiography as an aid in extra-enteric gastrointestinal bleeding due to visceral aneurysm. Ann Surg 187:357–361

Klemperer P, Otani S (1931) Malignant nephrosclerosis (Fahr). Arch Pathol 11:60–117

Lambert A, Hyde G (1960) Intrapancreatic aneurysm: report of a case with obstructive jaundice and portal hypertension. JAMA 174:72–74

Lazarus SS, Volk BW (1961) The pancreas in maturity-onset diabetes: pathogenic considerations. Arch Pathol 71:44–59

Lazarus SS, Volk BW (1962) Idiopathic diabetes. In: The pancreas in human and experimental diabetes. Grune and Stratton, New York, pp 196–233

Lennie RA, Sheehan HL (1942) Splenic and renal aneurysms complicating pregnancy. J Obstet Gynaecol Br Emp 49:426–436

Lung JA, Schow PD, Knight L (1980) Splenic artery aneurysm-pancreatic duct fistula. Am J Surg 139:430–431

McKay JW, Baggenstoss AH, Wollaeger EE (1958) Infarcts of the pancreas. Gastroenterology 35:256–264

Michels NA (1962) The anatomic variations of the arterial pancreaticoduodenal arcades: their import in regional resection involving the gall bladder, bile ducts, liver, pancreas and parts of the small and large intestines. J Int Coll Surg 37:13–40

Moberg A, Svenhamn K, Wagermark J (1968) Acute "idiopathic" pancreatitis. Acta Surg Scand 134:369–372

Moschcowitz E (1951) The relation of hyperplastic arteriosclerosis to diabetes mellitus. Ann Intern Med 34:1137–1162

Moschcowitz E (1956) The pathogenesis of the hyalinization of the islets of Langerhans. Arch Pathol 61:136–142

Owens MP, Wolfman EF (1973) Pancreatic trauma: management and the presentation of a new technique. Surgery 73:881–886

Pfeffer RB, Lazzarini-Robertson A, Safade D, Mixter G, Secoy CF, Hinton JW (1962) Gradations of pancreatitis, edematous, through hemorrhagic, experimentally produced by controlled injections of microspheres into blood vessels in dogs. Surgery 51:764–769

Pollak OJ (1968) Human pancreatic atherosclerosis. Ann N Y Acad Sci 149:928–939

Popper HL, Necheles H, Russell KC (1948) Transition of pancreatic edema into pancreatic necrosis. Surg Gynecol Obstet 87:79–82

Probstein JG, Joshi RA, Blumenthal HT (1957) Atheromatous embolization, an etiology of acute pancreatitis. Arch Surg 75:566–572

Proud G, Chamberlain J (1978) Aneurysm formation on the small pancreatic arteries in association with coeliac axis compression. Ann R Coll Surg Engl 60:294–297

Rob C (1965) Diseases of the coeliac and mesenteric arteries. Bibl Gastroent 8:149–167

Schuster NH (1937) Aneurysms of splenic artery in Osler–Weber–Rendu syndrome. J Pathol Bacteriol 44:29–39

Shallow TA, Herbut PA, Wagner FB (1946) Abdominal apoplexy secondary to ruptured "congenital" aneurysm. Surgery 19:177–185

Sheehan HL, Moore HC (1952) Renal cortical necrosis and the kidney of concealed accidental haemorrhage. Blackwell, Oxford, pp 79–91

Spittel JA, Fairbairn JF, Kincaid OW, Re Mine WH (1961) Aneurysm of the splenic artery. JAMA 175:452–456

Stamm BH (1984) Incidence and diagnostic significance of minor pathologic changes in the adult pancreas at autopsy: a systematic study of 112 autopsies in patients without known pancreatic disease. Hum Pathol 15:677–683

Sturim HS (1966) The surgical management of pancreatic injuries. Surg Gynecol Obstet 122:133–140

van Way CW, Michael CJ, Riddell DH, Foster JH (1971) Arteriovenous fistula in the portal circulation. Surgery 70:876–890

Volk BW, Wellmann KF (1977) The diabetic pancreas. Baillière Tindall, London, pp 231–260

Walter JF, Chuang VP, Brookstein JJ, Reuter SR, Cho KJ, Pulmano CM (1977) Angiography of massive hemorrhage secondary to pancreatic disease. Radiology 124:337–342

Warren S, Le Compte PM, Legg MA (1966) The pathology of diabetes mellitus, 4th edn. Henry Kimpton, London, pp 53–89

West JE, Bernhardt H, Bowers RF (1968) Aneurysms of the pancreaticoduodenal artery. Am J Surg 115:835–839

White AF, Baum S, Buranasiri S (1976) Aneurysms secondary to pancreatitis. Am J Roentgenol 127:393–396

Woodburne RT, Olsen LL (1951) The arteries of the pancreas. Anat Rec 111:255–270

6 The Pancreas in Diabetes Mellitus and Haemochromatosis

In the great majority of cases of human diabetes mellitus, the syndrome is primary and idiopathic, but diabetes has long been known to be an inevitable consequence of complete excision of the pancreas, or sometimes even of partial destruction of the pancreas by injury or disease, while, in experimental animals, selective toxic destruction of the islets of Langerhans will cause diabetes mellitus. Diabetes may also develop as a secondary consequence of over-function of the cortex or medulla of the suprarenal glands, the anterior pituitary and the thyroid gland, or secretory neoplasms of any of these endocrine organs.

In idiopathic diabetes mellitus the variations in the morphology of the pancreas are so indefinite that a confident diagnosis of diabetes mellitus on the morphology of the pancreas alone is unreliable. Much work has been done, and laborious quantitative studies of the pancreas, especially of the islets, have been carried out, but the information obtained has been unspectacular and has contributed less to the understanding of diabetes than the information obtained by biochemical, clinical and experimental studies. Thus it was the development of methods for the estimation of glucose in the blood, combined with experiments upon animals, that made the discovery of insulin possible; it was the development of methods for the estimation of insulin in the blood that made it clear that idiopathic diabetes mellitus included at least two different forms of the disease.

Idiopathic diabetes has for some time been recognised to occur in two, more or less, distinct types: type I and type II. Type I usually occurs in young people, especially in children and juveniles. The insulin level in the blood is characteristically reduced, or insulin may be undetectable in the blood. In type II, the patients are mature or elderly at the onset of the disease; in these patients, the blood insulin is normal, or even higher than normal. There are, however, many cases that are difficult to identify as either type I or type II and, after taking advice from various groups concerned with aspects of diabetes, the World Health Organization in 1980 suggested the following classification:

1. "Insulin-dependent" diabetes mellitus (IDDM), or type I diabetes mellitus;
2. "Non-insulin-dependent" diabetes mellitus (NIDDM), or type II diabetes mellitus, viewed as a heterogeneous entity, in which at least two subclasses are to be considered depending on whether or not obesity is present (obese NIDDM and non-obese NIDDM);
3. A third group comprising a great variety of conditions and syndromes associated with diabetes mellitus that includes diseases of the pancreas that are primarily of the exocrine pancreas, diseases primarily of endocrine glands other than the islets of Langerhans, the effects of various drugs or toxic substances, deficiencies of insulin receptors, genetic syndromes and other rare conditions. Finally the World Health Organization (1985) recommended the recognition of an additional subclass of "tropical diabetes" or "malnutrition-related diabetes".

Although animal experiments and immunohistochemistry have established beyond any doubt that it is the beta cells of the islets of Langerhans that produce insulin, there has been difficulty in correlating recognisable changes in the pancreas with either of the two main types of diabetes. By 1981, Gepts, in a review of the islet changes in human diabetes, expressed the opinion that some correspondence between lesions of the pancreas and the two types of diabetes was beginning to emerge. The following lesions have been described by Gepts and by various other workers.

Insulin-Dependent Diabetes Mellitus (Type I Diabetes)

Macroscopic Appearance of the Pancreas

Macroscopically, the pancreas of juvenile diabetics is abnormally small, for, although the weight is normal at the onset of the illness (Gepts 1965), the disease seems to prevent further growth of the organ (Doniach and Morgan 1973) and, within a year of the onset of the disease, the weight of the pancreas may be only half the normal weight (Rahier 1988). In patients in whom there has been survival for many years, fibrosis may cause some increased firmness, but there is really nothing characteristic about the gross appearance, nor is there any correlation between the weight of the pancreas, the age at onset of the disease or its duration. Atrophy of the pancreas is limited to the part derived from the dorsal primordium, while the part derived from the ventral primordium (a lobe rich in pancreatic polypeptide (PP) cells, which accounts for 10% of the weight of the normal pancreas) accounts for over 20% of the weight of the pancreas of chronic juvenile-onset diabetics (Rahier 1988). An ultrasonic study of living diabetic patients (Fonseca et al. 1985) has also shown that their pancreases were significantly smaller than those of healthy controls, and that the patients with insulin-dependent diabetes had significantly smaller pancreases than the patients with non-insulin-dependent disease.

Microscopic Appearance of the Pancreas

Microscopically in chronic cases, the firmness that may be recognised when the pancreas is handled in the autopsy room is reflected by an intralobular and perilobular fibrosis, while, in acute disease, local lesions of necrotising pancreatitis are common. Such lesions are usually centred around distended

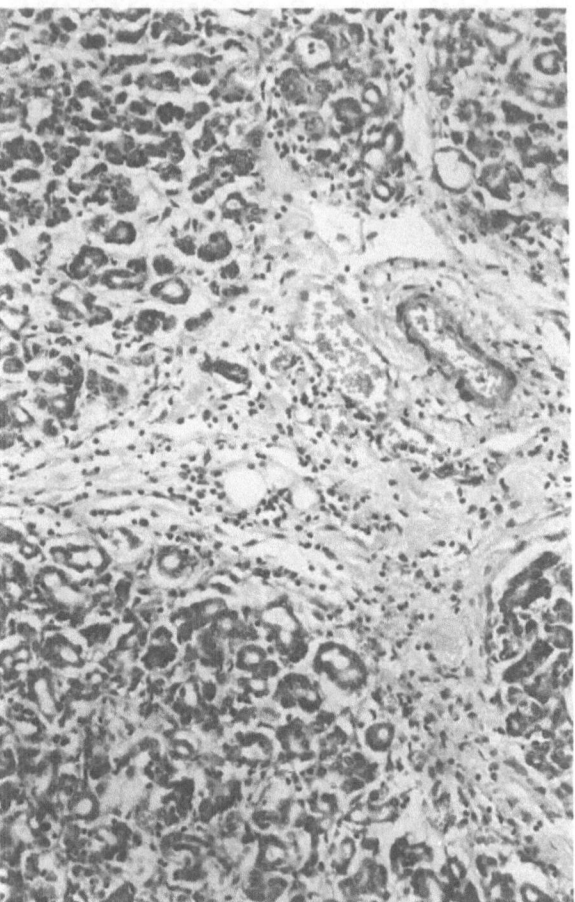

Fig. 6.1. Type I diabetes. Terminal non-specific interstitial pancreatitis with acinar ectasia in a 16-year-old diabetic who died in coma. H&E, × 150

ducts and, according to Gepts (1981), probably develop terminally because of dehydration in comatose patients (Fig. 6.1). When the disease has been present for many years, Gepts also found that the acinar cells are usually small and have relatively few zymogen granules, an observation that tallies with the reduction in exocrine pancreatic function that has been observed in insulin-dependent diabetics by workers such as Frier et al. (1976) and Dandona et al. (1984), while the lesions of arteriosclerosis and of arteriolosclerosis are common.

Quantitation of the Islets

It is, of course, the changes in the islet tissue and in the beta cells of the islets that have received most study. Quantitation of the islets is difficult because they are distributed throughout a large exocrine gland to whose volume they contribute no more than between 0.5% and 5% and because the number and size of the islets are not the same in different parts of the pancreas. Moreover, the various types of endocrine cells are present in varying proportions in the islets in different parts of the pancreas. Nevertheless, investigators who have undertaken the task of quantitating the islets in diabetes have found that the number is reduced in most patients, although there is a considerable overlap when the numbers of islets in groups of diabetics patients are compared with the numbers in the pancreases of matched groups of non-diabetic subjects.

Reduction of Insulin-Secreting Cells

The development of immunocytochemical methods has greatly improved the specificity with which the various cells in the islets can be identified, but, even with such methods, the results obtained by different groups of workers have varied somewhat. Thus, Orci et al. (1976) were unable to find any insulin-secreting cells in the islets of two chronic type I diabetics, while Gepts and De Mey (1978), who studied the cells in the islets of 58 insulin-dependent diabetics in whom the disease had developed before the age of 40, found significant numbers. They identified beta cells in 14 of 16 patients with recent-onset diabetes, seven of 14 in whom the disease had been present for less than 11 years, and in five of 28 who had had the disease for longer. In all these subjects, the number of beta cells was well below normal. The cytological features, such as an increase in cytoplasmic RNA of the remaining beta cells, suggested an increase of functional activity; this was an observation in keeping with the ability of some insulin-dependent diabetics to secrete a certain amount of insulin for a number of years after the clinical onset of the disease (Faber et al. 1976), and with reported histological appearances that suggested the formation of new islets (Maclean and Ogilvie 1955; Gepts 1981). With the passage of time, the distribution of the insulin-secreting cells was inclined to become more and more irregular, while the scanty remaining beta cells tended to occur as single cells among the exocrine cells rather than within recognisable islets (Gepts 1981). Fig. 6.2 illustrates such a scattering of insulin-positive cells. In a few cases of quite recent onset, Gepts and De Mey (1978) recognised focal regeneration of beta cells, but in those in which the disease had been present longer, regeneration became atypical with the production of islets that consisted entirely of PP-secreting cells. More recent work, in the studies by Rahier et al. (1983) and Klöppel et al. (1984), for example, confirm that the syndrome of

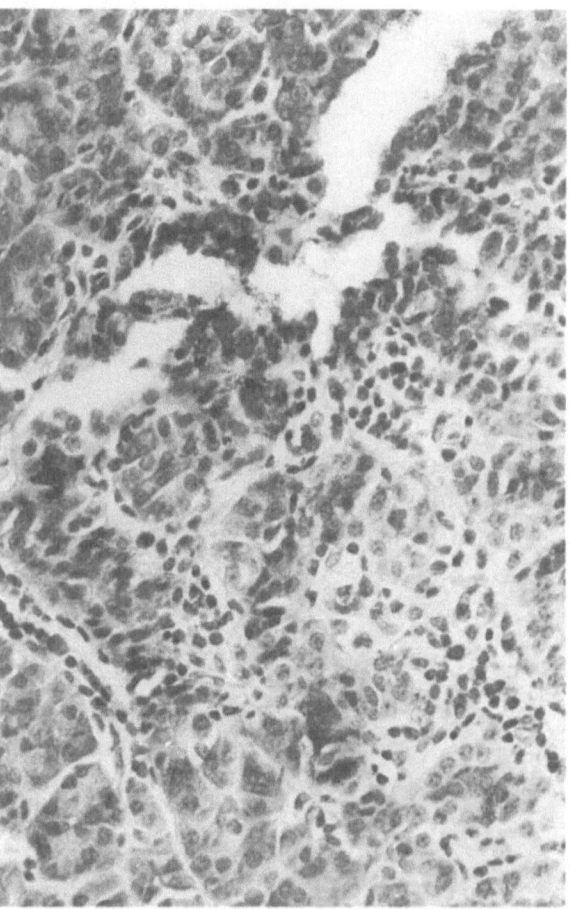

Fig. 6.2. Type I diabetes. The groups of dark cells have reacted positively in an indirect peroxidase–antiperoxidase preparation for insulin. The reacting cells are not in recognisable islets. The section is from the pancreas of the 7-year-old child whose islet is illustrated in Fig. 6.4. (Courtesy of Dr Anne Clark) × 375

insulin-dependent diabetes can be attributed to an insufficient number of pancreatic beta cells with at least a fivefold reduction of the beta cell mass at the clinical onset of the disease when compared with non-diabetic controls, while, though the islets of the diabetic cases may seem "atrophic", they still contain A, D and PP cells in proportions similar to the controls. Some beta cells that have escaped destruction may be found in about 40% of patients (Löhr and Klöppel 1987).

Inflammatory Infiltration of the Islets (Insulitis)

Inflammatory infiltration of the islets occurs only in juvenile diabetics (see Figs 6.3–6.6). This type of lesion was noted as long ago as 1909 by Cecil, and

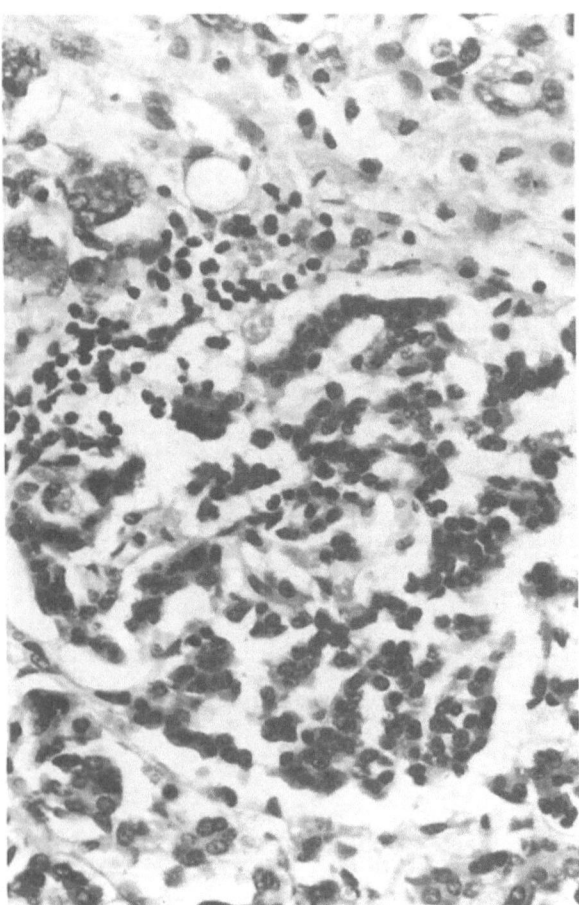

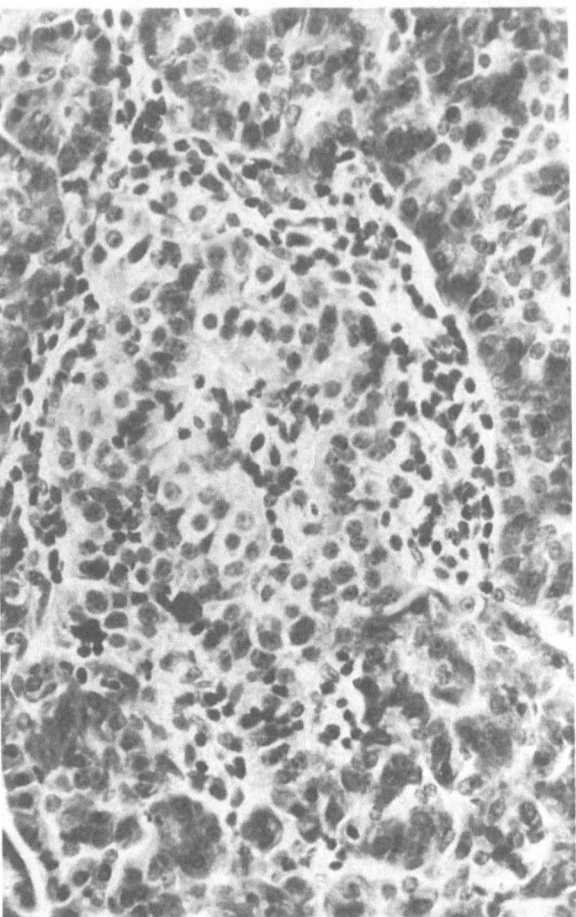

Fig. 6.3. Type I diabetes. Lymphocytic infiltration around part of the periphery of an islet. The patient was a boy aged 16, who had a fatal cardiac arrest while in diabetic coma. H&E, × 375

Fig. 6.4. Type I diabetes. Lymphocytic infiltration of an islet in a child aged 7, who died in diabetic coma. A number of the islet cells have the clear empty-looking cytoplasm (hydropic change) that is sometimes a feature of these cells in diabetes. The patient is likely to have received intravenous infusions of glucose. The photomicrograph is from an indirect peroxidase–antiperoxidase preparation for glucagon that was only faintly positive. (Courtesy of Dr Anne Clark) × 375

later by Warren and Root (1925), Stansfield and Warren (1928), and von Meyenburg (1940), but it was Le Compte (1958) who recognised that cellular infiltration, usually lymphocytic, of the islets of Langerhans was encountered most often in children in whom diabetes had developed acutely and had soon been followed by death. He attributed the rarity of the lesion to the infrequency with which such cases come to autopsy. That there is some uncertainty about the rarity, or otherwise, of the lesion is reflected by the findings of different workers. Thus Gepts (1965) found lymphocytic infiltration of the islets in 15 of 22 type I diabetics who died within 6 months of the first symptoms of the disease, but Doniach and Morgan (1973) found no examples, although seven of the 13 cases that they studied had had the disease, as judged by the presence of symptoms, for only 4 weeks or less. One of their photomicrographs, however, illustrates an islet

that contains shrunken cells with darkly staining nuclei, which create an appearance that might be interpreted as lymphocytic infiltration. However, Junker et al. (1977) found lymphocytic infiltration of the islets (insulitis) in six of 11 young diabetics who died within 2 months of onset of the disease.

An even higher incidence of insulitis was found by Foulis and Stewart (1984). Their material consisted of 11 cases of type I diabetes in children, nine of whom had had symptoms of the disease for less than 12 weeks. Insulitis was present in eight of these nine cases; it was not found in the two in which the disease had been present for 2 years and 6 years respectively. An important finding was that, in the pancreases of the cases in which the disease was of

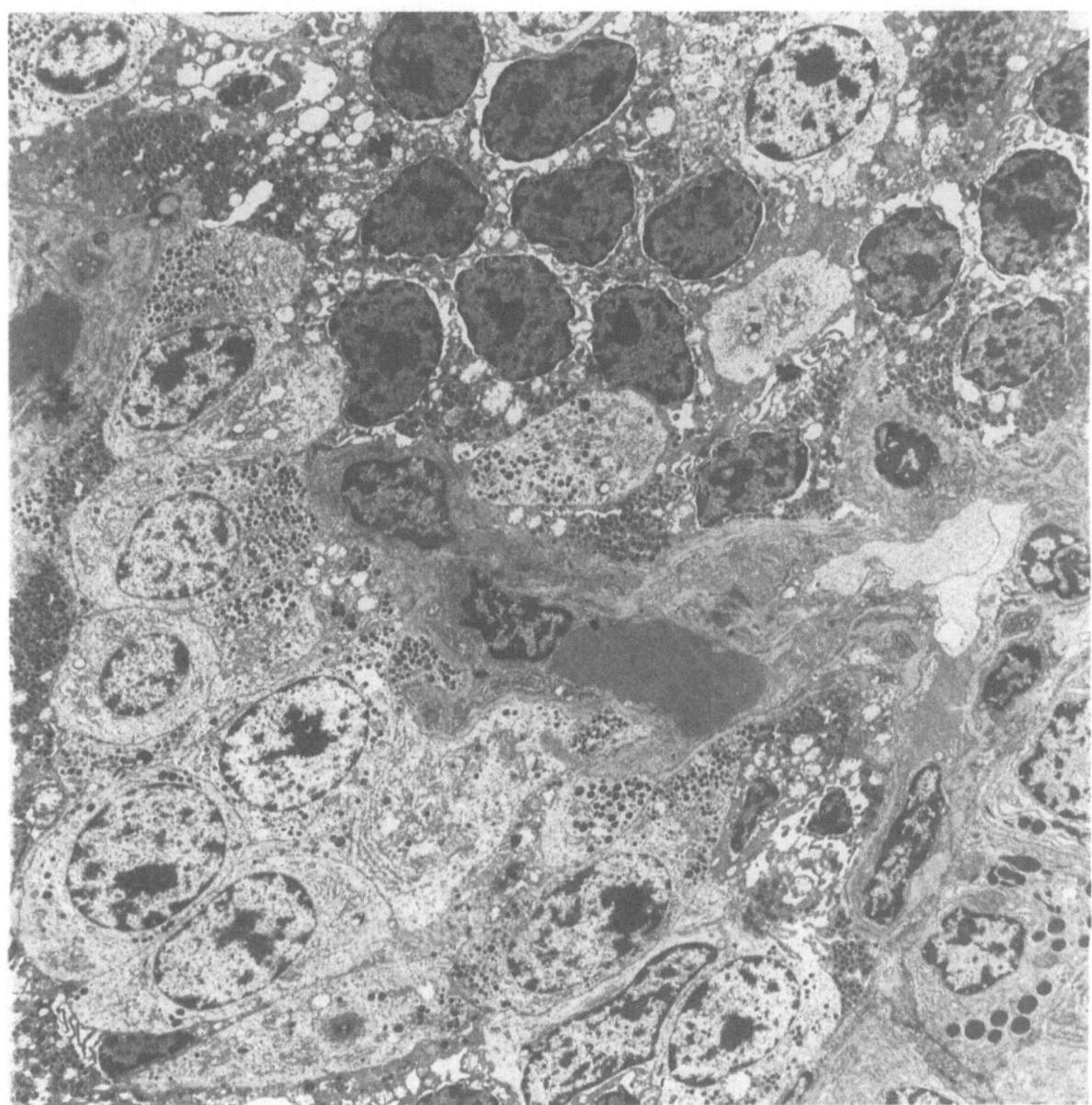

Fig. 6.5. Type I diabetes. Electron micrograph of the lymphocytes that infiltrated the islet in Fig. 6.4. No beta cells are recognisable. (Courtesy of Dr Anne Clark) × 3300

recent onset, 18% of islets in which insulin-containing cells were present had insulitis, while only 1% of insulin-deficient islets were affected. They also noted that the insulin-deficient islets were surrounded by atrophic exocrine glandular acini, while the insulin-containing islets were surrounded by normal acinar tissue. These exocrine changes were attributed to the effects of the islet–exocrine vascular connections and the associated effects of the islet hormones upon the pancreatic acini. Insulitis has

also been found in patients whose diabetes was cured temporarily by pancreatic transplantation, but who developed recurrent diabetes. In four such patients (three with isografts and one with an identical HLA allograft) reported by Foulis et al. (1992) there was insulitis in the grafts. No insulitis was present in the grafted pancreases of patients who had not developed recurrent diabetes.

When insulitis is present, it tends to be inconspicuous and to involve only certain of the islets, the

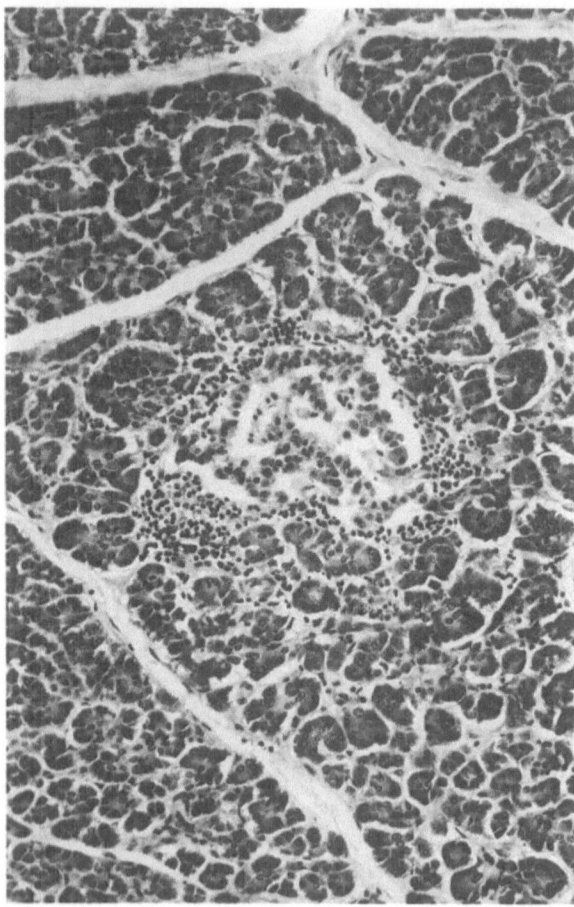

Fig. 6.6. Type I diabetes. Lymphocytic infiltration around, and within, an islet in the pancreas of a child who died in diabetic coma while suffering from varicella-zoster infection. (Courtesy of Dr J. Bouton) H&E, × 150

others being unaffected. The reasons for such patchiness seems to be related to the type of endocrine cells that the islets contain. When Gepts and De Mey (1978) carried out an immunocytochemical study of the islets in juvenile diabetes mellitus in which they could identify beta cells (insulin-secreting), alpha cells (glucagon-secreting), D cells (somatostatin-secreting) and PP cells (pancreatic polypeptide-secreting), they found that the majority of the islets, even in recent onset cases were devoid of beta cells (Fig. 6.5). There was insulitis in 11 of the 16 recent onset cases, and in one of these the lymphocytic infiltration was found only in islets that contained beta cells; it was strikingly absent in the islets composed of glucagon-secreting, somatostatin-secreting and PP-secreting cells. Most of the inflammatory cells in the affected islets are lymphocytes, but some larger mononuclear cells may be present. These

larger cells were identified as macrophages by Foulis et al. (1991) by the use of a monoclonal antibody (KPI) that reacted with phagocytic cells in paraffin sections of routinely processed tissues. They found that in 87 islets with insulitis the ratio of lymphocytes to macrophages was 9.7 : 1. They also found, when they used an antiserum against interferon-gamma, that 40% of the lymphocytes contained interferon-gamma.

Another observation by Foulis and his colleagues (1987a) was that there was hyperexpression of class II major histocompatibility complex molecules by beta cells and hyperexpression of class I major histocompatibility complex molecules by insulin-containing islets. The latter seemed to precede the onset of insulitis. Some of these findings were confirmed by Hanafusa et al. (1990) but, although Foulis et al. (1986) had found lymphocytic infiltration of the islets in 47 of 60 (78%) of cases that had died soon after the onset of type I diabetes, the Japanese authors found no lymphocytic infiltration of the islets in their specimens. The apparent discrepancy is almost certainly attributable to the small specimens examined by Hanafusa et al., who had obtained pancreatic biopsies laparoscopically from early cases of type I diabetes and thus did not have the relatively large autopsy specimens examined by Foulis and his colleagues. Moreover, the seven Japanese patients, although the duration of their diabetes was only 4 months or less, were relatively old. Their ages ranged from 24 to 49 years, and insulitis occurs mainly in young diabetics less than 15 years old (Rahier 1988).

When type I diabetes has been present for many years, islets become difficult to recognise. Insulin-secreting cells cannot usually be demonstrated, although clumps of glucagon-positive cells may be present (Fig. 6.7).

Aetiology

The reasons for the onset of type I diabetes are not fully understood, but the information available at present indicates that an interaction of genetic, infective and immunological factors may be concerned, although the selective toxic effect of certain substances upon the islets of susceptible subjects cannot be ruled out completely. There is also a substantial body of evidence, collected by an international research group (Diabetes Epidemiology Research International 1987), that environmental factors may be important, while the work on nutrition during foetal life and infancy in relation to the later development of diabetes has been reviewed by Wilkin (1993).

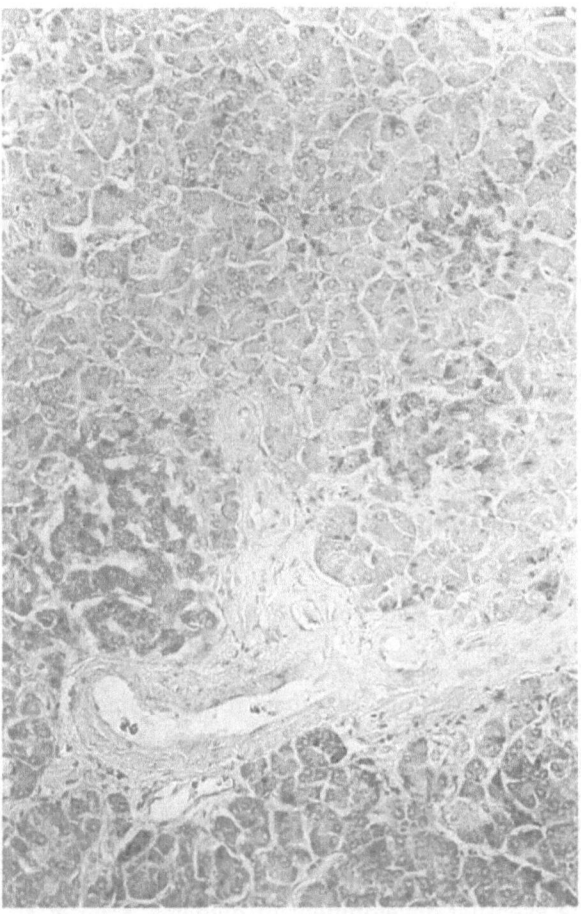

Fig. 6.7. Type I diabetes. Groups of dark glucagon-positive cells in an indirect peroxidase–antiperoxidase preparation of the pancreas of a type I diabetic, who died after having had insulin-dependent diabetes for 40 years. The adjacent section from the same block was negative for insulin-secreting cells. (Courtesy of Dr Anne Clark) × 150

Genetic Factors

The recognition of genetically susceptible subjects depends upon the association of the predisposing genetic material with the histocompatibility antigens. The genes that predispose to diabetes are located on chromosome 6, close to the histocompatibility complex, about which information can be obtained by the study of the surface antigens of human leucocytes. These human leucocyte antigens are usually referred to by the initial letters HLA. The human histocompatibility complex is divided into four principal gene loci, known as A, B, C and D. The A, B and C loci are concerned with the development of humoral antibodies and can be identified serologically by antisera to the human leucocytic antigens (HLA typing). These loci constitute the

class I molecules of the major histocompatibility complex (MHC) and they are expressed on most nucleated cells and on platelets. The D locus is concerned with cellular immunity and DP, DQ and DR loci have been identified. These proteins make up class II of the major histocompatibility proteins. They are found mainly on monocytes and on activated B and T lymphocytes. A fluorescein-labelled monoclonal antibody was used by Alviggi et al. (1984) to recognise HLA-DR-positive lymphocytes.

Each gene locus is composed of two alleles, one from each parent, and there are numerous possible variants of each allele. These are differentiated by numbers following the letters of the gene loci, for example A1, A2 and so on. The small letter "w" is put between the letter and the number in the case of alleles that have received only provisional acceptance.

Susceptibility to type I diabetes is conferred by genes in the HLA-D region of the major histocompatibility complex. The HLA-DR4 allele is strongly associated with type I diabetes in all ethnic groups, whereas the HLA-DR3 allele is associated with type I diabetes only in Caucasians and certain black populations. In the Japanese, for example, other HLA-DR alleles may substitute for the HLA-DR3 allele. The highest risk of developing type I diabetes is carried by heterozygotes with both HLA-DR3 and HLA-DR4 alleles.

Although genetic influences are powerful, instances where only one of a pair of identical twins has developed the disease (Barnett et al. 1981) occur more frequently than the known small genetic differences between identical twins (Johnston et al. 1983) would predict. This indicates that something in addition to genetic predisposition is required to precipitate the onset of the disease, and there is a good deal of evidence that points to viral infection as the precipitating cause.

Virus Infections

A number of different virus infections in man and in animals may cause lesions in the pancreas. Jenson et al. (1980) examined the pancreases of 250 children who had died during 14 different types of viral infection. They found signs of viral damage in the islets of four of seven cases of coxsackie B virus infection, 20 of 45 cases of cytomegalovirus infection, two of 14 cases of varicella-zoster infection, and two of 45 cases of congenital rubella. Destruction of beta cells and acute and chronic inflammation was most marked in those with coxsackie B virus infection. In one, 25%–30% of the islets were infiltrated by lymphocytes, macrophages and neutrophil polymorphonuclear leucocytes. Fewer islets were infiltrated in the remainder, but in all the cases there was some lysis of islet cells; many islets contained cells with deeply staining eosinophilic cytoplasm, while there were varying degrees of degranulation of the islet cells. In the cytomegalovirus cases, the characteristic inclusion bodies were present in two or more islets per section but mild inflammatory infiltration was found in only one. In the two cases of varicella-zoster with islet cell damage, there were four to five islets per slide with intranuclear inclusions, usually adjacent to cells that had undergone lysis or had pyknosis or karyorrhexis of nuclei.

Also in 1980, Ujevich and Jaffe found that, in fatal cases of neonatal coxsackie encephalomyocarditis, four of their five cases had varying degrees of damage, up to total necrosis, in the pancreatic islets. They were puzzled by their finding that non-beta cells in the islets had suffered necrosis as well as the beta cells. They suggested that the selective reduction of beta cells that is characteristic of insulin-dependent diabetes might be explained by post-necrotic regeneration of the non-beta cells without regeneration of the beta cells.

Although mumps is suspected of being associated with the onset of insulin-dependent diabetes, because it may cause pancreatitis, no lesions of the islets were found by Jenson et al. in their single fatal case of mumps, nor was any damage to the islets mentioned by Boström (1968) in her report of a fatal case of mumps, in which there was mild interstitial inflammation of the pancreas. No damage to the islets was found by Jenson and his colleagues in their 14 cases of viral hepatitis, although Oli and Nwokolo (1979) have published indirect evidence that diabetes may result from pancreatic damage during infectious hepatitis. Thus, of the viruses that may attack the pancreas, the coxsackie B virus seems to be particularly liable to damage the islets of Langerhans and a remarkable example of its selective attack upon the islet cells was reported by Yoon et al. in 1979. Their case was a previously healthy boy aged 10, who developed diabetic ketoacidosis within 3 days of the onset of a flu-like illness. He died 7 days later; lymphocytic infiltration of the islets and necrosis of beta cells was found at autopsy. A virus related to a diabetogenic variant derived from coxsackie B4 was obtained from homogenates of the pancreas; when this virus was inoculated into mice it caused hyperglycaemia, inflammatory infiltration of the islets of Langerhans and beta-cell necrosis, while viral antigens in the beta cells were demonstrated when sections of the mouse pancreas were stained with fluorescein-labelled antiviral antibody. A rising titre of neutralising antibody against the virus that had been

isolated could be demonstrated in samples of serum obtained from the patient during his illness. Two years later, Ahmad and Abraham (1982) found striking islet cell damage in an infant who had died of coxsackie B5 virus infection, a strain of the virus not previously associated with islet cell injury.

The following case, though less thoroughly investigated, is almost certainly another example of acute diabetes due to a viral infection, in this instance, infection by varicella-zoster virus. A girl aged 7 became acutely diabetic while suffering from chicken pox and died with severe brain damage. Although no convincing intranuclear inclusions were found in her organs, the diagnosis of varicella-zoster was confirmed serologically. In her pancreas there was pyknosis and karyorrhexis of nuclei in the islets of Langerhans, with well-marked lymphocytic infiltration around the islets and, to some extent, within the islets (Figs 6.6, 6.8). Two sections from different parts of her pancreas contained 122 islets, of which 45 had some degree of lymphocytic infiltration.

In such patients, the diabetes appears to have been the result of a direct necrotising effect of the virus upon the beta cells, but there is much evidence that infection by a virus with an affinity for beta cells may do no more than alter the beta cells sufficiently to initiate an auto-immune process, which leads to humoral and cellular immune reactions that cause progressive loss of beta cells with the eventual development of diabetes. King et al. (1983), for example, looked for serological evidence of previous coxsackie B infection in children with recently diagnosed insulin-dependent diabetes. Although islet cell cytoplasmic antibodies and complement fixing islet cell antibodies were detected in 15 of 18 sera tested, only six were positive for coxsackie B virus-specific IgM. In a larger group of children with insulin-dependent diabetes of recent onset, Banatvala et al. (1985) looked for serological evidence, not only of previous infection by the coxsackie B group of viruses, but also for evidence of previous infection by mumps, rubella and cytomegalovirus. They found evidence of recent infection by coxsackie B viruses in a significant number of the diabetic patients compared with controls, but found no evidence of previous infection by mumps, rubella or cytomegalovirus. A further study to evaluate the role of coxsackie B viruses in the pathogenesis of insulin-dependent diabetes was carried out by Schernthaner et al. (1985). They compared coxsackie B virus-specific IgM responses, complement-fixing islet cell antibodies and HLA-DR antigens with C-peptide secretion (C-peptide secretion was used in preference to estimations of serum insulin because it reflects the secretion of endogenous

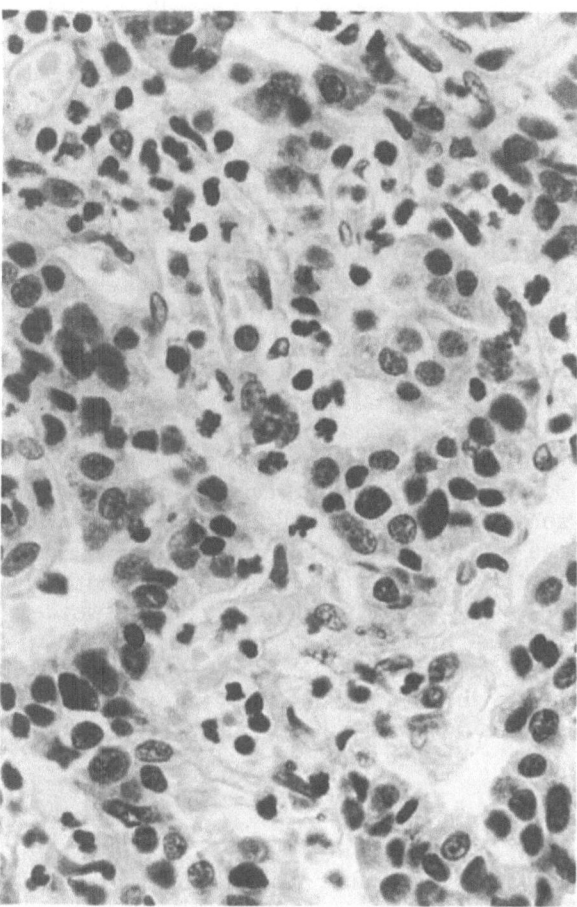

Fig. 6.8. Type I diabetes. Pyknotic nuclei in an islet in the pancreas of a child who died in diabetic coma associated with varicella-zoster infection. (Courtesy of Dr J. Bouton) H&E, × 600

insulin and is unaffected by insulin that has been injected). They found that coxsackie B-specific IgM responses correlated with HLA-DR3 and/or DR4 antigens as well as with complement-fixing islet cell antibodies and with low C-peptide levels.

The appearance of islet cell antibodies and insulin auto-antibodies in association with common viral infections other than coxsackie virus infections was observed by Bodansky et al. (1986). The study was a prospective one and patients with mumps, rubella, chickenpox and measles were followed for 6 months. There were 21 cases of mumps, 11 of rubella, 16 of chickenpox and seven of measles, in all of whom the clinical diagnosis was confirmed by serology. Insulin auto-antibodies appeared in serum samples from many of the patients, especially after chickenpox, IgM insulin auto-antibodies being more common than IgG insulin auto-antibodies. Islet cell antibodies were detected in only two subjects, one of whom had had rubella and another who had had measles, having previously had rubella, and who had a family history of auto-immunity. Islet cell antibodies did not appear in the serum of the patients who had had mumps.

A method for the detection of previous viral infection in insulin-dependent diabetes was that used by Foulis et al. (1987b) in their immunohistochemical study of 37 pancreases obtained at autopsy on patients who had died of insulin-dependent diabetes. They looked for the presence of immunoreactive interferon-alpha in the cases in which residual beta cells were still present in the islets; in 33 of 34 the beta cells were positive for alpha-interferon. They concluded that chronic viral infection of beta cells might underlie the pathogenesis of some cases of insulin-dependent diabetes.

Yet another approach to the question of the viral aetiology of autoimmune type I diabetes was used by Pak et al. (1988). They investigated the association of cytomegalovirus infection with type I diabetes in 59 newly diagnosed patients by examining lymphocytes for the presence of human cytomegalovirus genome, using molecular hybridisations with a human cytomegalovirus specific probe. They found a strong correlation between cytomegalovirus genome and islet cell auto-antibodies in the diabetic patients when compared with normal controls, which suggested to them that persistent cytomegalovirus infections may be relevant to the pathogenesis of some cases of type I diabetes.

In addition to the virological studies on human patients, some of which have been referred to in the preceding paragraphs, there is a substantial body of experimental work on the induction by viruses of diabetes in susceptible strains of laboratory animals. The results of such work have been reviewed by Leiter and Wilson (1988), but they do little to clarify the relationship between viral infection and the onset of clinical diabetes in man, and, as has been pointed out by Leslie (1983), there is unusually little serological evidence of a preceding viral infection at the time when most cases of insulin-dependent diabetes are diagnosed clinically.

Auto-immunity in Insulin-Dependent Diabetes Mellitus

Cellular Immune Reactions

Many immunological observations suggest that auto-immunity may be the main cause of type I diabetes. Cellular and humoral mechanisms are involved, and activity by such processes is usually detectable when the disease is diagnosed clinically. Even more significantly, if apparently normal people whose HLA-DR status indicates that they are vulnerable to diabetes are monitored, it has been found that signs of auto-immunity may be detected months or years before clinical diabetes develops. The antigen that initiates the auto-immune process has not been identified; molecular mimicry in which a foreign antigen (bacterial or viral) provokes an immune response that cross-reacts with a similar epitope on an endogenous antigen has been suggested (Lancet 1990) but only as a plausible hypotheses. The immunological activity that may precede the onset of diabetes does not inevitably lead to clinical disease. In some subjects, especially if the signs of activity are weak, the activity may subside before diabetes has developed (Leslie and Pyke 1991).

The cellular component of diabetic auto-immunity is seen in the pancreatic islets in "insulitis", which has already been described, but this cannot be monitored in the pre-diabetic period, and death followed by expert immunohistochemical examination of the pancreas of a patient with diabetes of recent onset is unusual. In insulitis, however, the infiltrating cells are mainly lymphocytes and studies with monoclonal antisera have shown that most of these are of the T-cytotoxic/suppressor phenotype and that some are positive for HLA-DR antigen, an indication that they are active in an immune reaction (Bottazzo et al. 1985). In 1984 Alviggi et al. demonstrated raised levels of activated T lymphocytes in the blood of 14 of 15 patients with recently diagnosed type I diabetes, while only seven of 28 with long-standing insulin-dependent diabetes had similar levels. Even the long-standing cases, however, had significantly higher levels of activated lymphocytes than non-insulin-dependent diabetics and healthy controls. When the unaffected co-twins of recently diagnosed insulin-dependent diabetics were examined, five of seven such twins had high levels of activated T cells. The increase persisted for 6 months in two, and during that time impaired glucose tolerance developed. The authors concluded that there is an active cellular immune response in newly diagnosed insulin-dependent diabetics and that it may precede the disease. Experiments of a different type in which the role of cytotoxic T cells in the pathogenesis of type I diabetes was reported in a preliminary communication by de Beardinis et al. in 1988. Their results showed that a CD4-positive T-cell clone could lyse HLA class II matched islet cells.

A possible target antigen in the autoimmune pathogenesis of type I diabetes was investigated by Roep et al. (1991). They had found that proliferation of CD4 T cells from a newly diagnosed patient with type I diabetes occurred in response to a 38 kDa polypeptide obtained from insulin-secretory-granule membranes of a transplantable rat insulinoma; they considered that the granular localisation of antigen might imply that exposure of beta-cell-specific determinants to components of the immune system might be related to the exocytosis of insulin. To find out whether similar T-cell reactivity was usually present at the onset of insulin-dependent diabetes, they tested T-cells lines from a series of children with newly diagnosed diabetes against a series of healthy controls matched for age and HLA antigens. The cell lines from 14 of the 19 patients responded to an islet cell antigen prepared from a rat beta-cell tumour, compared with a positive reaction in only two of the cell lines from the 16 normal controls. Reactivity to the 38 kDa fraction of insulin-secretory-granule membranes was then tested. Positive reactions were found with the cell lines only from patients that had responded to the crude antigen, being positive in eight of the ten responders tested. The workers found their results to be highly significant statistically and claimed that they had demonstrated an ongoing autoimmune T-cell response in newly diagnosed type I diabetics.

Effects of Interleukin-1

The possible importance of interleukin-1 in the initiation of insulitis and in the destruction of beta cells has been the subject of experiments and speculation by Nerup et al. (1988). Interleukin-1 is a polypeptide cytokine produced primarily by phagocytic cells, such as blood monocytes and tissue macrophages, but also by various other cells involved in inflammatory and immune responses. Its many functions and effects have been described by authors such as Dinarello (1984). It has been found in vitro to have selective adverse effects upon human and rat beta cells. Nerup et al. have suggested that the steps involved in the in vivo destruction of beta cells may be the release of beta-cell antigen, processed and presented by macrophages to T-helper lymphocytes with the initiation of what they described as "a self-perpetuating and self-limiting circuit of cytokine production", in which interleukin-1 is cytotoxic to the beta cells, the amount of interleukin-1 production being under the control of HLA-D genes.

Serological Signs of Auto-immunity

Much of the work on the recognition and significance of circulating antibodies in type I diabetes has been reviewed and summed up by Lernmark et al. (1988). These workers point out that such antibodies are most often found in newly diagnosed patients with insulin-dependent diabetes, they may be present for several years before the clinical onset of the disease, and they tend to decrease both in incidence and in titre as the established disease progresses. When titres of antibodies against islet cells are high, the loss of endogenous insulin production, as measured by C-peptide levels, tends to be rapid. Moreover, the finding of circulating antibodies in patients with non-insulin-dependent diabetes may be an indication that insulin-dependent diabetes is imminent. Nevertheless, the finding of circulating antibodies, in the unaffected monozygotic twin of a diabetic child for example, does not necessarily mean that diabetes in the unaffected twin is inevitable, especially if the titres are low, for antibodies have been found to disappear in such a twin, who then does not develop diabetes. Antibodies have also been reported by Lernmark et al. (1988) to decrease in titre during treatment of newly diagnosed cases of type I diabetes with cyclosporin A, although a rebound occurred when the treatment was stopped.

The complexity of the humoral immune process involved in the pathogenesis of type I diabetes has been pointed out by various authors, for example by Bottazzo (1984); he has suggested that type I diabetes, like type II diabetes, may not have a common auto-immune pathogenesis and that different mechanisms may be involved in apparently similar cases.

Insulin Auto-immune Antibodies

Anti-insulin antibodies that cannot be attributed to the therapeutic administration of exogenous insulin are commonly found, along with islet-cell antibodies, when type I diabetes is first diagnosed. They may be present before the clinical onset of the disease and thus may be valuable markers of people at risk; they probably indicate that insulitis is in progress. They can be demonstrated and measured by enzyme-linked immunosorbent assay or by radioimmunoassay; different techniques may account for some of the discrepancies in the frequency with which they are reported. They are generally believed to be a result, rather than a cause, of insulitis, but why endogenous insulin should become antigenic is not known.

Islet-Cell Antibodies

Auto-immune antibodies against islet cells are more likely than insulin antibodies to injure beta cells.

The methods for their detection and measurement are difficult, and varying techniques have been used by different groups of workers. Antibodies that will attach themselves to the surfaces of cells in the islets can be demonstrated by an indirect immunofluorescence test that requires fresh frozen sections of blood group O human pancreas. The sections are dried onto slides and are then incubated with the serum to be tested. After careful rinsing, the sections are incubated with a second antibody reagent that is fluorescent and will also bind to human immunoglobulin. If immunoglobulin has become attached to the islet cells, a fluorescent reaction can be seen in the islets with a fluorescence microscope and epi-illumination. Unless the serum sample contains islet-cell antibodies, the islets will not be visible. The supply of suitable human pancreatic material must in itself be a problem for those using this technique, and if, by chance, the test section of pancreas contains no islets there will be a false negative result. The islet-cell antibodies detected by this technique are known as cytoplasmic islet-cell antibodies.

The mere attachment of antibody to the islet cells does not necessarily mean that the antibody will injure the cells, and techniques have been developed to recognise the presence of cytotoxic islet-cell antibodies. Most of the methods for the assay of cytotoxic islet-cell antibodies involve single cell preparations of islet cells from human or rodent insulinomas. The process of cytotoxicity involves the activation of the complement cascade and the consumption of complement is an indication of a positive test. If rodent islet cells are used, steps to overcome the species difference are necessary. Quantitative methods for the assessment of the damage to the target cells have also been devised. For example, the target cells may be labelled with radioactive chromium, and measurement of the release of the isotope will provide an accurate assessment of the degree of cytotoxicity of the serum being tested. The methods for the recognition and assessment of islet-cell antibodies have been reviewed by Lernmark et al. (1988).

The identification of the particular molecule, other than insulin, within the beta cell, which may be the antigen that causes the specific auto-immune reaction against beta cells in type I diabetes, has received much attention. The work involves the labelling of the beta-cell proteins by metabolic labelling in vitro, followed by immunoprecipitation of the labelled proteins with sera from patients with type I diabetes. Similar work can be done using genetically diabetic BB (BioBreeding) rats. These rats are inbred Wistar rats developed in the Worcester Mass. colony. Between 40%–80% of such

rats will suddenly develop insulin-dependent diabetes when they are 16–120 days' old, with an auto-
immune type of diabetes that includes well-marked
insulitis in their pancreases. Such studies (e.g. those
of Atkinson et al. 1990) suggested that antibodies
against a dimeric glycoprotein with a molecular
weight of approximately 64K might be an important
early indicator of beta-cell auto-immunity. In the
same year, Baekkeskov et al. (1990) identified this
64K antigen as glutamic acid decarboxylase (GAD),
an enzyme capable of converting glutamic acid into
gamma-aminobutyric acid, an inhibitory neuro-
transmitter found in pancreatic beta cells and in a
subpopulation of central nervous system neurons.

In 1992, Atkinson et al. selected this substance
from amongst other pancreatic islet-cell antigens
and tested the proliferative response of peripheral
blood mononuclear cells to this antigen in newly
diagnosed insulin-dependent diabetics, relatives of
diabetic patients known to have islet-cell antibodies
and normal controls. They found that the likelihood
of a positive response was substantially greater
among the diabetic patients and relatives positive
for islet-cell auto-antibodies than among subjects at
low risk of diabetes (normal controls and relatives
negative for islet-cell antibodies). They suggested
that GAD might have a pathogenic role in insulin-
dependent diabetes.

The presence of auto-antibodies against GAD in
the blood of subjects at risk of insulin-dependent
diabetes was confirmed by Harrison et al. (1993).
They measured immunity to GAD in 31 first-degree
relatives of insulin-dependent diabetic patients in
whom islet-cell antibodies had been found. Their
results showed that, in most of the subjects, the
auto-immunity to GAD was either predominantly
humoral or predominantly cellular. High concentrations of circulating auto-antibodies that precipitated
native GAD activity were associated with low proliferation of peripheral blood T cells to recombinant
GAD while, conversely, low concentrations of auto-
immunity to GAD were associated with high T-cell
proliferation to GAD. Such results indicated hetero-
geneity within at-risk relatives that might have
prognostic importance. They postulated that, if
GAD were a pathogenic auto-antigen, sensitisation
to beta GAD is more likely to cause insulin-dependent diabetes when the immune response deviates
towards the expansion of autoreactive T cells rather
than towards generation of auto-antibodies. They
considered such an idea to be consistent with evidence that beta-cell destruction is mediated by T
cells and that high concentrations of GAD antibodies are associated with slower progression to clinical
disease.

The probable importance of GAD as an auto-
antigen in the pathogenesis of insulin-dependent
diabetes is supported by studies of non-obese diabetic (NOD) mice, one of the animal models for the
human disease. In this genetic strain of mice, spontaneous insulin-dependent diabetes develops by the
age of 12 weeks, as a result of insulitis in which T
lymphocytes selectively destroy the beta cells of the
islets. Using this strain of mice, Kaufman et al.
(1993) were able to show that a T-helper-1 response
to GAD developed along with the onset of insulitis.
At first the response was provoked only by a special
region of the molecule, but intramolecular spread
led to the development of reactivity to beta-cell antigens other than GAD. Prevention of the spontaneous response of reactive T cells could be obtained
by the induction of tolerance to GAD. This was
achieved by the intravenous injection of GAD when
the mice were 3 weeks old, an age at which the GAD-
reactive T cells were not yet spontaneously primed
to respond to GAD. The development of GAD tolerance prevented the initiation of the cascade of T-cell
responses to the other beta-cell antigens involved in
the development of insulitis and diabetes.

Support for the conclusions reached by Kaufman
and his colleagues was provided by Tisch et al.
(1993), who determined the temporal sequence of T-
cell and antibody responses in NOD mice to a panel
of five murine beta-cell antigens. They found that
antibody and T-cell responses specific for the two
isoforms of GAD appeared first in 4-week-old NOD
mice. This GAD-specific reactivity was the earliest
response to the islet cell extracts they tested, and it
coincided with the onset of insulitis. In addition, if
the mice were given intrathymic injections of GAD
at the age of 4 weeks, there was marked reduction
of their T-cell proliferation responses to GAD and
to the other beta-cell antigens tested; in particular,
they remained free from diabetes.

Destruction of Beta Cells by Toxins

It has been found experimentally in animals that
certain drugs and toxins, in appropriate doses,
have a specific lethal effect upon the beta cells of
the pancreatic islets and that diabetes can be
caused. Alloxan and streptozotocin are such drugs,
while the rat poison Vacor, when taken suicidally
or accidentally by man, has caused acute ketoacidosis along with a toxic neuropathy, and, in three
fatal cases, destruction of the beta cells of the pancreatic islets (Karam et al. 1980). Although the diabetogenic effects of alloxan in experimental

animals have been known since the work of Dunn et al. (1943), and those of streptozotocin since 1963 (Rakieten et al. 1963), it has never been shown that such toxins play any part in the pathogenesis of natural diabetes mellitus in man. The possible importance of a toxin is, however, suggested by the studies of Helgason and his colleagues in Iceland (Helgason and Jonasson 1981; Helgason et al. 1982). Their observations and experiments suggest that mutton cured by smoking may contain a toxin that will induce diabetes in the progeny of parents that have been using this in their diet at the time of the conception of the progeny.

Even coffee consumption has been suggested, on circumstantial evidence, to be a possible trigger for insulin-dependent diabetes mellitus in childhood (Tuomilehto et al. 1990).

Various therapeutic substances have been reported to have caused diabetes; this was transient is some patients and ceased when the therapy was changed. In 1968, Bryceston attributed diabetes to the use of pentamidine in the treatment of leishmaniasis; additional cases of leishmaniasis that developed diabetes during treatment with pentamidine mesylate were reported briefly by Belehu and Naafs (1982). No diabetes occurred amongst the patients who were treated with pentamidine isethionate. Pancreatic material from human cases of pentamidine-induced diabetes does not appear to have been studied, but in laboratory studies such as those described by Pipeleers et al. (1988), pentamidine, in appropriate concentrations, will cause selective necrosis of rodent beta cells. Thus, the use of pentamidine preparations in the prophylaxis or treatment of *Pneumocystis carinii* pneumonia in AIDS, carries a risk of adding diabetes to the patients' problems. Another therapeutic substance reported to have caused transient diabetes in a patient given a renal allograft is cyclosporin A (Bending et al. 1987), while it has been suggested (Bhatnagar et al. 1984) that nifedipine, widely used to treat angina pectoris and hypertension, is, at least potentially, diabetogenic. A single patient, in which type I diabetes mellitus developed during interferon-alfa therapy for cryptogenic chronic hepatitis, has also been reported (Fabris et al. 1992).

Insulin-Independent Diabetes Mellitus (Maturity-Onset, Type II Diabetes)

Many changes have been described in the pancreas in type II diabetes, but no satisfactory correlation between the changes and the clinical syndrome has yet been established; nearly all the changes described have been found also in the pancreases of elderly non-diabetic subjects. Because the amount of insulin in the blood is often normal and because insulin can be extracted from the pancreases of type II diabetics in an amount similar to that extractable from non-diabetic pancreases, it might seem that deficiency of insulin plays no part in the pathogenesis of type II diabetes, but there is some evidence that the secretion of insulin is not always appropriate for the level of glucose in the blood in these patients. Some patients with type II diabetes are actually hyperinsulinaemic; this is attributed to an increase of resistance to the action of insulin upon the liver and muscles. The role of insulin resistance has been discussed in a review by Cerasi (1988), whose conclusion was that glucose intolerance and diabetes develop in subjects with limited beta-cell function, either when insulin release deteriorates further, or when "additional factors", such as insulin resistance, aggravate the insulin deficiency of the subject. A similar conclusion was expressed in a leading article in the Lancet (1989), in which the author gave the opinion that insulin resistance is a necessary prelude to non-insulin-dependent diabetes, but that hyperglycaemia will not develop unless there is also a defect in insulin secretion. Once hyperglycaemia has developed, it has been found experimentally (Leahy et al. 1988) that the hyperglycaemia itself causes further deterioration in beta-cell function.

The pancreatic lesions that have been described include reduced pancreatic size, which has been confirmed by ultrasonic studies in living patients (Fonseca et a. 1985), pancreatic fibrosis, changes in the appearances of the islet cells, and gradual replacement of the islets by hyaline material, which has been found to be a type of amyloid tissue. The latter change, though long recognised, has received much recent study.

Hyaline Change (Amyloidosis) in the Islets

Lesions of the islets of Langerhans were noted to be associated with diabetes over 20 years before the

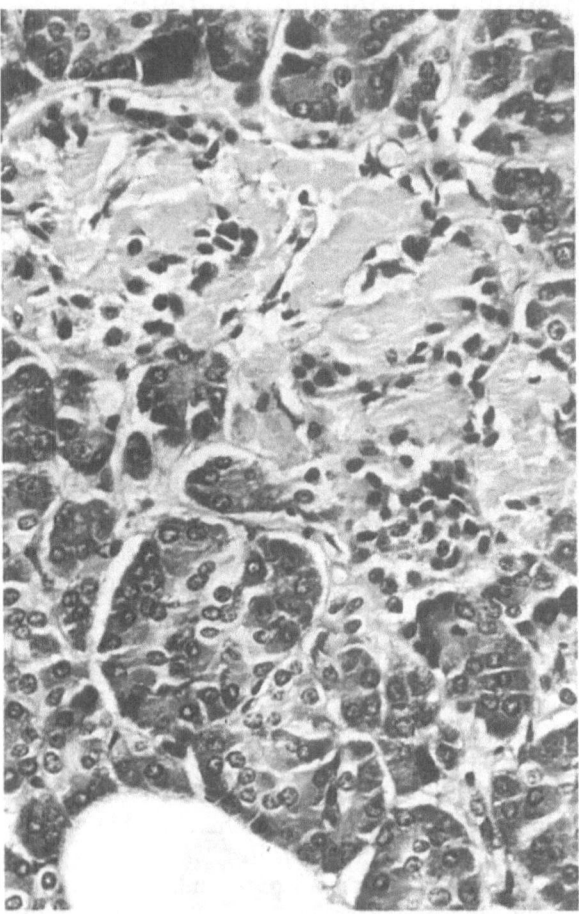

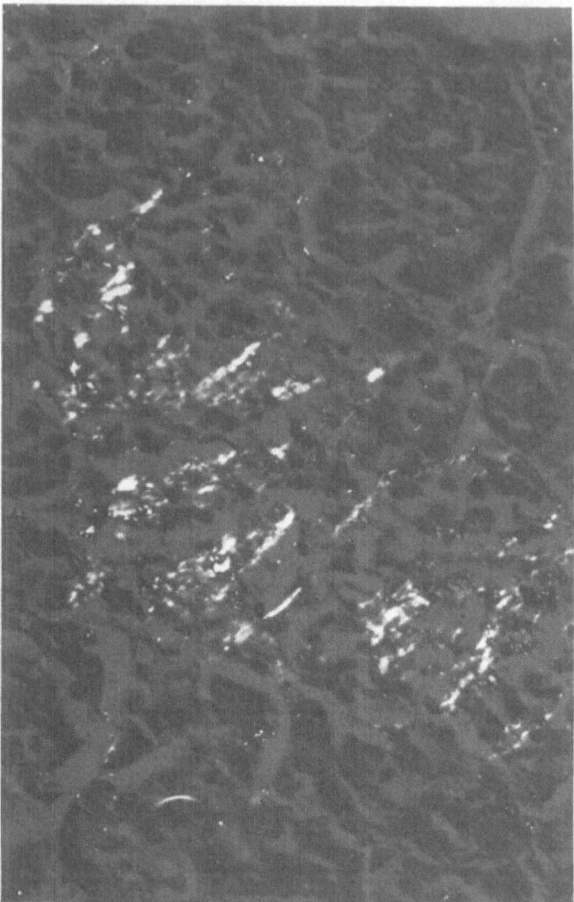

Fig. 6.9. Type II diabetes. Hyaline change (amyloid) in a pancreatic islet in a man aged 65, who had had mild diabetes for at least 9 years. He died of purulent bronchitis following a cerebral infarct. H&E, × 375

Fig. 6.10. Type II diabetes. Amyloid change in the islet shown in Fig. 6.9, stained with Congo red and photographed with crossed prisms. × 375

discovery of insulin. Opie (1900–1901) in America and, independently, Weichselbaum and Stangl (1901) in Vienna, associated a hyaline change (Fig. 6.9) in the islets of Langerhans with diabetes mellitus, but this lesion is found in the islets of only a proportion of cases with a history of diabetes. It has been found also in the islets of people who have not suffered from diabetes; the change is, however, much less common in the absence of a history of diabetes (Bell 1959; Melato et al. 1977). Much of the work on the relationship of hyaline islets to diabetes has been reviewed by Clark (1989). Her analysis confirmed the association between islet amyloidosis and type II diabetes, and showed that the amount of amyloid material increases, not only with age, but also with increasing severity of the disease, as indicated by the development of a need for insulin, as sometimes happens in patients with type II diabetes.

The resemblance of the hyaline change to amyloid degeneration was noted by the early workers, but Opie, for example, could not obtain the characteristic staining reactions in the alcohol-hardened material with which he was working, and could find no hyaline changes in the various organs most commonly affected by amyloidosis. Much more recently, however, it was found by Westermark (1976) that the hyalinosis of the islets found in elderly subjects, especially in those with maturity-onset diabetes, is, in fact, a type of amyloid (Fig. 6.10). It differs from most other types of amyloid by lacking significant amounts of tryptophan, which suggested to Westermark that the amyloid of hyaline islets might be similar to the amyloid sometimes found in endocrine tumours (Pearse et al. 1972). This suggestion was in keeping with the results of experiments by Linke et al. (1976), who found that fibrils with the characteristic staining reactions of amyloid could be produced in vitro from both insulin and glucagon. Moreover, such fibrils had the electron microscopic, X-ray crystallographic and infra-red spectroscopic characteristics of amyloid fibrils. Thus, it seemed to these workers that either insulin or glucagon might be the source of the amyloid in hyaline islets of Langerhans and the amyloid sometimes found in insulinomas. Unfortunately for such an attractive suggestion, the deposition of amyloid material in senile subjects is not usually confined to the pancreatic islets, but is found also in the aorta, heart, lung and prostate (Ishii et al. 1983). Ishii et al., unlike Westermark, also found that in senile amyloidosis, including senile amyloidosis with involvement of the islets of Langerhans, the amyloid material contained tryptophan and thus differed significantly from the amyloid of the endocrine tumours studied by Pearse et al. They could recognise no correlation between ageing, diabetes mellitus and pancreatic insular amyloidosis in their own material, but did not feel prepared to dismiss the possibility of the existence of some complex relationship between such factors.

Further studies by Westermark and his associates (1987) have shown that a peptide with a structural resemblance to calcitonin gene-related peptide could be purified from amyloid deposits in an insulinoma and from any amyloidosis of the islets of Langerhans. This polypeptide, which they have named islet amyloid polypeptide, has been found to be a constituent of normal beta cells. In type II diabetes, the islet amyloid polypeptide reactivity of the beta cells is diminished, while the same polypeptide is being laid down as amyloid fibrils in the islets of Langerhans. Although they could not suggest a normal function for the peptide they felt that their study had demonstrated that, in type II diabetes, this normal product of beta cells had an altered metabolic fate. In 1987 and 1988, similar results were obtained by Clark et al., who found that amyloid deposits in the islets in cases of type II diabetes contained a peptide that seemed to originate from beta cells. They suggested that the accumulation of amyloid material in the pancreatic islets might be important in the development of type II diabetes.

Further work (Leighton and Cooper 1988; Cooper et al. 1988) showed that islet amyloid polypeptide (amylin in their terminology) might be a hormone that influenced the metabolism of glycogen in skeletal muscle. This led Johnson et al. (1989) to suggest that type II diabetes might be the result of a combination of impaired function of the islet cells due to amyloid deposits, preceded by resistance to the effects of insulin on the metabolism of skeletal muscle because of over-secretion of islet amyloid

polypeptide. Since that time, van Jaarsveld et al. (1990) have demonstrated islet amyloid polypeptide in the plasma of normal subjects as well as in that of patients with type I and type II diabetes. These authors found no difference in fasting concentrations of the polypeptide between the three groups, but, after stimulation with glucagon, the concentration of islet amyloid polypeptide rose significantly in the normal controls and patients with type II diabetes, but not in those with type I diabetes. The authors interpreted their results as supporting the suggestion that islet amyloid polypeptide is secreted by pancreatic beta cells but, because the polypeptide can be measured in the blood of patients with insulin-dependent diabetes, they concluded that cells other than pancreatic beta cells must be able to secrete it. Further evidence for the co-secretion of insulin and islet amyloid polypeptide has been supplied by Hartter et al. (1990), who suggest that type II diabetes may, at least partially, be a result of dysregulation of the physiologically sensitive co-secretion of insulin with its agonist islet amyloid polypeptide.

In her review of islet amyloid and type II diabetes, Clark (1989) states that, in severe islet amyloidosis in type II diabetes, up to 88% of the islets may be affected and that the deposits occupy up to 80% of the islet space created by the loss of islet cells. The affected islets are not distributed uniformly throughout the pancreas for, as islet amyloid polypeptide is produced by beta cells, amyloid deposits are not found in the area of the head of the pancreas where the islets contain cells that secrete little other than pancreatic polypeptide.

It has been shown that the beta cells of several species, such as the cat, dog, rat and mouse, contain islet amyloid polypeptide and amyloidosis of the islets has been found in these animals. Certain non-human primates also develop spontaneous type II diabetes, but experimentally-induced diabetes in animals is not associated with amyloidosis of the islets.

In humans, type II diabetes has a strong hereditary component, although, unlike the inheritance of type I diabetes, it is not linked with the genes of the major histocompatibility region. In certain apes, type II diabetes is hereditary, and familial type II diabetes in a colony of Macaca nigra monkeys has been monitored by Howard (1986). In spite of the species difference, his findings suggest that something similar may occur in human type II diabetes. Pancreatic biopsies were carried out on 18 of the monkeys before they became diabetic and the islets were assessed morphologically, after which the metabolism of the animals was monitored for between 4 and 10 years, when a second biopsy or autopsy was carried out. Metabolic deterio-

ration correlated with the development of islet amyloidosis. In the islets, there was a gradual loss of
secretory cells with concurrent amyloid deposition.
As non-diabetic monkeys with 0% to 3% of islet
amyloid progressed to 20%–40% of affected islets,
the insulin secretion and glucose clearance were both
significantly decreased, while blood glucose and
glucagon levels increased. The impaired monkeys
progressed to overt diabetes when islet amyloid
exceeded 50%–60%; they had hyperglycaemia with
impaired insulin secretion and glucose clearance. The
importance of this work is that a minor degree of
amyloidosis was shown to precede any metabolic
deterioration, but, as the lesions progressed, metabolic deterioration developed and eventually became
overt type II diabetes mellitus. The above observations on non-human primates have been quoted in
some detail to support the suggestion that, in
human pathology, the islet amyloidosis found in
older, clinically non-diabetic subjects probably represents a pre-diabetic lesion.

The electron microscopic appearances of islet
amyloidosis have been described by Clark et al.
(1987). They found the amyloid material to be situated between the capillaries and the hormone-
producing cells; it was not present between islet
cells. Thick strands of amyloid fibrils lay within
deep invaginations into the insulin-containing beta
cells, and also closely adjacent to the plasmalemmal
membranes of the other types of endocrine cells.
Fragments of cytoplasm containing ribosomes and
nuclei were identifiable within the amyloid. There
was no evidence of capillary damage or thickening
of the basement membrane.

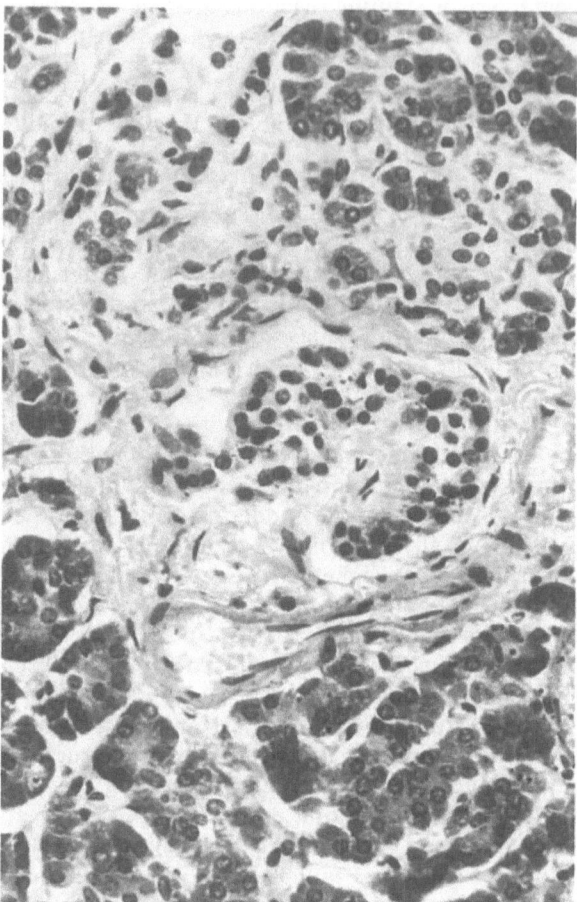

Fig. 6.11. Type II diabetes. Fibrosis of an islet in the pancreas of
a woman aged 76, who had had non-insulin-dependent diabetes for 10 years. H&E, × 375

Fibrosis of the Pancreas with Involvement of the Islets

Fibrosis of the pancreas in relation to involvement
of the islets and diabetes has received much attention in the past, and the publications up to 1977 have
been cited and discussed by Volk and Wellmann
(1977). More recently, Clark et al. (1988) found that
type II diabetic subjects had increased exocrine
fibrosis in the corpus region, but not in the head.
They took this fibrosis to be secondary to disor-
dered islet cell function. On the whole there seems
to be little definite correlation between interlobular
or interacinar fibrosis and fibrous replacement of
the islets except in the cases of very marked fibrosis.
In such cases, the fibrous tissue may surround and
extend into the islets along the course of the capillaries. This may be quite marked but tends to be
focal and patchy. There seems, however, to be
general agreement that intra-insular fibrosis (Figs

6.11–6.14) is found in the older diabetes but this was
not confirmed by Clark et al. (1988) whose 15 cases
of type II diabetes were almost all elderly. In some
there may be hyaline change in the islets as well as
fibrosis, either in different islets or with both lesions
in the same islets. Various degrees of fibrosis of the
islets have also been observed in the pancreases of
babies of mothers with diabetes (Hultquist and
Olding 1975).

The progressive fibrosis of chronic calcifying pancreatitis of the type seen in Europe by Sarles and his
colleagues (Sarles et al. 1979) is associated with the
onset of overt diabetes in one-third of cases and
with impaired glucose tolerance in another third. A
very similar incidence of diabetes (34%) was found
in America by Owens and Howard (1958) in patients
with chronic alcoholic pancreatitis. They noted also
that radiologically recognisable calcification of the
pancreas and the onset of diabetes tended to occur
at about the same stage of the illness. In India, there

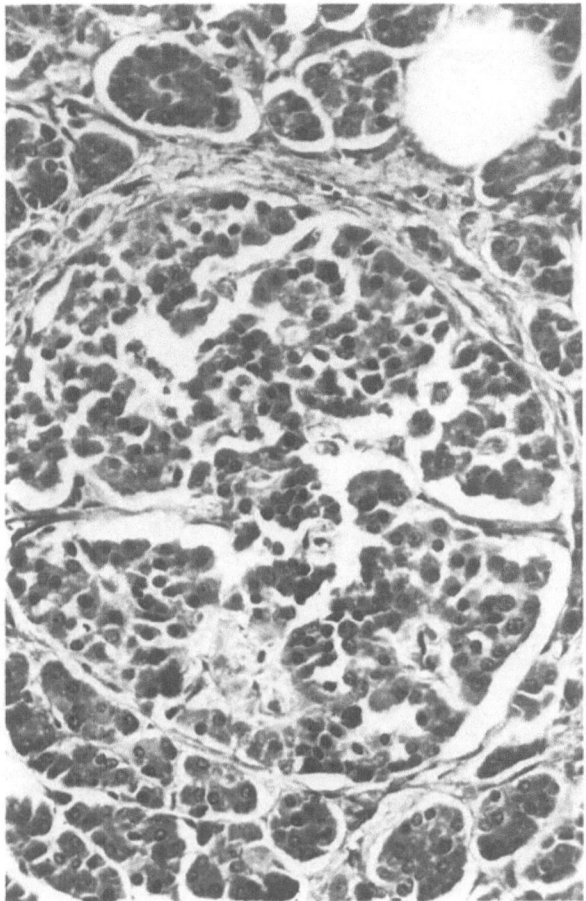

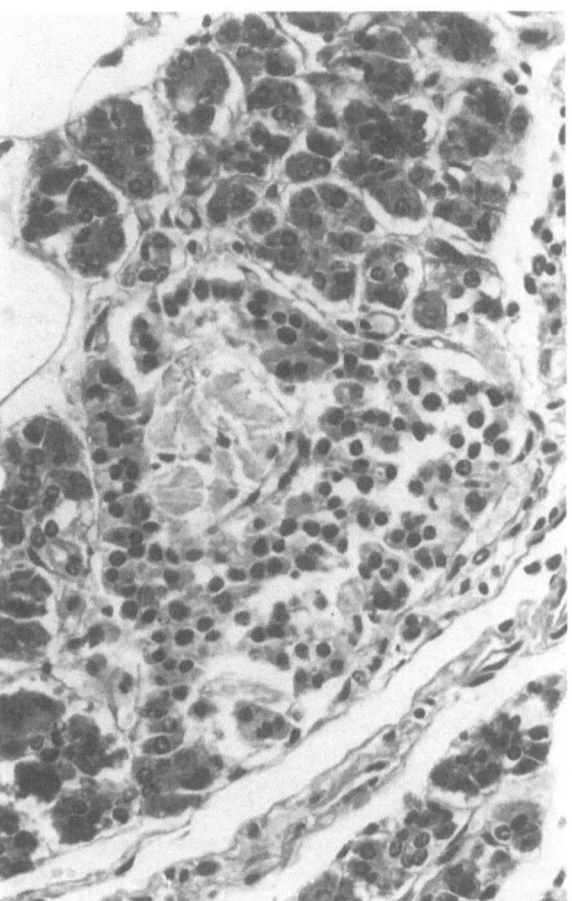

Fig. 6.12. Type II diabetes. Fibrosis around the periphery of an islet in the same pancreas as that in Fig. 6.11. Gomori's trichrome stain, × 300

Fig. 6.13. Type II diabetes. A partially hyaline islet in the pancreas shown in Fig. 6.12. H&E, × 375

is said to be a high incidence of diabetes in young adults with the type of chronic pancreatitis attributed to infantile malnutrition (Sarles et al. 1979). Diabetes attributable to the residual effects of acute pancreatitis is relatively unusual for, according to figures quoted by Dürr (1979), it develops in only 10%, or less, of patients that have recovered from acute pancreatitis.

Hydrops of Beta Cells

This lesion, originally noted by Weichselbaum and Stangl (1901), has been studied by various workers, whose publications have been reviewed by Volk and Wellmann (1977). The hydrops is the result of the replacement of the granules of the beta cells by vacuoles that increase in size until they occupy most of the cytoplasm. The nuclei remain intact

and are surrounded by glycogen, while basophilic bodies, which have been shown to be RNA, may appear in the cytoplasm. The lesion is relatively infrequent in diabetic pancreases (Warren et al. 1966) and may be present in the beta cells of non-diabetic pancreases; it may also be simulated by post-mortem change, and has been found when prolonged administration of glucose has preceded death in non-diabetic subjects.

Haemorrhage into the Islets

This has been described as a microscopic feature of the pancreas in diabetes but it is now generally attributed to autolysis (Fig. 6.15). Haemorrhagic islets (peliosis) have been reported in a non-diabetic woman with the MEN-1 syndrome which included multihormonal pancreatic islet cell tumours, hyper-

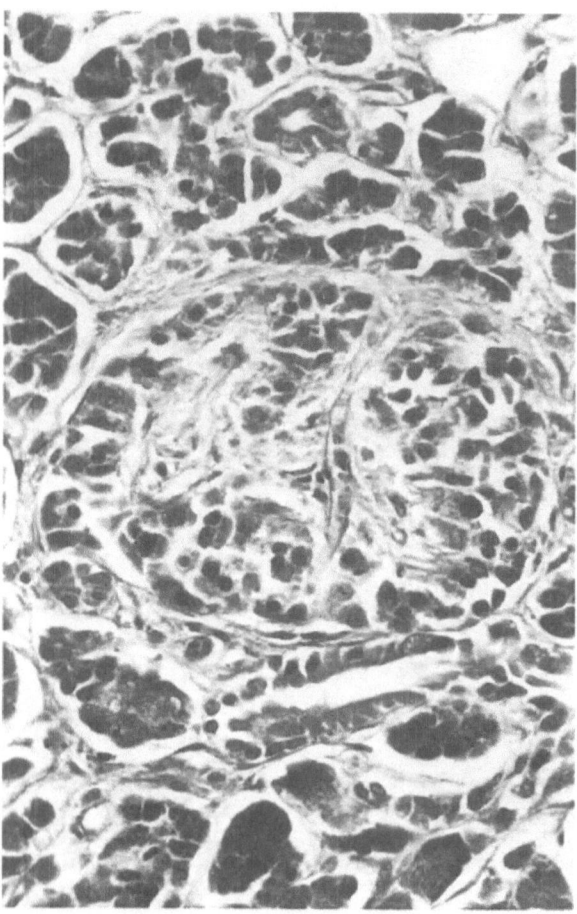

Fig. 6.14. Type II diabetes. Perivascular fibrosis in a pancreatic islet in a man who developed glycosuria at the age of 72, and who died of coronary arterial disease after an abdominal operation. Gomori's trichrome stain, × 375

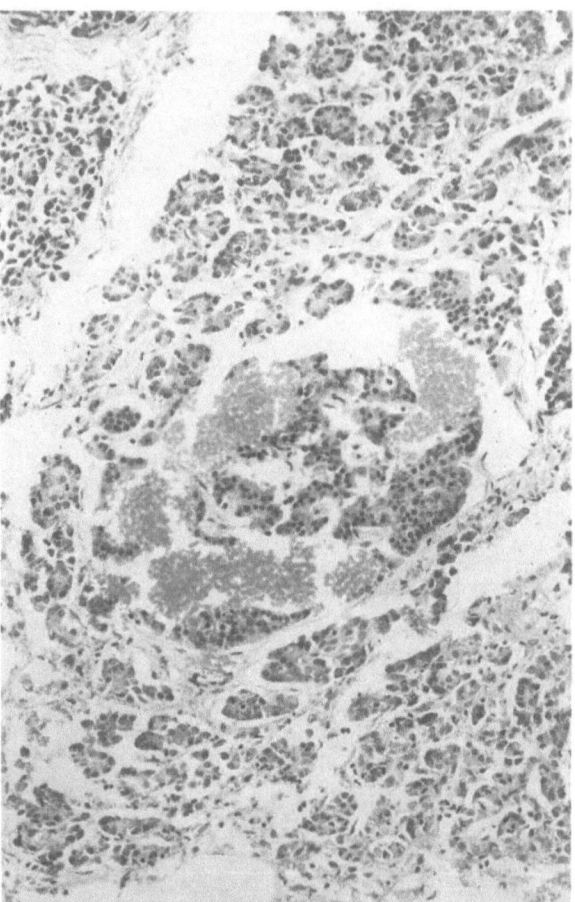

Fig. 6.15. Haemorrhage into an islet of Langerhans in the pancreas from a non-diabetic subject. Such haemorrhage has been noted occasionally in diabetics, but is generally believed to be a post-mortem phenomenon. Autolysis was marked in other parts of the pancreas. H&E, × 150

parathyroidism and a pituitary adenoma (Kovacs et al. 1986) and, as an incidental autopsy finding in a pancreatic islet cell adenoma (Pernicone and Lie 1987).

Calcium Deposits in the Islets

References to this rare lesion of the islets in diabetes are quoted by Volk and Wellmann (1977). The deposition of calcium may be associated with enlargement of the islets, which makes them visible with the naked eye, and with hyalinisation.

Congenital Absence of the Islets of Langerhans

This rare cause of fatal diabetes in a new-born infant has been described by Dodge and Laurence (1977).

Islet Cell Necrosis in the Neonatal Pancreas

Three patients with this rare condition, associated with antepartum haemorrhage, anoxia, shock and intravascular coagulation, were reported by Roberts (1987); he was able to refer to three previous reports. It is not known whether any non-fatal cases have survived with diabetes mellitus.

Tropical Diabetes or Nutrition-Related Diabetes Mellitus

The pancreatic lesions of this type of diabetes are described in the chapter on non-infective chronic pancreatitis (pp. 286–290).

The Pancreas in Haemochromatosis

The word, Hämochromatose, the German equivalent of haemochromatosis, was used first by von Recklinghausen, and the disease is sometimes referred to as von Recklinghausen–Appelbaum disease (*Butterworths Medical Dictionary*, 2nd edn, 1978), but various observers had noted the association of bronzing of the skin with glycosuria before von Recklinghausen's publication. All the early publications have been reviewed by Sheldon (1935) in his monograph, *Haemochromatosis*. At that time, there were reports of 345 cases, of which 311 were considered by Sheldon to be true examples of the condition. There have been many publications since 1935, and it is now believed by many that, in addition to the primary, idiopathic type, an anatomically indistinguishable secondary type may develop.

In the primary idiopathic form there is an unexplained abnormality of the metabolism of iron, in which the absorption of iron from the intestine is in such excess of the normal requirements of the body that the iron-containing pigment, haemosiderin, accumulates within cells in various organs in amounts sufficient to cause cellular damage and a fibrous reaction. The diabetes that is part of the syndrome of primary haemochromatosis is probably an associated metabolic abnormality, but, in the past, the diabetes has usually been attributed to iron-induced damage to the beta cells of the pancreatic islets. Iron accumulates in many organs, but the toxic effects are usually most marked in the liver, myocardium and pancreas, while selective deposition of iron in the gonadotrophic cells of the anterior pituitary gland may lead to secondary testicular atrophy and hypogonadism (Stremmel et al. 1988). The bronzing of the skin is not, however, due to deposition of haemosiderin, but to the presence of a non-iron pigment. Only small amounts of haemosiderin are found in the skin, in the vicinity of the apocrine glands.

Secondary haemochromatosis is the result of such severe and prolonged haemosiderosis that damage similar to that of idiopathic haemochromatosis occurs in the same organs that are involved in primary haemochromatosis. Clinical diabetes is not a feature of secondary haemochromatosis, but there is often some impairment of glucose tolerance.

The review of Powell et al. (1980) gives an account of the transport and storage of iron in haemochromatosis, along with the possible mechanisms of iron toxicity. It also suggests methods for the early detection of overloading with iron as well as the genetic nature of idiopathic haemochromatosis. The latter has become much better understood as a result of HLA typing (Kidd 1979; Dadone et al. 1982; Finlayson 1990), and it has now been established that idiopathic haemochromatosis is inherited as an autosomal recessive trait with partial expression in some heterozygotes.

The idiopathic type of haemochromatosis is rare in women, only about one-tenth of the patients being female (Finch and Finch 1955), the suggested explanation being that menstruation and pregnancy reduce the accumulation of the excessively absorbed iron. It is not usually recognised before the age of 10 years; most cases are diagnosed between the ages of 40 and 60 years (Volk and Wellmann 1985), but Witzleben and Uri (1989) have described a type of heavy iron accummulation, resembling that of haemochromatosis, in perinatal infants who had died of severe subacute or chronic liver disease of unknown aetiology.

Macroscopic Features

The appearance of the pancreas in haemochromatosis have been described many times. By 1935, Sheldon was able to refer to 125 case reports that included a description of the pancreas. Such reports made it clear that the pancreas was invariably pigmented, having a deep brown colour in which there was usually a reddish or rusty tint. The glands described were usually slightly enlarged, the average weight, based upon 34 cases in which the weight was recorded, being 123 g. It is true that this is above the average normal weight, but it is within the range of the variation in the weights of normal pancreases.

In many subjects the amount of fat was said to be markedly increased, with replacement of the atrophic gland by fat, but the marked variability of the amount of fat associated with normal pancreases makes replacement by fat of little value in the naked eye appraisal of a pancreas.

Rusty-looking lymph nodes, lighter in colour than the pancreas, perhaps due to the absence of the non-iron pigment, haematoidin, are often conspicuous near the pancreas.

The colour of the pancreas is due to the presence of haematoidin and haemosiderin; it is the latter pigment that has toxic effects. Once the pancreas has been damaged, the pancreatic injury alone seems to enhance the further absorption of iron (Davies 1961).

Microscopic Features

Microscopically, the haemosiderin granules are a golden-brown when they are small, but the larger granules are almost black. They are found in the cyto-

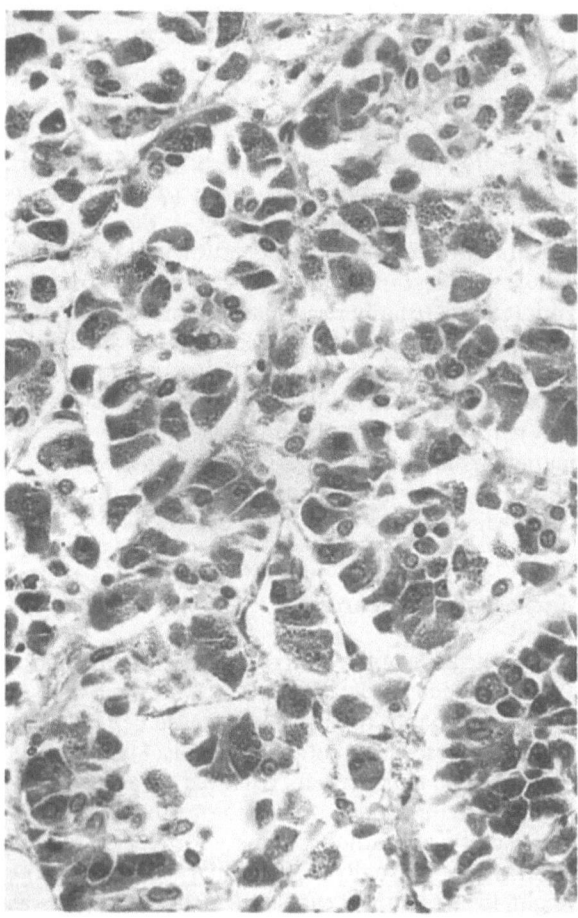 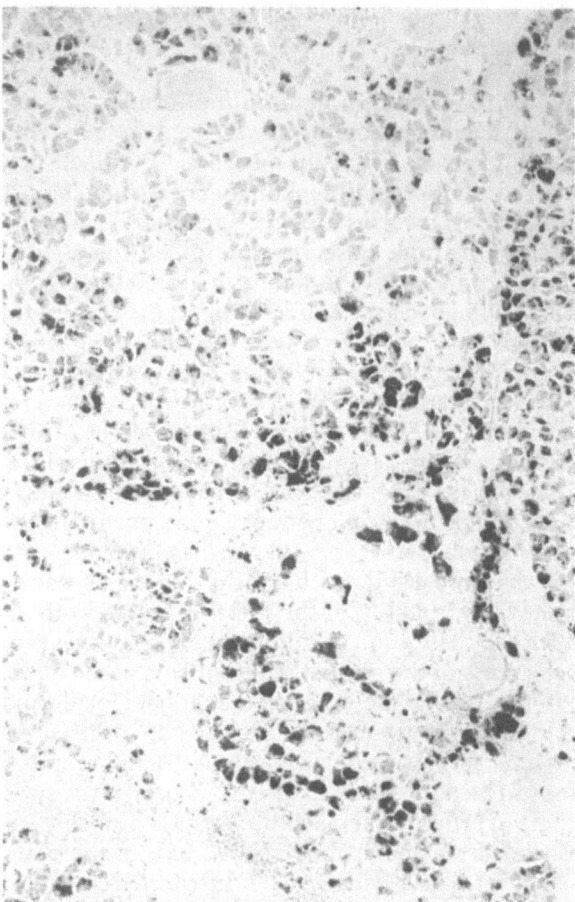

Fig. 6.16. Secondary haemochromatosis. Inconspicuous granules of haemosiderin are present in the acinar cells of the pancreas; there is no fibrosis. A man aged 76 had received many blood transfusions for a chronic refractory sideroblastic anaemia during the 13 years that preceded his death. His skin became pigmented and he developed cirrhosis of the liver and diabetes. H&E, × 375

Fig. 6.17. Secondary haemochromatosis. The haemosiderin granules in the pancreas shown in Fig. 6.16, stained by the method of Perls. × 150

plasm of the epithelium of the ducts, within the acinar and islet cells, and also embedded in fibrous tissue (Figs 6.16, 6.17). An increase of fibrous tissue is characteristic, but the degree of fibrosis and the amount of haemosiderin do not always correspond. It seems that the most severely pigmented glandular cells eventually disintegrate and become an amorphous pigmented mass. The granules of haemosiderin within the islet cells are usually smaller than those within the exocrine glandular cells; in some of the reported cases the islet cells have been found to contain no pigment. An attempt to recognise the type of islet cells that were most liable to become pigmented was made by McGarvan and Hartroft in 1956. They studied ten cases of

haemochromatosis and 13 cases of transfusional siderosis, and found that in both conditions the haemosiderin seemed to have a predilection for the beta cells. At that time, of course, islet cells could not be classified with the accuracy that the modern immunocytochemical methods have made possible and, at that time also, it was not accepted that transfusional siderosis might progress to become secondary haemochromatosis. Nevertheless, the limiting of the deposition of iron to the cytoplasm of the beta cells, with sparing of the other islet endocrine cells in haemochromatosis with diabetes, has since been confirmed by Warson and Gepts (unpublished observations: cited in Gepts 1981) and by Rahier et al. (1987).

Iron Content of the Pancreas

Estimations of the iron content of the pancreas have been undertaken by various investigators. The results available in 1935 were tabulated by Sheldon (on p 207 of that publication); it varied from less than 1% to 5%, with an average of 1.89%. When compared with a normal central figure of 0.0178%, the average iron content of the pancreas in haemochromatosis was thus roughly 100 times greater than normal.

Electron microscopy has shown that haemosiderin consists of aggregates of ferritin, a complex of colloidal ferric hydroxide–phosphate within a protein shell. The light and electron microscopic study carried out in 1962 by Scheuer et al. upon liver biopsies from the relatives of patients with haemochromatosis indicates that, at least in the liver, lipofuscin, the non-iron brown pigment that tends to accumulate in ageing cells, may form a basis in which ferritin, itself too soluble to remain in sections prepared for light microscopy, may develop into granules of haemosiderin.

The Islets

In some of the reported cases collected by Sheldon there were said to be no recognisable islets, while in others they were unusually large and conspicuous. Diabetes has not, of course always developed at the time when patients die with haemochromatosis, for death may be caused by the hepatic or cardiac effects of the haemochromatosis, or by unrelated disease, before the onset of diabetes.

In the pancreases of the diabetic patients with primary or secondary iron overload studied by Rahier et al. (1987), the islets seemed normal in sections stained by haemalum and eosin but, in a method in which the Prussian blue reaction was combined with immunoperoxidase staining, it was found that the beta cells contained iron granules, while the other types of islet cells contained none. By electron microscopy, the iron-containing beta cells were seen to have progressive loss of their endocrine granules, but the granules of the other endocrine cells were normal. The authors expressed the opinion that the islets did not have the atrophic appearance of the islets found in type I diabetes, and they did not see the amyloid material that is characteristic of type II diabetes.

An increase of fibrous tissue in the pancreas is usual; in some cases, possibly the less advanced, it may be focal, but in others, probably the more advanced, the whole gland is involved. Microscopically the fibrosis is mainly interlobular

(Fig. 6.18), but there is also some fibrosis within the lobules, and sometimes the fibrosis can be recognised to involve the islets by forming a fibrous capsule around the islets (Volk and Wellmann 1985).

Islet-Cell Adenomas and Transfusional Iron Overload

Examples of the above association have been reported by Sale and Lerner (1977), Sidi et al. (1984), and Sale (1985).

The Pancreas in Diabetes Mellitus Associated with Other Endocrine Diseases

The occasional association of diabetes with non-neoplastic overactivity, or with functioning neoplasms of the pituitary, adrenal or thyroid glands, has already been mentioned, but there are few reports of the condition of the pancreas in secondary diabetes of this type; what reports there are, do not record any consistent abnormalities.

Hormonally-induced diabetes may also be due to inappropriate secretion of a hormone by a neoplasm in an organ other than those ordinarily regarded as endocrine glands. An example of such secretion was reported by Soler (1973) in a patient in which the acute onset of diabetes was induced by an oat-cell carcinoma of the bronchus that secreted adrenocorticotrophic hormone. In most cases of hyperadrenocorticism in man, according to Volk and Wellmann (1985), there is insufficient evidence of damage to the islets of Langerhans to account for the diabetic state. In acromegaly and in thyrotoxicosis, as well as in phaeochromocytoma associated with diabetes, the few available studies have not shown any consistent relationship between the histological appearances of the islets and the presence, or otherwise, of diabetes. As the diabetes is usually insulin resistant, the abnormality is suspected to be in the insulin receptors of peripheral cells throughout the body.

Genetic Syndromes Associated with Glucose Intolerance

Some 40 distinct genetic disorders associated with glucose intolerance or clinical diabetes have been tabulated by Rotter and Rimoin (1981), but pancreatic lesions have been recognised in only a few of

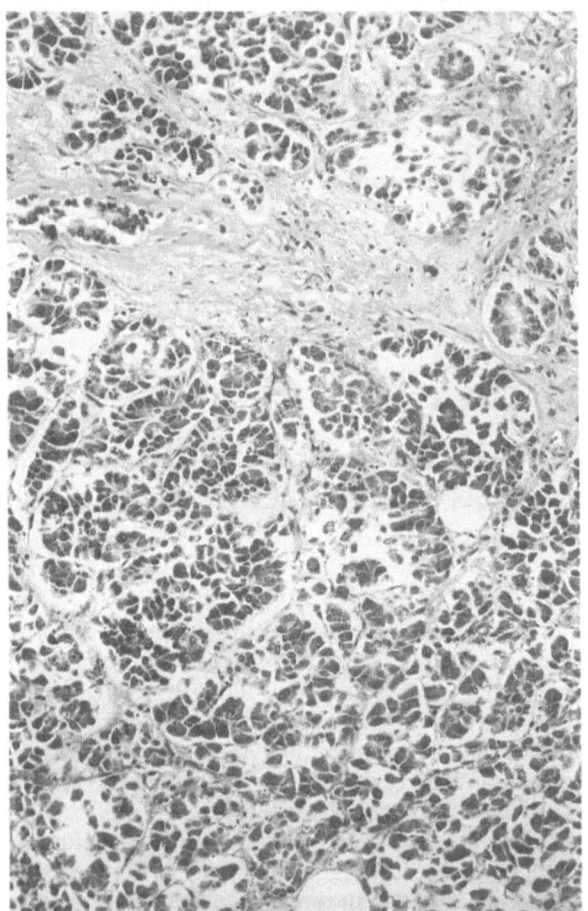

Fig. 6.18. Interstitial fibrosis in the case of secondary haemochromatosis shown in Fig. 6.16. and 6.17. H&E, × 150

mation about the condition of the pancreas in such people. Auto-antibodies against the insulin receptors known to be present upon the surface of fat cells, monocytes and other cells, have also been found in certain patients in whom there was glucose intolerance and marked insulin resistance (Kahn et al. 1976). Such patients had pigmentation of the skin due to acanthosis nigricans, and hyperinsulinaemia. Another form of insulin resistance with glucose intolerance has been attributed by the same workers to a primary defect in insulin receptors upon the surface membranes of peripheral cells, but no observations have been made upon the state of the endocrine or exocrine pancreatic tissue in such patients.

Stiff-Man Syndrome with Insulin-Dependent Diabetes Mellitus

The rare condition known as the stiff-man syndrome is a severe disease of the central nervous system, in which insulin-dependent diabetes mellitus may be part of the clinical picture. Solimena et al. (1990) have presented findings that support the hypothesis that the syndrome is an auto-immune disease in which GAD is the primary auto-antigen. The diabetes mellitus sometimes associated with the syndrome is additional evidence to support the importance of GAD as a primary antigen in type I diabetes as discussed on pp. 101–102.

these conditions. The syndromes in which there are pancreatic lesions include cystic fibrosis of the pancreas associated with general mucoviscidosis, hereditary relapsing pancreatitis, and haemochromatosis. The pancreatic lesions of mucoviscidosis are described in Chap. 4, and hereditary pancreatitis is discussed in Chaps. 12 and 13. In the latter condition, diabetes occurs only occasionally, while only about 10% of cases of mucoviscidosis develop diabetes.

Insulin-Resistant Diabetes Mellitus

In subjects with established auto-immunity, but without established diabetes, auto-antibodies against human insulin have been demonstrated (Wilkin and Nicholson 1984); such subjects may be in a pre-diabetic state. There is no available infor-

References

Ahmad N, Abraham A (1982) Pancreatic isletitis with coxsackie virus B5 infection. Hum Pathol 13 : 661–662

Alviggi L, Hoskins PJ, Pyke DA et al. (1984) Pathogenesis of insulin-dependent diabetes; a role for activated T lymphocytes. Lancet ii : 4–6

Atkinson MA, Maclaren NK, Scharp DW, Lacy PE, Riley WJ (1990) 64 000 Mr autoantibodies as predictors of insulin-dependent diabetes. Lancet 335 : 1357–1360

Atkinson MA, Kaufman DL, Campbell L et al. (1992) Response of peripheral-blood mononuclear cells to glutamate decarboxylase in insulin-dependent diabetes. Lancet 339 : 458–459

Baekkeskov S, Aanstoot H-J, Christgau S et al. (1990) Identification of the 64K autoantigen in insulin-dependent diabetes as the GABA-synthesizing enzyme glutamic acid decarboxylase. Nature 347 : 151–156

Banatvala JE, Bryant J, Schernthaner G et al. (1985) Cosackie B, mumps, rubella, and cytomegalovirus specific IgM responses in patients with juvenile-onset insulin-dependent diabetes mellitus in Britain, Austria, and Australia. Lancet i : 1409–1412

Barnett AH, Leslie RGD, Pyke DA (1981) Diabetes in identical twins: a study of 200 pairs. Diabetologia 20 : 87–93

Belehu A, Naafs B (1982) Diabetes mellitus associated with pentamidine mesylate. Lancet i : 1463–1464

Bell ET (1959) Hyalinization of the islets of Langerhans in nondiabetic individuals. Am J Pathol 35:801–805

Bending JJ, Ogg CS, Viberti GC (1987) Diabetogenic effect of cyclosporin. Br Med J 294:401–402

Bhatnagar SK, Amin MMA, Al-Yusuf AR (1984) Diabetogenic effects of nifedipine. Br Med J 289:19

Bodansky HJ, Grant PJ, Dean BM et al. (1986) Islet-cell antibodies and insulin autoantibodies in association with common viral infections. Lancet ii:1351–1353

Boström K (1968) Path-anatomical findings in a case of mumps with pancreatitis, myocarditis, orchitis, epididymitis, and seminal vesiculitis. Virchows Arch [A] 344:111–117

Bottazzo GF (1984) B-cell damage in diabetic insulitis: are we approaching a solution? Diabetologia 26:241–249

Bottazzo GF, Dean BM, McNally JM, McKay EH, Swift PGF, Gamble DR (1985) In situ characterization of autoimmune phenomena and expression of HLA molecules in the pancreas in diabetic insulitis. N Engl J Med 313:353–360

Bryceston ADM (1968) Pentamidine-induced diabetes mellitus. East Afr Med J 45:110–117

Cecil RL (1909) A study of the pathological anatomy of the pancreas in ninety cases of diabetes mellitus. J Exp Med 11:266–290

Cerasi E (1988) Insulin secretion in diabetes mellitus. In: Lèfebvre PJ, Pipeleers DG (eds) The pathology of the endocrine pancreas. Springer, Berlin, pp 191–218

Clark A (1989) Islet amyloid and type 2 diabetes. Diabetic Medicine 6:561–567

Clark A, Cooper GJS, Lewis CE et al. (1987) Islet amyloid formed from diabetes-associated peptide may be pathogenic in type-2 diabetes. Lancet ii:231–234

Clark A, Wells CA, Buley ID et al. (1988) Islet amyloid, increased A-cells, reduced beta cells and exocrine fibrosis: quantitative changes in the pancreas in type 2 diabetes. Diabetes Res 9:151–159

Cooper GJS, Leighton B, Dimitriadis GD et al. (1988) Amylin found in amyloid deposits in human type 2 diabetes mellitus may be a hormone that regulates glycogen metabolism in skeletal muscle. Proc Natl Acad Sci USA 85:7763–7766

Dadone MM, Kushner JP, Edwards CQ, Bishop DT, Skolnick MH (1982) Heredity and hemochromatosis: analysis of laboratory expression of the disease by genotype in 18 pedigrees. Am J Clin Pathol 78:196–205

Dandona P, Freedman DB, Foo Y et al. (1984) Exocrine pancreatic function in diabetes mellitus. J Clin Pathol 37:302–306

Davies AE (1961) Relationship of disturbed pancreatic function to haemosiderosis. Lancet ii:749–751

de Beardinis P, Londei M, James RFL, Lake SP, Wise PH, Feldmann M (1988) Do CD4-positive cytotoxic T cells damage islet beta cells in type I diabetes? Lancet ii:823–824

Diabetes Epidemiology Research International (1987) Preventing insulin dependent diabetes mellitus: the environmental challenge. Br Med J 295:479–481

Dinarello CA (1984) Interleukin-1 and the pathogenesis of the acute-phase response. N Engl J Med 311:1413–1418

Dodge JA, Laurence KM (1977) Congenital absence of islets of Langerhans. Arch Dis Child 52:411–413

Doniach I, Morgan AG (1973) Islets of Langerhans in juvenile diabetes mellitus. Clin Endocrinol 2:233–248

Dunn JS, Sheehan HL, McLetchie NGB (1943) Necrosis of islets of Langerhans produced experimentally. Lancet i:484–487

Dürr GH-K (1979) Acute pancreatitis. In: Howatt HT, Sarles H (eds) The exocrine pancreas. Saunders, London, pp 352–401

Faber OK, Binder C, Lauritzen T, Heding LG (1976) Preserved beta-cell function and blood glucose control in insulin dependent diabetes mellitus [abstract]. Diabetes 25:362

Fabris P, Betterle C, Floreani A et al. (1992) Development of type 1 diabetes mellitus during interferon alfa therapy for chronic

HCV hepatitis [letter]. Lancet 340:548

Finch SC, Finch CA (1955) Idiopathic hemochromatosis, and iron storage disease. Medicine 34:381–430

Finlayson NDC (1990) Hereditary (primary) haemochromatosis. Br Med J 301:350–351

Fonseca V, Berger LA, Beckett AG, Dandona P (1985) Size of pnacreas in diabetes mellitus: a study based on ultrasound. Br Med J 291:1240–1241

Foulis AK, Farquharson MA (1986) Aberrant expression of HLA-DR antigens by insulin-containing beta-cells in recent-onset type 1 (insulin-dependent) diabetes mellitus [abstract]. J Pathol 148:92–93A

Foulis AK, Stewart JA (1984) The pancreas in recent-onset type 1 (insulin-dependent) diabetes mellitus: insulin content of islets, insulitis and associated changes in the exocrine acinar tissue. Diabetologia 26:456–461

Foulis AK, Liddle CN, Farquharson MA, Richmond JA, Weir RS (1986) Pancreas in type 1 (insulin-dependent) diabetes mellitus: 25 yr review of deaths in patients under 20 yr of age in United Kingdom [abstract]. J Pathol 148:93A

Foulis AK, Farquharson MA, Hardman R (1987a) Aberrant expression of class II major histocompatibility complex molecules by B cells and hyperexpression of class I major histocompatibility complex molecules by insulin containing islets in type 1 (insulin-dependent) diabetes mellitus. Diabetologica 30:333–343

Foulis AK, Farquharson MA, Meager A (1987b) Immunoreactive gamma-interferon in insulin-secreting beta-cells in type 1 diabetes mellitus. Lancet ii:1423–1427

Foulis AK, McGill M, Farquharson MA (1991) Insulitis in type 1 (insulin-dependent) diabetes mellitus in man – macrophages, lymphocytes, and interferon-gamma containing cells. J Pathol 165:97–103

Foulis AK, McGill M, Sutherland DER, Sibley RK (1992) Immunological phenomena associated with recurrent diabetes in pancreatic transplants [abstract]. J Pathol 167 (Suppl):136 A

Frier BM, Saunders JHB, Wormsley KG, Bouchier IAD (1976) Exocrine pancreatic function in juvenile onset diabetes mellitus. Gut 17:685–691

Gepts W (1965) Pathologic anatomy of the pancreas in juvenile diabetes mellitus. Diabetes 14:619–633

Gepts W (1981) Islet changes in human diabetes. In: Cooperstein SJ, Watkins D (eds) The islets of Langerhans. Academic Press, New York, pp 321–356

Gepts W, De Mey J (1978) Islet cell survival determined by morphology: an immunocytochemical study of the islets of Langerhans in juvenile diabetes mellitus. Diabetes 27:251–261

Hanafusa T, Miyazaki A, Miyagawa J et al. (1990) Examination of islets in the pancreas biopsy specimens from newly diagnosed type 1 (insulin-dependent) diabetic patients. Diabetologia 33:105–111

Harrison LC, Honeyman MC, De Aizpurua HJ et al. (1993) Inverse relation between humoral and cellular immunity to glutamic acid decarboxylase in subjects at risk of insulin-dependent diabetes. Lancet 341:1365–1369

Hartter E, Svoboda T, Lell B et al. (1990) Reduced islet-amyloid polypeptide in insulin-dependent diabetes mellitus [letter]. Lancet 335:854

Helgason T, Jonasson MR (1981) Evidence for a food additive as a cause of ketosis-prone diabetes. Lancet ii:716–720

Helgason T, Ewen SWB, Ross IS, Stowers JM (1982) Diabetes produced in mice by smoked/cured/mutton. Lancet ii:1017–1022

Howard CF (1986) Longitudinal studies on the development of diabetes in individual Macaca nigra. Diabetologica 29:301–306

Hultquist GT, Olding LB (1975) Pancreatic-island fibrosis in young infants of diabetic mothers. Lancet ii:1015–1016

Ishii T, Hosoda Y, Ikegami N, Shimada H (1983) Senile amyloid deposition. J Pathol 139:1–22

Jenson AB, Rosenberg HS, Notkins AL (1980) Pancreatic islet-cell damage in children with fatal viral infections. Lancet ii: 354–358

Johnson HK, O'Brien TD, Jordan K, Westermark P (1989) Impaired glucose tolerance is associated with increased islet amyloid polypeptide (IAPP) immunoreactivity in pancreatic beta cells. Am J Pathol 153: 245–250

Johnston C, Pyke DA, Cudworth AG, Wolf E (1983) HLA-DR typing in identical twins with insulin-dependent diabetes: difference between concordant and discordant pairs. Br Med J i: 253–255

Junker K, Egeberg J, Kromann H, Nerup J (1977) An autopsy study of the islets of Langerhans in acute-onset juvenile diabetes mellitus. APMIS [A] 85: 699–706

Kahn CR, Flier JS, Bar RS et al. (1976) The syndromes of insulin resistance and acanthosis nigricans: insulin-receptor disorders in man. N Engl J Med 294: 739–745

Karam JH, Lewitt PA, Young CW et al. (1980) Insulinopenic diabetes after rodenticide (Vacor) ingestion: a unique model of acquired diabetes in man. Diabetes 29: 971–978

Kaufman DL, Clare-Salzler M, Tian J et al. (1993) Spontaneous loss of T-cell tolerance to glutamic acid decarboxylase in murine insulin-dependent diabetes. Nature 366: 69–72

Kidd KK (1979) Hemochromatosis [editorial]. N Engl J Med 301: 209–210

King ML, Shaikh A, Bidwell D, Voller A, Banatvalla JE (1983) Coxsackie-B-virus-specific IgM responses in children with insulin-dependent (juvenile-onset; type 1) diabetes mellitus. Lancet i: 1397–1399

Klöppel G, Drenck CR, Oberholzer M, Heitz PU (1984) Morphometric evidence for a striking B-cell reduction at the clinical onset of type 1 diabetes. Virchows Arch [A] 403: 441–452

Kovacs K, Horvath E, Asa SL, Murray D, Singer W, Reddy SSK (1986) Microscopic peliosis of pancreatic islets in a woman with MEN-1 syndrome. Arch Pathol Lab Med 110: 607–610

Lancet (1989) Type 2 diabetes or NIDDM: looking for a better name [leading article]. i: 589–591

Lancet (1990) The 64K question in diabetes [editorial]. 336: 597–598

Leahy JL, Bonner-Weir S, Weir GC (1988) Rat models of non-insulin-dependent diabetes mellitus: evidence that mild increases in plasma glucose play an important role in pathogenesis. In: Lèfebvre PJ, Pipeleers DG (eds) The pathology of the endocrine pancreas in diabetes. Springer, Berlin, pp 285–309

Le Compte PM (1958) "Insulitis" in early juvenile diabetes. Arch Pathol 66: 450–457

Leighton B, Cooper GJS (1988) Pancreatic amylin and calcitonin-gene-related peptide cause resistance to insulin in skeletal muscle in vitro. Nature 335: 632–635

Leiter EH, Wilson GL (1988) Viral interactions with pancreatic B-cells. In: Lèfebvre PJ, Pipeleers DG (eds) The pathology of the endocrine pancreas in diabetes. Springer, Berlin, pp 85–105

Lernmark A, Markholst H, Baekkeskov S (1988) Circulating signs of autoimmune islet disease. In: Lèfebvre PJ, Pipeleers DG (eds) The pathology of the endocrine pancreas in diabetes. Springer, Berlin, pp 53–70

Leslie RDG (1983) Causes of insulin dependent diabetes. Br Med J iii: 5–6

Leslie RDG, Pyke DA (1991) Escaping insulin-dependent diabetes. Br Med J 302: 1103–1104

Linke RP, Eanes ED, Termine JD, Bladen HA, Glenner GG (1976) Formation of amyloid-like fibrils from insulin and glucagon in vitro. In: Wegelius O, Pasternack A (eds) Amyloidosis. Academic Press, London, pp 371–373

Löhr M, Klöppel G (1987) Residual insulin positivity and pancreatic atrophy in relation to duration of chronic type 1 (insulin-dependent) diabetes mellitus and microangiopathy. Diabetologia 30: 757–762

Maclean N, Ogilvie RF (1955) Quantitative estimation of the pancreatic islet tissue in diabetic subjects. Diabetes 4: 367–376

McGarvan MH, Hartroft W (1956) The predilection of pancreatic beta cells for pigment deposition in hemochromatosis and hemosiderosis [abstract]. Am J Pathol 32: 631

Melato M, Antonutto G, Ferronato E (1977) Amyloidosis of the islets of Langerhans in relation to diabetes mellitus and aging. Beitr Pathol 160: 73–81

Nerup J, Mandrup-Poulsen T, Molvig J, Spinas G (1988) Immune interactions with islet cells: implications for the pathogenesis of insulin-dependent diabetes mellitus. In: Lèfebvre PJ, Pipeleers DG (eds) The pathology of the endocrine pancreas in diabetes. Springer, Berlin, pp 71–84

Oli JM, Nwokolo C (1979) Diabetes after infectious hepatitis: a follow-up study. Br Med J ii: 926–927

Opie EL (1900–1901) On the relation of chronic interstitial pancreatitis to the islets of Langerhans and to diabetes mellitus. J Exp Med 5: 397–428

Orci L, Baetens D, Rufener C et al. (1976) Hypertrophy and hyperplasia of somatostatin containing D-cells in diabetes. Proc Nat Acad Sci USA 73: 1338–1342

Owens JL, Howard JM (1958) Pancreatic calcification: a late sequel in the natural history of chronic alcoholism and alcoholic pancreatitis. Ann Surg 147: 326–338

Pak CY, Eun H-M, McArthur RG, Yoon J-W (1988) Association of cytomegalovirus infection with autoimmune type 1 diabetes. Lancet ii: 1–4

Pearse AGE, Ewen SWB, Polak JM (1972) The genesis of apud-amyloid in endocrine polypeptide tumours: histochemical distinction from immunamyloid. Virchows Arch [B] 10: 93–107

Pernicone PJ, Lie JT (1987) Isolated peliosis of pancreatic islet cell adenoma. Arch Pathol Lab Med 111: 690–691

Pipeleers DG, Veld PAI, Van De Winkel M (1988) Death of the pancreatic B-cell. In: Lèfebvre PJ, Pipeleers DG (eds) The pathology of the endocrine pancreas in diabetes. Springer, Berlin, pp 106–124

Powell LW, Bassett ML, Halliday JW (1980) Hemochromatosis: 1980 update. Gastroenterology 78: 374–381

Rahier J (1988) The diabetic pancreas: a pathologist's view. In: Lèfebvre PJ, Pipeleers DG (eds) The pathology of the endocrine pancreas in diabetes. Springer, Berlin, p 22

Rahier J, Goebbels RM, Henquin JC (1983) Cellular composition of the human diabetic pancreas. Diabetologica 24: 366–371

Rahier J, Loozen S, Goebbels RM, Abrahem M (1987) The haemochromatotic human pancreas: a quantitative immuno-histochemical and ultrastructural study. Diabetologia 30: 5–12

Rakieten N, Rakieten ML, Nadkarni MV (1963) Studies on the diabetogenic action of strepozotocin (NSC-37917). Cancer Chemother Rep 27: 91–98

Roberts PF (1987) Islet cell necrosis in the neonatal pancreas: a report of three cases. J Clin Pathol 40: 1206–1211

Roep BO, Kallan AA, Hazenbos WLW et al. (1991) T-cell reactivity to 38 kD insulin-secretory-granule protein in patients with recent onset type 1 diabetes. Lancet 337: 1439–1441

Rotter JI, Rimoin DL (1981) The genetics of the glucose intolerance disorders. Am J Med 70: 116–126

Sale GE (1985) Multiple islet cell adenomas in a patient with secondary hemochromatosis [letter]. Arch Pathol Lab Med 109: 795

Sale GE, Lerner KG (1977) Multiple tumors after androgen therapy. Arch Pathol Lab Med 101: 600–603

Sarles H, Sahel J, Staub JL, Bourry J, Laugier R (1979) Chronic pancreatitis. In: Howat HT, Sarles H (eds) The exocrine pancreas. Saunders, London, pp 402–439

Schernthaner G, Banatvala JE, Scherbaum W et al. (1985)

Coxsackie-B-virus-specific IgM responses, complement-fixing islet-cell antibodies, HLA-DR antigens, and C-peptide secretion in insulin-dependent diabetes mellitus. Lancet ii: 630–632

Scheuer PJ, Williams R, Muir AR (1962) Hepatic pathology in relatives of patients with haemochromatosis. J Pathol Bacteriol 84: 53–64

Sheldon JH (1935) Haemochromatosis. Oxford University Press, London

Sidi Y, Liban E, Solomon F, Pinkhas J, Tikva P (1984) Multiple islet cell adenomas in a patient with secondary hemochromatosis. Arch Pathol Lab Med 108: 690–692

Soler NG (1973) Acute onset diabetes due to an ACTH secreting oat cell carcinoma of the bronchus. Postgrad Med J 49: 928–929

Solimena M, Folli F, Aparisi R, Pozza G, De Camilli P (1990) Autoantibodies to GABA-ergic neurons and pancreatic beta cells in stiff-man syndrome. N Engl J Med 322: 1555–1560

Stansfield OH, Warren S (1928) Inflammation involving the islands of Langerhans in diabetes. N Engl J Med 198: 686–687

Stremmel W, Niederau C, Berger M, Kley H-K, Krüskemper H-L, Strohmeyer G (1988) Abnormalities in estrogen, androgen, and insulin metabolism in idiopathic hemochromatosis. Ann NY Acad Sci 526: 209–223

Tisch R, Yang X-D, Singer SM, Liblau RS, Fugger L, McDevitt HO (1993) Immune response to glutamic acid decarboxylase correlates with insulitis in non-obese diabetic mice. Nature 366: 72–75

Tuomilehto J, Tuomilehto-Wolf E, Virtala E, LaPorte R (1990) Coffee consumption as trigger for insulin-dependent diabetes mellitus in childhood. Br Med J 300: 642–643

Ujevich MM, Jaffe R (1980) Pancreatic islet cell damage: its occurrence in neonatal coxsackievirus encephalomyocarditis. Arch Pathol Lab Med 104: 438–441

van Jaarsveld BC, Hackeng WHL, Nieuwenhuis MG, Erkelens DW, Geerdink RA, Lips CJM (1990) Islet-amyloid polypeptide in human plasma [letter]. Lancet 335: 60

Volk BW, Wellmann KF (1977) Idiopathic diabetes. In: Volk BW, Wellmann KF (eds) The diabetic pancreas. Baillière Tindall, London, pp 231–260

Volk BW, Wellmann KF (1985) Hemochromatosis and diabetes. In : Volk BW, Arquilla ER (eds) The diabetic pancreas, 2nd edn. Plenum, New York, pp 327–336

von Meyenburg H (1940) Ueber "insulitis" bei diabetes. Schweiz Med Wochenschr 21: 554–557

Warren S, Root HF (1925) The pathology of diabetes with special reference to pancreatic regeneration. Am J Pathol 1: 415–430

Warren S, Le Compte PM, Legg MA (1966) The pathology of diabetes mellitus, 4th edn. Henry Kimpton, London, p 85

Weichselbaum A, Stangl E (1901) Zur Kenntniss der feineren Veränderungen des Pankreas bei Diabetes mellitus. Wien Klin Wochenschr 14: 968–972

Westermark P (1976) The nature of amyloid in islets of Langerhans in old age. In: Wegelius O, Pasternack A (eds) Amyloidosis. Academic Press, London, pp 533–541

Westermark P, Wilander E, Westermark GT, Johnson KH (1987) Islet amyloid polypeptide-like immunoreactivity in the islet B cells of type 2 (non-insulin-dependent) diabetic and nondiabetic individuals. Diabetologia 30: 887–892

World Health Organization (1980) Expert committee on diabetes mellitus: second report. WHO, Geneva, pp 1–80 (World Health Organization Technical Report Series 646)

World Health Organization (1985) Report of a study group. WHO, Geneva, pp 1–113 (Technical Report Series 727)

Wilkin TJ (1993) Early nutrition and diabetes mellitus: nutrition during fetal life and infancy may be crucial to the development of diabetes mellitus. Br Med J 306: 283–284

Wilkin TJ, Nicholson S (1984) Autoantibodies against human insulin. Br Med J i: 349–352

Witzleben CL, Uri A (1989) Perinatal hemochromatosis: entity or end result? Hum Pathol 20: 335–340

Yoon J-W, Austin M, Onodera T, Notkins AL (1979) Virus-induced diabetes mellitus: isolation of a virus from the pancreas of a child with diabetic ketoacidosis. N Engl J Med 300: 1173–1179

7 Pancreatic Transplantation

Pancreatic transplantation is the subject of much current research; the progress in such research, up to 1989, was reviewed by Sells and Leslie (1989). The present clinical application of pancreatic transplantation is mainly in the management of patients with insulin-dependent diabetes mellitus in whom diabetic renal failure has progressed to a stage at which renal transplantation becomes necessary. It was soon recognised that diabetic patients who received a renal transplant alone seldom did as well as the patients that received a transplanted kidney for renal failure unrelated to diabetes, and methods for the simultaneous transplantation of a donor's kidney and pancreas were devised. There were, of course, failures amongst such cases and the reasons for such failures were reviewed by Sibley and Sutherland (1987). They carried out an immunohistological and histopathological examination of 100 pancreatic grafts, on material obtained by biopsy, at pancreatectomy, or at autopsy, to ascertain why such grafts had functioned inadequately or had failed. Obstructive lesions and infections accounted for a substantial number of the failures, but even in cases where such factors were important, signs of rejections were also recognised.

A difficult technical problem was the disposal of the exocrine secretion of the grafted pancreas. Drainage of the ducts into the alimentary canal of the recipient seemed to favour the onset of acute pancreatitis in the graft and leakage from anastomoses also caused failures. Attempts to cause exocrine atrophy of the donor pancreas by the injection of its ducts with substances such as Prolamine or Silastic were also unsatisfactory because of the foreign body type of inflammation that occurred in the graft. Oddly, drainage of the exocrine pancreatic secretion into the urinary bladder, though much less

physiological than drainage into the alimentary canal, was found to be more satisfactory technically and to have the advantage that pancreatic function could be monitored by estimations of the amount of amylase in the urine. The operative procedure, as developed by Nghiem and Corry (1987) and by D'Allesandro et al. (1989), involves the removal of the donor pancreas along with the segment of duodenum that receives its duct, the closure of the cut ends of the duodenal segment, and the making of a side-to-side anastomosis between the duodenal segment and the vault of the bladder; the donor kidney is transplanted during the same operation. A blood supply for the transplanted pancreas is provided by anastomoses from the iliac vessels on one side of the pelvic cavity and for the transplanted kidney from the iliac vessels on the other side. It is said by Sells and Leslie (1989) that this technique has almost abolished the leakage of exocrine secretion and wound sepsis, although the risk of pancreatic vessel thrombosis is still about 10%. Occasional complications have been duodenal erosions or ulceration, that made duodenal excision and reanastomosis necessary, acidosis secondary to renal impairment, and cystitis. Immunosuppression depends mainly on the use of cyclosporin, but if there are clinical signs of rejection azathioprine, or prednisone, or both, may be necessary.

Rejection

The pathological signs of rejection, as described by Sibley and Sutherland in pancreases studied by biopsy, after pancreatectomy or at autopsy, consist of extensive focal, or even diffuse, infiltration of the exocrine tissues by small and large lymphocytes, usually in association with signs of acute or chronic vascular rejection. Acute vascular rejection is indicated by mononuclear infiltration of the endothelial region of vessels or by fibrinoid necrosis. In more chronic rejection, there is fibromyointimal proliferation with narrowing of the lumen of the vessels. Sometimes there is also mononuclear cell infiltration around the peripancreatic nerves. It is of interest that, in most cases, the islets were normal and had abundant beta cells. In such cases the graft failure could not be attributed to beta-cell loss.

Recurrence of Diabetes

In some of the pancreatic grafts between the best matched recipients and donors, for example, between HLA identical siblings or identical twins, Sibley and Sutherland found selective destruction of beta cells associated with mononuclear cell infiltration of the islets. When destruction of the beta cells became complete, the inflammatory infiltration disappeared. The resemblance to the stages in the pathogenesis of type I diabetes suggested that the auto-immune process, responsible for the original damage to the recipient's own beta cells and the onset of diabetes, had remained sufficiently active to destroy also the beta cells of the pancreas grafted from the well-matched donor. The appearances were not those of rejection and these patients redeveloped clinical and biochemical diabetes. Further studies of the recurrence of diabetes with insulitis and eventual disappearance of insulin-secreting beta cells in pancreases grafted into patients with type I diabetes have been reported by Foulis et al. (1992), who found that, in 90 of 143 insulin-containing cells, there was hyperexpression of class I major histocompatibility molecules while none of these changes were seen in grafts that did not develop recurrent diabetes. Another study of recurrent diabetes after an apparently successful pancreatic graft was carried out by Santamaria et al. (1992). These workers made a detailed characterisation of the T lymphocytes that were present in the antigen-identical graft that had caused an apparent cure for 8 years in a diabetic patient before the diabetes recurred. Although such information contributes towards an understanding of type I diabetes, much still remains to be explained.

Transplantation of Islets

The technical difficulties of transplanting the entire pancreas with its exocrine components, as well as its islets, could be avoided if islets alone could be grafted; the progress towards this end, achieved in various research centres, has been described by Karcher (1989). The present aim of such work is to find how a suspension of islets, or even of beta cells alone, obtained from homogenates of living pancreatic tissue, can be prepared for intravenous injection. It has been found that the islets in a homogenate of pancreatic tissue will stain selectively with neutral red without apparent loss of vitality, and, after fluorescence of the neutral red has been induced, automatic sorting can be carried out. At present, the yield of islets is small and it has been calculated that 100 000–200 000 islets would have to be injected. The immunologically matched islets would then be trapped in vascular organs, such as the liver or spleen, where they would survive and provide an adequate replacement of insulin. Some success in experimental procedures of this type has been reported in primates by Gray et al. (1986), and in a few human patients by Tzakis et al. (1990). In the patients treated by the latter authors, upper abdominal exenteration had had to be carried out because of otherwise unresectable neoplasms; this was followed by liver transplantation combined with islet transplantation. The team who carried out these formidable procedures claims that at least one of their patients, who requires neither parenteral alimentation nor insulin, is the first example of successful clinical islet cell transplantation.

As with whole pancreatic grafts, however, immunological difficulties remain to be overcome in the transplantation of pancreatic islets or beta cells. Nevertheless, it is the opinion of Sells and Leslie (1989) that: "A successful combination of techniques allowing a high yield of pure human islets, together with a uniformly successful method for reducing their immunogenicity, would provide a new method of treating diabetes with enormous clinical potential."

Some progress towards such an achievement has since been claimed by Gores et al. (1993). By the use of a new immunosuppressive agent, 15-disoxyspergualin, combined with antilymphocytic globulin and followed later by azathioprine, prednisone and cyclosporin, they produced insulin-independence after the transplantation of unpurified islets from a single donor. The unpurified islets were transplanted concomitantly with a kidney in two uraemic diabetic patients. Islet function has been sustained in both; one of the patients remained insulin-independent and euglycaemic for more than 6 months after transplantation.

References

D'Alessandro AM, Sollinger HW, Stratta RJ, Kalayoglu M, Pirsch JD, Belzer FO (1989) Comparison between button and duodenal segment in pancreas transplantation. Transplantation 47:120–122

Foulis AK, McGill M, Sutherland DER, Sibley RK (1992) Immunohistological phenomena associated with recurrent diabetes in pancreatic transplants [abstract]. J Pathol 167 Suppl:136A

Gores PF, Najarian JS, Stephanian E, Lloveras JJ, Kelley SL, Sutherland DER (1993) Insulin independence in type I diabetes after transplantation of unpurified islets from single donor with 15-deoxyspergualin. Lancet i:19–21

Gray DWR, Warnock GL, Sutton R, Peters M, McShane P, Morris PJ (1986) Successful autotransplantation of the isolated islets of Langerhans in the cynomolgus monkey. Br J Surg 73:850–853

Karcher HL (1989) New sorting machine for islet cells. Br Med J 298:1413

Nghiem DD, Corry RJ (1987) Technique of simultaneous renal pancreatoduodenal transplantation with urinary drainage of pancreatic secretion. Am J Surg 153:405–406

Santamaria P, Nakhleh RE, Sutherland DE, Barbosa JJ (1992) Characterization of T lymphocytes infiltrating human pancreas allograft affected by isletitis and recurrent diabetes. Diabetes 41:53–61

Sells RA, Leslie D (1989) Pancreas transplantation. In: Sells RA, Leslie D (eds) Organ transplantation: current clinical and immunological concepts. Baillière Tindall, London, pp 119–136

Sibley RK, Sutherland DER (1987) Pancreas transplantation. An immunohistologic and histopathologic examination of 100 grafts. Am J Pathol 128:151–170

Tzakis AG, Ricordi C, Alejandro R et al. (1990) Pancreatic islet transplantation after upper abdominal exenteration and liver replacement. Lancet 336:402–405

8 Cystic Pancreatic Neoplasms

Most cystic neoplasms of the pancreas arise from the exocrine components of the gland. Such lesions are much less common than solid exocrine carcinomas. Cystic change in endocrine tumours of the pancreas is unusual (see p. 208), and cystic vascular tumours of the pancreas are even more unusual. The lesions to be considered in this chapter are:

The serous cystadenomas, also known as microcystic, glycogen-rich cystadenomas. Such tumours are nearly always benign.

A type of mucin-secreting cystic tumour with much larger loculi that may behave, even for years, as a benign cystadenoma, but which has, nevertheless, a malignant potential.

A mucin-secreting cystadenocarcinoma that seems, in most cases, to be the result of malignant change in part, or parts, of the wall of a pre-existing mucinous cystic tumour.

In addition, there will be a short review of the published cases, along with the authors' own experience, of a type of partially solid and partially cystic tumour of the pancreas that occurs mainly, but not invariably, in young women or adolescent girls. Names suggested for this tumour include: solid and papillary tumour, papillary and cystic neoplasm, and Frantz's tumour. In many of the published cases of this type of tumour, early surgical removal has been curative, but, as in the case of cystic mucinous tumours, there is an undoubted potential for malignant behaviour.

Other much less common cystic lesions to be discussed include the recently recognised condition of mucinous ductal ectasia, caused by papillary intraductal epithelial hyperplasia, and cavernous lymphangioma of the pancreas.

Incidence

There can be no question about the rarity of cystic neoplasms of the pancreas, but the true incidence is difficult to estimate because such tumours are difficult to pick out of hospital records where they tend to be classified into a heterogeneous group of "pancreatic cysts", a type of lesion whose true nature may be as difficult to determine now as it was over a century ago (Virchow 1887). It has been estimated however, that cystadenomas and cystadenocarcinomas account for at least 12% of pancreatic cysts (Becker et al. 1965)

In the Merseyside region of England, a conurbation with a population of 1.56 million people, Campbell and Cruickshank (1962) scanned the records for the previous 30 years in the hospitals and public mortuaries of the region and could find notes of, and preserved material from, only six cases of serous cystadenoma, eight cases of mucinous cystic pancreatic tumours and three cases of cystadenocarcinoma. In American hospitals the incidence was also low. There were, for example, ten pancreatic cystadenomas among 23 551 surgical specimens at the Presbyterian Hospital in New York (Frantz 1959), 44 patients among about 2.4 million admissions to the Mayo Clinic (Cullen et al. 1963) and 11 cases in the records of four New Orleans hospitals with a total of over 2 million admissions during a 27-year period (Becker et al. 1965). By 1978, however, Compagno and Oertel (1978 a, b) were able to find 75 cases listed as cystadenoma or cystadenocarcinoma of the pancreas in the files of the Armed Forces Institute of Pathology in Washington DC. An analysis of this relatively large collection, from many parts of North America, made it clear, as had been suspected by earlier authors with fewer cases, that, until that time the diagnosis of cystadenoma of the pancreas had encompassed two neoplasms with different pathological characteristics, one of which was entirely benign while the other was potentially or actually malignant. They called the benign tumours "microcystic adenomas" ("glycogen-rich cystadenomas") and entitled the other type "mucinous cystic neoplasms of the pancreas with overt and latent malignancy (cystadenocarcinoma and cystadenoma)". Their series included 34 cases of the benign type of tumour and 41 of the malignant, or potentially malignant, mucinous cystic neoplasms. This classification is now generally accepted. Thus in 1985, Chen and Baithun, in their analysis of 391 cases of exocrine tumours of the pancreas recorded in the Department of Morbid Anatomy of the London Hospital, found only four cases of serous cystadenoma, all of which were incidental autopsy findings, and ten cases of cystadenocarcinoma. They classified none of these as examples of mucinous cystadenomas, but Warshaw et al. (1990) found 15 apparently benign mucinous cystic neoplasms in their series of 67 patients with cystic pancreatic neoplasms treated in the Massachusetts General Hospital in Boston, MA.

Serous Cystadenoma, Microcystic Adenoma (Glycogen-Rich Cystadenoma)

The above titles have been used for the type of cystic neoplasms in which the cystic spaces contain serous fluid and in which the risk of malignant behaviour is almost negligible. It is a rare tumour, but between 1978 and 1991 no less than 211 cases were reported (Pyke et al. 1992).

Age

In Compagno and Oertel's (1987a) series of 34 cases, the ages of the patients ranged from 34 to 88 years, with both a mean and median age of 68 years; 28 (82%) of the patients were over the age of 60 years. One of the present authors (AHC) has now had personal experience of 12 serous microcystic adenomas. The specimens were obtained from patients whose ages ranged from 53 years to 90 years, with a mean of 71 years.

Sex

In most of the publications before 1978 (e.g. those by Mozan (1951), Campbell and Cruickshank (1962), Becker et al. (1965)), female patients with pancreatic cystadenomas substantially outnumbered males, but, when Compagno and Oertel (1978a, b) had separated the microcystic adenomas from the mucinous tumours, they found that 21 of the patients with microcystic tumours were female and 13 were male. They considered this difference in the sex incidence to be unimportant. Nevertheless, in 12 examples of microcystic serous cystadenomas of the pancreas collected by one of the present authors, only one of the tumours was found in a man, only one of the eight studied by Shorten et al. (1986) was from a male, while all four of the microcystic tumours studied by Yamaguchi and Enjoji (1987) were from women. Likewise, the three serous cystadenomas in the series reported by Kerlin et al. (1987) were all from women, and 11 of the 14 serous cystadenomas collected by Alpert et al. (1988) were also from women, as were the two cases reported by Doberstein et al. (1990); moreover, 72% of the examples collected by Warshaw et al. (1990) were from females.

Pathology

Macroscopically, these tumours are usually well circumscribed, but, especially with the larger tumours, there may be some fibrous adhesions to adjacent organs. They are roughly spheroidal and, although their size varies, they seldom exceed 10 cm in diameter. Amongst those studied by the authors, the largest measured 13 x 10 x 10 cm, but Becker et al. (1965) reported one that was 20 cm in diameter. When these tumours are bisected, they do not collapse and can be seen to contain loculi that seldom exceed 2 cm in diameter, from which thin serous fluid escapes. The loculi give the cut surface a honeycomb appearance, especially peripherally, the central region tending to be myxoid and non-cystic (Fig. 8.1). The central solid tissue is white and glistening; it radiates irregularly towards the periphery, reaching the capsule in places. It may be slightly gritty, a quality that seems to prevent the specimen from collapsing when it is bisected and may explain why no important reduction in the size of the tumour can be obtained by aspiration of fluid. The capsule is thin and translucent and is well defined as far as adjacent organs are concerned, but becomes difficult to recognise where the cystadenoma is attached to normal pancreatic tissue. The cystic spaces do not contain macroscopically recognisable

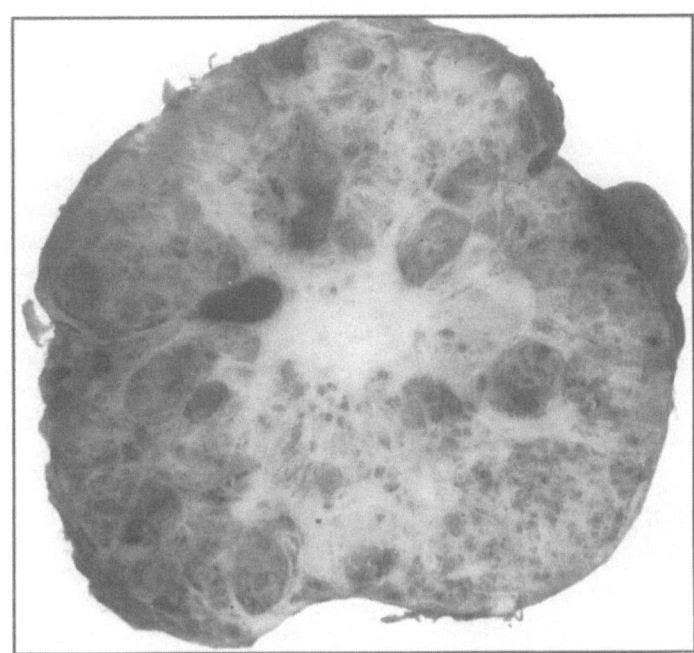

Fig. 8.1. A cystadenoma of the small locular type from the front of the head of the pancreas in a 78-year-old woman. The cystic spaces lie in a myxomatous stroma. (Courtesy of the editor of the *Journal of Clinical Pathology*) Natural size

papillary processes. The gross appearances from tumour to tumour are remarkably similar, as has been pointed out by Becker et al. (1965). The predominant colour is whitish, but areas of recent haemorrhage are quite common and loculi containing brown fluid and with rust-like material on their walls are attributable to old haemorrhage. In one case in our experience there was fatal intraperitoneal haemorrhage from a serous cystadenoma of the pancreas. No communication between the cystic loculi and the pancreatic ducts has been demonstrated in autopsy specimens or by retrograde pancreatography during life (Warshaw et al. 1990).

Microscopically, the loculi are lined by cuboidal or flattened epithelium (Fig. 8.2). The degree of the epithelial flattening seems to be determined by the amount of dilatation of the cystic loculi and, in the routinely stained sections of their three cases of serous cystadenoma, Bogomoletz et al. (1980) were able to recognise a change of pattern in different areas of the sections. In one of the patterns there were collections of small undilated cysts in a loose myxoid stroma that did not form septa between the cystic spaces. They named this the "porous" pattern; in such areas, the cysts were lined by cuboidal cells with abundant clear cytoplasm. In the other pattern, larger cystic spaces were separated from each other by thin definite septa. They named this the "spongy" pattern; in these areas, the spaces were lined by

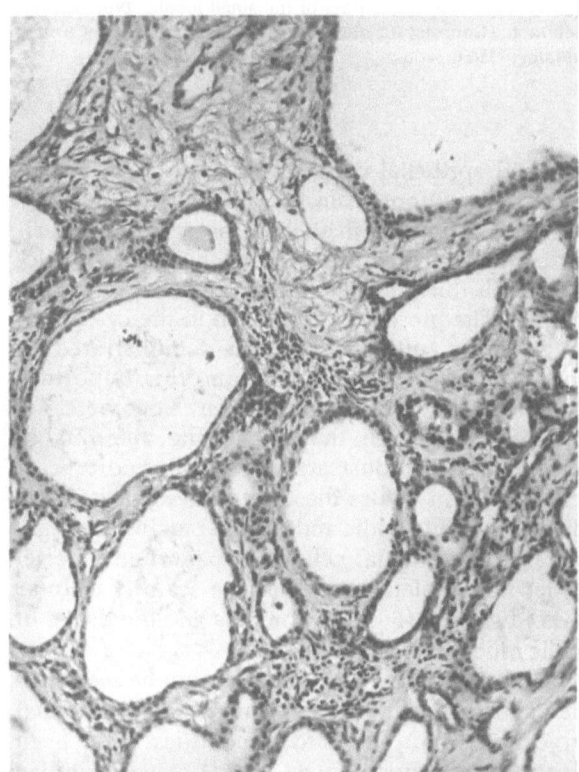

Fig. 8.2. Small locular type of cystadenoma. The spaces are lined by low epithelium that is not secreting mucus. (Courtesy of the editor of the *Journal of Clinical Pathology*) H&E, × 120

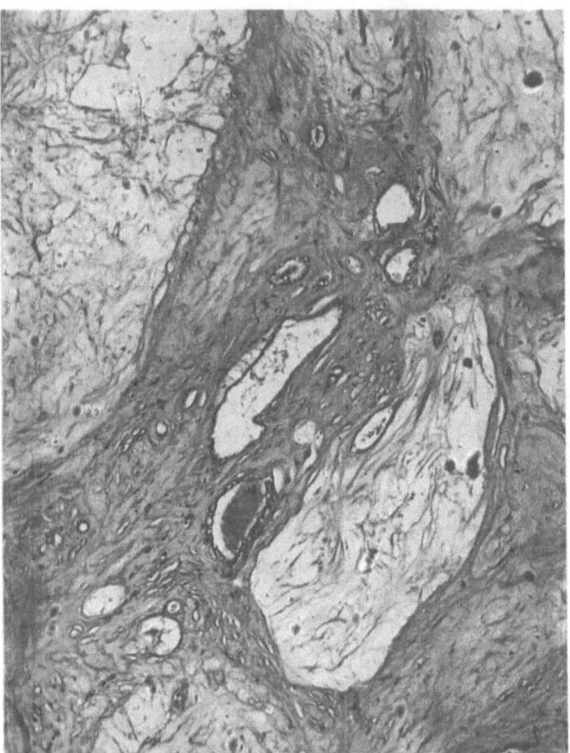

Fig. 8.3. Myxomatous stroma of the small locular type of cyst-adenoma. (Courtesy of the editor of the *Journal of Clinical Pathology*) H&E, × 60

flattened epithelial cells that had an endothelioid aspect. Transitions from the porous to the spongy pattern were present in all their cases. In our experience, the spongy pattern has been the more conspicuous, with thick fibrous trabeculae between groups of cysts. The presence of glycogen in the cytoplasm of the lining epithelial cells was demonstrated by Compagno and Oertel (1978a) and this important diagnostic feature was confirmed by Bogomoletz et al. (1980), although they found the amounts of glycogen, as demonstrated by the periodic acid-Schiff reaction before diastase, somewhat variable. Mucin stains for acidic and neutral mucins are negative in the epithelial cells (Compagno and Oertel 1978a; Bogomoletz 1992), but the scantily cellular myxoid stroma (Fig. 8.3) contains an abundance of acidic mucopolysaccharide.

Although papillary processes cannot be seen with the naked eye, there may be microscopic epithelial projections into the cystic spaces; these have been illustrated by Bogomoletz (1992). Such papillae consist of small tufts of projecting epithelial cells without definite fibrovascular cores. In these, the epithelial cells form a single layer and appear cyto-

logically to be entirely bland. In many of the spaces, however, the epithelial lining has been lost to a variable extent; this was found by Warshaw et al. (1990) to have been misleading in biopsies carried out during operations. The epithelial lining includes no goblet cells, and no argentaffin or argyrophilic cells.

Becker et al. (1965) seem to have been the first to suggest that the epithelium that lines the loculi is centro-acinar epithelium. Centro-acinar cells are difficult to recognise on routine examination of the pancreas except as nuclei surrounded by pale-staining cytoplasm in the central part of an acinus, but they have been identified as the cells of the tiny duct that drains the acinus. These cells tend to be more or less invaginated into the lumen of the acinus on one of its sides (Ham 1974), hence the name that has been given to them. Because such cells are so inconspicuous, the origin of the small acinar type of cyst-adenoma from such cells is not obvious, but the suggestion seems to be the best explanation for the origin of this sort of tumour. The light and ultra-structural studies carried out by Lo et al. (1977) on a cystadenoma of the microcystic type, showed the similarity between the cells that lined the cystic spaces and the centro-acinar cells of the normal pancreas. These workers noted the presence of glycogen granules in the cytoplasm of the cells and pointed out that this was a feature of foetal, though not adult, centro-acinar cells. Compagno and Oertel (1978a) also found the ultrastructure of the cells to be compatible with that of centro-acinar cells, while Bogomoletz et al. (1980) found, in the two microcystic adenomas that they were able to study with the electron microscope, that the neoplastic cells were fairly similar to the centro-acinar cells of the normal pancreas. Further ultrastructural studies that have been summarised by Bogomoletz (1992) support an origin from centro-acinar cells. He has also reviewed the recent immunohistochemical studies and states that the epithelial cytoplasm expresses cytokeratin and epithelial membrane antigen, and that no immunoreactivity for carcinoembryonic antigen, or for endocrine peptide markers, has been demonstrated. The presence of myoepithelial cells, first reported by Nyongo and Huntrakoon (1985) in their ultrastructural studies has not been confirmed by Kim et al. (1990). The latter found, instead, that vimentin-positive cells, which they took to be pericytes, were present within the interstitial space incorporated closely with the basal lamina of the cyst wall.

Patchy calcification may occur in the stroma (Fig. 8.4). This is usually recognisable only microscopically and may be associated with some formation of bone, but it was reported radiologically before operation by Haukohl and Melamed (1950),

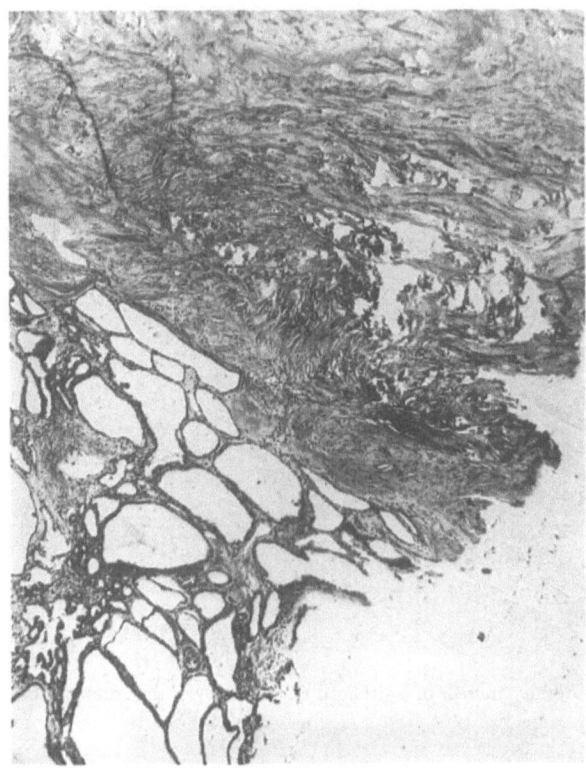

Fig. 8.4. Small locular type of cystadenoma, in which darkly staining calcium in the fibrous wall has caused fragmentation of the section. von Kossa, × 32

and was so marked in one of their cases that the excised tumour was difficult to cut. Both the cases reported by Haukohl and Melamed were, as is illustrated by their photomicrographs, of the small locular type. Calcification was present in 18% of Mozan's (1951) collected cases, but was mentioned in only 10% of the reports of the cases reviewed by Becker et al. (1965). Using a computed tomographic technique, Johnson et al. (1988) found that radiological calcification was present in 38% of their 16 serous cystadenomas. The appearances of a central scar with sunburst calcification, however, though previously taken to be highly suggestive of the serous type of cystadenoma, was seen in only two of the 18 serous cystadenomas examined by Warshaw et al. (1990), who also used computed tomographic scans.

A cystadenoma of the pancreas was reported by Davison et al. in 1936, in association with the cystic pancreatic lesions of the von Hippel–Lindau syndrome; their illustrations show the cystadenoma to be of the small locular serous type. Since that time it has become accepted that this type of pancreatic cystadenoma may, occasionally, be a component of

the von Hippel–Lindau syndrome (Fishman and Bartholomew 1979; Lamiell et al. 1989; Maher et al. 1990; Neumann et al. 1991). Other pancreatic components of the syndrome are discussed in relation to congenital lesions of the pancreas (pp. 43–44).

A multicentric type of microcystic serous cystadenoma of the pancreas has been recognised by Kim et al. (1990). These authors found that two of the three cases of microcystic adenoma that they reported were multicentric within the pancreas. This led them to speculate that confluence of such tumours might lead to the formation of a single larger tumour. Such confluence of multiple serous cystadenomas appears to have occurred in two of the cases reported by Fishman and Bartholomew (1979).

Serous Cystadenocarcinoma

In 1989, George et al. reported what they believed to be the first recorded case of serous cystadenocarcinoma of the pancreas. At that time, these authors were able to find reports of 113 cases of serous cystadenoma in the English literature and none of these tumours had behaved malignantly. In their case, however, a tumour with naked eye, microscopic and ultramicroscopic appearances of a serous cystadenoma, situated at the tail of the pancreas in a man aged 70 years, had infiltrated the splenic vein and the spleen itself as well as the wall of the stomach. Death was caused by severe haemorrhage during an operation in which splenectomy, distal pancreatectomy, partial gastrectomy and a wedge resection of the liver had been carried out. The resected wedge of liver contained a metastatic tumour deposit, 1.5 cm in diameter, and five or six similar metastatic nodules were found in the liver at autopsy. Metastases were not found elsewhere and no primary cancer was found in the other organs.

Mucinous Cystic Neoplasm with Latent Malignancy, Mucinous Cystadenoma, Large Locular Cystadenoma

The macroscopic appearances of this type of tumour are illustrated in Fig. 8.5. In this type of cystadenoma, the sizes of the loculi vary much more than in the small locular type. Some loculi may be only 1 cm in diameter, while others may be 6 or 8 cm; some tumours may consist of only one cystic cavity. The contents of the loculi are mucoid, thick

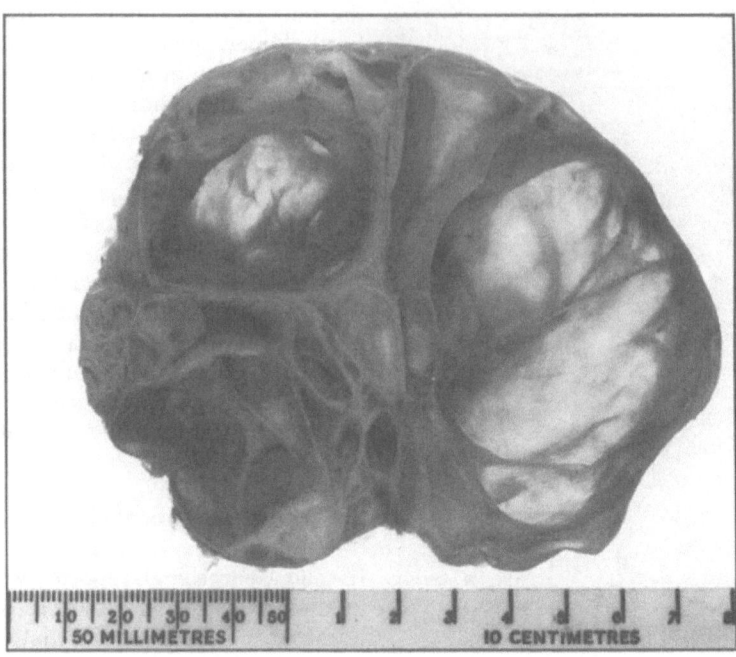

Fig. 8.5. Large locular cystadenoma removed surgically from the body of the pancreas of a girl aged 13. (Courtesy of the editor of the *Journal of Clinical Pathology*)

and viscid; papillary projections into the loculi may be seen with the naked eye in some, but not in all, of these tumours. This type of tumour tends to be larger than the small locular type and is more liable to be adherent to adjacent organs. The mucoid contents are usually grey and opaque but may be blood stained or brownish. The resemblance of this type of cystadenoma to a multilocular mucin-secreting cystadenoma of the ovary may be so close that, during an operation upon a woman, it is only when the attachments have been defined that the two types of tumour can be differentiated. Adhesions to the stomach, transverse colon and spleen are common, and can sometimes be recognised as being due to the granulomatous pseudomyxomatous type of reaction that occurs around mucus that has escaped into the tissues. When the tumours are bisected, the contents escape and the larger loculi, whose walls are usually thin, collapse. The fibrous septa between the loculi are also more delicate that those in the small locular type of cystadenoma and this too favours the collapse of the incised tumour. As in the small locular type, some calcification may be present in the capsule and septa. A peripheral rim of calcification found by tomographic scanning may be a danger signal; Warshaw et al. (1990) found, to their surprise, that, in six mucinous tumours with this sign,

there was malignancy when the excised tumours were examined pathologically.

Microscopically (Fig. 8.6), the loculi of this type of tumour are lined by tall columnar epithelial cells, with basal nuclei and clear vacuolated cytoplasm that stains with both mucicarmine and alcian blue. The fibrous septa, unlike those of the small locular type of tumour, give no reaction with stains for mucins. Papillary epithelial projections are marked, especially in the smaller loculi. Glycogen is not found; goblet cells and a few Paneth cells may be present. When immunoperoxidase methods were used, Warshaw et al. (1990) found neuroendocrine cells in the majority of their 15 apparently benign mucinous cystadenomas. There is also strong immunostaining for carcinoembryonic antigen in the epithelium; it also accumulates in the cyst contents (Yu and Shetty 1985).

The appearances of the epithelial lining of the spaces suggest that the tumours are derived from the mucus-secreting epithelium that lines the larger pancreatic ducts. Such epithelium is also found in the gall bladder and bile ducts, and cystadenomas similar to the large locular type of cystadenoma have been reported in relation to the biliary passages (Edmondson 1958; Corrin 1962). Neuroendocrine cells have been recognised in the epithelium of the larger pancreatic ducts. A mucus-

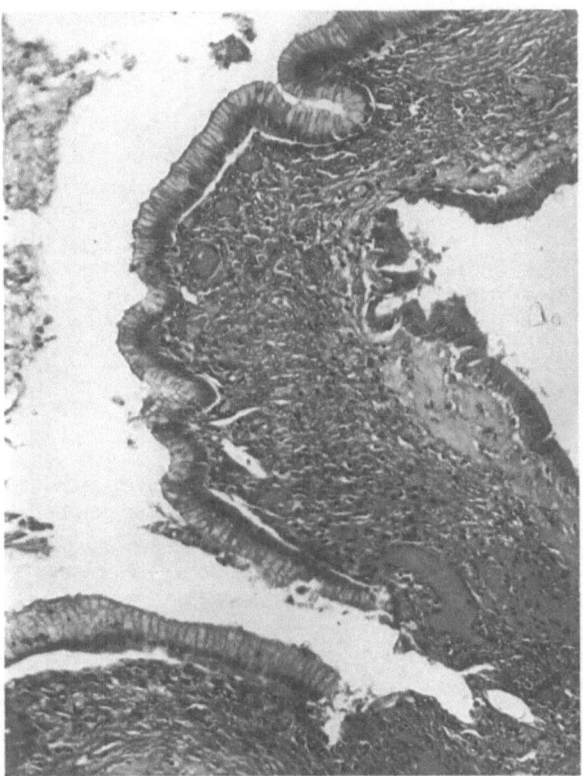

Fig. 8.6. Mucus-secreting epithelium lining the loculi of the large locular type of cystadenoma removed surgically from a woman aged 37. (Courtesy of the editor of the *Journal of Clinical Pathology*) H&E, × 120

secreting cystadenoma with many islands of argentaffin cells in its walls, and a carcinoid tumour in the wall of the cyst, has been reported by Persaud and Walrond (1971).

The large locular, mucin-secreting type of cystadenoma is potentially, or actually, malignant. The risk of malignancy may, at first, be very low, but, as has been emphasised by Compagno and Oertel (1978b), virtually all of these neoplasms will, given sufficient time, form foci that are histologically identifiable as carcinoma; it is necessary to take many samples from different parts of these tumours to avoid missing foci of malignancy. Total excision is necessary, as remnants left by procedures such as marsupialisation or internal drainage will lead to recurrence and possible metastasis. There have been several reports of eventual carcinomatous behaviour by the remnants of incompletely removed mucinous cystadenomas (Speese 1915; Judd et al. 1931; Young 1937; Campbell and Cruickshank 1962; Grosfield et al. 1970). In cases diagnosed as cystadenocarcinoma, too, there is often clinical or anatomical evidence of a pre-existing mucus-secreting cystadenoma

(Becker et al. 1965; Hodgkinson et al. 1978b). More recently, Albores-Saavedra et al. (1987), in their study of 20 mucinous cystadenocarcinomas of the pancreas, found that six of their specimens had been diagnosed originally as cystadenomas.

Anatomical Site

It has been said (Hoover et al. 1991) that the serous microcystic adenomas are most likely to be found in the head of the pancreas, while the mucinous tumours tend to occur in the body or tail of the gland, but cystadenomas of either type may develop in any part of the pancreas, although the region of the tail seems to be the area most likely to be affected. The bigger tumours often involve adjacent parts of the pancreas or may replace the whole gland (Becker et al. 1965).

A cystadenoma of the mucinous type within the spleen was described by Satake et al. (1979). The tumour, which was near the hilum of the spleen but was completely separated from the tail of the pancreas, was thought to have arisen in heterotopic pancreatic tissue within the spleen.

Clinical Effects

Cystadenomas of either type seem seldom to be associated with symptoms, unless they are more than about 5 cm in diameter. Smaller tumours have usually been incidental findings, either at autopsy or during operations for non-pancreatic disease, especially during surgery for biliary disease. The effects of large tumours are probably due to pressure upon adjacent structures; the splenic vein seems particularly liable to compression. Many descriptions of pancreatic cystadenomas mention their vascularity, and slight or moderate splenomegaly may be produced by venous congestion. Congestion of the area of gastric mucosa draining to the splenic vein by the vasa brevia may cause bleeding into the stomach (Grunberg et al. 1952), and there are usually haemorrhagic loculi within both types of cystadenoma. Episodes of haemorrhage into these tumours may account for the pain recorded in the case histories of many of the reported cystadenomas, although certain patients have had only a symptomless mass in the epigastrium or left upper abdominal quadrant. Severe haemorrhage into a papillary cystadenoma of the pancreas, with leakage of blood into the lesser sac of the peritoneum and through the foramen of Winslow into the general peritoneal cavity, caused an abdominal emergency in a girl aged 17 (Mallory 1941). Rupture of a haemorrhagic

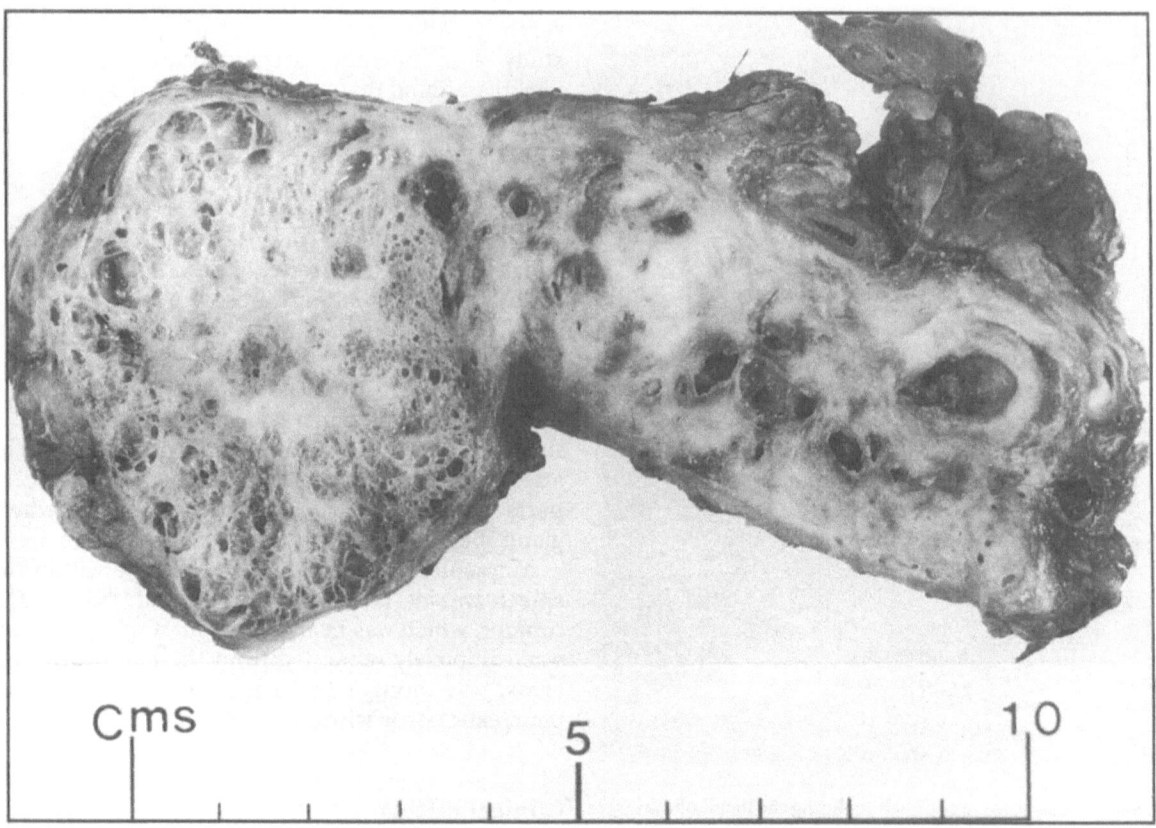

Fig. 8.7. An unusual effect of the microcystic cystadenoma in the head of this pancreas is that it appears to have caused dilatation of the ducts in the body and tail of the gland. The patient had complained of severe abdominal pain. (Courtesy of Dr Kathleen Lodge)

loculus that had become adherent to the stomach, with discharge of blood into the stomach, was suggested to have occurred in one of the cases reported by Campbell and Cruickshank (1962) to explain the episodes of severe haematemesis and melaena associated with a cystadenoma of the large locular type. Although the part of the stomach to which the tumour was adherent was removed along with the cystadenoma, the specimen was too fragmented to be informative, but a reduction in the size of the abdominal swelling, observed after one of the preoperative episodes of haemorrhage, was taken to be due to the escape of blood into the stomach following ulceration of the stomach and the establishment of a communication through which the haemorrhagic contents of the cystadenoma escaped. In a more recent patient in the experience of one of the authors, a serous cystadenoma of the pancreas in a women aged 76 years caused fatal intraperitoneal bleeding.

In many patients, the pain, which is rarely severe, is difficult to explain pathologically. Partial obstruction of the common bile duct in cystadenomas in the head of the pancreas with associated biliary disease is a possible cause of pain. Disease of the biliary tract is associated in 12% of patients according to Becker et al. (1965), but jaundice due to the effects of a cystadenoma of the head of the pancreas is rare. In one of the Merseyside cases (Campbell and Cruickshank 1962), in which there was a cystadenoma of the small locular type, 7 cm in diameter, in the head of the pancreas, there was fat necrosis in the body of the pancreas and an abscess at the tail. In the case illustrated in Fig. 8.7, a microcystic cystadenoma in the head of the pancreas can be seen to be associated with obstructive dilatation of the pancreatic duct. The patient had had abdominal pain for a few months before her admission to hospital. The pain, which was felt in the hypochondrium, had become severe during the 2 weeks immediately before her admission.

Diabetes mellitus is present in only a few patients (8% according to Becker et al. 1965), and is probably incidental and unrelated, but transient glycosuria or hyperglycaemia is not uncommon post-operatively when a cystadenoma has been removed.

In a series of 30 cases of pancreatic cystadenoma reported by Soloway in 1965, there was a high incidence of associated tumours, both benign and malignant, while in the female patients, who substantially outnumbered the males, a spontaneous or induced premature menopause often preceded the appearance of the pancreatic lesion by many years. This was not, however, the experience of Hodgkinson et al. (1978a) in their series of 45 cases.

Differential Diagnosis

As has been mentioned already, the true nature of cystic lesions of the pancreas may be obscure. The lesions most likely to be confused pathologically with cystadenoma of the pancreas are cystic carcinomas and carcinomas that have caused obstruction of the pancreatic ducts with resulting dilatation; such dilatation is, however, seldom sufficiently marked to simulate a cystadenoma. In cystadenomas of the large locular type with many papillary epithelial processes, whose malignant potential is well known, a dogmatic microscopic distinction between simplicity and malignancy may scarcely be justified, although, if metastatic spread has not occurred and the tumour has been removed completely, a good prognosis is justified. Immunohistochemical tests, such as the demonstration of carcinoembryonic antigen reactivity, may be useful indicators of malignant potential. The use and interpretation of such tests has been described and discussed by Yamaguchi and Enjoji (1987) and by Warshaw et al. (1990).

The recognition of pseudocysts and their differentiation from cystadenomas is mainly by chemical examination of the contents of the cysts. The contents of pseudocysts include an abundance of pancreatic enzymes, while only insignificant amounts are present in the contents of cystadenomas. Microscopically, an epithelial lining is absent from the walls of a pseudocyst, but a substantial loss of the epithelial lining may occur in a cystadenoma. The development of a pseudocyst is usually preceded by a history of trauma or of pancreatitis; such causes do not contribute to the development of a cystadenoma.

In the small locular type of cystadenoma, the endothelial appearance of the lining epithelium may suggest a diagnosis of lymphangioma. If there is doubt, the demonstration of glycogen within the cystoplasm of the lining of the cells may help to establish the diagnosis of cystadenoma.

The congenital cystic lesions of the pancreas in the von Hippel–Lindau syndrome may be almost indistinguishable from those of the small locular pancreatic cystadenoma and may be accompanied by cystadenoma of either type. In such cases, the effects of the hamartomatous lesions of the central nervous system dominate the clinical illness, the symptomatic effects of the pancreatic lesions being insignificant.

In fibrocystic disease of the pancreas associated with mucoviscidosis, the cysts are seldom large enough (even in a child who has survived for 10 or more years), or sufficiently localised, to resemble a cystadenoma.

Retroperitoneal dermoid cysts in the vicinity of the pancreas have been reported (Kerr 1918; Dennis 1923); in such cysts the presence of hair in the greasy material characteristic of dermoid cysts appears to have been important in establishing the diagnosis.

The pancreas is a very rare site for the hydatid cysts of *Echinococcus granulosus*, and, as was reported by Kattan (1975), the Casoni test may be negative. However, the macroscopic appearances at laparotomy are usually characteristic. The complement-fixation test is helpful if the diagnosis is suspected pre-operatively (Anderson and Peebles Brown 1959–1960). The pancreatic duct may communicate with the cyst and its secretion may give the hydatid fluid and daughter cysts an unusually milky colour.

In some older publications, for example Hueper (1928), cysts due to the retention of secretion are mentioned, and the condition of the ranula pancreatica, a beaded type of dilatation of the pancreatic duct, is attributed to obstruction of the pancreatic duct with retention of secretion in chronic pancreatitis. This type of lesion seems unlikely to be confused with a cystadenoma of the pancreas, and the idiopathic dilatation of the pancreatic duct, of which four cases were noted by White in 1897, and which has occurred in the experience of the authors, is obviously a lesion of the duct and has no resemblance to a cystadenoma (see Fig. 3.16). The authors have no personal experience of the cystic dilatation of the pancreatic duct that may be caused by intraductal mucin-hypersecreting neoplasms of the pancreas, but publications, such as that by Rickaert et al. (1991), suggest that the clinical diagnosis depends upon endoscopic retrograde pancreatography.

Cystadenocarcinoma

The recognition of cystadenocarcinoma and its distinction from solid carcinoma of the pancreas is of importance because, while the prospects of a cure by excision of a solid carcinoma in any part of the pancreas are poor, even large cystadenocarcinomas that have not extended to adjacent important organs, can be cured by resection (Becker et al. 1965).

Incidence

Cystadenocarcinoma is even rarer than cystadenoma, the incidence being about half that of cystadenoma, but, by 1965, Becker et al. were able to collect reports of 63 cases to which they added two of their own. They tabulated the available information about these 65 cases and, when they had analysed the information, they were able to offer some useful generalisations about the disease. In 1968, Warren and Hardy published their study of 17 cases of cystadenocarcinoma collected from amongst 993 pancreatic operations carried out at the Lahey Clinic Foundation in Boston. In 1978, Compagno and Oertel (1978b) searched the files of the Armed Forces Institute of Pathology for tumours listed as cystadenoma or cystadenocarcinoma; of the 75 tumours so classified, they selected 41 mucinous cystic tumours that they considered to have overt or latent malignancy.

Also in 1978, Hodgkinson et al. (1978b), in their study of 21 cases from the files of the Mayo Clinic, were impressed by the relatively low grade of malignancy in most of them, along with signs that the cystadenocarcinomas were the result of malignant change in pre-existing mucinous cystadenomas. More recent results such as those of ReMine et al. (1987) and Warshaw et al. (1990), indicate that, while some cystadenocarcinomas may be of low histopathological malignancy, having only foci in which cells are piled up without individual cell contact with the basement membrane, a substantial number of others are of high clinical and histological malignancy by the time they are diagnosed.

Sex

As with cystadenoma, there is usually a marked female preponderance; about three-quarters (76%) of the cases reviewed by Becker et al. were women. A slightly less marked, but still substantial, female preponderance was evident in the cases collected by Warren and Hardy (1968), 11 of these patients being women, while Compagno and Oertel's (1978b) cases included 35 women and six men. In the Mayo Clinic series, however, the numbers of men and women were almost equal (Hodgkinson et al. 1978b); this was also so in the 11 cases of ReMine et al. 1987.

However, in the 27 cases in the series studied by Warshaw et al. (1990), 74% of the patients were women.

Age

Of the 55 cases reviewed by Becker et al. (1965), in which the age was given, 28 patients, just under half the series, were less than 50 years old; the youngest was 18 and the oldest was 76. The ages of Warren and Hardy's (1968) patients ranged from 23 to 77, the average age being 52 years, while Compagno and Oertel's (1978b) cases had an age range of 20–82 years, with a mean age of 49. In their cases there was a striking difference between the ages of the two sexes, the mean age of the women being 45 years while that of the men was 70. In the cases of ReMine et al. (1987) the age distributions were similar in the two sexes, with an average age of 60 years; in Warshaw et al.'s cases the average age was 63 years. A 17-year-old girl with a cystadenocarcinoma of the pancreas was reported by Corrente in 1980. Four years earlier this patient had received a blunt epigastric injury, sufficiently severe to cause her admission to the hospital, and it was suggested that a traumatic pseudocyst might have been complicated by the development of cystadenocarcinoma.

Macroscopic Appearances

Cystadenocarcinomas resemble their benign counterparts, the large locular mucinous type of cystadenoma, and their position in the pancreas is similar, the majority of the tumours being in the tail or body, although, in the 17 cases studied by Warren and Hardy (1968), this was not so, the distribution being equal in the three regions of the pancreas. Cystadenocarcinomas tend to be larger than cystadenomas, varying from about 5 cm in diameter to 25–30 cm, and usually have a papillary structure that is more obvious than that of the large locular cystadenoma (Fig. 8.8). The papillae may, however, be limited to parts of the wall, the remainder of the wall being smooth (Fig. 8.9). The outer parts of the walls are fibrous and are usually about 0.5 cm thick; calcification may be marked in the fibrous tissue (Cornes and Azzopardi 1959–1960; Warshaw et al. 1990) and large amounts of haemosiderin may be present (Campbell and Cruickshank 1962). Local invasiveness seems to precede metastatic spread, at least in some cases, and a cystadenocarcinoma at the tail of the pancreas may invade the spleen. Of more importance as far as symptoms are concerned is the invasion of the stomach or the colon, with the

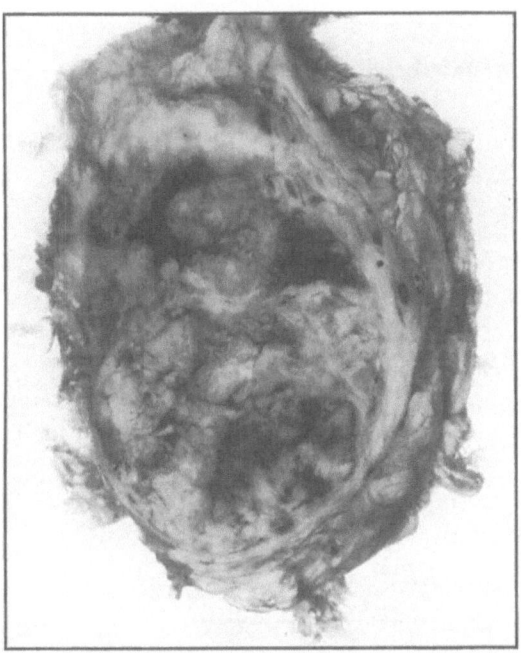

Fig. 8.8. A cystadenocarcinoma, 9 cm in diameter, removed surgically from a woman aged 59. (Courtesy of the editor of the *Journal of Clinical Pathology*)

formation of fistulas. Fistulas into both the stomach and the splenic flexure of the colon had developed in one of the cases reported by Campbell and Cruickshank (1962), although there was no involvement of lymph nodes or other evidence of metastatic spread. These tumours may be multilocular or consist of a single main cavity. In Warren and Hardy's 17 cases, nine of the cysts were multilocular and seven unilocular; in one case the information was not available.

The cyst contents are characteristically greyish mucoid material, which may be brownish or blood stained. Infection of the contents may occur and then the cyst becomes an abscess (Campbell and Cruickshank 1962). Fat droplets may be seen in the contents of uninfected tumours. As in the case of cystadenomas, only trivial amounts of pancreatic enzymes are present in the contents.

The external surface of excised tumours has smooth glistening areas that alternate with shaggy or haemorrhagic areas where adhesions have been divided.

If previous marsupialisation has been carried out, there is usually invasion of the abdominal wall. The behaviour of the fistula that follows this procedure

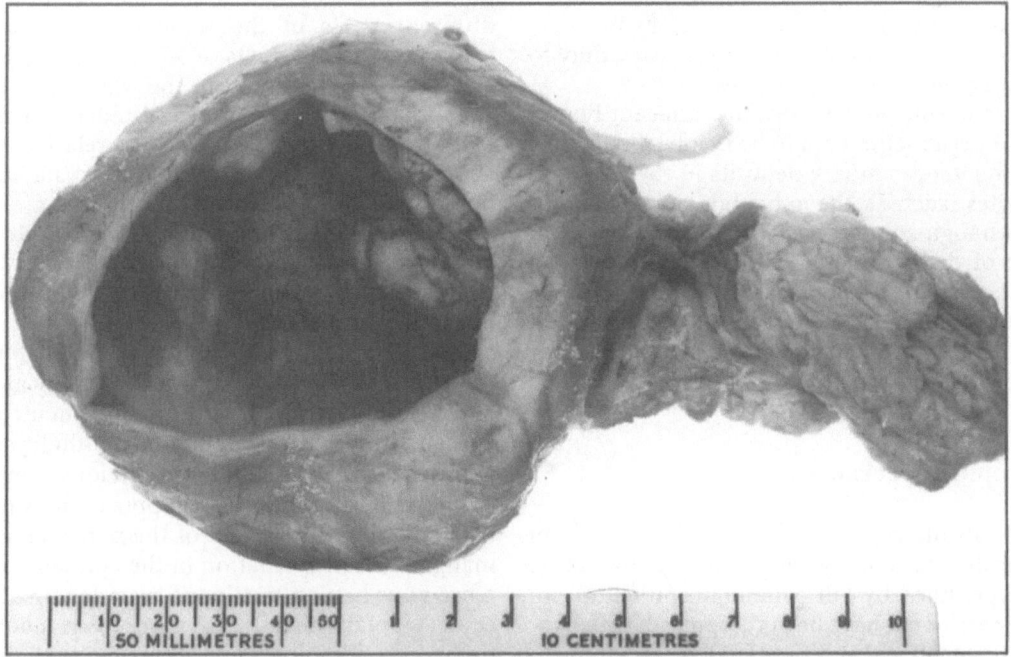

Fig. 8.9. A cystadenocarcinoma of the tail of the pancreas, with an opening in its posterior wall to show the carcinomatous thickening of part of the wall. (Courtesy of the editor of the *Journal of Clinical Pathology*)

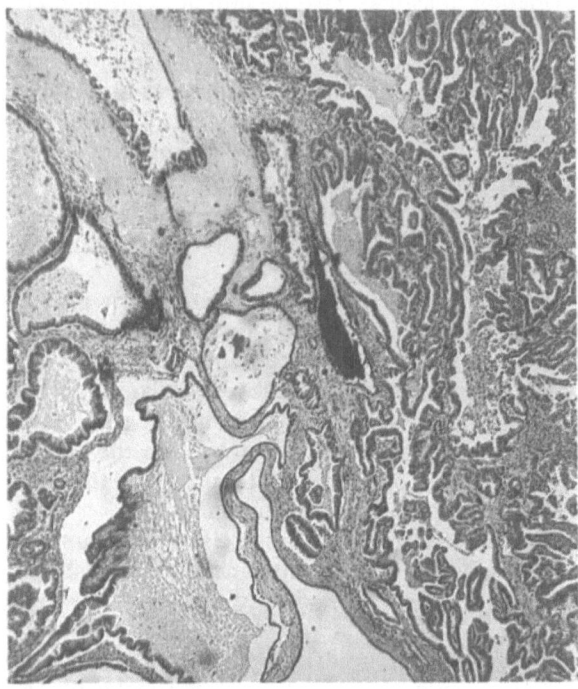

Fig. 8.10. Well-differentiated and less well-differentiated areas in a cystadenocarcinoma. (Courtesy of the editor of the *Journal of Clinical Pathology*) H&E, × 32

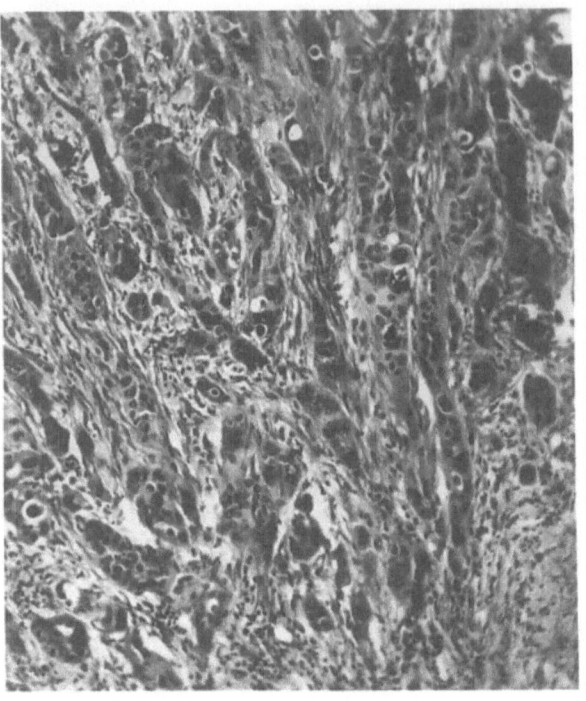

Fig. 8.11. Poorly differentiated area in the same cystadenocarcinoma as that shown in Fig. 8.9. (Courtesy of the editor of the *Journal of Clinical Pathology*) H&E, × 120

seems to reflect the gradual transformation of an originally benign mucus-secreting neoplasm into a cystadenocarcinoma, for the original fistula may close and cause no trouble for several years, only to recur as an obviously malignant lesion.

In patients with metastases, the adjacent lymph nodes and peritoneum tend to be involved relatively early, with later secondary deposits in the liver and distant sites, such as the subcutaneous tissues or brain. Although some reports refer to radiological evidence of displacement of the left kidney by a cystadenocarcinoma of the tail of the pancreas, the left kidney has not been recognised to have been invaded directly and is only an occasional site for metastatic deposits.

Microscopic Appearances

In almost all the reported cases, transitions from histologically benign cystadenoma of the large locular type, lined by tall columnar epithelium, to papillary carcinoma have been recognised, with progression to anaplastic undifferentiated carcinoma in some cases. Areas of histologically benign neoplastic

epithelium, well-differentiated carcinoma, and poorly differentiated carcinoma may be found in different parts of the same tumour. Pancreatic acinar tissue with ducts or islets of Langerhans can almost always be found in the walls. As a rule, the change from cystadenoma to cystadenocarcinoma is obvious (Figs 8.10, 8.11), but relatively subtle changes from cystadenoma to early cystadenocarcinoma have been illustrated by Cullen et al. (1963), and, because many of the tumours are quite large, it may be necessary to examine many samples from different parts of the tumour to avoid missing foci of malignancy in what may seem, if inadequately sampled, to be a mucinous cystadenoma. The dividing line between histological simplicity and histological malignancy may thus be difficult and the presence of well-differentiated epithelium, along with atypical epithelium and obviously malignant epithelium, in many cases supports the suggestion that cystadenocarcinoma of the pancreas is due to malignant transformation in the epithelial lining of a previous benign mucinous cystadenoma. ReMine et al. (1987) divided their 11 cases of cystadenocarcinoma into two subgroups according to their microscopic appearances. They classified five as of low malignancy and the remaining six as of high malignancy. The clinical courses of the two types showed some correspondence with the grade of malignancy assigned to them microscopically.

More elaborate microscopic studies were carried out by Albores-Saavedra et al. (1987) on material from 20 mucinous pancreatic cystadenocarcinomas, on which they used immunohistological stains and electron microscopy. Most of the tumours were highly heterogeneous with areas of benign-looking epithelium and other areas where the epithelium was cytologically malignant. The well-differentiated areas resembled colonic epithelium, both by light and electron microscopy. Goblet cells, argyrophil and argentaffin cells, and Paneth cells were identified. Immunohistochemically, endocrine cells were shown in 13 of the 20 tumours and were more numerous in the areas of poorly differentiated epithelium. Serotonin-containing cells were the most numerous endocrine cells, followed by somatostatin-containing cells and cells with immunoreactivity for pancreatic polypeptide and gastrin. None of these patients had had clinical effects attributable to these hormones, but the Zollinger–Ellison syndrome in association with a pancreatic cystadenocarcinoma has been reported by Margolis and Jang (1984), and the pancreatic cholera syndrome, due to a cystadenocarcinoma that secreted vasoactive intestinal polypeptide, has been described by Rood et al. (1988). Neuroendocrine cells, as confirmed by immunoperoxidase stains, were found by Warshaw et al. (1990) in 47% of their cystadenocarcinomas, but no clinical effects could be attributed to such cells.

Many of the features described earlier in the section on the mucinous type of cystadenoma can be recognised in parts of cystadenocarcinomas. It will be obvious that mucinous cystic tumours of the pancreas are very similar, both in their appearance and in their behaviour, to mucinous tumours of the ovary; Compagno and Oertel (1978b) even comment on the presence of a dense cellular stroma, resembling that of the ovary and containing scattered mast cells, located under the mucus-secreting epithelium but sufficiently well separated from it to exclude a desmoplastic reaction. There is also a report of the Zollinger–Ellison syndrome in association with a mucinous cystadenocarcinoma of the ovary (Cocco and Conway 1975), and pseudosarcomatous nodules, such as have been described in ovarian mucinous tumours, have been described in a pancreatic mucinous cystadenocarcinoma (Rego et al. 1991).

From the foregoing, it will be clear that cystadenocarcinoma of the pancreas is the result of the progression, from clinical and microscopic benignity in a mucinous cystadenoma, to aggression and, eventually, to invasive and metastasising malignancy. The cell of origin is, as is that of the mucinous cystadenoma, the epithelial cell of the large pancreatic ducts, which is akin to, and closely resembles, the epithelial cells of the biliary passages. The biliary passages too, may occasionally give rise to mucinous tumours, at first apparently benign, but, if incompletely removed, capable of eventual highly malignant behaviour (Cruickshank and Sparshott 1971). The similarities between carcinomas of the gall bladder and mucinous cystadenocarcinomas of the pancreas have been studied by Albores-Saavedra et al. (1988), who attribute the presence of endocrine cells in these tumours to intestinal differentiation. In the pancreas, however, unlike in intrahepatic biliary tumours, pre-existing cystic malformations do not seem to be aetiological factors, and, although preceding chronic pancreatitis has been reported (Dreiling 1959), most patients with mucinous cystic neoplasms do not appear to have suffered from acute or chronic pancreatitis; there is usually no history of alcoholic injury to the pancreas. The marked preponderance of women patients suggests that the female sex hormones may have an influence on the development of these tumours, but there is no definite evidence of any hormonal aetiology.

In common with other types of adenocarcinoma, cystadenocarcinoma of the pancreas may produce carcinoembryonic antigen, and Ferrer et al. (1978) have reported the case of a 40-year-old woman with a serum level of 200 ng/ml of carcinoembryonic antigen, which fell to normal when a mucinous retroperitoneal tumour, thought to be pancreatic, had been removed. The cyst fluid contained carcinoembryonic antigen 100 000 times in excess of the normal blood level.

Acinar Cell Cystadenocarcinoma

A single example of an acinar cell cystadenocarcinoma of the pancreas was reported by Cantrell et al. in 1981; at that time these authors could find no report of a similar tumour. The tumour, in a 64-year-old man, was very large (weight 7 kg) and replaced the body and tail of the pancreas. It had caused secondary peritoneal implants. The acinar characteristics of the carcinoma cells in the cystic and solid parts of the tumour were recognised by light microscopy; zymogen granules, together with the other characteristic features of acinar cells, were demonstrated within the cells by electron microscopy. In 1987, another acinar cell cystadenocarcinoma was recorded by Stamm et al. That was also a large multicystic mass, weighing 2 kg and being 25 cm in diameter, in the body and tail of the pancreas in a male patient. Unlike the tumour described by Cantrell et al., it had caused no recognisable metastases when it was removed, but a solitary hepatic metastasis had to be excised 16 months later. The diagnosis of acinar cell cystadenocarcinoma was based on the ultrastructural demonstration of zymogen granules in the tumour cells.

"Ductectatic" Cystadenoma and Cystadenocarcinoma (Intraductal Papillary Neoplasms of the Pancreas)

An account of some of the reports of a type of pancreatic lesion in which cystic dilatation of the main duct, or a large tributary, caused by a combination of hypersecretion of viscid mucus with partial obstruction by papillary hyperplasia of the epithelial lining of the duct is included here because authors such as Itai et al. (1986) have called this lesion cystadenoma or cystadenocarcinoma of the "ductectatic" type. Itai and his colleagues described five examples of the condition. The abnormality was recognised by endoscopic retrograde pancreatography and all five patients were treated by pancreaticoduodenectomy. In four of the five pathological specimens, the lining epithelium of the dilated ducts was found to be indistinguishable from the epithelial lining of mucinous cystadenomas while, in the fifth specimen, the lining epithelium resembled that of a cystadenocarcinoma. By 1991, some 70 similar pancreatic lesions had had described, mostly by Japanese authors (Rickaert et al. 1991).

An example of such a report is that by Morohoshi et al. (1989). They gave the results of a clinicopathological study of six patients, three of each sex, aged between 64 and 79 years. Three had had a long history of symptoms that suggested chronic pancreatitis. In the others, the pancreatic lesions were found incidentally; one of these had had diabetes for 11 years but had no other symptoms that suggested pancreatic disease. In all six patients, the pancreas was thickened, nodular and hard. The ducts were dilated with mucus and contained solitary or multiple small sessile tumours that were soft, grey-white in colour, and liable to crumble. They did not extend beyond the wall of the duct and did not involve lymph nodes. The pancreatic parenchyma was fibrotic. Microscopically, these tumours had a well-differentiated papillary or papillotubular pattern, in which fibrovascular stalks were covered by columnar epithelial cells with oval basal nuclei. Mitoses were infrequent, but in the three specimens with the papillotubular pattern, there were foci of carcinoma in situ. There was no invasion; acinar fibrosis and the absence of metastases in the lymph nodes was confirmed. Most of the epithelial cells secreted mucus that stained by the periodic acid-Schiff method and with alcian blue. The secretion of mucus was also noted by electron microscopy.

In 1991, Rickaert et al. described the clinical and pathological features of eight additional patients, five men and three women, in whom there were intraductal mucin-hypersecreting neoplasms, with extreme dilatation of the main pancreatic duct. Their ages ranges from 47 to 85 years, and five of them had a history of episodes of pancreatitis with raised levels of serum amaylase. In six of the pathological specimens, there was extreme dilatation of the entire pancreatic duct, and of the tail segment in the remaining two, but, unlike the specimens described and illustrated by Morohoshi et al. (1989), no papillary lesions within the ducts were visible with the naked eye. The dilated segments of the ducts contained viscous mucin; microscopically they were lined by well-differentiated mucin-secreting cells, forming papillary foldings with occasional cellular atypia. None of the specimens contained invasive tumour or metastases, and the six patients who were followed up after their lesions had been resected did well. The authors suggested a common pathogenesis for their cases (to which they gave the name "intraductal mucin-hypersecreting neoplasms of the pancreas"), and those previously described as intraductal papillary neoplasms of the pancreas. They pointed out how such cases differed from true cystadenoma and cystadenocarcinoma of the pancreas.

Such cases are, however, very similar histologically to the condition known as mucinous or multicentric biliary papillomatosis (Veloso et al. 1983; Padfield et al. 1988). The condition is one in which multiple papillomas are found in the intrahepatic and extrahepatic bile ducts. Although nuclear atypia is marked, these tumours are not invasive, at least for several years, and one of the authors (EWB) has seen an example of this rare condition in which papillomas in the common channel at the ampulla of Vater appeared to have contributed to the development of chronic pancreatitis. In mucinous biliary papillomatosis, however, as was noted by Veloso et al., the lesions do not extend into the pancreatic duct proper. Thus, in spite of similarities, intraductal papillary lesions of the pancreas and mucinous biliary papillomatosis are probably separate entities.

Solid and Papillary, Papillary and Cystic Epithelial Neoplasm of the Pancreas (Frantz's Tumour)

A characteristic type of pancreatic tumour of low malignancy, and with a special tendency to occur in young women, has become recognised since 1979, when Compagno et al. found 52 examples in the files of the Armed Forces Institute of Pathology in Washington. Only occasional reports of this rare type of tumour had appeared before that time, although as was suggested by Compagno and his colleagues, examples are likely to have been misclassified in the past.

A list of earlier reports of what would now be classified as this tumour has been prepared by Todani et al. (1988); the list includes: non-functioning islet-cell tumour, acinar-cell carcinoma, papillary cystadenocarcinoma and infantile pancreatic carcinoma. The title that Todani and his colleagues used was "Frantz's tumour". This has the merit of brevity; Virginia Frantz included three examples of this type of tumour in her contribution to the *Atlas of Tumor Pathology*, 1st series, published by the US Armed Forces Institute of Pathology in 1959, and drew attention to the uncertainty about its malignancy.

Another early report is that of Hamoudi et al. in 1970. They used the name papillary epithelial neoplasm of the pancreas and described an escapsulated tumour that was excised radically from the head of the pancreas of a 12-year-old black girl; there was no sign of recurrence 16 months after the pancreaticoduodenectomy. From the ultrastructure of the cells, the authors concluded that the tumour might have been derived from ductular epithelium.

From their collection of cases, Compagno et al. (1979) were able to state that such tumours have a microscopically distinctive solid and papillary epithelial structure and are usually large (the mean diameter of their specimens was 10 cm). The tumours appear macroscopically to be encapsulated, but capsular invasion is seen on microscopic examination. They are found predominantly in the tail of the pancreas and the majority have been found in young women (mean age 24 years); they are often haemorrhagic. In spite of the histological signs of local aggression, follow-up, with a mean time of over 7 years, confirmed the low grade of malignancy. Only one patient died of metastasis; none of the others developed a recurrence. Like Hamoudi and his colleagues, Compagno et al. could find no secretory granules on electron microscopy,

and found that the cells resembled those of the small pancreatic ducts.

In 1980, Cubilla and Fitzgerald were able to add that this type of tumour might be cystic and papillary. In a patient of their own, there was a recurrence in the pancreatic area 7 years after the first operation, and, although complete excision of the recurrence was not possible, the patient was alive 5 years later, 12 years after the original diagnosis.

In 1981, Schlosnagle and Campbell reported two examples of this type of tumour. They too, attributed the tumours to an origin from the cells of small ducts, but found that neurosecretory granules were present in the cells of the tumour from one of their patients. They attributed the granules to partial differentiation of the ductular cells towards endocrine cells. Klöppel (1984), however, in his discussion of this type of tumour gave the opinion, based on his own studies, that these tumours originate from acinar cells. Bombi et al. (1984) also attributed the origin of the tumour to acinar cells, while Learmonth et al. (1985), after ultrastructural and histochemical studies on their two cases, discussed possible acinar differentiation but did not commit themselves further.

Histologically, Klöppel (1984) described the solid areas as resembling endocrine tumours, but felt confident that they could be differentiated from endocrine tumours by the presence of widespread foci of cystic necrosis with haemorrhage and cholesterol granulomas. In various places the tumour cells are arranged around myxoid fibrovascular stalks that give a papillary appearance, but true papillae are not formed. No ductular structures are present. The cytoplasm of the tumour cells may be either clear or eosinophilic, and occasional PAS-positive granules may be present, but these resist digestion with diastase, and glycogen has not been demonstrated. There may be microscopic calcification in the fibrous tissue around areas of necrosis; capsular calcification was a marked radiological feature in one of the papillary cystic tumours in the series of cystic pancreatic tumours reviewed by Warshaw et al. (1990). The nuclei of the tumour cells are regular ovoid and have a delicate but distinct chromatin pattern. Mitotic figures, though present, are scarce. Frantz's tumour is demonstrated in Figs 8.12–8.15.

The more recent ultrastructural studies have been summarised by Bogomoletz (1992), who found that most authors have described closely packed polygonal cells with clear cytoplasm, rounded or indented nuclei, and eccentric nuceoli, and that mitochondria are numerous, but Golgi apparatus and rough endoplasmic reticulum are sparse. Oncocytic change has been described by Rode et al. (1988). Most authors have found electron-dense bodies but there is no

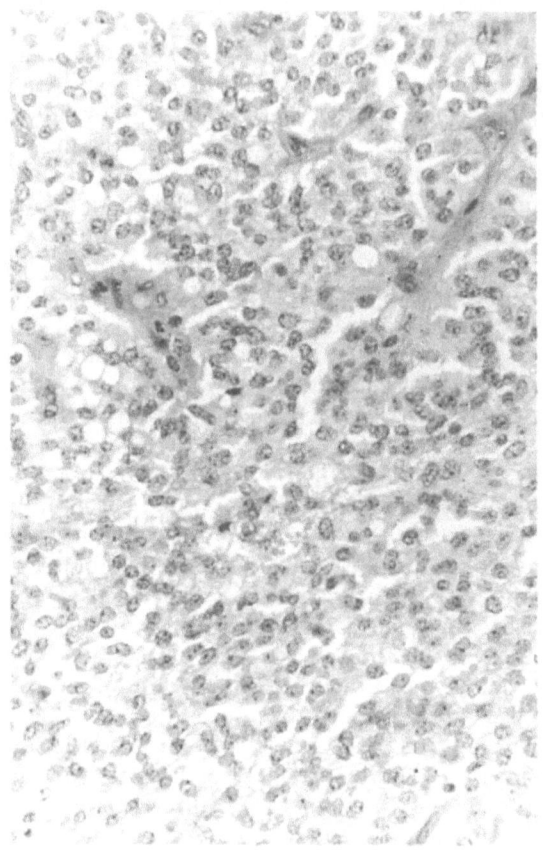

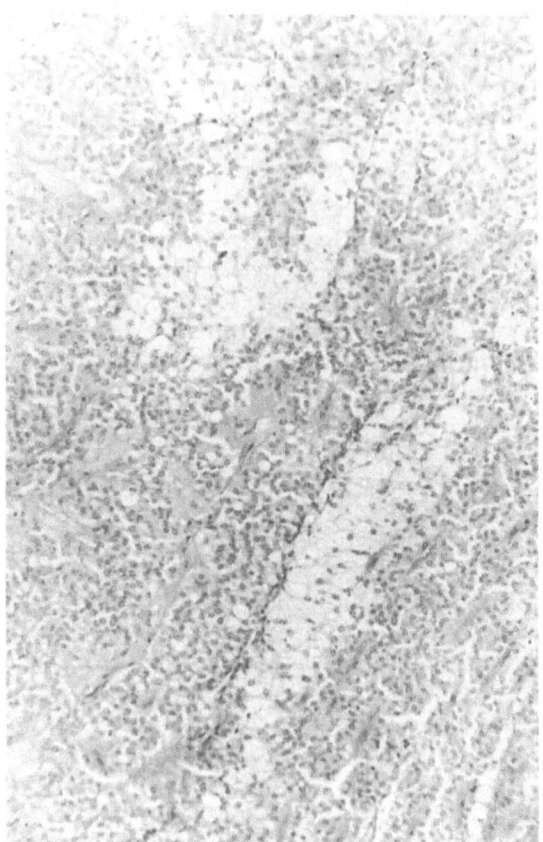

Fig. 8.12. A solid cellular area of a Frantz's tumour, 12 cm in diameter, from the head of the pancreas in a woman aged 19. H&E, × 375

Fig. 8.13. Another solid area from the tumour shown in Fig. 8.12. Clumps of tumour cells with small nuclei and abundant clear cytoplasm are present. H&E, × 150

agreement as to whether, or not, these are neuro-secretory granules. Zymogen-like granules have been taken to indicate acinar cell differentiation.

Immunohistochemical results by various workers, using material from different cases, have also varied somewhat. Klöppel (1984), for example, interpreted results obtained by himself and colleagues as indicating an origin from, and differentiation towards, acinar cells. They obtained positive reactions for alpha$_1$-antitrypsin in some of the cells and sometimes for pancreatic enzymes, such as amylase and lipase, in others. Klöppel suggested that the cystic areas of the tumour might be the result of the digestive effects of the latter enzymes.

Yagihashi et al. (1988), in their two cases, found there was diffuse positivity for neuron-specific enolase in both, with positive reactions also for Grimelius's stain, insulin, glucagon and somatostatin; however, there was some variation in the numbers of positive cells between the two cases. They concluded that both tumours were non-

functioning islet cell tumours, yet other workers (Miettinen et al. 1987) found only foci of endocrine differentiation in their three cases, while Stömmer et al. (1991), in their study of ten cases of the tumour, interpreted their results as indicating the presence of both endocrine and exocrine differentiation.

Oestrogen and progesterone receptors have been demonstrated by Ladanyi et al. (1987) in the two tumours they studied. They included these estimations in their study because of the marked preponderance of these tumours in young women, but, since then, Klöppel et al. (1991) have reported two additional examples of the solid-cystic (papillary-cystic) tumour in young men. The male patients described by these workers were both 25 years old. In one, the large tumour (13 x 11 x 7 cm) was found in the body and tail of the pancreas. In the other, the tumour, which was 7–8 cm in diameter, was extra-pancreatic, but lay retroperitoneally behind the head of the pancreas; there was no connection to, or infiltration of, adjacent organs, and it was removed

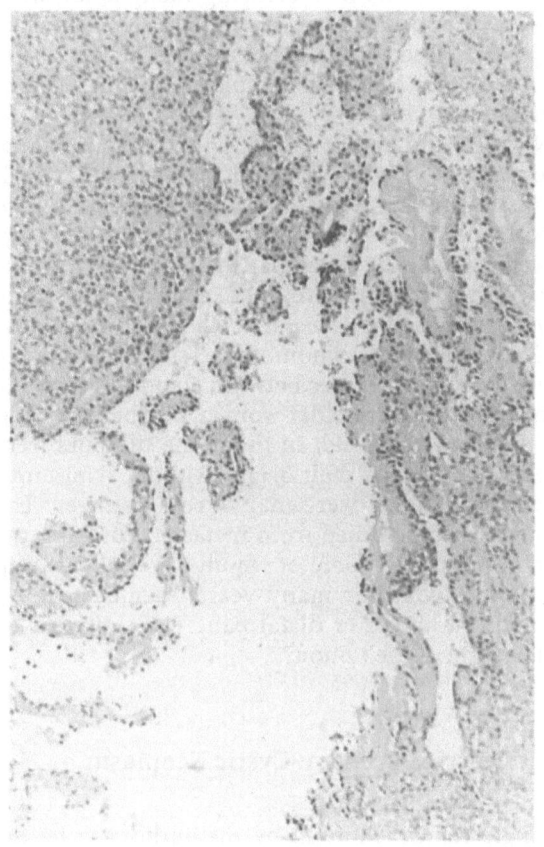

Fig. 8.14. Part of a cystic area in the tumour shown in Figs 8.12. and 8.13. The cystic change has caused papilla-like projections. H&E, × 150

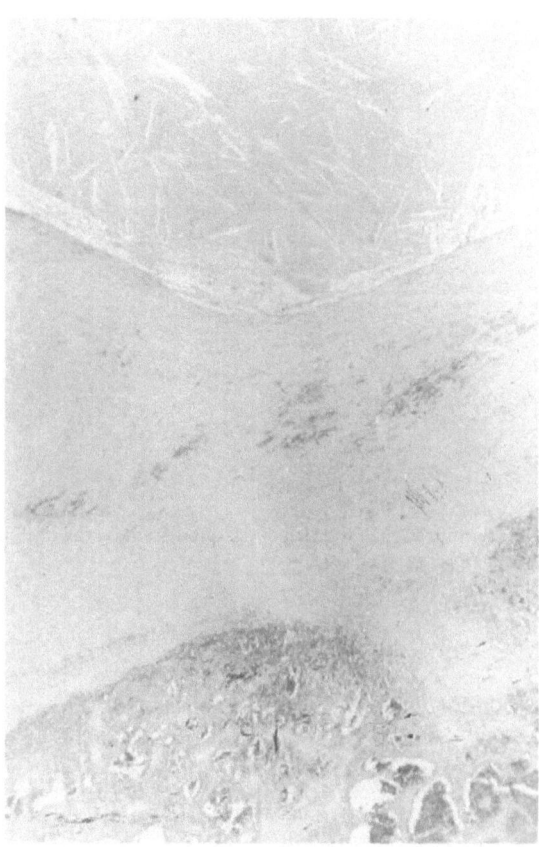

Fig. 8.15. An area of the tumour shown in Figs 8.12.–8.14. Dense, patchily calcified, fibrous tissue separates angiomatous-like blood filled spaces from a collection of old blood, in which there are cholesterol clefts. H&E, × 37.5

without difficulty. On microscopic examination, some ductal structures resembling pancreatic ducts were found in the fibrous capsule of the tumour and an origin from ectopic pancreas was suggested. In other respects the macroscopic and microscopic appearances of the two tumours were those of solid-cystic (papillary-cystic) tumours. Immunostaining was (at least focally) positive for Lu 5 (a broad spectrum keratin marker), vimentin and alpha$_1$-antitrypsin. The tumours were negative for neuroendocrine markers (except for neuron-specific enolase), pancreatic hormones and enzymes, pancreatic stone protein, carcinoembryonic antigen, CA 19-9, and nuclear oestrogen and progesterone receptors. The authors' conclusion was that these results did not support the suggestion that the tumours were female sex hormone-dependent, because, as in most cases of the solid-cystic (papillary-cystic) tumour in young women, both the male patients made good post-operative recoveries and seemed to be cured.

Malignant Potential

Various reports (Sanfey et al. 1983; Bombi et al. 1984; Kuo et al. 1984; Learmonth et al. 1985) have indicated that, if complete exicision is possible, a permanent cure can be expected, and that recurrence or metastasis occurred only in patients in whom complete excision had not been possible. Complete removal may sometimes be difficult to achieve, for it is not uncommon to find microscopic infiltration beyond the capsule when excision has seemed, macroscopically, to have been complete (Figs 8.16, 8.17). Such capsular penetration is a clear indication of the malignant potential of these tumours but, even when excision has been known to be incomplete, there is usually a long interval before recurrence or metastasis becomes apparent. Thus, the progression of the malignancy would seem to be slow. In the patient reported by Hernandez-Maldonado et al. (1989), however, carcinomatosis had already developed by the time the tumour was removed.

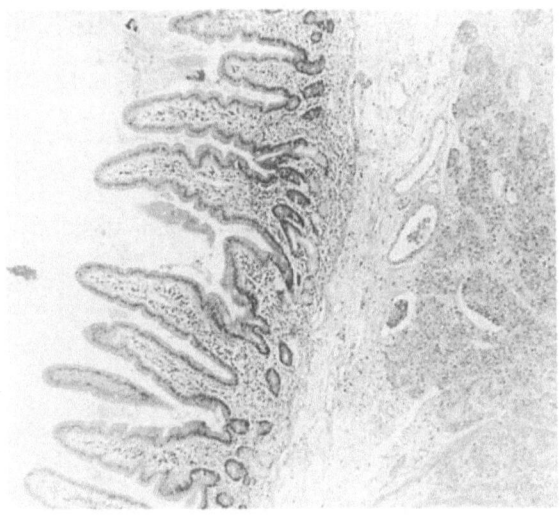

Fig. 8.16. Infiltration of the wall of the duodenum by the tumour shown in Figs 8.12.–8.15. H&E, × 60

Microscopic signs of increasing malignancy were noted by Cappellari et al. (1990) in three successive biopsy specimens, taken at intervals of two years, from a patient in whom complete excision had not been possible.

Necrosis and haemorrhage in these tumours may cause acute symptoms but, in the absence of such events, quite large tumours may be painless. The experience of Matsunou and Konishi (1990), however, makes it clear that the absence of symptoms, other than the presence of a palpable lump, should not delay excision. They reported nine patients, seven of whom were characteristically young women with ages between 8 and 24 years; the remaining two were older women, one being 47 and the other 60 years old. In these, the tumours were known to have had their origin, without symptoms, when the patients were many years younger. The two older women died from metastatic disease; the younger patients, some of whom were followed up post-operatively for many years, seemed to have been cured by either distal pancreatectomy or by enucleation of the tumour.

Multicentric Papillary-Cystic Neoplasm

A single report, thought by the authors to be the first example of two distinct papillary-cystic neoplasms in the same pancreas, has been published by Orlando et al. (1991). The patient was a 26-year-old black woman, who developed sharp right upper abdominal pain that radiated to the right shoulder; she also had jaundice and pruritus, and had been vomiting. She was in the first trimester of pregnancy, which was terminated when an upper abdominal mass was found and was shown by computed tomography to be within the head of the pancreas and to be causing extrahepatic and intrahepatic biliary obstruction. An exploratory laparotomy with frozen section biopsy of the mass established a diagnosis of cystic-papillary neoplasm and, 2 weeks later, a Whipple's procedure, with total pancreatectomy and splenectomy, was carried out. On examination of the excised pancreas a second, separate, smaller tumour was found in the tail, 7 cm from the larger tumour in the head. Both tumours were identical microscopically and had the light microscopic and ultrastructural features of papillary-cystic tumours. There was associated chronic obstructive pancreatitis. Post-operatively there was, of course, a lack of pancreatic function but no evidence of recurrent or metastatic disease was found 9 months after the patient's discharge from hospital.

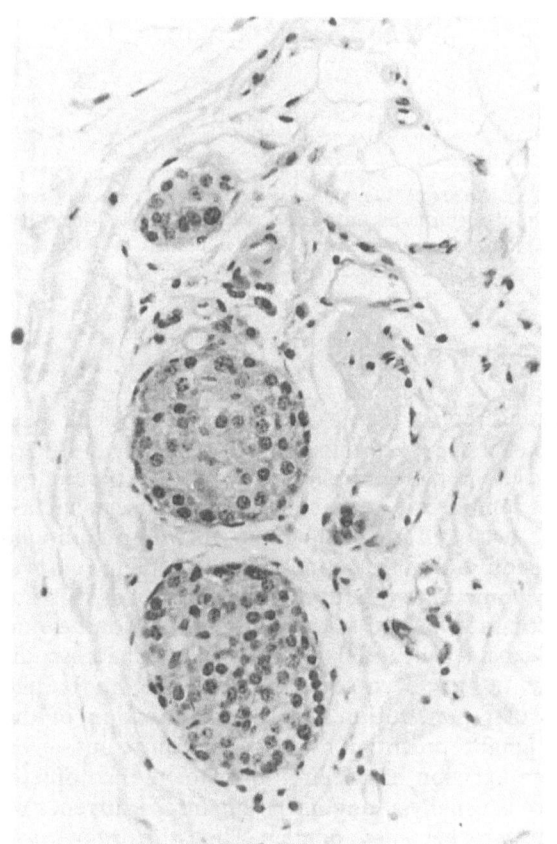

Fig. 8.17. Permeation of lymphatics by tumour cells in the section shown in Fig. 8.16. H&E, × 375

Cavernous Lymphangioma

The pancreas is a rare site for a lymphangioma and the study of 32 cases of lymphangioma in children, including lesions in rare sites, by Singh et al. (1971) contains no example of lymphangioma in the pancreas. Nevertheless, there have been reports of pancreatic lymphangiomas, nearly always of single cases. It must be noted, however, that, if the diagnosis depends upon the microscopic appearances of a small biopsy, it is usually impossible to make a confident differential diagnosis between lymphangioma and serous cystadenoma of the pancreas. In 1946, Porter described a lymphangioma in the region of the head of the pancreas that caused obstructive jaundice in a 66-year-old man. The diagnosis depended upon the softness of the tumour when it was handled during a laparotomy, and upon a biopsy in which multilocular cavernous spaces with an endothelial lining were described. A lymphangioma of the pancreas was also reported by Pack et al. (1958), but when the illustrations of the gross and microscopic appearances of that tumour are compared with those in more recent publications, there can be little doubt that that tumour would now be diagnosed as serous cystadenoma. In 1969, Dodds et al. suggested that the radiological appearances of a cavernous lymphangioma might be characteristic. Their patient was a Caucasian woman, 81 years old, whose chief complaint was of an abdominal mass that had been present for 5 years and was enlarging. The radiological appearances were that mutiple, non-movable and amorphous phlebolith-like calcifications were present in the upper abdomen. At surgery, a multinodular mass (15 × 15 cm) involved the entire pancreas; numerous small cystic structures were scattered over its surface. Resection was considered to be unwise, but tissue was removed for histology. The microscopic appearances were of a multicystic structure with delicate collagenous, highly vascularised walls. Each of the cystic spaces was completely encircled by a thin layer of smooth muscle cells. The surfaces of the cysts were lined by small columnar cells consisting of clear cytoplasm and oval peripheral nuclei. Red cells were seen in some of the larger cysts. Several small areas of cylindrical cells suggested ductal epithelium. Following the operation, recovery was uneventful, and, when the patient was followed up 7 years later, now at the age of 88 and generally weak, the abdominal mass had not changed in size. Although the pathological diagnosis was that the tumour was a cavernous lymphangioma, many of the features mentioned in the histological description are compatible also with a diagnosis of serous cystadenoma. It is true that the smooth muscle cells that were described as encircling the cystic spaces are not usually seen in serous cystadenomas, but myoepithelial cells have been seen ultramicroscopically by certain authors (e.g. Nyongo and Huntrakoon 1985).

In 1975, Epstein and Berman reported a lesion that they described as a mesenteric and pancreatic lymphangioma, presenting as a right adnexal mass in a young woman. At operation, the mass was found to be cystic and to be attached by a twisted stalk, 35 cm long, to the subdiaphragmatic and pancreatic regions. Enucleation involved omentectomy and partial pancreatectomy. The pathological diagnosis was that the cyst was a mesenteric and pancreatic lymphangioma, with focal acute inflammation and fat necrosis. The mesentery is known to be a site in which lymphangiomas may be found (Singh et al. 1971) but involvement of the pancreas is unusual.

Epstein and Berman did not give an opinion about whether the lesion had originated primarily in the mesentery, or in the pancreas, or simultaneously in both. Two years later, Hanelin and Schimmel (1977) exhibited a radiological lesion with the features that had been described by Dodds et al. (1969) as a calcifying lymphangioma of the pancreas, but which, as the patient was followed over a 15-year period, developed appearances that became those of a cystadenoma.

What appears to have been a true lymphangioma of the pancreas was the subject of a case report by Dubois (1981). The patient was a boy aged 7, who developed abdominal pain that was only temporarily relieved by the removal of a normal-looking appendix. The abdominal pain recurred a few days later and was associated with pain and oedema of the left side of the scrotum. A left abdominal mass, which was shown radiologically and by ultrasound to be cystic, was palpable, and at operation a large multilocular cyst was found lying anterior to the colon and attached to the tail of the pancreas. There were loose adhesions to the small intestine and mesentery. The cystic mass contained clear viscid fluid with some brown staining. After removal and microscopic examination, the walls of the cysts were reported to be of connective tissue lined by flattened cells; there were some areas of chronic inflammation. A photomicrograph showed a close association between the cystic loculi and the pancreatic glandular tissue. The author attributed the oedema of the scrotum to pressure by the cystic mass upon the left renal vein.

A thorough review of the published cases of vascular tumours of the pancreas was carried out by Letoquart et al. (1989). They found that the literature previously contained accounts of 30 cases of cystic connective tissue tumours of the pancreas to which they added their own example of a cystic lymphangioma. Their list contained 27 lymphangiomas, three haemolymphangiomas, and a single haemangioma. Their list did not include cases in which vascular lesions of the pancreas had been incidental findings at autopsy. Their own patient was a woman aged 54, whose past history included replacement of a heart valve. The cystic lesion involved the head of the pancreas and the adjacent duodenum and, to remove it, cephalic duodenopancreatectomy had to be combined with right hemicolectomy. The patient was well when she was reviewed 3 months later. Microscopically, the specimen had the characteristics of a cystic lymphangioma and the adjacent pancreatic tissue had only minor abnormalities. The cystic cavities were lined by flattened cells similar to vascular lining cells and the adjacent connective tissue contained curved bundles of smooth muscle cells.

References

Albores-Saavedra J, Angeles-Angeles A, Nadji M, Henson DE, Alvarez L (1987) Mucinous cystadenocarcinoma of the pancreas: morphological and immunocytochemical observations. Am J Surg Pathol 11:11–20

Albores-Saavedra J, Nadji M, Henson DE, Angeles-Angeles A (1988) Entero-endocrine cell differentiation in carcinoma of the gall bladder and mucinous cystadenocarcinomas of the pancreas. Pathol Res Pract 183:169–175

Alpert LC, Truong LD, Bossart MI, Spjut HJ (1988) Microcystic adenoma (serous cystadenoma) of the pancreas: a study of 14 cases. Immunohistochemical and electronmicroscopic correlation. Am J Surg Pathol 12:251–263

Anderson GS, Peebles Brown DA (1959–1960) A case of hydatid cyst of the pancreas. Br J Surg 47:147–149

Becker WF, Welsh RA, Pratt HS (1965) Cystadenoma and cystadenocarcinoma of the pancreas. Ann Surg 161:845–863

Bogomoletz WV (1992) Cystic tumours of the exocrine pancreas. In: Anthony PP, MacSween RNM (eds) Recent advances in histopathology. Churchill Livingstone, Edinburgh, pp 141–155

Bogomoletz WV, Adnet JJ, Widegren S, Stavrou M, McLaughlin JE (1980) Cystadenoma of pancreas: a histological histochemical and ultrastructural study of seven cases. Histopathology 4:309–320

Bombi JA, Milla A, Badal JM, Piulachs J, Estape J, Cardesa A (1984) Papillary-cystic neoplasm of the pancreas. Cancer 54:780–784

Campbell JA, Cruickshank AH (1962) Cystadenoma and cystadenocarcinoma of the pancreas. J Clin Pathol 15:432–437

Cantrell BB, Cubilla AL, Erlandson RA, Fortner J, Fitzgerald PJ (1981) Acinar cell cystadenocarcinoma of human pancreas. Cancer 47:410–416

Cappellari JO, Geisinger KR, Albertson DA, Wolfman NT, Kute TE (1990) Malignant papillary cystic tumour of the pancreas. Cancer 66:193–198

Chen J, Baithun SI (1985) Morphological study of 391 cases of exocrine pancreatic tumours with special reference to the classification of exocrine pancreatic carcinoma. J Pathol 146:17–29

Cocco AE, Conway S (1975) Zollinger-Ellison syndrome associated with ovarian mucinous cystadenocarcinoma. N Engl J Med 293:485–486

Compagno J, Oertel JE (1978a) Microcystic adenomas of the pancreas (glycogen-rich cystadenomas): a clinicopathologic study of 34 cases. Am J Clin Pathol 69:289–298

Compagno J, Oertel JE (1978b) Mucinous cystic neoplasms of the pancreas with overt and latent malignancy (cystadenocarcinoma and cystadenoma): a clinicopathological study of 41 cases. Am J Clin Pathol 69:573–580

Compagno J, Oertel JE, Kremzar M (1979) Solid and papillary epithelial neoplasm of the pancreas, probably of small duct origin: a clinico-pathologic study of 52 cases. (International Academy of Pathology (United States – Canadian Division) 68th annual meeting, San Francisco, 5–9 March, 1979) Lab Invest 40:248–249

Cornes JS, Azzopardi JG (1959–1960) Papillary cystadenocarcinoma of the pancreas with report of two cases. Br J Surg 47:139–144

Corrente RF (1980) Cystadenocarcinoma of the pancreas. Am J Surg 139:265–267

Corrin B (1962) Cystadenoma of the liver. J Pathol Bacteriol 84:441–443

Cruickshank AH, Sparshott SM (1971) Malignancy in natural and experimental hepatic cysts: experiments with aflatoxin in rats and the malignant transformation of cysts in human livers. J Pathol 104:185–190

Cubilla AL, Fitzgerald PJ (1980) Cancer (non-endocrine) of the pancreas: a suggested classification. In: Fitzgerald PJ, Morrison AB (eds) The pancreas. Williams and Wilkins, Baltimore, pp 82–110

Cullen PK, ReMine WH, Dahlin DC (1963) A clinicopathological study of cystadenocarcinoma of the pancreas. Surg Gynecol Obstet 117:189–195

Davison C, Brock S, Dyke C (1936) Retinal and central nervous hemangiomatosis with visceral changes (von Hippel-Lindau's disease). Bull Neurol Inst New York 5:72–93

Dennis WA (1923) Dermoid cyst of the pancreas. Surg Clin North Am 3:1319–1322

Doberstein C, Kirchner R, Gordon L, Silberman AW, Morgenstern L, Shapiro S (1990) Cystic neoplasms of the pancreas. Mt Sinai J Med 57:102–105

Dodds WJ, Margolin FR, Goldberg HI (1969) Cavernous lymphangioma of the pancreas. Radiol Clin Biol 38:267–270

Dreiling DA (1959) Cystadenocarcinoma of the pancreas in a patient with long-standing chronic relapsing pancreatitis and pancreatic calcinosis. J Mt Sinai Hosp 26:589–593

Dubois JD (1981) Lymphangioma of the pancreas masquerading as acute appendicitis and torsion of the left testis. Br J Surg 68:799–800

Edmondson HA (1958) Tumors of the liver and intrahepatic bile ducts. (Atlas of tumor pathology, Section 7, Fascicle 25) Armed Forces Insititute of Pathology, Washington, DC, pp 24–28

Epstein HS, Berman R (1975) Mesenteric and pancreatic lymphangioma presenting as a right adnexal mass. Am J Obstet Gynecol 121:1117–1118

Ferrer JP, Hensley G, Kalser MH, Zappa R (1978) Cystadenocarcinoma and carcinoembryonic antigen. Cancer 42:632–634

Fishman RS, Bartholomew LG (1979) Severe pancreatic involvement in three generations in von Hippel-Lindau disease. Mayo Clin Proc 54:329–331

Frantz VK (1959) Tumors of the pancreas. Armed Forces Institute of Pathology, Washington, DC, p 32 (Atlas of tumor pathology, section 7, fascicles 27, 28)

George DH, Murphy F, Michalski R, Ulmer BG (1989) Serous cystadenocarcinoma of the pancreas: a new entity? Am J Surg Pathol 13:61–66

Grosfield JL, Clatworthy HW, Hamoudi AB (1970) Pancreatic malignancy in childhood. Arch Surg 101:370–375

Grunberg A, Blair JL, St Hill CA (1952) Congestive splenomegaly due to pancreatic cystadenoma. Br Med J ii:265–266

Ham WA (1974) Histology, 7th edn. Lippincott, Philadelphia, pp 682–683

Hamoudi AB, Misugi K, Grosfeld JL, Reiner CB (1970) Papillary epithelial neoplasm of pancreas in a child: report of a case with electron microscopy. Cancer 26:1126–1134

Hanelin LG, Schimmel DH (1977) Lymphangioma of the pancreas exhibiting an unusual pattern of calcification. Radiology 122:636

Haukohl RS, Melamed A (1950) Cystadenoma of the pancreas: a report of two cases showing calcification. AJR 63:234–245

Hernandez-Maldonado JJ, Rodriguez-Bigas MA, Gonzalez DePesante A, Vazquez-Quintana E (1989) Papillary cystic neoplasm of the pancreas: a report of a case presenting with carcinomatosis. Am J Surg 55:552–559

Hodgkinson DJ, ReMine WH, Weiland LH (1978a) Pancreatic cystadenoma: a clinicopathological study of 45 cases. Arch Surg 113:512–519

Hodgkinson DJ, ReMine WH, Weiland LH (1978b) A clinico-pathologic study of 21 cases of pancreatic cystadenocarcinoma. Ann Surg 188:679–684

Hoover E, Natesha R, Dao A, Adams CZ, Barnwell S (1991) Proliferative pancreatic cysts: pathogenesis and treatment options. Am J Surg 162:274–277

Hueper WC (1928) Cystadenoma of the pancreas. Arch Pathol 5:261–266

Itai Y, Ohhashi K, Nagai H et al. (1986) "Ductectatic" mucinous cystadenoma and cystadenocarcinoma of the pancreas. Radiology 161:697–700

Johnson CD, Stephens DH, Carboneau JW, Carpenter HA, Welch TJ (1988) Cystic pancreatic tumors – CT and sonographic assessment. AJR 151:1133–1138

Judd ES, Mattson H, Mahorner HR (1931) Pancreatic cysts: report of forty-seven cases. Arch Surg 22:838–849

Kattan YB (1975) Hydatid cysts in pancreas. Br Med J iv:729–730

Kerlin DL, Frey CF, Bodai BI, Twomey PL, Ruebner B (1987) Cystic neoplasms of the pancreas. Surg Gynecol Obstet 165:475–478

Kerr AA (1918) Cysts and pseudocyst of the pancreas, with report of cases. Surg Gynecol Obstet 27:40–44

Kim YI, Seo JW, Suh JS, Lee KU, Choe KJ (1990) Microcystic adenomas of the pancreas: report of three cases with two of multicentric origin. Am J Clin Pathol 94:150–156

Klöppel G (1984) Pancreatic, non-endocrine tumours. In: Klöppel G, Heitz PU (eds) Pancreatic pathology. Churchill Livingstone, Edinburgh, pp 101–102

Klöppel G, Maurer R, Hofmann E et al. (1991) Solid-cystic (papillary-cystic) tumours within and outside the pancreas in men: report of two patients. Virchows Archiv [A] 418:179–183

Kuo T-T, Su I-J, Chien C-H (1984) Solid and papillary neoplasm of the pancreas: report of three cases from Taiwan. Cancer 54:1469–1474

Ladanyi M, Mulay S, Arseneau J, Bettez P (1987) Estrogen and progesterone receptor determination in the papillary cystic neoplasm of the pancreas with immunohistochemical and ultrastructural observations. Cancer 60:1604–1611

Lamiell JM, Salagar FG, Hsia YE (1989) Von Hippel-Lindau disease: affecting 43 members of a single kindred. Medicine 68:1–29

Learmonth GM, Price SK, Visser AE, Emms M (1985) Papillary and cystic neoplasm of the pancreas: an acinic cell tumour? Histopathology 9:63–79

Letoquart JP, Marcorolles P, Lancien G et al. (1989) Un nouveau cas de lymphangiome kistique du pancréas. J Chir (Paris) 126:650–658

Lo JW, Fung CHK, Yonan TN, Martinez N (1977) Cystadenoma of the pancreas: an ultrastructural study. Cancer 39:2470–2474

Maher ER, Yates JRW, Harries R et al. (1990) Clinical features and natural history of von Hippel-Lindau disease. Q J Med New Ser 77 (283):1151–1163

Mallory TB (1941) Case records of the Massachusetts General Hospital: Case 27262. N Engl J Med 224:1112–1114

Margolis RM, Jang N (1984) Zollinger-Ellison syndrome associated with pancreatic cystadenocarcinoma. N Engl J Med 311:1380–1381

Matsunou H, Konishi F (1990) Papillary-cystic neoplasm of the pancreas: a clinicopathologic study concerning the tumor aging and malignancy of nine cases. Cancer 65:283–291

Miettinen M, Partanen S, Fräki O, Kivilaskso E (1987) Papillary cystic tumor of the pancreas: an analysis of cellular differentiation by electron microscopy and immunohistochemistry. Am J Surg Pathol 11:855–865

Morohoshi T, Kanda M, Asanuma K, Klöppel G (1989) Intraductal papillary neoplasms of the pancreas: a clinico-pathologic study of six patients. Cancer 64:1329–1335

Mozan AA (1951) Cystadenoma of the pancreas. Am J Surg 81:204–214

Neumann HPH, Dinkel E, Brambs H et al. (1991) Pancreatic lesions in the von Hippel-Lindau syndrome. Gastroenterology 101:465–471

Nyongo A, Huntrakoon M (1985) Microcystic adenoma of the pancreas with myoepithelial cells: a hitherto undescribed morphological feature. Am J Clin Pathol 84:114–120

Orlando CA, Bowman RL, Loose JH (1991) Multicentric papillary-cystic neoplasm of the pancreas. Arch Pathol Lab Med 115:958–960

Pack GT, Trinidad SS, Lisa JR (1958) Rare primary somatic tumors of the pancreas. Arch Surg 77:1000–1003

Padfield CJH, Ansell ID, Furness PN (1988) Mucinous biliary papillomatosis: a tumour in need of wider recognition. Histopathology 13:687–694

Persaud V, Walrond RE (1971) Carcinoid tumour and cystadenoma of the pancreas. Arch Pathol 92:28–30

Porter HW (1946) Case of lymphangioma in the region of the head of the pancreas causing an obstructive jaundice. Br J Surg 34:217–218

Pyke CM, van Heerden JA, Colby TV, Sarr MG, Weaver AL (1992) The spectrum of serous cystadenoma of the pancreas: clinical, pathologic, and surgical aspects. Ann Surg 215:132–139

Rego JAG, Ruvira LV, Garcia AA, Freijanes MPS, Penaranda JMS, Soto JMR (1991) Pancreatic mucinous cystadenocarcinoma with pseudosarcomatous mural nodules: a report of a case with immunohistochemical study. Cancer 67:494–498

ReMine SG, Frey D, Rossi RL, Munson JL, Braasch JW (1987) Cystic neoplasms of the pancreas. Arch Surg 122:443–446

Rickaert F, Cremer M, Devière J et al. (1991) Intraductal mucin-hypersecreting neoplasms of the pancreas: a clinicopathologic study of eight patients. Gastroenterology 101:512–519

Rode J, Dhillon AP, Hamid Q, Polak JM, Moss E (1988) Solid and cystic tumour of the pancreas [abstract]. J Pathol 155:351A

Rood RP, DeLellis RA, Dayal Y, Donowitz M (1988) Pancreatic cholera syndrome due to a vasoactive intestinal polypeptide-producing tumor: further insights into the pathophysiology. Gastronterology 94:813–818

Sanfey H, Mendelsohn G, Cameron JL (1983) Solid and papillary neoplasm of the pancreas: a potentially curable surgical lesion. Ann Surg 197:272–275

Satake K, Uchima K, Yamashita K, Yashimoto T, Umeyama K (1979) Pancreatic cystadenoma of the spleen. Am J Surg 137:670–672

Schlosnagle D, Campbell WG (1981) The papillary and solid neoplasm of the pancreas. Cancer 47:2603–2610

Shorten SD, Hart WR, Petras RE (1986) Microcystic adenomas (serous cystadenomas) of pancreas: a clinicopathologic investigation of eight cases with immunohistochemical and ultrastructural studies. Am J Surg Pathol 10:365–372

Singh S, Baboo M, Pathak I (1971) Cystic lymphangioma in children: report of 32 cases including lesions at rare sites. Surgery 69:947–951

Soloway HB (1965) Constitutional abnormalities associated with pancreatic cystadenomas. Cancer 18:1297–1300

Speese JJ (1915) Cystadenoma of the pancreas with extension to the abdominal wall ten years after drainage of a pancreatic cyst. Ann Surg 61:759–761

Stamm B, Burger H, Hollinger A (1987) Acinar cell cystadenocarcinoma of the pancreas. Cancer 60:2542–2547

Stömmer P, Kraus J, Stolte M, Giedl J (1991) Solid and cystic pancreatic tumors: clinical, histochemical, and electron microscopic features in ten cases. Cancer 67:1635–1641

Todani T, Shimada K, Watanabe Y, Toki A, Fujii T, Kagawa NU (1988) Frantz's tumor: a papillary and cystic tumor of the pancreas in girls. J Pediatr Surg 23:116–121

Veloso FT, Ribeiro AT, Teixeira AA, Ramalhão J, Saleiro J, Serrãs D (1983) Biliary papillomatosis: report of a case with five year follow-up. Am J Gastroenterol 78:645–648

Virchow R (1887) Ueber Ranula pancreatica and Über Pleuritis retrahens. Berl Klin Wochenschr 24:248–250

Warren KW, Hardy KJ (1968) Cystadenocarcinoma of the pancreas. Surg Gynecol Obstet 127:734–736

Warshaw AL, Compton CC, Lewandrowski K, Cardenosa G, Mueller PR (1990) Cystic tumors of the pancreas: new clinical, radiologic, and pathologic observations in 67 patients. Ann Surg 212:432–445

White WH (1897) Diseases of the pancreas. Guy's Hosp Reports 54 (39 3rd series):17–63

Yagihashi S, Sato I, Kaimori M, Matsumoto J, Nagai K (1988) Papillary and cystic tumor of the pancreas: two cases indistinguishable from islet cell tumor. Cancer 61:1241–1247

Yamaguchi K, Enjoji M (1987) Cystic neoplasms of the pancreas. Gastroenterology 92:1934–1943

Young EL (1937) Pancreatic cyst: report of a case. N Engl J Med 216:334–339

Yu HC, Shetty Y (1985) Mucinous cystic neoplasm of the pancreas with high carcinoembryonic antigen. Arch Pathol Lab Med 109:375–377

Carcinoma of the pancreas is a disease in which surgery can offer little more than palliation and in which other forms of therapy are equally unsatisfactory. In America, for example, Elmer-Dewitt (1992), using figures obtained from the National Cancer Institute, has shown that only 3.1% of patients diagnosed as having cancer of the pancreas between 1981 and 1987 were alive 5 years from the time of the diagnosis. Moreover, this dreadful disease is becoming more common.

Increasing Incidence

In 1958, Rodney Smith wrote: "Malignant tumours of the pancreas are relatively uncommon. Carcinoma is the only one encountered with any frequency and even this accounts for only 1%–2% of all carcinoma." By 1973, however, cancer of the pancreas had become the fourth commonest cause of death from cancer in the United States (Levin and Connelly 1973), its incidence having trebled since 1930, while in England and Wales its incidence had approximately doubled during a similar period (Adelstein 1977). Now, in most Western countries, there is an annual incidence of between 9 and 10 cases per 100 000 of the whole population. The number of cases reported to the Mersey Regional Cancer Registry are probably typical: in 1971 there were 12.9 male cases and 9.2 female cases per 100 000; in 1972 the corresponding figures were 13.6 males and 8.2 females; and in 1973 the numbers were 10.4 males and 9.0 females. The accuracy of

this has been confirmed more recently by Dr Ruth Hussey, who found an annual incidence of between 10.6 and 12.7 per 100 000 between 1983 and 1987 (personal communication).

The Mersey Cancer Registry receives registrations, not only from the industrial areas of Merseyside, but also from the mainly rural areas of Clwyd, Gwynedd and the Isle of Man. In people over 75 years of age the incidence is said to rise towards 100 per 100 000 of this population (Levison 1979). The increase affects both sexes (Adelstein 1977) and is probably world-wide. Japan is not, of course, representative of the other Eastern countries, for there the diagnostic facilities and vital statistics are as reliable as in the United States (Wynder 1975), but in Japan there has been a fourfold increase in the incidence during the past 25 years (Segi et al. 1969). Figures collected by the World Health Organization were quoted in an anonymous note in the *Lancet* (1978) that drew attention to an alarming increase in the incidence in the northern European countries, for example Scotland, or Sweden where, in 1972, the incidence was 16.6 per 100 000.

A more recent study of the epidemiology of pancreatic cancer is that of Fontham and Correa (1989), where it is pointed out that, although death rates for pancreatic cancer in the USA have risen steadily since about 1930, there has been a recent levelling off. In Britain it has been estimated that over 6000 are killed by the disease every year, but, at least in England and Wales, the graphs for cancer deaths published by Davis et al. (1990) show a levelling off in the number of deaths from pancreatic cancer in both sexes in recent years.

Statistics such as those that have just been quoted include all cases registered as pancreatic cancer and take no account of the microscopic structure of the cancers. Only a proportion of the registered cases have had the diagnosis confirmed by microscopic examination, but carcinoma that has originated from epithelium of the pancreatic ducts is so overwhelmingly preponderant among the microscopic types that the statistics almost certainly reflect the incidence of this type of carcinoma rather than that of the rarer types. The statistics also depend entirely upon the diagnosis, often unconfirmed by an autopsy, of the cause of death (Höpker 1987). It is well known that certified causes of death, particularly without an autopsy, are very unreliable (Cochrane and Moore 1981; Kircher et al. 1985).

Aetiology

Geographical, Racial and Social Factors

The results of attempts to find associations between such factors and the incidence of cancer of the pancreas have been reviewed by Levison (1979). No clear pattern could be recognised amongst the inhabitants of the various parts of the USA when the age-adjusted death rates for cancer of the pancreas were correlated by sex and race with demographic and industrial information, except that the rates were higher in urban areas, especially in males (Blot et al. 1978). The study just mentioned did not indicate any association with socioeconomic or industrial conditions, although an earlier study (Krain 1971) had suggested that there was an inverse relationship between socioeconomic class and pancreatic cancer, while Fraumeni, in 1975, had found that the rising frequency within the USA was in males and in blacks, the increased incidence in the blacks having become recognisable only after 1950. Although there are marked differences between the incidence in various racial groups both in the USA and internationally, no satisfactory explanation has been offered. The possible effect of migration, however, may be significant, for people who move from areas where the incidence of pancreatic cancer is low to areas where is it high seem to be particularly at risk (Haenszel and Kurihara 1968; Mancuso and Sterling 1974); thus change of environment, possibly because of an associated change in dietary habits, seems to be important.

In general, comparisons of the incidence of the disease in different parts of the world point to its being a disease of the industrialised western countries, in which the diet tends to have a high content of fat or cholesterol, or both fat and cholesterol (Wynder 1975). Many epidemiological findings about the incidence of carcinoma of the pancreas, however, remain unexplained, while some, for example the observation by Williams and Horm (1977) that there is a positive association between college attendance (but not income) and cancer of the pancreas in American males, seems inexplicable.

Smoking and Environmental Influences

As long ago as 1796 Erasmus Darwin wrote: "The unwise custom of chewing and smoking tobacco for many hours in a day not only injures the salivary glands, producing dryness in the mouth when this drug is not used, but I suspect that it also produces schirrhus of the pancreas." Darwin's idea received some support from the anonymous author of a letter to the *Lancet* published in 1829, but it was not until the 1970s that the results of investigations into the aetiology of cancer of the pancreas began to suggest that there might be an important association between cigarette smoking and pancreatic carcinoma.

In several epidemiological studies, for example those of Krain (1970), Wynder et al. (1973) and Williams and Horm (1977), the association could be demonstrated, and Wynder (1975) has suggested ways in which cigarette-derived carcinogens may reach the pancreas, or how changes in the blood lipids induced by smoking may affect the development of pancreatic cancer. In 1989, after a comprehensive review of the epidemiological publications on possible risk factors in the development of pancreatic cancer, Fontham and Correa came to the conclusion that cigarette smoking was the best established risk factor in the aetiology of the disease.

Experimental work by Longnecker and Curphey (1975) and by Pour et al. (1975) has shown that carcinogens injected into rats and hamsters induce exocrine pancreatic hyperplasia, adenomas and carcinomas while the alimentary adminstration of N-methyl-N-nitrosourea to inbred guinea pigs by Reddy and Rao (1975) induced pancreatic adenocarcinoma. Thus the entry of carcinogens, whether through the lungs from cigarette smoke, or from atmospheric pollution, followed by distribution through the bloodstream to act eventually upon the pancreas, may be aetiologically important, while entry of remotely acting carcinogen by the alimentary route has also been shown experimentally to be a possibility that cannot be excluded from the potential aetiology of the human disease.

Age

The incidence of carcinoma of the pancreas increases with increasing age and, as has been pointed out by Hartveit and Maartmann-Moe (1982) and Karwinski et al. (1989), in the aged the disease may be atypical clinically and may thus be unrecognised in the absence of an autopsy. It is unusual before the age of 45, but becomes relatively common above that age. From figures from the Mersey Regional Cancer Registry, published by the Mersey Regional Health Authority (1977), for the years 1971–1973, the incidence in males over the age of 75 varied between 93 and 127 per 100 000 of the population during these years, while the corresponding figures for women varied between 53 and 62 per 100 000. Cases below the age of 20 years are liable to be written up and published as rarities; only 42 such cases had been recorded up to 1974, when Tavassoli and Lynch reviewed the published cases and added one of their own. Occasional cases have been published since that time, for example those of Horie et al. (1977), Benjamin and Wright (1980), Rich et al. (1986), and McWhirter et al. (1989), but at least some of these tumours differ conspicuously on microscopic examination from the ductal adenocarcinomas of adults: the name pancreaticoblastoma, rather than adencarcinoma has been suggested for such tumours (Cubilla and Fitzgerald 1980).

Sex

In most countries, the incidence in males is almost double that in females; the figures that have been quoted above in relation to age illustrate this difference between the sexes in at least a part of England and parts of Wales and the Isle of Man, during the years 1971–1973, and although the incidence of the disease has increased in both sexes the ratio of males to females at that time was very similar to that in the figures tabulated by Cliffton (1956) in an article in which he reviewed most of the publications relating to carcinoma of the pancreas that had appeared during the preceding century. In more recent figures for the Mersey Region, however, there has been a change. During the years 1983–1987, the incidence of pancreatic carcinoma in all ages in men was 11.6 per 100 000, while the comparable figure for women was 12.2. It

remains to be seen whether the change is an isolated and temporary one, or the beginning of a trend.

Diet

The possible importance of diet in the aetiology of carcinoma of the pancreas had been discussed by Morgan and Wormsley (1977), who refer to work that shows the increased incidence of carcinoma of the pancreas in Japan has coincided with an increase of fat and animal protein in the national diet. They go on to suggest that the increased functional demands upon the pancreas caused by a diet rich in fat and protein may increase cell turnover in the pancreas, with the resulting increased susceptibility of the gland to environmental or dietary carcinogens. Such a suggestion is in keeping with the results of experiments carried out by themselves and their colleagues (Morgan et al. 1977), in which it was found that a diet containing raw soya bean flour greatly increased the sensitivity of the pancreas of rats to the carcinogenic action of azaserine. Morgan and Wormsley (1977) also speculated about the existence, and possible mode of action, of dietary carcinogens in relation to carcinoma of the pancreas in man. It is of interest that a high consumption of vegetarian products rich in protein such as beans, lentils, peas and dried fruits, was found by Mills et al. (1988) to be associated with a low incidence of pancreatic cancer.

A possible association between the consumption of coffee and carcinoma of the exocrine pancreas aroused the interest of medical statisticians, and caused some public anxiety in 1981 when MacMahon et al. published the results of a study that they undertook to reinvestigate the relationship of cancer of the pancreas to smoking and the use of alcohol. Between 1974 and 1979 these workers interviewed 369 patients with histologically confirmed carcinoma of the pancreas and, in addition to asking questions about their smoking habits and their use of alcoholic drinks, they enquired about how many cups of tea and coffee each of the patients had been in the habit of consuming during a typical day before the onset of their illness. Similar questions were put to 644 controls drawn from patients with diseases other than pancreatic carcinoma, in the same group of New England hospitals. The patients and the controls were all white Americans less than 79 years of age. An unexpected result on analysis of the answers was that there was a strong association between coffee consumption and carcinoma of the pancreas, and that, when the figures for the two sexes were combined, there was a significant dose-response relationship. A weak association with cigarette smoking was also found and a correction for this was introduced in assessing the association with coffee drinking. No association was found between the smoking of cigars, pipes or the drinking of tea or alcohol with carcinoma of the pancreas.

An association between the consumption of coffee and cancer of the pancreas had been noted earlier by Stocks (1970) in his study of cancer mortality in relation to the use by various nations of cigarettes, solid fuel, tea and coffee. He had found that coffee consumption was positively related to cancer of the pancreas, to cancer of the prostate and with leukaemia in men; and with cancer of the ovary and with leukaemia in women. Little interest had been aroused by these findings in 1970, but, shortly before the publication by MacMahon et al., a report of simultaneous cancer of the pancreas in a husband and wife had been published (Ferguson and Watts 1980). The husband and wife lived on a bizarre diet that included copious amounts of margarine and coffee, which they had enhanced by adding a liquid concentrate of coffee before percolating their ground coffee. This paper added to the interest aroused by the work of MacMahon and his colleagues and helped to cause the publication of articles and letters that either supported, refuted or suggested other explanations for the findings of the MacMahon group. Jick and Dinan (1981), for example, in a similar study in the same part of the world and on a similar population, could not confirm an association between coffee consumption and carcinoma of the pancreas, while Nomura et al. (1981), from a cohort study of 8000 men of Japanese ancestry in Hawaii, tentatively supported a positive association between coffee intake and pancreatic cancer. A study by Kinlen et al. (1984) in England, where coffee is usually *Coffea robusta* instead of the *Coffea arabica* usually used in America, could demonstrate no association between cancer of the pancreas and coffee consumption, while in Norway, Heuch et al. (1983), in an investigation of the use of alcohol, tobacco and coffee in relation to the risk of pancreatic cancer, found no association with coffee drinking. They found, however, that there was a clear association with the chewing of tobacco or the use of snuff; there was a weaker association with cigarette smoking. The results of these epidemiological studies seem to leave the possible role of coffee in the aetiology of pancreatic carcinoma as an indefinite one. In reviewing the evidence available in 1982, Benarde and Weiss concluded that, although a rise or fall in coffee consumption per person in the USA was associated with a rise and fall in the incidence of pancreatic cancer after a lag of 10 years, there were inconsistencies that cast doubt upon the possibility that the relationship might be one of cause and effect. The numerous studies carried out to test the existence of a relationship between the consumption of coffee and the risk of pancreatic cancer were reviewed by Fontham and Correa (1989). They concluded that there was insufficient evidence to support a causal association.

Diabetes

It has often been stated that pancreatic carcinoma is more frequent in the diabetic than in the general population. The numerous publications on the subject up to 1971 were reviewed by Volk and Wellmann (1977), but an important publication not quoted by them is that of Kessler (1970), who carried out a study of cancer mortality among 21 447 diabetic patients in a large clinic for diabetics in Boston, Massachusetts. He concluded that diabetics, especially females, have a significantly increased risk of death from pancreatic cancer. Kessler's conclusions have not been accepted without reservations by Levison (1979), who refers to studies of the English statistics (Armstrong et al. 1976; Fuller and Goldblatt, cited as a personal communication in Levison 1979), which, he states, do not bear out Kessler's conclusions. Levison's reservations about Kessler's conclusions depend upon Kessler's criteria for the diagnosis of diabetes, which may not have been sufficiently strict; carcinoma of the pancreas, in common with malignancy in many other organs, may cause a diabetes-like impaired tolerance of carbohydrates (Volk and Wellmann 1977) that is not true diabetes mellitus. Mills et al. (1988), however, in their study of the dietary habits and past medical history as related to fatal pancreatic cancer among 34 000 Seventh-Day Adventists in California, found that a history of diabetes was associated with an increased risk of death from cancer of the pancreas. A similar association with diabetes and gall bladder disease was also reported by Cuzick and Babiker (1989).

Other Possible Aetiological Factors

Alcoholism has been suggested to be important by Burch and Ansari (1968), but this was not confirmed by the more recent study by Wynder (1975). Chronic pancreatitis of the alcoholic type does not seem to predispose to cancer of the pancreas (Wynder 1975), although a few cases in which the two conditions coincided have been reported (Robinson et al. 1970).

Hereditary factors can have importance in that MacDermott and Kramer (1973) reported adenocarcinoma of the pancreas in four siblings, and Foster (1972) stated that cancers of the pancreas tend to occur in families in which hereditary pancreatitis occurs, though not necessarily in the members with pancreatitis. The increased incidence of pancreatic carcinoma in such families has also been emphasised by Barkin and Fayne (1986).

In his epidemiological studies of cancer of the pancreas, Wynder (1975) found that in women there was a positive correlation with cholecystectomy, but, as the finding was based on relatively few cases, he recommended that this should be confirmed by further studies. Partial gastrectomy, too, has been found to have some association with pancreatic cancer (Offerhaus et al. 1987) but it is agreed by the authors that further study is required.

The suggestion that endogenous oestrogen production might have some protective effect, as was suggested by Bourhis et al. (1987), was not confirmed by Devesa and Silverman (1988). By collation, a history of tonsillectomy was found by Gold et al. (1985) to be associated with a reduced risk and this received some support from Mills et al. (1988). The use of psoralen and ultraviolet A radiation in the treatment of skin disorders was found by Lindelöf et al. (1991) to be associated with a significant increase of pancreatic cancer in males, and therapeutic radiation for ankylosing spondylitis was found by Court-Brown and Doll (1965) to be associated with an increased risk of pancreatic cancer, as well as increased risks of cancer in other organs within the irradiated regions.

Occupational factors in relation to pancreatic cancer were studied by Norell et al. (1986) by two approaches: a population based case control study and a retrospective cohort study based on registered information. Both approaches found an association between pancreatic cancer and exposure to petroleum products. There were also less definite associations with exposure to paint thinner, paint and varnish, detergents, floor cleaning agents and window cleaning. There was also an association with exposure to refuse. Alderson (1987) published a table that showed an increased risk of pancreatic cancer in chemists and workers in the aluminium and petrochemical industries, and the study by Foster et al. (1993) led the authors to suggest an aetiological relationship between elevated levels of drug-metabolising enzymes of the P-450 family, and the subsequent development of chronic pancreatitis and pancreatic cancer.

Fontham and Correa (1989) have drawn attention to the completely divergent findings in relation to pancreatic cancer and industrial exposure to radiation that different groups have published. For example, excess deaths have been observed among workers exposed to radiation at a large atomic plant in the USA, but no excess of pancreatic cancer was found in workers at the British Nuclear Fuels plant at Sellafield, and there is no evidence of excess risk among the Japanese survivors of the atomic bomb.

A study of the mortality amongst doctors in different occupations was published by Doll and Peto in 1977; one of their tables showed that amongst anaesthetists there was more than the expected number of cases of pancreatic cancer. This prompted Neil et al. (1987) to undertake a study of the mortality of male anaesthetists in the UK between 1957 and 1983. A cohort of 3769 male anaesthetists was followed up for a total of 51 431 person years of observation. They found no evidence of a significant excess of cancer, and, in particular, the small excess of cancer of the pancreas reported previously could not be confirmed.

Causes of Symptoms

Pain, jaundice and loss of weight are the most important symptoms of carcinoma of the pancreas.

Pain

Although the presence or absence of jaundice in relatively early carcinoma of the pancreas depends very much on whether the carcinoma is in the head or elsewhere in the pancreas, carcinoma in any part of the pancreas causes pain.

It is often stated that pain is characteristically absent, and that painless jaundice is the most typical manifestation of carcinoma of the head of the pancreas, but in almost all the studies in which there have been careful attempts to explain the symptoms of carcinoma of the pancreas in the light of the anatomical findings, pain has been important (Berk 1941; Thompson and Rodgers 1952; Cliffton 1956; Gullick 1959; Salmon 1966; Hall and Krementz 1968; Walker 1970). Pain is usually in the upper abdomen at first but, as the disease progresses, there is often associated pain in the lumbar region. Pain may be the only symptom in patients with carcinoma of the body or tail of the pancreas (Cliffton 1956); it is very persistent (Brown et al. 1952).

The cause of the pain, especially of the persistent type, is usually attributed to invasion of the perineural lymphatics of nerves in and around the pancreas; such invasion has been demonstrated by Drapiewski (1944). In 1951 J.R. Miller et al. found carcinomatous involvement of the perineural lymphatics in 73% of 202 autopsy cases of carcinoma of the pancreas, with a marginally higher incidence (78%) in carcinoma of the head of the gland, while, in the same year E.M. Miller et al. reported that the perineural lymphatics of the duodenum, pancreas and common bile duct were invaded in 18 of 27 surgically resected specimens of carcinoma of the head of the pancreas. These authors could not, however, correlate the presence or absence of perineural lymphatic infiltration with the presence or absence of pain in the clinical histories of the patients.

The pancreas is innervated by sympathetic and parasympathetic fibres of the autonomic nervous system. Parasympathetic sensory neurons pass from the pancreas via the vagus nerves but, in man, vagal afferent fibres do not appear to be involved in pain sensation from the pancreas (Ray and Console 1949; Rack and Elkins 1950). It seems that sympathetic fibres convey the sensations of pancreatic pain centrally, but, although relief of the pain of chronic relapsing pancreatitis is reported to have been obtained by procedures such as unilateral and bilateral sympathectomy, coeliac ganglionectomy and selective division of sympathetic fibres, only transient relief can be produced in cancer of the pancreas (Ray and Console 1949; Yoshioka and Wakabayashi 1958). The afferent pathway from the pancreas passes to the coelic plexus and then, by the right and left splanchnic nerves, to the right and left 6th–11th sympathetic ganglia (Bliss et al. 1950). Thus pain from the head of the pancreas tends to be experienced in the epigastrium to the right of the midline, pain from the body of the pancreas is felt in the mid-epigastrium while pain from the tail of the pancreas is felt in the left epigastrium. This information, which was obtained by stimulation of the pancreas by electrodes introduced during elective operations on the biliary tract, fits well with the clinicopathological observation of Duff (1939) that carcinoma of the body and tail are associated with pain that radiates to the left of the upper abdomen, while, according to Gullick (1959), carcinoma of the head is liable to cause right-sided pain. The lateralisation is not absolute (Bliss et al. 1950) but it is probable that most fibres from the head pass to the right side and most from the tail to the left (British Medical Journal 1976). Kune et al. (1975) found that the injection of absolute alcohol, through a needle introduced under X-ray control into the region of the splanchnic nerves anterolateral to the first lumbar vertebra on each side, produced relief of pain in ten of 12 patients with proved pancreatic carcinoma.

Direct involvement of nerves within, or around, the pancreas may not necessarily be the only, or the most important, cause of pain in carcinoma of the pancreas; the dilatation of ducts, either biliary or pancreatic, behind an obstructing carcinoma is liable to cause pain. Drainage of a dilated pancreatic duct produced dramatic relief of pain in the patient with carcinoma of the pancreas reported by Apalakis et al. (1977), who remained free from pain until his death 3 months later. Apart from the pressure that may be caused by a dilated duct, some degree of pancreatitis is often associated with obstruction of the pancreatic duct. In the study of Haunz and Baggenstoss (1950), in which the effects of obstruction of the pancreatic ducts by carcinoma of the head of the gland received particular attention, there were variable degrees of pancreatitis in 16 of the 25 specimens that were examined in detail.

Pancreatitis is usually painful, and it has been stated (Braganza and Howat 1972) that, in the early stages of cancer of the pancreas, the pain does not differ from that of chronic relapsing pancreatitis. Thus, inflammation associated with carcinoma of the pancreas may be responsible, at least in part, for the pain of carcinoma of the pancreas. The numerous and large corpuscles of Vater–Pacini that are present in and around the pancreas appear to play no part in causing the pain of pancreatic disease.

Jaundice

Obstructive jaundice is nearly always, though not invariably, associated with carcinoma of the head of the pancreas. It is normally absent in cases of carcinoma of the body and tail, at least until the terminal phase of the illness when metastatic tumour has reached the liver. Slight jaundice appeared terminally in eight of the 16 cases of carcinoma of the body and tail of the pancreas studied by Duff (1939).

Carcinoma of the head is more common than carcinoma of the body and tail (J.R. Miller et al. 1951; Cliffton 1956; Frantz 1959; Salmon 1966) and almost 90% of patients with carcinoma of the head of the pancreas become jaundiced (Levison 1979). In almost 90% of those with jaundice there is invasion of the common bile duct by carcinoma (J.R. Miller et al. 1951), for, as was pointed out by Kaplan and Angrist (1943), it is invasion of the duct rather than compression that causes the obstruction. In some cases the duct may be plugged by papillary projections of carcinoma into its lumen but this is more characteristic of carcinoma of the distal end of the common bile duct and of the ampulla of Vater than of carcinoma of the pancreas itself. When the carcinoma has arisen in the pancreas, and has then infiltrated the wall of the common bile duct, it is the fibrous reaction provoked by the carcinoma cells that forms the malignant stricture that obliterates

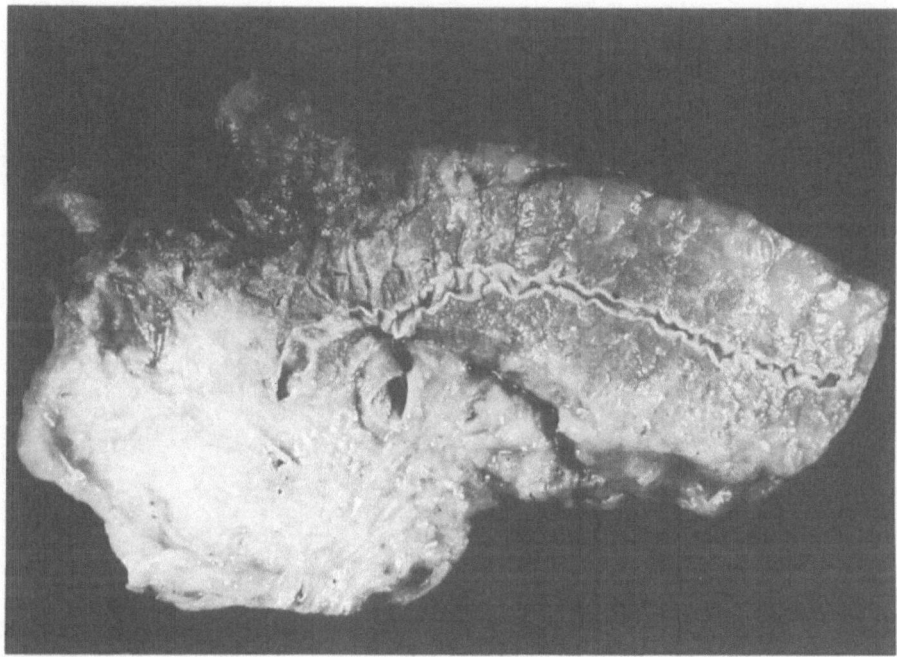

Fig. 9.1. Carcinoma of the head of the pancreas causing only slight dilatation of the duct behind the tumour. The tumour caused obstructive jaundice in an obese man aged 69. Palliative choledochoduodenostomy was carried out because the tumour was attached to the portal vein and was considered to be inoperable. The patient collapsed and died soon after the operation. No secondary carcinoma was found at the autopsy.

the lumen. This is by far the most common mechanism by which carcinoma of the pancreas causes obstructive jaundice.

Loss of Weight

It is difficult to explain from the anatomical findings, either at operation or after death, why carcinoma of the pancreas, either in the head or elsewhere in the gland, should cause the marked loss of weight that is often an early symptom of the disease (Berk 1941; Thompson and Rodgers 1952; Cliffton 1956; Gullick 1959; Collure et al. 1974). It is only in advanced cases that invasion of the duodenum or of the stomach has taken place and it is said that malabsorption and steatorrhoea do not correlate with, or account for, the early loss of weight. As with some of the other systemic effects, such as the depression and anxiety that are said to be very marked (Cliffton 1956; Fras et al. 1967), the loss of weight has no structural explanation. It has been said, moreover, that loss of weight alone does not necessarily indicate advanced disease (Gullick 1959). Some of the main types and anatomical effects of exocrine carcinoma of the pancreas are illustrated in Figs 9.1–9.10.

Venous Thrombosis and Thrombotic Endocarditis

As long ago as 1865 Armand Trousseau, when discussing "phlegmatia alba dolens" with his students, remarked that he had long been struck by the frequency of painful oedema in cancer sufferers, whatever the site of the cancer. He distinguished such thrombotic episodes from those that might follow cancerous invasion of veins and attributed them to the "cancerous diathesis". He stated that if cachexia could not be attributed to tuberculosis or to the puerperal state as the cause of such episodes, then it was very probable that a cancerous tumour existed in some part of the body. Amongst his illustrative examples he referred to the case of one of the professors of the Faculty, whose gastric symptoms were attributed to peptic ulceration by his doctors. When Trousseau learned however, that the patient had developed a painful venous thrombosis he did not hesitate to predict that the patient would succumb to cancer, as, indeed, he did. Trousseau's illustrative examples did not, at least in the 1865 edition of his *Clinique Médicale*, include cases of carcinoma of the pancreas, but, by the 1930s, it was being noted that carcinoma in the body or tail of the pancreas, sites notorious for harbouring obscure or unsuspected

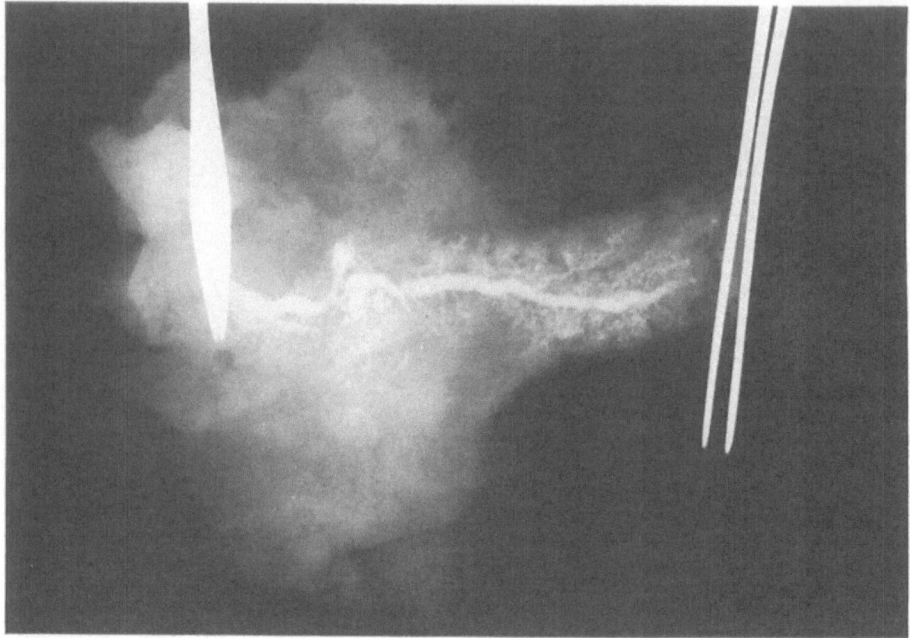

Fig. 9.2. Radiograph of the ducts in the specimen shown in Fig. 9.1. after injection with barium. An obstruction of the main duct is present but an accessory duct appears to be unobstructed.

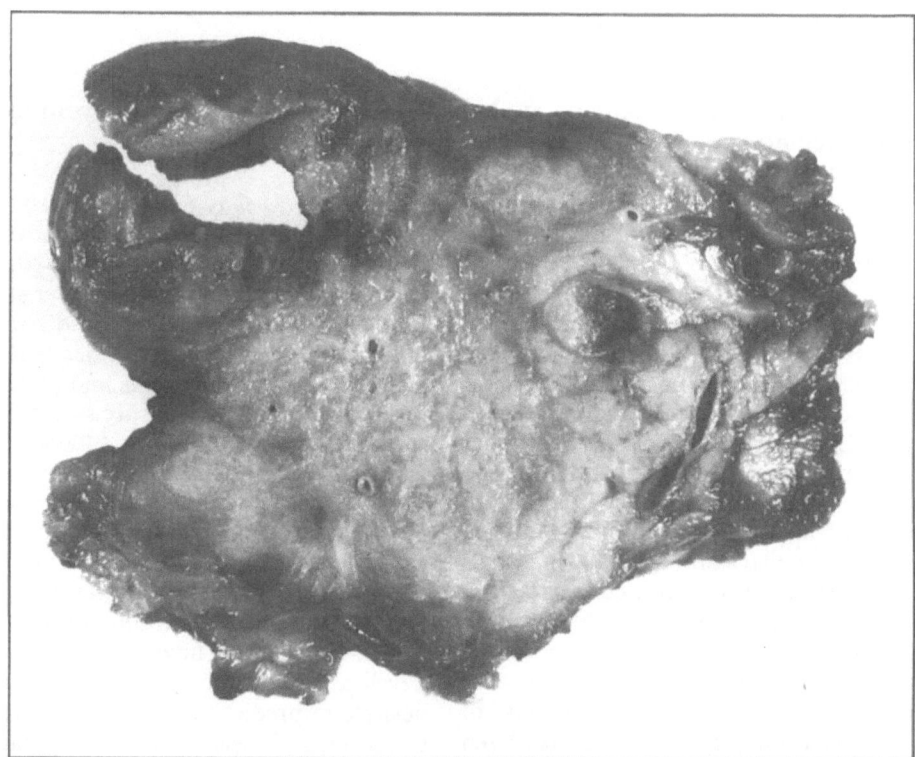

Fig. 9.3. A surgically resected carcinoma of the head of the pancreas that caused jaundice and had ulcerated into the duodenum distal to the papilla. The patient was a man aged 56. Microscopically the tumour was a ductal adenocarcinoma that was forming some mucin.

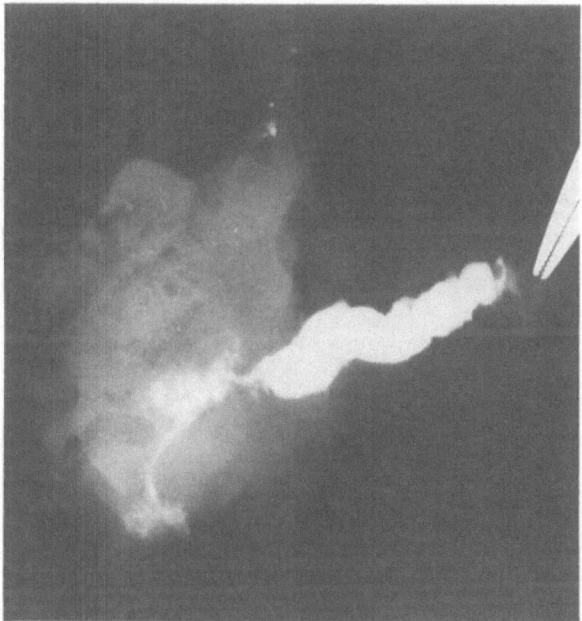

Fig. 9.4. The obstructive effect upon the duct of the pancreas demonstrated by the injection of Urografin in carcinoma of the head of the pancreas in a woman aged 65 who died with secondary carcinomatous deposits in the liver, lungs and kidneys associated with multiple venous thromboses and multiple pulmonary emboli. There was also cerebral infarction, non-bacterial thrombotic endocarditis and chronic pyelonephritis. Microscopically, the carcinoma was a poorly differentiated adenocarcinoma that secreted mucus and had caused a fibrous reaction.

carcinoma, was a relatively frequent cause of what has become known as Trousseau's syndrome. In 1938 Sproul published the results of her study of the association between thrombosis in any part of the circulatory system and the associated pathological findings in a series of 4258 consecutive necropsies. She found that a carcinoma was the most common cause of thrombosis in veins in the neck, abdomen, pelvis and the extremities, and that, in 56.2% of the cases of carcinoma in the body or tail of the pancreas, at least a single thrombus was present, while in 31.3% there was widely disseminated venous thrombosis; carcinoma of the head of the pancreas was associated with multiple thromboses in 9.7%.

In addition to venous thrombosis in association with carcinoma, Sproul also noted that non-bacterial vegetations, capable of embolising viscera and causing infarcts, might be present on the heart valves. Such vegetations, previously regarded as terminal and of no clinical significance (Libman and Sacks 1924; Gross and Friedberg 1936) received further attention during the 1950s (Oelbaum and Strich 1953; Smith and Yates 1955; MacDonald and Robbins 1957), while emboli from inconspicuous cardiac vegetations of this type may help to explain the observations by Thompson and Rodgers (1952) that, in their analysis of the autopsy records of 157 cases of carcinoma of the pancreas, there was a higher incidence of arterial thromboses than of venous thrombosis; they found this surprising.

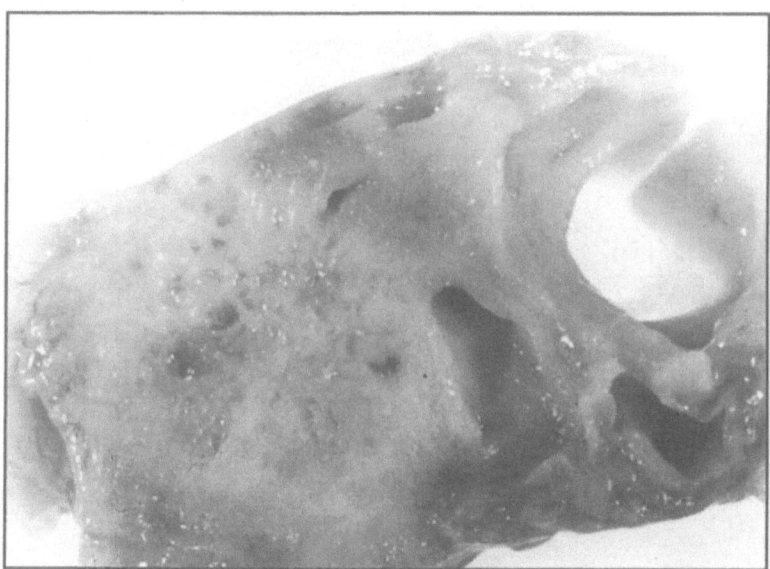

Fig. 9.5. Carcinoma of the head of the pancreas that caused no obstruction of the common bile duct but caused very marked dilatation of the pancreatic duct. Part of the dilated duct is included. The dilatation of the duct in the body of the pancreas is shown in Fig. 9.6. The pancreatic lesions were incidental findings in the body of a man of 65 whose sudden and unexpected death was explained by extensive myocardial fibrosis associated with atheromatous occlusion of the coronary arteries. Microscopically the tumour was a well-differentiated adenocarcinoma. No metastases were found.

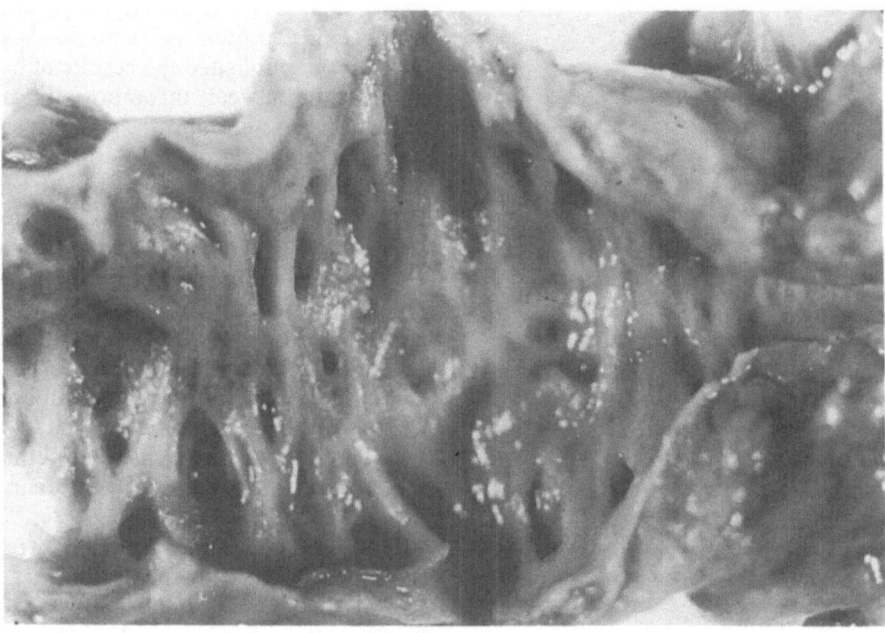

Fig. 9.6. The dilatation of the main duct and its tributaries in the body of the pancreas caused by the carcinoma of the head of the pancreas illustrated in Fig. 9.5.

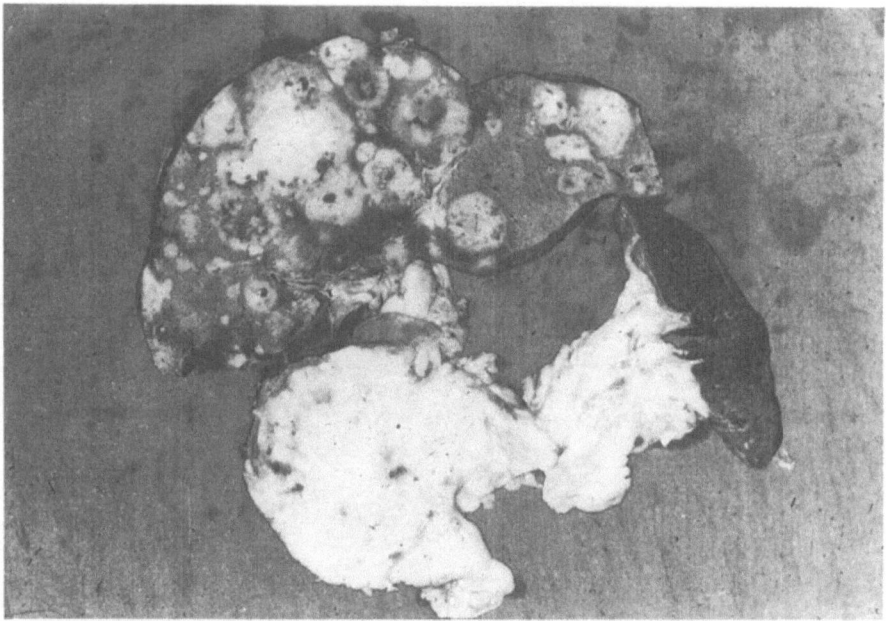

Fig. 9.7. Carcinoma of the head of the pancreas that caused the death of a man aged 63. At laparotomy, an inoperable pancreatic mass had been found. Microscopically it was a mucin-secreting adenocarcinoma. At autopsy, carcinoma of the head of the pancreas had invaded the first part of the duodenum and had caused thrombosis of the splenic and portal veins with many metastatic tumours in the liver. There was also thrombosis of both iliac veins and an infarct of the upper lobe of the right lung that was attributed to pulmonary embolism.

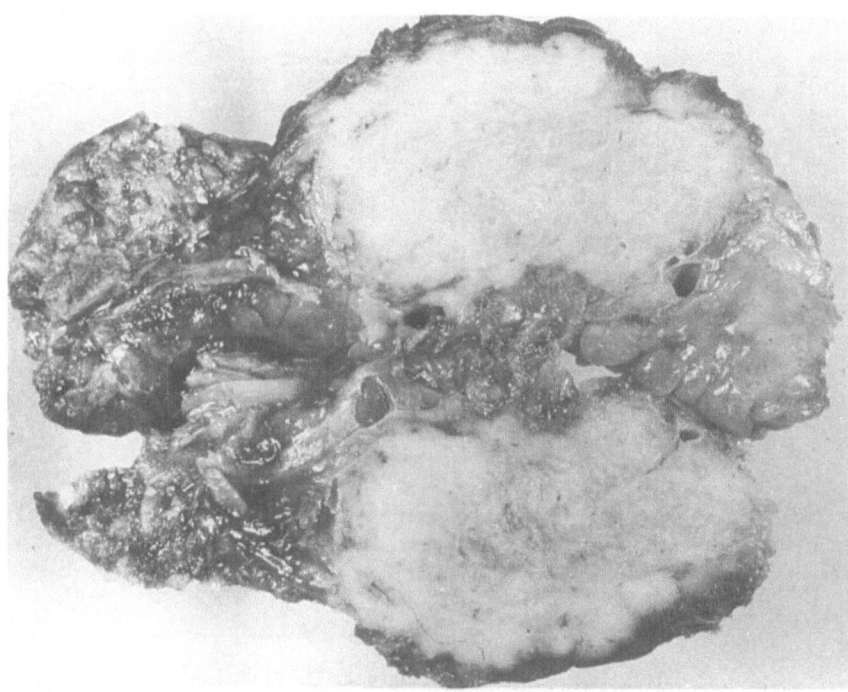

Fig. 9.8. This carcinoma appeared to have originated in the body of the pancreas, which was replaced by a firm infiltrative tumour that had spread into the tail of the gland and slightly into the head, but not sufficiently to obstruct the common bile duct. There was secondary carcinoma in the liver and the immediate cause of death was bronchopneumonia. The patient was a man aged 79 who had lost weight and who had had back pain for 13 weeks before his admission to hospital. Radiological examination of the alimentary system had demonstrated no abnormality and biopsy of a palpable lymph node in the groin was uninformative. Microscopically, the carcinoma was a poorly differentiated adenocarcinoma that had caused a fibrous reaction. It was forming some extracellular mucus, and intracellular mucus caused the presence of signet-ring cells. Phagocytosis of carcinoma cells by other carcinoma cells was seen, and there was well-marked invasion of the sheaths of nerves. Some calcification in one of the secondary tumours in the liver was demonstrated by the von Kossa method.

There now seems little doubt that, in some patients at least, non-bacterial thrombotic vegetations may cause clinical effects by embolising and causing infarcts in the brain or other viscera (British Medical Journal 1978). In his review of the cases of venous thromboses associated with cancer up to 1961, Gillam found that the pancreas was the most frequent site for the carcinoma; this is borne out in the more recent publications of Sack et al. (1977).

The thrombotic vegetations (Fig 9.11) occur principally on the mitral and aortic valve cusps, or less commonly on the tricuspid cusps, along the lines where they come into contact with each other during closure of the valves; they are very similar to the vegetations of rheumatic fever. Unlike this condition, however, they have been reported on the cusps of the pulmonary valve by Fayemi and Deppisch (1977), who also attributed myocardial infarction to embolism of the coronary arteries by fragments of vegetation.

The abnormality of the clotting process that produces Trousseau's syndrome and non-bacterial thrombotic endocarditis has not been fully determined as yet. Hypofibrinogenaemia, thrombocytopenia, fibrinogen–fibrin degradation products with or without increased fibrinolytic activity, increased prothrombin time, decreased Factors V, VIII and X, microangiopathic haemolytic anaemia, and the presence of cryoprotein, have been reported; the condition seems to be one of chronic disseminated intravascular coagulation (Sack et al. 1977). It has been suggested (Levison 1979) that in carcinoma of the pancreas, as in pancreatitis, the C5 component of complement may be activated to cause aggregation of neutrophils in the microcirculation, endothelial damage and microvascular coagulation.

It must be stressed that the majority of patients with carcinoma of the pancreas have neither a history of venous thromboses during their last illness nor recognisable thrombi post-mortem. Venous thrombosis was associated with the carcinoma in only 56 of the 194 cases of pancreatic carcinoma in which J.R. Miller et al. (1951) considered

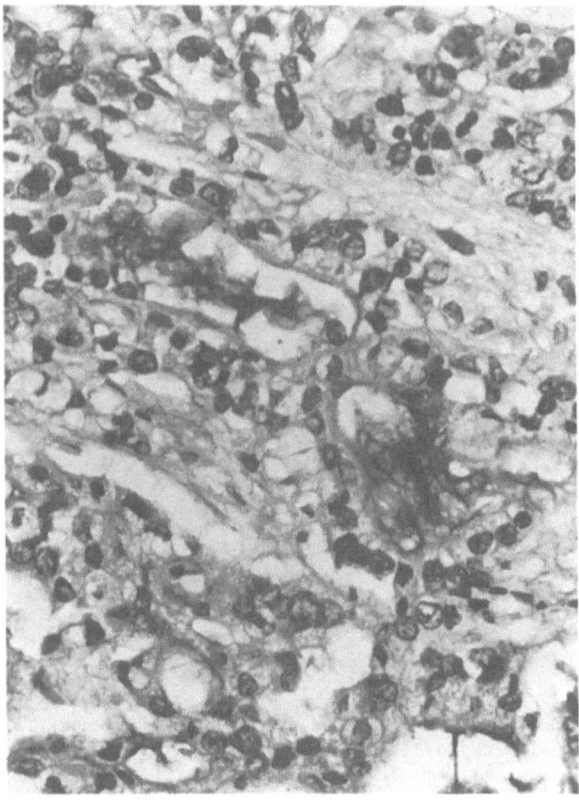

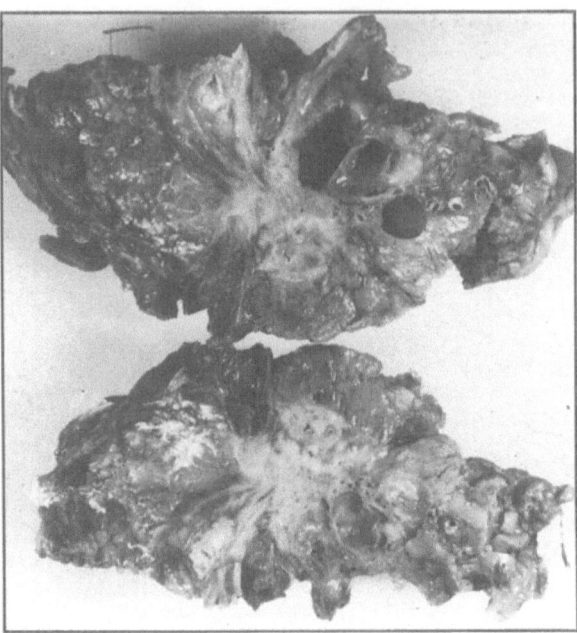

Fig. 9.9. Collections of extracellular mucus in the poorly differentiated carcinoma of the pancreas illustrated in Fig. 9.8. H&E, ×375

Fig. 9.10. The two halves of a bisected specimen of a carcinoma of the body of the pancreas, with cystic areas of dilated duct in the vicinity of the carcinoma. The cystic areas filled when the duct was injected. The specimen was obtained from a man aged 81. There were many hepatic metastases and there was thrombosis of the portal vein. Hyaline vegetations were present on the cusps of the aortic valve and there were patches of fibrous replacement of the left ventricular myocardium. The man was said to have been diabetic. Microscopically the pancreatic tumour and its metastases were adenocarcinomatous and there was some secretion of mucus. Invasion of nerve sheaths was marked.

that adequate information was available. They found it was more frequently associated with carcinoma of the body of the pancreas than with the head. They did not consider the histological type to be of importance in relation to venous thrombosis, although acinar-cell carcinomas were associated with a slightly higher incidence of thrombosis than were ductal carcinomas. The tumours with the highest histological grades of malignancy were, however, associated with the highest incidence of venous thrombosis. In a later study, Lafler and Hinderman (1961) found that, when carcinomas of the pancreas contained areas in which there was differentiation into structures that resembled pancreatic islets or acini, there was a high incidence (31%) of multiple thrombi, while, when the carcinoma consisted of undifferentiated neoplastic ductal epithelium in both the primary site and in metastatic deposits, the incidence of multiple thrombi was no greater than with carcinoma of the stomach. In 23 of 25 cases of pancreatic carcinoma that had multiple thrombi, these authors classified the micro-

scopic structure of the carcinoma as being of a "differentiating" ductal type. Such "differentiating" carcinomas tended to occur in the body and tail of the pancreas (Figs 9.8–9.17).

Other writers (Rohner et al. 1966; Chaudhuri 1971) have found an association between the secretion of mucus by a carcinoma, in any site, and venous thrombosis with non-bacterial vegetations on the heart valves, while yet others (Dreiling et al. 1955) have stressed that a tendency to thrombophlebitis occurs, not only in cases of pancreatic neoplasm, but also in inflammatory disease of the pancreas.

It seems unlikely that the tendency to thrombosis depends upon the liberation of pancreatic enzymes because cancers in many non-pancreatic sites have been associated with the syndrome and the mechanism remains obscure. The pathogenesis of the arterial lesions is also obscure in many cases, for it is almost impossible, even at autopsy, to be confident whether the arterial thrombi and the associated infarcts are a result of primary arterial thrombi, whether they are due to emboli from

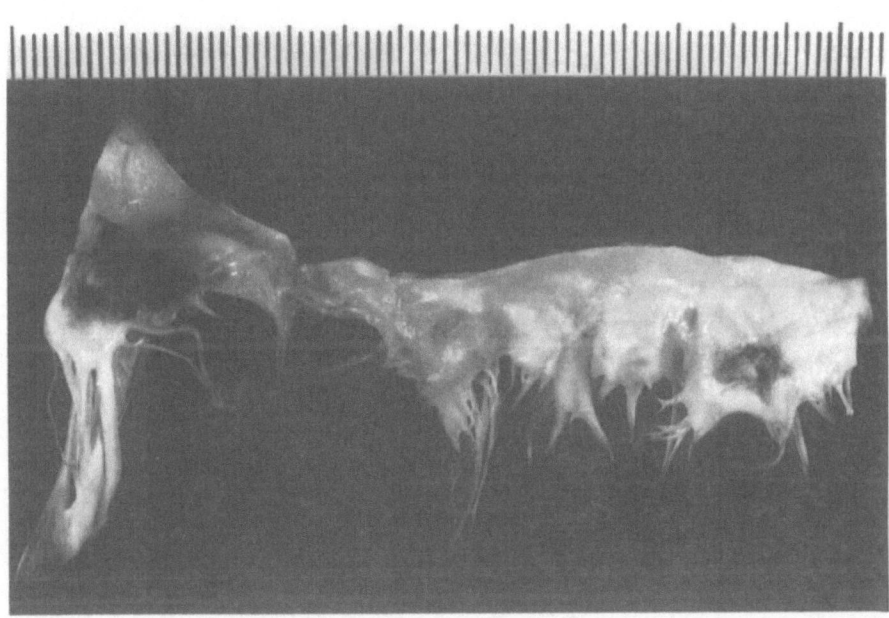

Fig. 9.11. Non-bacterial thrombotic vegetations on the mitral valve cusps of a man aged 65, who had generalised arteriosclerosis that caused intermittent claudication. After death, thrombi were found in the right coronary, femoral and carotid arteries, along with an atheromatous aneurysm of the abdominal aorta. Thrombi were also present in the veins of both legs and there was thrombotic endocarditis of the mitral valve. An unsuspected carcinoma in the tail of the pancreas had caused secondary carcinoma in lymph nodes and in the liver. Microscopically, the carcinoma was an adenocarcinoma in which there was some secretion of mucus with the formation of areas that resembled pancreatic islets in the secondary deposits in the liver. × 1.5

cardiac vegetations, or whether both embolic infarcts and infarcts due to non-embolic arterial thrombi are part of the syndrome. Attempts also to associate the syndrome with any type of histological differentiation in the carcinoma tend also to depend very much upon the subjective assessment of individuals. Acinar differentiation is easily overlooked (Webb 1977) and mixed histological patterns are common in carcinomas of the pancreas and in their metastatic deposits. In large masses of primary tumour with many metastases the determination of the predominant pattern might require more sampling and more searching than would be possible in most routine laboratories.

In 1983 Rickles and Edwards reviewed the clinical, histological, pharmacological and pathophysiologi-

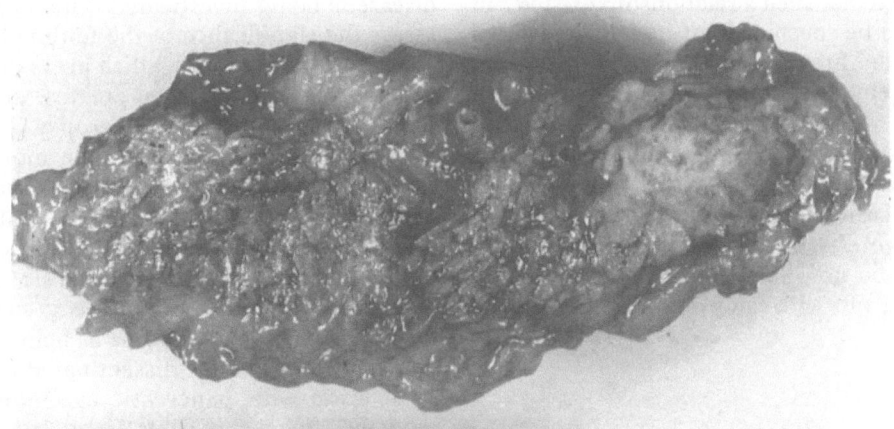

Fig. 9.12. The carcinoma in the tail of the pancreas from the case illustrated in Fig. 9.11, in which thrombosis of veins, thrombotic endocarditis and advanced degenerative arterial disease were also present.

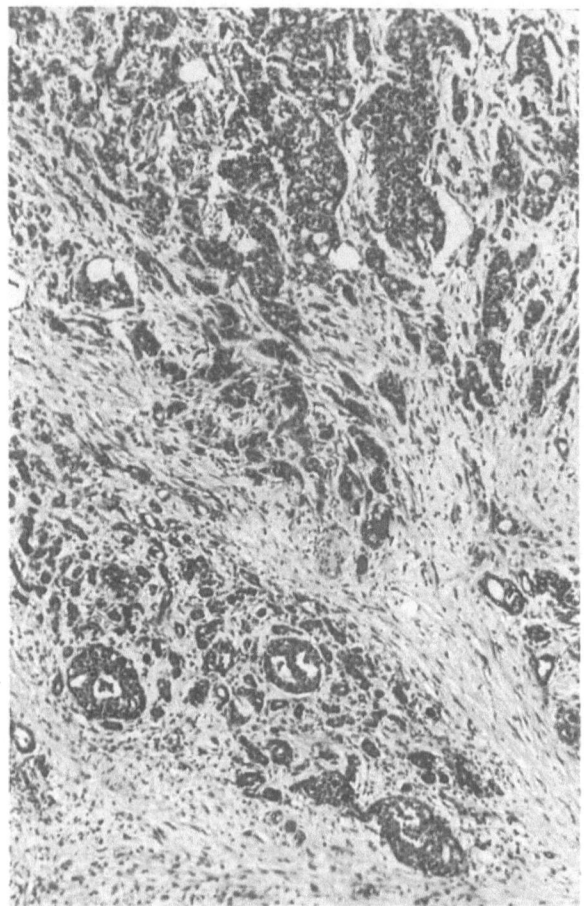

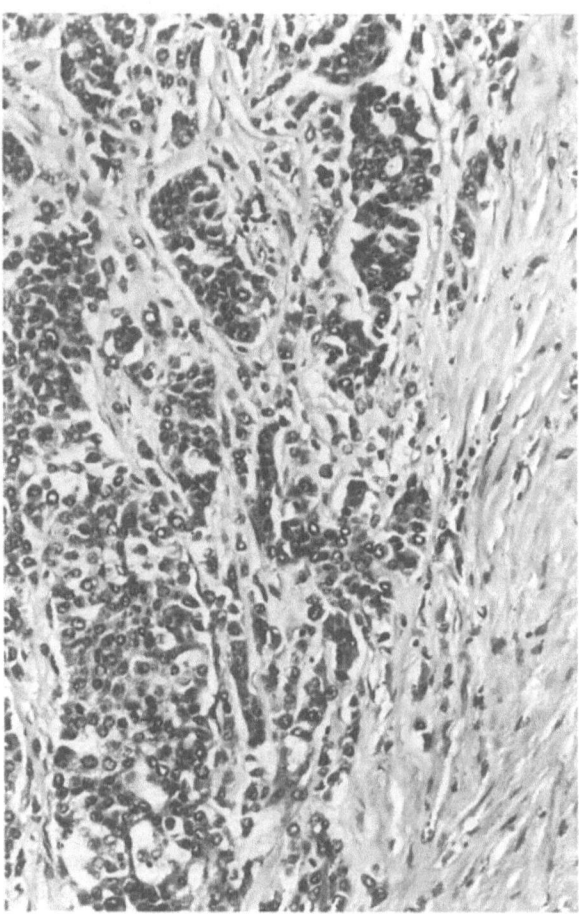

Fig. 9.13. A low-power view of the carcinoma illustrated in Fig. 9.12. Much of the carcinoma is poorly differentiated but islet-like structures are also present. H&E, × 60

Fig. 9.14. Higher-power view of the poorly differentiated area of the adenocarcinoma illustrated in Fig. 9.13. H&E, × 150

cal evidence that supported a relationship between cancer and abnormalities of blood coagulation. They concluded that such a relationship existed but were unable to be specific about its nature. It is of interest that the first of their tables showed that cancer of the pancreas was second only to cancer of the lung in being associated with thrombo-embolism. More recently (1989), Mellor et al. found that blood from patients with cancer of the breast or with colorectal cancer was abnormally vulnerable to the coagulative effects of endotoxin stimulation. Their studies did not, however, include samples of blood from patients with cancer of the pancreas.

Fat Necrosis

Foci of fat necrosis in and around the pancreas are commonplace in the bodies of patients who have died of non-pancreatic disease; this complicates the interpretation of fat necrosis when pancreatic disease is being investigated. Thus it is difficult to assess the significance of the finding by J.R. Miller et al. (1951) that small whitish areas of fat necrosis, usually less than 5 mm in greatest diameter, were found in 56 of their 202 necropsy cases of carci-noma of the pancreas, and even more difficult to assess the significance of their observation that fat necrosis was associated more commonly with acinar carcinomas than with those of the ductal type. They did not find fat necrosis, except in the vicinity of the pancreas, in the 27 cases in which they classified the carcinoma as being of the acinar type. However, widely disseminated fat necrosis in association with pancreatic carcinoma has been reported, for example by Auger (1947), in whose case a highly differentiated acinar cell carcinoma of the tail of the pancreas, in which the tumour cells

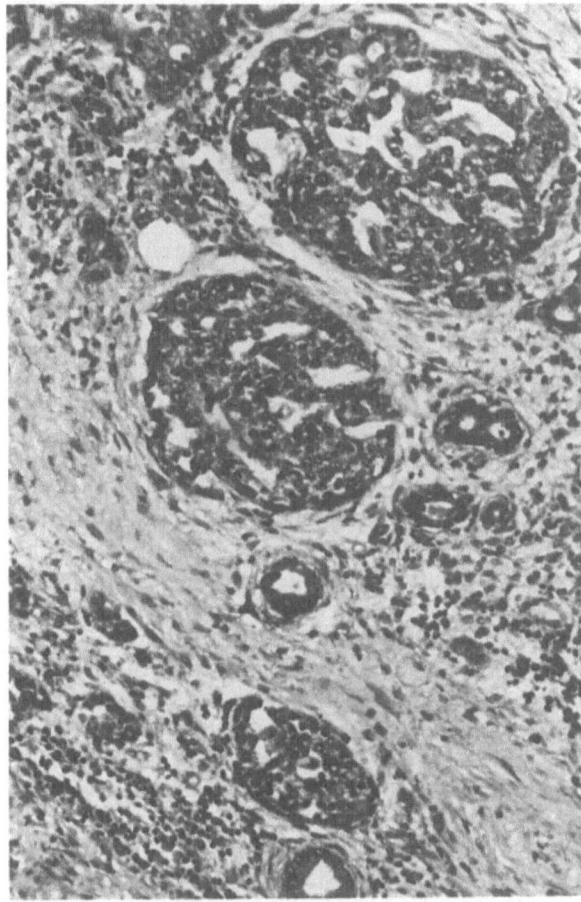

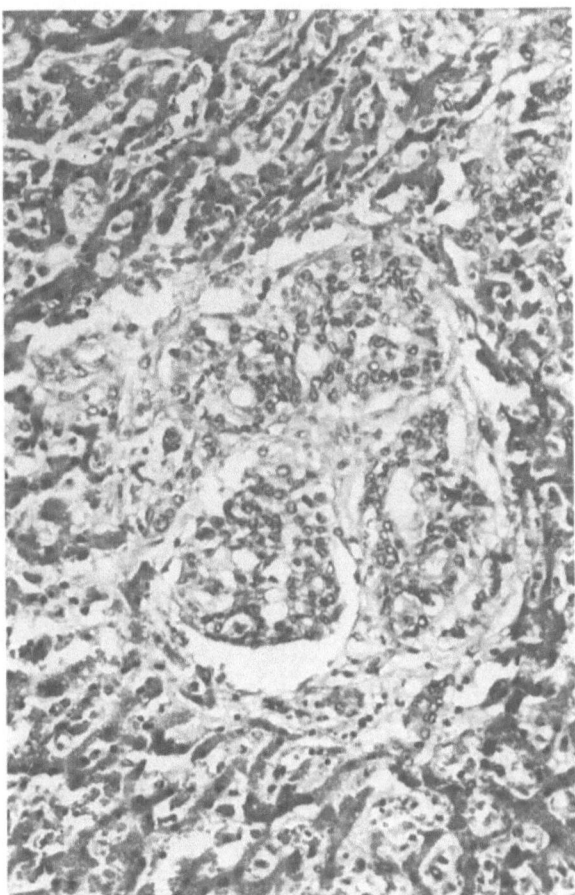

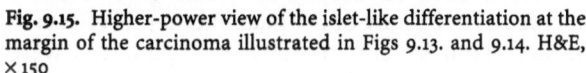

Fig. 9.15. Higher-power view of the islet-like differentiation at the margin of the carcinoma illustrated in Figs 9.13. and 9.14. H&E, ×150

Fig. 9.16. Islet-like differentiation in a deposit of secondary carcinoma in the liver from the pancreatic carcinoma illustrated in Figs 9.12–9.15. H&E, ×150

contained zymogen granules, had caused hepatic metastases; there were areas of fat necrosis in the subcutaneous tissues and in the epicardial fatty tissues, as well as in the peritoneal and retroperitoneal collections of fat. Auger concluded that the tumour cells must have been secreting lipase and liberating it into the circulation. In 1950 Osborne reported a similar case and referred to several earlier records, while, by 1970, Robertson and Eeles were able to find nine previously published cases when they described one of their own, in which they were able to show that the serum lipase was increased to about four times the normal level. Similar markedly raised serum lipase was present in the case published by Burns et al. (1974), who also demonstrated histochemically and biochemically that the carcinomatous tissue, obtained postmortem, had abundant lipase activity. More recently, Hubran et al. (1987) have described a neo-

plasm with both pancreatic and hepatocellular differentiation that caused subcutaneous fat necrosis. The neoplasm was taken originally to be a hepatocellular carcinoma, but at autopsy a small tumour in the tail of the pancreas was interpreted by the authors, mainly on biochemical evidence, to be the primary cancer.

Disseminated fat necrosis, it must be emphasised, is a rare phenomenon in carcinoma of the pancreas, even in cases in which the tumour has a well-differentiated acinar cell structure. Many cases of carcinoma of the pancreas have some elevation of the serum lipase (Braganza and Howat 1979) but disseminated fat necrosis is only rarely associated. Moreover, fat necrosis was not found in any of the 11 patients with acinar cell carcinoma studied by Webb (1977); it was absent also in his case in which the pancreas contained an adenoma of acinar cells. Moreover, disseminated fat necrosis

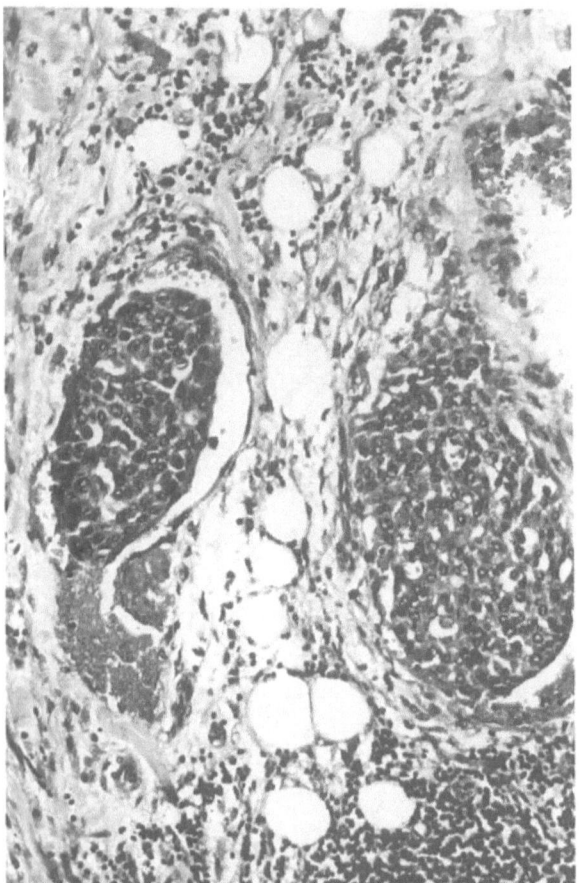

Fig. 9.17. Invasion of small blood vessels, associated with some thrombosis, by the carcinoma illustrated in Figs 9.12–9.15. The vessels are in the connective tissue around the pancreas. H&E, × 150

can occur in non-neoplastic pancreatic disease, especially in pancreatitis (Scarpelli 1956; Lièvre 1974). When there is disseminated fat necrosis, it is often associated with a clinical syndrome in which polyarthritis is a conspicuous feature, along with fever, some increase of eosinophil granulocytes in the blood, and the cutaneous lesions of Weber–Christian disease (i.e. relapsing, nodular, non-suppurative panniculitis). In this syndrome, many of the features are without satisfactory explanations. Fat necrosis in the bone marrow is sometimes present in disseminated fat necrosis, but this seems unlikely to be the cause of the eosinophilia and, while cases of Weber–Christian disease with fat necrosis in deep visceral sites have been reported by, for example, Milner and Mitchinson (1965), most cases of Weber–Christian disease have fat necrosis only in the subcutaneous

fat, and there is no evidence that the pancreas plays any part in the pathogenesis of this disease.

Effects of Pancreatic Carcinoma upon the Splenic and Superior Mesenteric Blood Vessels

In 1963, Bauerlein and de la Vega published a note that they had heard a highly localised bruit in the left upper abdominal quadrant in two patients, both of whom proved at surgery to have cancer of the body of the pancreas; in one of these, narrowing of the splenic artery by the carcinoma was demonstrated post-mortem. The value of this sign was confirmed by Serebro (1965), who reported that the bruit had been heard in eight of 21 cases of carcinoma of the body, or body and tail, but was heard in only one of the 34 patients with carcinoma of the head of the pancreas, while Arlen and Brockunier (1967) also found the bruit to be of value, in combination with other evidence, in the diagnosis of carcinoma of the tail of the pancreas. If a bruit is heard, coeliac angiography is likely to be of value in differentiating between carcinoma of the body or tail of the pancreas and other causes of a bruit, for example an aneurysm or exaggerated tortuosity of the splenic artery.

The splenic vein is particularly vulnerable to compression, thrombosis and invasion when there is carcinoma of the tail or body of the pancreas and the results of a study of the haemodynamic effects of its occlusion by carcinoma of the pancreas were reported by Ku et al. in 1989. They found that, if the occlusion was only partial, neither gastric varices nor splenomegaly developed. If the occlusion was complete while the splenic artery remained patent, both gastric varices and moderate splenomegaly were produced (in their illustrative case of this type the patient had had episodes of severe haematemesis). If however, occlusion of the splenic artery became superimposed upon the occlusion of the splenic vein, varices would shrink and splenomegaly would disappear.

The superior mesenteric artery may also be constricted by carcinoma of the pancreas. Our own experience of this was in a 70-year-old man who was admitted to hospital because of upper abdominal pain that he had had for 5 months. Two days after his admission he had a severe haemorrhage from his rectum and died. Post-mortem he was found to have infarction of his small intestine because of the occlusion of the superior mesenteric artery by scirrhous carcinoma of the body and tail of the pancreas. Microscopically the cancer was a poorly differentiated adenocarcinoma; it had widely infiltrated the mesentery of the small intestine and there was secondary carcinoma in the liver.

Alimentary Haemorrhage

Gastrointestinal bleeding is usually a late manisfestation of carcinoma of the pancreas. In eight of Duff's (1939) 16 cases of carcinoma of the body and tail of the pancreas there was a history of haematemesis, and in six others gross or occult blood had been observed in the stools. Duff attributed such bleeding to invasion with ulceration of the stomach or duodenum by the cancer rather than to haemorrhage from gastric varices.

Splenomegaly

Palpable splenomegaly is rare in pancreatic carcinoma. In the observations of Ku and his colleagues referred to above, the splenomegaly was detected by scanning or at laparotomy. Splenomegaly was present in only three of the 100 cases of pancreatic carcinoma reviewed by Grieve (1973).

Constipation and Diarrhoea

Either constipation or diarrhoea, or alternating constipation and diarrhoea, are not uncommon symptoms in the clinical histories of patients with carcinoma of the pancreas, but it is rare to find an anatomical explanation for these symptoms.

Vomiting

Vomiting is an early symptom in some patients with pancreatic carcinoma, especially when the tumour is in the head of the gland (Gullick 1959; Braganza and Howat 1972). It is much less common as an early symptom of the disease when the carcinoma is in the body or tail of the gland. The effects of the carcinoma in the head of the gland upon the adjacent duodenum are the obvious explanation for the difference in the incidence and, even in patients where a carcinoma of the head of the pancreas has been deemed to be resectable, invasion of the muscularis of the duodenum, or even mucosal involvement, is commonly found in the surgically removed specimen, while palliative procedures very often have to include gastrojejunostomy along with drainage of the obstructed biliary passages. Direct invasion of the stomach is liable to occur in the late stages of carcinoma of the body or tail of the pancreas (Duff 1939).

Ascites

Ascites is seldom the presenting symptom in carcinoma of the pancreas, but involvement of the peritoneal cavity is very common as the disease progresses. Ascites due to peritoneal spread of the carcinoma was present in ten of the 16 cases of carcinoma of the body and tail studied by Duff (1939).

Steatorrhoea

Although atrophy of the body and tail of the pancreas is sometimes extreme when a carcinoma has obstructed the main pancreatic duct, steatorrhoea is rare. A case of cancer of the body of the pancreas in a woman aged 61, in whom the presenting symptom was steatorrhoea, has however, been described by Braganza and Howat (1972).

Osteomalacia

In a case examined post-mortem by one of the authors, very marked atrophy of the pancreas caused by a small carcinoma in the head of the gland that had obstructed the main pancreatic duct without obstructing the common bile duct, was associated with advanced osteomalacia in a woman aged 94. It seemed that deficiency of pancreatic secretion must have prevented the absorption of vitamin D and caused the osteomalacia. Osteomalacia in association with a mucin-secreting carcinoma of the pancreas was present also in a case discussed by Whitfield (1968) at a clinicopathological conference at the Royal Postgraduate Medical School and later published in the *British Medical Journal.*

Autonomic Dysfunction

Thomas and Shields (1970) described the case of a man aged 68, in whom carcinoma of the pancreas was associated with sodium depletion due to increased sodium excretion and postural hypotension. The authors suggested that a defect of aldosterone secretion had been induced by impairment of the renin–angiotensin mechanism, due to damage to the sympathetic nerve supply to the kidneys. No post-mortem examination was permitted, but the presence of carcinoma, with metastic deposits in the liver, had been found at laparotomy during which the adrenal glands were found to be normal.

Renal Failure

Acute renal failure may develop in association with carcinoma of the pancreas in two different ways. Hobbs et al. (1974) described the case of a man of 43 who became anuric. When peritoneal dialysis was begun he was found to have ascitic fluid that contained mucus-secreting adenocarcinoma cells; laparotomy confirmed that he had peritoneal carcinomatosis. At necropsy, he was found to have carcinoma of the body and tail of the pancreas. His renal failure was shown convincingly to have been due to renal tubular obstruction by mucoproteins that had been released into the ascitic fluid from a mucus-secreting carcinoma of the pancreas that had caused many secondary deposits within the peritoneal cavity. The mucoproteins were believed to have entered the patient's serum and to have been filtered through the renal glomeruli to form very viscous casts in the renal collecting tubules, with consequent oliguria.

Another type of renal failure associated with pancreatic carcinoma is the result of diffuse intravascular coagulation. A case of this type has been described by Lorge and Richards (1976), whose patient, a woman aged 57, was being treated for thrombosis of the arteries to her right arm and hand when she became anuric and died. At necropsy, there was bilateral renal cortical necrosis with fibrin thrombi in the afferent glomerular arterioles. Thrombi were also present in the lungs, portal vein and submucosal veins of the colon, as well as in the right subclavian and brachial arteries. The pancreas contained a scirrhous mucus-secreting adenocarcinoma that replaced most of the head and body of the gland and had metastasised widely throughout the abdomen.

Abnormal Immunity and Pancreatic Carcinoma

There are reports of at least two cases in which there was thought to be a possibly significant association between states of abnormal immunity and carcinoma of the pancreas. In one, an unsuspected adenocarcinoma was found post-mortem in a 17-year-old girl with leukaemia who had been treated by immunosuppression (Tavassoli and Lynch 1974), while Cibull et al. (1978) have recorded the case of a 53-year-old man in whom immunoblastic lymphadenopathy developed 5 months before he was recognised to have an anaplastic adenocarcinoma of the pancreas.

Neurofibromatosis and Pancreatic Carcinoma

The case history of a woman aged 27, who suffered from von Recklinghausen's neurofibromatosis and who developed adenocarcinoma of the pancreas, has been published by Keller and Logan (1977).

Lipomatous Pseudohypertrophy and Pancreatic Carcinoma

Two examples of the association of these two conditions have been recorded by Salm (1960, 1968).

Skin Changes

A generalised increase in skin pigmentation occurred during the illness of a woman whose case was discussed by Fraser at a clinicopathological conference published in 1963. After death, the patient was found to have a poorly differentiated adenocarcinoma of the pancreas that had infiltrated the adjacent vertebral bodies. Such pigmentation is not uncommon in diseases associated with emaciation and is quite non-specific.

The pigmentation that occurs in acanthosis nigricans, however, is more specifically associated with deep-seated, sometimes unsuspected, malignancy. Acanthosis nigricans is a paraneoplastic syndrome and is one of the so-called skin markers of malignancy. There is evidence that it is a form of ectopic hormone production in which circulating molecules closely related to epidermal growth factor become bound to epidermal growth factor receptors on keratinocytes (Ellis et al. 1987). It is more characteristic clinically than microscopically and forms brownish patches on the skin of the axillae, neck, genital or submammary regions. If this type of pigmentation appears for the first time in an adult (the juvenile form has no sinister significance), and is unassociated with signs of endocrine disease, such as insulin-resistant diabetes mellitus or the polycystic ovarian syndrome, it is reputed (Curth et al. 1962) to indicate that a person has, or shortly will have, an adenocarcinoma. The most common site for the adenocarcinoma is the stomach, but, amongst the 42 cases of acanthosis nigricans studied by Curth et al., there were three in whom the adenocarcinoma was in the pancreas. The specificity of the association between the carcinoma and the dermatosis is that the dermatosis regresses after removal of the primary tumour and recurs when metastases develop (Sneddon 1963). Acanthosis nigricans is a rare manifestation of carcinoma in any site, and a very rare manifestation of carcinoma of the pancreas.

In 1964, Boyd published a case report of the association of pemphigoid of the skin with a mucus-secreting adenocarcinoma that involved the body and tail of the pancreas, and referred to nine previously reported cases in which pemphigoid of the skin had been associated with malignant tumours. It has, of course, since been shown that necrolytic migratory erythema of the skin is an important component of the syndrome caused by glucagon-secreting carcinomas of the pancreas, but such tumours are undoubtedly endocrine tumours of the pancreas (Higgins et al. 1979), not exocrine carcinomas.

Ectopic Hormone Production

ACTH

The association of hyperplasia of the suprarenal cortices with carcinoma of the pancreas was first noted by Kepler in 1933 in a woman with muscular weakness, altered appearance, facial hair, loss of weight, glycosuria, amenorrhoea and subcutaneous oedema. The removal of what was thought to be a carcinoma of the left suprarenal gland did not relieve her symptoms and when she died she was found to have a carcinoma of the entire head of the pancreas with metastases in the liver, lymph nodes and peritoneum. The right superarenal gland was identical, both macroscopically and microscopically, to the previously removed left suprarenal gland. Reports of similar cases followed, and by 1977 Davis and Hipkin estimated that, amongst the great variety of tumours incriminated in the ectopic ACTH syndrome, about 10% of the reported cases had been caused by carcinoma of the pancreas, although not all these carcinomas have been exocrine, for islet cell carcinomas and carcinoid tumours of the pancreas may also cause the syndrome.

ADH

This syndrome is usually discovered following routine serum electrolyte estimations showing that a patient has hypontraemia. Further investigations of the type carried out by Marks et al. (1968) and by Vorherr et al. (1968) have demonstrated that the antidiuretic hormone has had its origin in a carcinoma. Such carcinomas are most commonly "oat cell" carcinomas of the lung, but, in the case studied by Marks et al., although cancer of the lung was present, the source of the antidiuretic hormone was demonstrated to be an unrelated adenocarcinoma of the pancreas. Nine of the ten cases reported by Vorherr et al. had carcinoma of the lung, but in the remaining case the antidiuretic hormone was secreted by an adenocarcinoma of the pancreas.

Hypercalcaemia

A case of intractable hypercalcaemia associated with squamous cell carcinoma of the pancreas has been reported by Brayko and Doll (1982). The patient had normal parathormone levels during the illness and was found at autopsy to have normal parathyroid glands and to have no skeletal deposits of secondary carcinoma. Hypercalcaemia has also been found in a patient with a small cell carcinoma of the pancreas by Hobbs et al. (1984). The pancreatic tumour was similar histologically to an oat cell carcinoma of the lung, with which hypercalcaemia is well known to be associated, but no tumour was present in the lung.

Macroscopic Features

Site

The importance of whether a carcinoma is situated in the head of the pancreas, or elsewhere in the gland, has already been mentioned in relation to jaundice. In all the largest studies of the subject, the head is the commonest site. The figures given by Gullick (1959) are typical: amongst 100 cases, the carcinoma was in the head in 60, in the head and adjacent body in another five, in the body alone in 14, in the body and tail in ten, and in the tail alone in two; in nine, the site of the cancer was not determined. Very similar figures are those given by Mikal and Campbell (1950), who classified the site only as the head, body or tail. They found that in 100 consecutive autopsy cases of carcinoma of the pancreas, 67 of the carcinomas were located in the head, 19 in the body and 14 in the tail; thus about two-thirds of carcinomas of the pancreas occur in the head and one-third in the body and tail. Such precise localisation to arbitrary anatomical parts of the pancreas is very difficult in practice, for carcinoma may be diffusely distributed (Salmon (1966) classified 22 of his 336 cases as diffuse), or there may be multiple tumour nodules (Grauer 1939). As far as symptoms are concerned, it has been pointed out by Frantz (1959) that there are only three important sites: the head, the rest of the pancreas, and heterotopic pancreatic tissue, which, according to Barbosa et al. (1946) may give rise to carcinomas. If a carcinoma that has arisen in aberrant pancreatic tissue is an islet cell tumour, its origin is relatively easily recognised, but, if it is a carcinoma of the exocrine component, its true origin is likely to be missed and the tumour classified as an adenocarcinoma of the stomach, duodenum or small intestine, depending on the site of the heterotopia.

Size

In autopsy material, carcinomas of the head tend to be smaller than carcinomas of the body and tail, probably because their obstructive effect upon the biliary tree tends to cause death more rapidly than non-obstructive carcinomas in the body or tail, but the difference in size is not very marked. Mikal and Campbell (1950) found the average diameter of carcinoma of the head to be 5.7 cm, that of carcinoma of the body to be 7.3 cm and that of the tail to be 6.9 cm, while carcinoma of the ampulla of Vater was only about 1 cm in diameter.

In living patients, the prognostic implications of the diameter of carcinomas of the head of the pancreas were studied by Nix et al. (1991) in 220 cases. In these, the diameter of the tumours ranged from 0.5 to 15.0 cm. As was to be expected, the small tumours without hepatic or other metastases were associated with the greatest chance of curative operation and, on average, had the longest survival. Small tumours, however, with liver or other metastases carried a worse prognosis than large tumours with liver or other metastases. If tumours were found to be unresectable at operation, the size of the tumour did not affect survival.

Features

Some abnormality of the surface of the pancreas is usually recognisable, but the presence of a tumour is more easily recognised by palpation; most tumours are very hard. When the gland is incised, the carcinoma becomes obvious as grey, whitish or creamy areas with ill-defined margins. Small cystic spaces are quite common on the cut surface and it is sometimes difficult without microscopic examination to identify a small carcinoma that may have caused much dilatation of ducts in its vicinity. It has been pointed out by Bowden (1958) that, in carcinoma of the head of the pancreas, the mass in the gland may be appreciably greater than the true size of the actual neoplasm. In autopsy specimens, there has very often been some previous operation during which some palliative procedure, usually cholecystenterostomy, has been carried out to relieve biliary obstruction; a gastrojejunostomy may also have been constructed to relieve duodenal obstruction. If no effective palliative operation has been carried out, a carcinoma of the head is usually associated with dilatation of the biliary passages, deep jaundice and secondary biliary cirrhosis; ulceration into the duodenum is common. Although carcinoma of the head of the pancreas usually causes some dilatation of the duct system in the body and tail of the gland, the degree of dilatation is very variable. Some haemorrhagic foci are not uncommon but large areas of gross haemorrhage and necrosis are rare. A gritty sensation on cutting the tumour is common, but calcification has not been recognised by the authors except in microscopic preparations. The presence of mucus is often recognised, but it is difficult with the naked eye to differentiate between the formation of mucus by the carcinoma and mucoid secretion that has been retained in obstructed ducts. The large acinar mucus-filled cystandenocarcinoma is discussed elsewhere (Chap. 8). Acinar carcinomas are said to be softer than the commoner ductal type (Levison 1979) and it is said also that, when carcinoma is associated with pancreatic lithiasis, there may be a cystic mass in which calculi of various sizes may be felt (Frantz 1959). Foci of fat necrosis within the pancreas and in the adjacent fat are common, but such foci, which appear to develop terminally in many moribund patients, may not be specifically related to the carcinoma. The obstructive effects of carcinoma of the head of the pancreas upon the ducts of the body and tail have been studied in detail by Haunz and Baggenstoss (1950). Gross cystic changes were present in only seven of the 25 cases they examined in detail, but they found that there was dilatation of the duct of Wirsung to an average of three and a half times the size of the normal duct, and that there was marked fibrous and fatty replacement of the acinar tissues, greatest in the cases in which the dilatation of the duct of Wirsung was most marked. An example of marked dilatation of the duct of Wirsung, with obvious dilatation of the ducts of the lobules, caused by a carcinoma of the head of the pancreas is illustrated in Fig. 9.6.

Since the introduction of endoscopic retrograde cholangiopancreatography the case reported by Mizumoto et al. (1988) has illustrated that the very earliest stages of the disease can be diagnosed by that method, and that a prompt operation may yield an apparently normal specimen in which invasive carcinoma can, nevertheless, be found microscopically.

In carcinoma of the head of the gland there is early invasion of the common bile duct and of the wall of the first, or more commonly, the second part of the duodenum. Probably later, although determining exact timing is impossible and the circumstances vary from case to case, there is invasion of the walls of the portal or superior mesenteric veins. In carcinoma of the body or tail of the gland the splenic vein tends to be invaded. In any of these veins, penetration of the wall may lead to thrombosis within the vein, but this is by no means invariable. In microscopic preparations of invaded veins, clumps of carcinoma cells in a background of cellular fibrous tissue can be seen to form rounded projections on the internal aspect of the vein with only a thin layer of thrombus on their surfaces. It is, no doubt, from such projections that emboli of carcinoma cells reach the liver. At a later stage, thrombosis of the veins occurs and the thrombus becomes permeated by carcinoma. The malignantly infiltrated thrombus may then extend along the portal venous system and into the liver.

In any carcinoma of the pancreas, especially of the body, there is early invasion of the retroperitoneal tissues, both directly and around the nerves and ganglia of the coeliac plexus (Fig. 9.18). The results of a clinicopathological study of neural invasion in cancer of the head of the pancreas has been reported by Nagakawa et al. (1992). In such studies it is important to distinguish between true neural invasion and the benign epithelial inclusions in pancreatic nerves described by Costa (1977). The findings in the 34 cases examined by Nagakawa et al. led them to recommend the en bloc resection of the retropancreatic nerve plexus and fatty tissue. The frequent involvement of the peripancreatic soft tissue has also been shown by the results of Willett et al. (1993). Invasion of the peritoneal cavity is liable to occur with carcinoma in any part of the pancreas and such invasion usually leads to

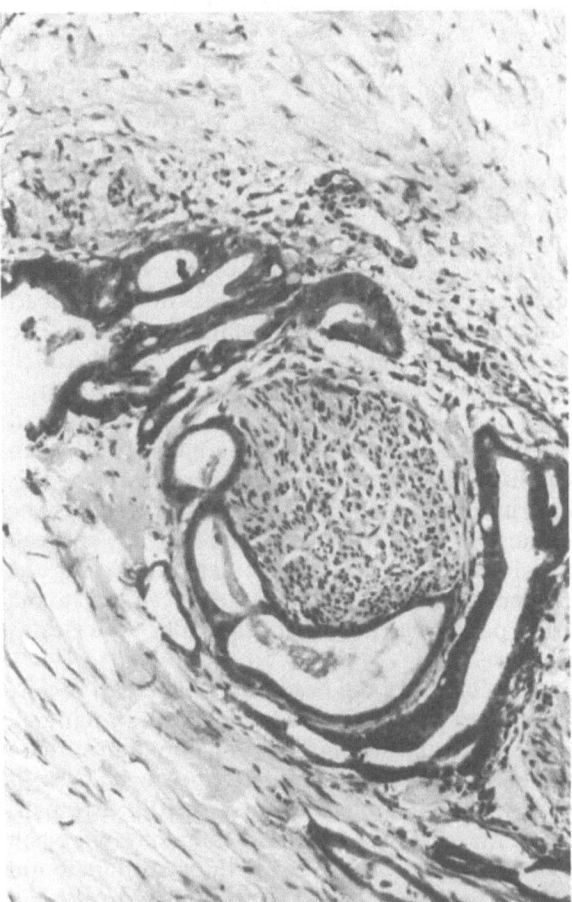

Fig. 9.18. Well-differentiated adenocarcinoma of the pancreas in a man aged 60. The carcinoma is spreading in the sheath of a nerve. In other parts of the tumour there was squamous differentiation of the carcinoma cells. H&E, × 150

transperitoneal spread and peritoneal carcinomatosis. If peritoneal carcinomatosis is caused by the spread of a mucin-secreting carcinoma of the pancreas, the mucin may provoke a granulomatous reaction that may obscure the presence of the carcinoma cells in a peritoneal biopsy (Chen and Brittin 1980).

In the advanced stages of the disease found in the post-mortem room, various effects of local invasion that have been noted include invasion and obstruction of the third part of the duodenum by carcinoma of the body of the pancreas, infarction of the spleen by occlusion of the splenic artery, invasion of the stomach by carcinoma of the body of the pancreas, invasion of the left adrenal gland and kidney by carcinoma of the tail of the pancreas, and infiltration of the transverse mesocolon by carcinoma of the body. In one of our own cases a carcinoma near the head of the pancreas in a man of 84 years had invaded the right kidney, although the cancer had not caused biliary obstruction. When there is extensive retroperitoneal spread it is impossible in the post-mortem room to distinguish between direct infiltration and spread that may originally have been to retroperitoneal lymph nodes with subsequent extension beyond the capsules of the nodes. Peritoneal spread, too, may involve retroperitoneal structures, as in one case of peritoneal carcinomatosis due to carcinoma of the tail of the pancreas in which, post-mortem, one of the authors found bilateral ureteric obstruction by the carcinoma. A case in which occlusion of the superior mesenteric artery by carcinoma of the body and tail of the pancreas caused infarction of the small intestine has already been described (p. 158). In arterial thrombosis of this type, unless invasion of the arterial wall can be demonstrated, it is difficult to differentiate between local invasive effects and the general thrombotic tendency that may accompany advanced carcinoma of the pancreas, and which may affect arteries as well as veins.

In carcinoma of the head of the pancreas, in particular, and in most cases in which the carcinoma has arisen from the epithelium of the ducts, there may be marked extension along the ducts, even in the absence of lymphatic involvement or extrapancreatic invasion, as has been pointed out by Matsui et al. (1979). In five such cases, these authors found that the cancer extended continuously to the tail along the ducts and had reached the end of the ducts in three. They attributed the recurrences amongst their cases (who had been treated by the Whipple's type of procedure), to the intraduct type of spread into the pancreatic remnant. The possibility that some carcinomas of the pancreas may consist of multiple foci of tumour has also been suggested to explain recurrences within the pancreatic remnant after subtotal pancreatectomy. The existence of multicentricity has been investigated by Motojima et al. (1993) using point mutations in the Kirsten-*ras* oncogene. They claim to have shown the existence of multicentricity in 6% of their 53 cases of carcinoma of the pancreas.

Direct invasion of the spleen may occur in carcinoma of the distal pancreas, but this is much less common than invasion of the stomach or duodenum, which had occurred in 20% of the 100 autopsy cases studied by Mikal and Campbell (1950).

Metastatic Spread

It is surprising that almost all the studies of carcinoma of the pancreas based upon the findings at necropsy, when advanced disease is to be expected, include cases in which no metastatic spread was recognisable. The figures quoted by Frantz (1959), in her review of such reports, varied between 13% and 18%, but, if the cancer is in the body or tail, metastatic spread has nearly always taken place; Silver and Lubliner (1948) found metastases in 95% of cases of carcinoma of the body and tail. In her review, Frantz collected a total of 850 cases from the published reports and was able to classify the freqency with which various sites were affected as: common, fairly common, uncommon and rare. The common sites were: liver, regional lymph nodes, peritoneum and lungs. The fairly common sites were: adrenals, duodenum, kidneys, stomach, gall bladder, intestines, spleen, bones (skull, vertebrae, ribs, sternum, mandible), pleura and diaphragm. In this group, she pointed out that some of the sites were liable to be involved by invasion as well as by metastasis. The group of uncommon sites included: brain, heart and pericardium, skin and subcutaneous tissue, ovaries, uterus, urinary bladder and thyroid. The rare sites were: testis, epididymis, prostate, ureter, spinal cord, oesophagus, skeletal muscles, parotid gland, breast, umbilicus and rectum.

The two very common sites for metastatic deposits are the liver and the lymph nodes in the immediate vicinity of the pancreas. Liver biopsy, either pre-operatively or during laparotomy or peritoneoscopy, is thus recommended by Bender and Brennan (1978) for all patients on whom pancreatic resection for carcinoma is being considered. The involvement of lymph nodes by carcinoma in the area of the head of the pancreas has been studied by Cubilla et al. (1978) in 33 pancreatectomy specimens amongst which there were 22 cases of adenocarcinoma of the pancreatic ducts. Pancreatic duct adenocarcinoma tended to metastasise to multiple lymph nodes above the head and body of the pancreas and to the pancreaticoduodenal lymph nodes behind the head of the pancreas. These nodes were involved in 88% of the cases studied. The results of a similar study carried out on autopsy specimens by Nagai et al. (1986) were, on the whole, similar. No lymphatic metastatic spread was found in two of their cases in which the primary tumour was less than 1 cm in diameter. They also found that, although lymphatic spread and perineural invasion were closely related, the two types of spread did not always coincide in the same specimen.

The tendency of exocrine carcinomas of the pancreas to spread is only slightly influenced by their microscopic structure; J.R. Miller et al. (1951) concluded that ductal carcinomas were more invasive than the less common acinar tumours, while Cihak et al. (1972) found that the uncommon microscopic variant with squamous cell components, the adenocanthoma, was as malignant and aggressive as the more common adenocarcinoma.

It has been pointed out by Willis (1952) that unsuspected carcinoma of the pancreas is not uncommonly the source of clinically obtrusive metastases. Willis reviewed the published accounts of cases of this type that had appeared between 1899 and 1948. He thought that cases with metastatic lesions of the nervous system, which were taken to be primary lesions until necropsy disclosed an unsuspected carcinoma of the pancreas, formed an important group. He referred to several published accounts and gave a short description of a case of his own. Metastasis to the nervous system is, however, much less common than it is to the lungs. Lisa et al. (1964), in their study of 104 autopsy cases, have drawn attention to the risks, previously noted by Hewer (1961), of mistaking pulmonary metastases from carcinoma of the pancreas for primary lung cancers. In Lisa et al.'s cases there were pulmonary metastases in 40%, and metastases in thoracic lymph nodes in 25%. In 12 of their cases, the clinical manifestations of the secondary tumours in the thorax simulated primary carcinoma of the lung, and in nine of these the diagnosis of lung cancer was thought to have been confirmed by biopsy specimens obtained from lymph nodes, or by bronchoscopy or thoracotomy. In the 12 cases that simulated lung cancer, the site of the primary pancreatic cancer involved the tail in eight. In two, the carcinoma was in the head and in two the head and body were involved. These authors concluded that metastatic pulmonary lesions from carcinoma of the pancreas may reproduce all the clinical manifestations of carcinoma of the lung, including the radiological appearances, cervical adenopathy, Horner's syndrome and superior vena caval compression.

As has been mentioned earlier, the skeleton is a relatively common site for secondary deposits; it is thus not surprising that a pathological fracture may be the presenting symptom, as is illustrated by the following case. A man aged 64 was admitted to the Liverpool Royal Infirmary because of a fracture of the left thigh. He died during an operation undertaken to fix the fracture. At the post-mortem examination it was found that a carcinoma, only 1 cm in diameter, was present in the head of the pancreas. The carcinoma had not caused jaundice but it had caused metastatic deposits in lymph nodes, the liver, the adrenal glands, the spine and in both femora, with a pathological fracture through the tumour in the left femur. Microscopically, the carcinoma was a mucin-secreting adenocarcinoma.

In the mandible, adenocarcinoma, metastatic from a carcinoma of the pancreas, has been found

by oral surgeons (Hayes et al. 1966), and a patient with metastases from adenocarcinoma of the pancreas presented himself to a department of otorhinolaryngology because of sudden deafness due to bilateral secondary tumours in the temporal bones (Igarashi et al. 1979). Another patient consulted an ophthalmologist because an unsuspected adenocarcinoma of the pancreas had produced a secondary deposit in the iris (Barsky 1978).

Ultimate Causes of Death

Because carcinoma of the pancreas is predominantly a disease of the old, it is usual in the post-mortem room to find unrelated conditions, prostatic enlargement for example, and lesions such as venous thrombosis with pulmonary embolism, or thrombosis of coronary or cerebral arteries, which, though possibly related to the thrombotic tendency associated with the carcinoma, are common in people without carcinoma. The effects of biliary obstruction in carcinoma of the head of the pancreas are often the immediate cause of death through secondary biliary cirrhosis or suppurative cholangitis. Sudden deterioration and death has, in our experience, been caused by rupture of a haemorrhagic secondary tumour in the liver causing haemoperitoneum in one patient, and rupture of a distended gall bladder with biliary peritonitis in another. As with all debilitating and immobilising diseases with pain requiring sedation, terminal bronchopneumonia is common. In certain cases of carcinomatosis with involvement of the pancreas, as well as other organs liable to be the site of a primary adenocarcinoma or an anaplastic carcinoma, although a pancreatic primary may be suspected, it may be impossible to exclude metastatic involvement of the pancreas.

Microscopic Features

Ductal Carcinomas

The great majority of cancers of the pancreas are adenocarcinomas, believed to be the result of neoplasia of the epithelial lining of the pancreatic ducts. J.R. Miller et al. (1951) classified 162 of 202 cases of carcinoma of the pancreas as adenocarcinomas of ductal origin, an incidence of 80.2%. In the even larger series of 406 cases of non-endocrine carcinoma of the pancreas studied by Cubilla and

Fitzgerald (1975), the figures were very similar, with 76% of the tumours classified as duct cell adenocarcinoma, to which might be added two other types of adenocarcinoma that they classified separately: microadenocarcinoma (4%), and mucinous adenocarcinoma (2%). They also found that cystandenocarcinoma made up 1% of their cases.

In 1983, Morohoshi et al. published the results of their histopathological examination of 264 exocrine pancreatic tumours (167 autopsy and 97 surgical) in the files of the Institute of Pathology of the University of Hamburg. They classified 250 of the 264 tumours as having originated from ducts. These they subdivided into well-differentiated adenocarcinomas and poorly differentiated. The poorly differentiated type predominated (81.1%), with variants such as pleomorphic giant cell carcinoma making up 5.3%, adenosquamous carcinoma 3.8%, and mucinous carcinoma accounting for 1.1%. With all these carcinomas the prognosis was poor. Serous cystadenomas made up 1.1% and mucinous cystic tumours 1.5%. There were two cases of intraductal papilloma (papillary adenoma).

The result of a somewhat similar study of both autopsy and surgical material collected in the London Hospital was published by Chen and Baithun in 1985. They found 391 primary exocrine pancreatic tumours and classified them histologically. Carcinoma accounted for 98.5% of these tumours, most of which were taken to be ductal adenocarcinomas, and the great majority of which were either moderately- or poorly differentiated; 78.8% were ductal adenocarcinomas. Pleomorphic carcinomas were classified separately and accounted for 7.2%, while spindle cell carcinoma made up 0.8%, small cell carcinoma 3.1%, mucinous carcinoma 2.1%, adenosquamous carcinoma 3.4%, and cystadenocarcinoma 2.6%. The collection included four cases of acinar cell carcinoma, one of which contained a component of carcinoid tumour. Three were classified as microadenocarcinomas, and one as an oncocytic carcinoma.

As non-neoplastic metaplasia to a squamous type of epithelium is not uncommon in the epithelial lining of the pancreatic ducts, it is not surprising that metaplasia of this type may occur when the epithelium of the ducts becomes neoplastic and J.R. Miller et al. classified 1.4% (three cases) of their ductal carcinomas as squamous cell carcinomas. Carcinomas of a purely squamous cell type are very unusual, but combinations of squamous cell carcinoma with adenocarcinoma, though rare, are much less unusual than purely squamous cell carcinomas of the pancreas (see Figs 9.18–9.20). Cubilla and Fitzgerald (1975) classified 14 (3.5%) of their 406 cases as adenosquamous, while Morohoshi et al.

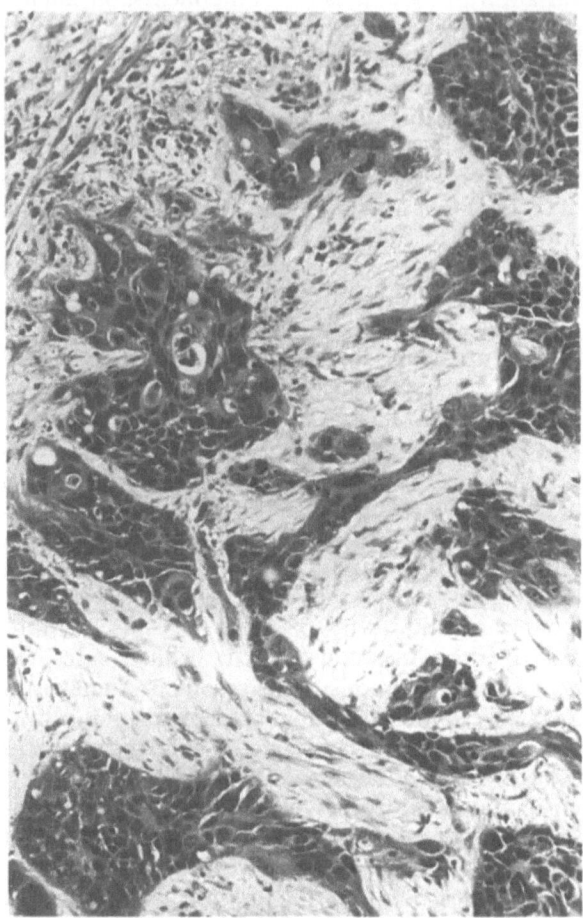

Fig. 9.19. Squamous differentiation in another area of the carcinoma illustrated in Fig. 9.18. H&E, × 150

(1983), in their 264 cases had 3.8% of adenosquamous tumours, and Chen and Biathun had 3.4%. None of these groups found pure squamous cell carcinomas; no doubt this can occur, but, as has been pointed out by Cihak et al. (1972), cases originally taken to be squamous cell carcinoma have been shown by examination of additional material to contain adenocarcinomatous areas.

The degree of differentiation of adenocarcinomas varies greatly. There are tumours that are so well differentiated that their malignancy is almost unrecognisable, while there are others that are so poorly differentiated that only traces of a tubular structure can be discerned. J.R. Miller et al. graded their series of tumours into four grades of malignancy, and felt that there was some correlation between this and the size of the tumours, the largest tumours being those with the most malignant-looking microscopic appearances. They thought

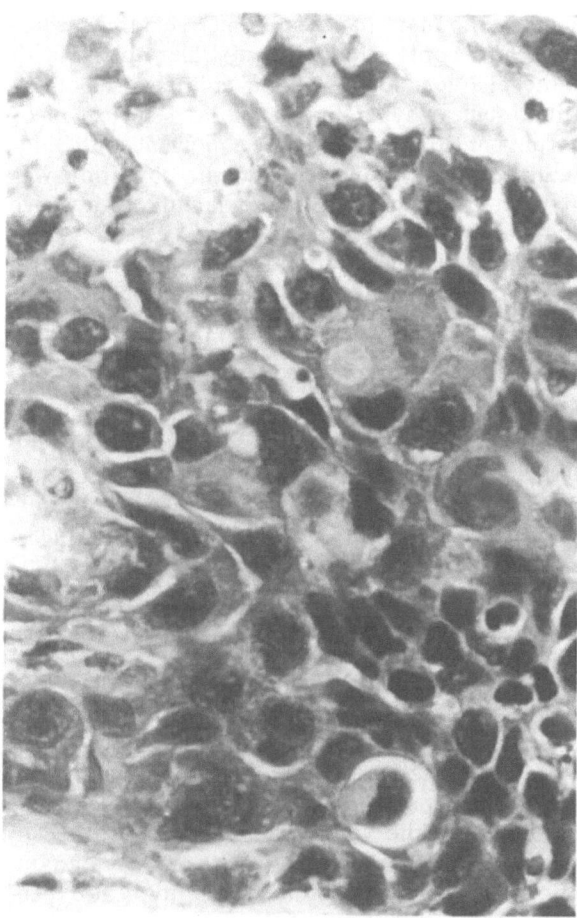

Fig. 9.20. Vacuoles of mucus in the squamous cells shown in Fig. 9.19 justify the term "mucoepidermoid carcinoma" used by Frantz (1959) for this type of pancreatic cancer. H&E, × 600

highly differentiated tumours (grade I) polarised tumour cells bordered a common luminal space and rested on a well-defined basal lamina. Secretion granules were concentrated in the apical cytoplasm and were discharged exclusively at the apical plasma membrane into the common luminal space. They assigned 20 of their tumours to grade I. In the intermediate grade, although duct-like structures were formed, these were combined with solid epithelial buds. There was a loss of cell polarity and mutiple bizarre lumina were seen within the cytoplasm of the tumour cells. The loss of cell polarity was combined with the disappearance of a regular basal lamina and its replacement by collagen fibres around and between the tumour cells. There were also appearances that the authors interpreted as secretion into the interstitial space. They assigned 25 of their 51 tumours to grade II. The least differentiated tumours (six of 51) were classed as grade III. These consisted of irregular aggregates of polymorphous cells without the formation of tubules. No basal laminae were seen and collagen fibres were diffusely distributed around aggregates of tumour cells, associated with widening of the intercellular spaces. Secretion appeared to be of the endocytic type. The nuclei in the tumour cells were large and irregular, sometimes highly segmented.

Ploidy, as determined by flow cytometry, has also been used as a guide to prognosis in pancreatic adenocarcinoma (Weger et al. 1987, 1990; Alanen et al. 1990). In work of this type, in which the nuclear DNA content of the tumour cells is analysed automatically after disintegration of sections from paraffin-embedded material, it has been shown that patients whose tumour cells are of the diploid type survived longer than patients whose tumour cells are of the non-diploid type (Alanen et al. 1990). The latter authors suggest that a study of the ploidy in biopsy specimens of pancreatic adenocarcinomas may be of value in the selection of patients for curative operations. Herrera et al. (1992), however, in a comparison of the DNA nuclear pattern in the pancreatic adenocarcinomas of a group of patients who had survived for 3 years or more with the pattern in a group who died within 12 months of pancreatic resection, found no differences in the DNA analysis of the cancer cells.

Lectin histochemistry has also been investigated as a possible guide to prognosis in pancreatic adenocarcinoma by Ching et al. (1988), for example, and by Lymboura and Leathem (1991), but no definite results have been obtained as yet.

Minor degrees of mucus formation are common in ductal adenocarcinomas, but the secretion of pools of cell-free mucus is unusual (2%, according to Cubilla and Fitzgerald 1975); "signet-ring" cells

also that metastases and thrombotic lesions were more common amongst the tumours they classified as having the higher grades of malignancy. Since that time, Kern et al. (1987) have added the fine structure of pancreatic adenocarcinomas to their light-microscopic appearances to obtain more accurate grading of malignancy. In a series of 51 cases of pancreatic adenocarcinoma they found that all the tumours consisted of one major type of cell. Cells of this type secreted mucoprotein and had ultrastructural features similar to those of the cells that lined the large interlobular ducts of the normal pancreas. At the ultrastructural level, the grading of the tumours was based upon the extent of the loss of cell polarity, combined with the degree of reduction in the association of the tumour cells with elements of the extracellular matrix (basal lamina). They classified the tumours into three grades of malignancy on the basis of these appearances. In the most

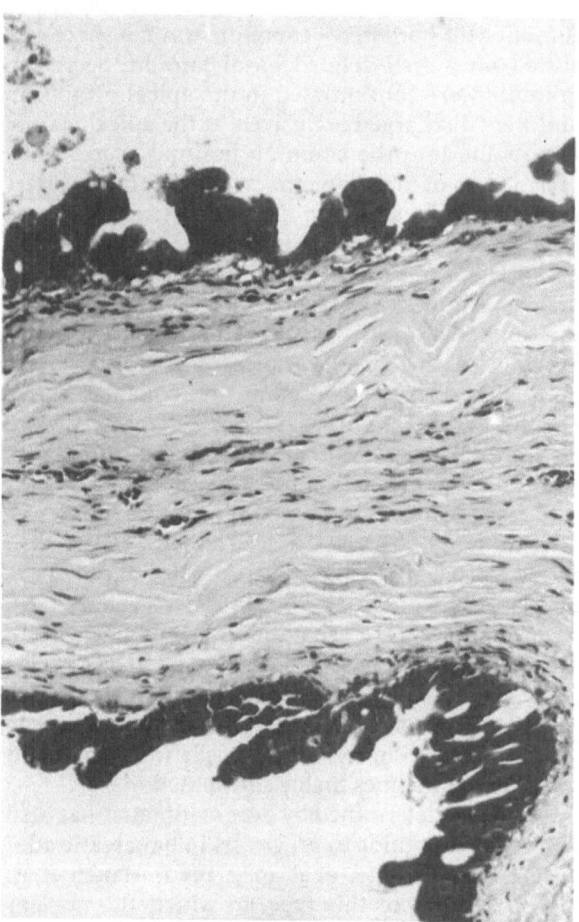

Fig. 9.21. Pre-invasive epithelial hyperplasia in dilated ducts distal to the carcinoma illustrated in Figs 9.18–9.20. H&E, × 150

ments of the main pancreatic duct, its larger tributaries and some of the intralobular ducts, with epithelial atypia, loss of normal epithelial cell orientation, nuclear hyperchromatism and nuclear pleomorphism. No invasion by the abnormal epithelium could be found, however, and the condition was interpreted as being in a stage of latent, pre-invasive malignancy.

Previous studies (Sommers and Meissner 1954; Kozuka et al. 1979) had indicated a probable relationship between epithelial hyperplasia in the ducts and pancreatic cancer, but, unless accompanied by invasive cancer, such hyperplasia, even of the atypical type, had not caused clinical symptoms. The marked inflammatory reactions associated with the epithelial changes described by Ferrari and his colleagues suggest that invasion may have been imminent. In the case reported by Mizumoto et al. (1988), hyperplasia of the epithelium of the ducts, carcinoma in situ and invasive carcinoma were found to coexist. Their patient, a Japanese woman aged 68, had complained of loss of appetite and loss of weight, but had had no pain for a year and a half before seeking medical advice.

Another study of the ductal epithelium in relation to the histogenesis of carcinoma of the pancreas is that of Chen et al. (1985). They examined the ductal epithelium in the vicinity of the tumours in 248 cases of carcinoma of the pancreas and came to the conclusion that both papillary and atypical hyperplasia of the epithelium of the ducts were pre-cancerous lesions, and that their results supported the ductal origin of most histological types of pancreatic carcinoma. Only acinar cell carcinoma and microadenocarcinoma were relatively infrequently associated with ductal epithelial hyperplasia.

Pour et al. (1982), who carried out thorough microscopic examinations of the pancreases of 83 military veterans in their study of hyperplastic, pre-neoplastic and neoplastic lesions, concluded that, even histologically, malignant tumours may remain clinically occult in certain patients; such tumours are found at autopsy when death has been caused by unrelated disease. They found hyperplasia of the epithelium of the ducts in 57% of their cases and of the epithelium of the ductules in 39%; squamous metaplasia of the ductules was present in 48%. Most of the lesions were found in the head of the pancreas. The occult malignant lesions they found were: two early cancers (one adenocarcinoma and one adenosquamous cell carcinoma), one ductal carcinoma in situ and seven ductal carcinomas in situ.

A reaction in which there is usually marked fibrosis is characteristic of ductal carcinoma of the pancreas, and this is responsible for the scirrhous sensation when these tumours are palpated. The

are also unusual. Papillary structures are not frequent, and tend to be limited to the lining of the dilated ducts behind an obstructing carcinoma (Fig. 9.21). Pre-invasive papillary hyperplasia with marked atypia has been observed by Cubilla and Fitzgerald (1975) in the ducts adjacent to a cancer in 19% of the cases in their large series. This they interpreted as suggesting that carcinoma in situ may precede, possibly for some time, the development of invasive carcinoma.

A case of atypical papillary hyperplasia of the pancreatic duct, without invasion, but with an associated inflammatory reaction, which, combined with the epithelial changes, caused an obstruction of the major pancreatic duct, has been described by Ferrari et al. (1979). The obstruction was demonstrated by endoscopic retrograde pancreatography and was interpreted as indicating a pancreatic carcinoma. Pancreaticoduodenectomy was carried out and there were areas of papillary hyperplasia in seg-

fibrous reaction is associated with a variable amount of lymphocytic infiltration, which is, however, seldom marked. More marked inflammation with histological evidence of significant pancreatitis was present in 26 of 255 consecutive patients with pancreatic and ampullary carcinoma studied by Gambill (1971), but carcinoma as a late sequel of long-standing relapsing pancreatitis with calculi, as in the cases described by Bartholomew et al. (1958), Paulino-Netto et al. (1960), Johnson and Zintel (1963) and Robinson et al. (1970), is sufficiently unusual to be published. In the great majority of cases of ductal carcinoma of the pancreas, the inflammation appears to be a reaction to the disease, or a complication, rather than an aetiological factor.

A very unusual stromal reaction that included well-formed osteoid elements was present in the highly pleomorphic carcinoma of the pancreas reported by Kay and Harrison (1969). These authors were not, however, able to ascribe the origin of the carcinoma to ductal or acinar cells, although they felt confident that the neoplasm was epithelial. One of the present authors has seen a pleomorphic carcinoma of the pancreas in which osteoid was seen in association with osteoclast-like giant cells (Newbould et al. 1992).

While the usual type of differentiation in ductal carcinomas is the formation of tubular structures, with or without the secretion of mucus, other types of differentiation have been recognised, and a collection of unusual carcinomas of the pancreas by Sommers and Meissner (1954) included three cases that they described as pleomorphic carcinoma. One of these tumours was atypical macroscopically in that it was surrounded by a large mass of haemorrhagic necrosis, but the other two were hard and had the usual grey-white appearance of scirrhous carcinoma. Microscopically, however, the appearances, which included many multinucleated and bizarre cells, suggested such diagnoses as: rhabdomyosarcoma, malignant melanoma, chorionepithelioma, hepatoma, angiosarcoma and giant cell thyroid carcinoma. In one of these, when further material was obtained at autopsy, areas of moderately well-differentiated adenocarcinoma were found, and such areas could be seen to undergo transitions to the atypical pleomorphic pattern. Sommers and Meissner also found a marked papillary pattern in two of their unusual carcinomas. These tumours were believed to be ductal in their origin and did not differ in their naked-eye appearances from usual ductal carcinomas. Cilia were found also as an unusual feature in one of the ductal adenocarcinomas studied by these authors, and have been found also by Frantz (1959), both in a primary ductal adenocarcinoma and in one of its

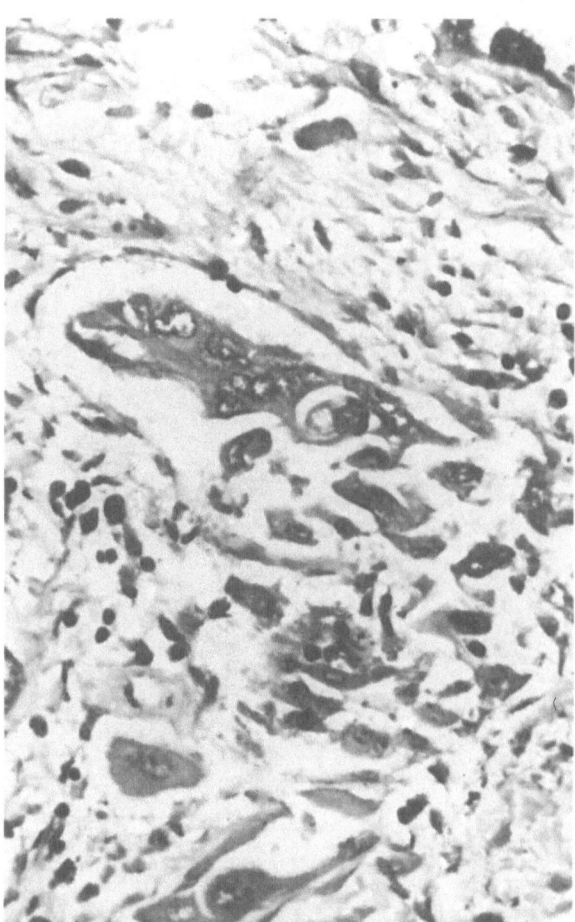

Fig. 9.22. A multinucleated giant cell in a poorly differentiated adenocarcinoma of the tail of the pancreas in a woman aged 81. There was direct invasion of the stomach, spleen, left kidney and left adrenal gland, with invasion of the splenic vein and thrombosis of the portal vein. Secondary carcinoma was present in the right lobe of the liver with involvement of the overlying diaphragm. Microscopic invasion of nerve sheaths was a marked feature. The multinucleated cell illustrated has phagocytosed another, probably a carcinoma cell. H&E, × 375

metastatic deposits in the liver. Mixtures of some of the unusual types they described were also recognised in four tumours by Sommers and Meissner.

A carcinoma of the pancreas, believed to be ductal, in which there was marked formation of oncocytes, has been reported by Huntrakoon (1983). This type of carcinoma has also been recognised by Chen and Baithun (1985). Unlike oncocytic tumours of the kidney, oncocytic carcinomas of the pancreas do not appear to be any less aggressive than other types of ductal carcinoma. Some of the variations in the cell type and microscopic structure of ductal carcinomas are illustrated in Figs 9.22–9.25.

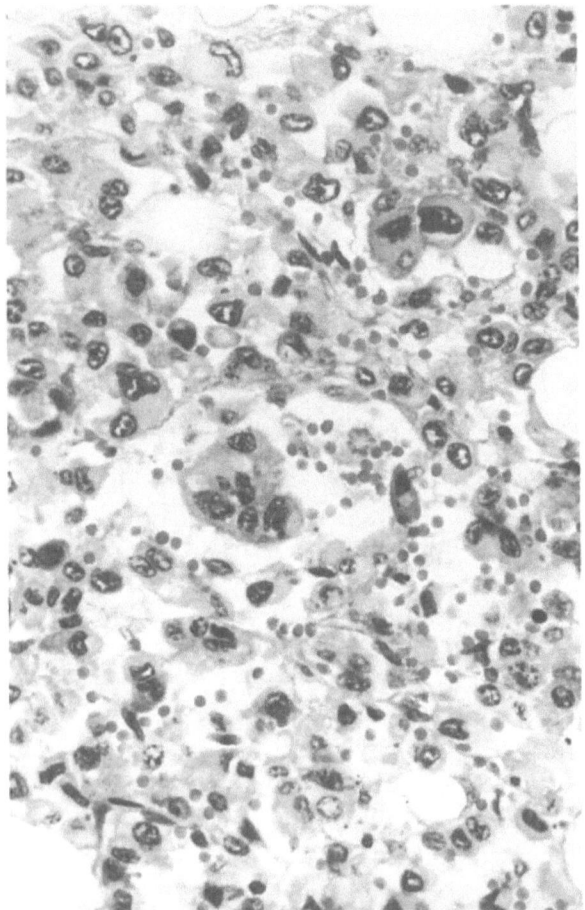

Fig. 9.23. Multinucleated cells in a poorly differentiated carcinoma of the body of the pancreas in a man aged 80. There was abdominal carcinomatosis and secondary carcinoma of the liver, from which fatal intra-abdominal haemorrhage occurred. H&E, × 375

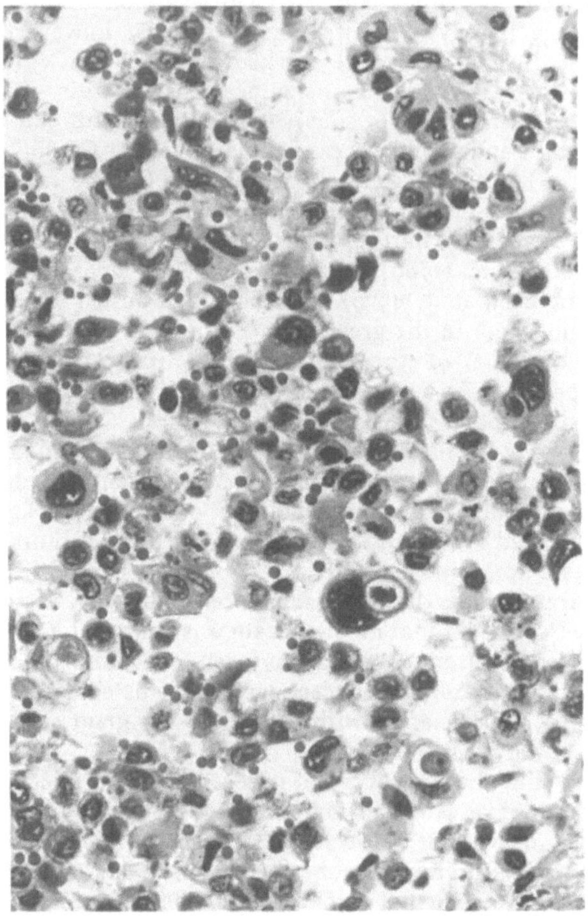

Fig. 9.24. Phagocytosis of other cells by carcinoma cells in the same tumour as that illustrated in Fig. 9.23. H&E, × 375

The capacity of ductal carcinomas to differentiate towards the formation of specialised structures has also been scrutinised by Lafler and Hinderman (1961). These authors concluded that ductal carcinomas, especially those in the head of the pancreas, seem to have only a limited capacity to differentiate, whereas others, especially in the body or tail, may produce variable amounts of glandular differentiation that resembles acini, or a type of differentiation that resembles the islets of Langerhans. It was this "differentiating ductal carcinoma", they claimed, that was most likely to be associated with the thrombotic complications of pancreatic carcinoma.

The possible role of growth factors in the genesis of ductal carcinomas of the pancreas has been studied by workers such as Barton et al. (1991) and Lemoine et al. (1992), by the use of immunohisto-chemical techniques on sections of paraffin-embedded stored material from cases of pancreatic cancer. These authors found that there is almost ubiquitous overexpression of epidermal growth factor receptor in pancreatic cancer and also in chronic pancreatitis. This led them to suggesting that an autocrine loop involving the epidermal growth factor receptor system may be involved in the genesis of pancreatic neoplasia, as well as in reactive hyperplasia of the pancreatic ductal epithelium.

The role of oncogenes in pancreatic carcinoma is also receiving much attention. About 80% of pancreatic cancers contain active *ras* oncogenes, but it is not yet known what human *ras* genes do except that they are involved in the transduction of growth-promoting signals (Lancet 1990).

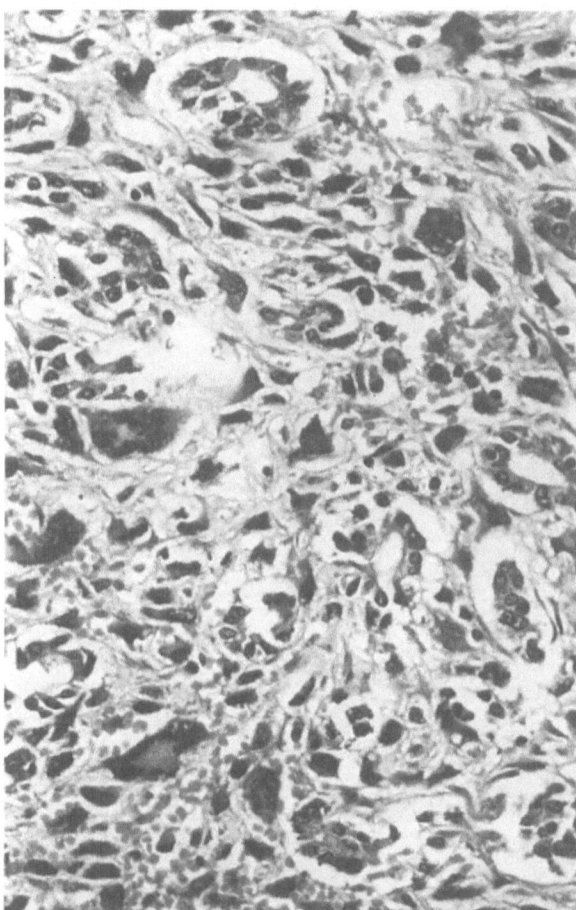

Fig. 9.25. A pleomorphic carcinoma that replaced the body and tail of the pancreas in a woman aged 62. Tubular structures are associated with spindle cells and multinucleated giant cells. Death was due to carcinomatosis with metastatic tumours in the abdominal lymph nodes, liver, lungs, spleen and kidneys. (Courtesy of Dr Al Jafari) H&E, × 375

Acinar Cell Carcinoma

The recognition of acinar cell carcinoma as a distinct type, except in rare instances, is difficult, as has been pointed out by Frantz (1959); this probably accounts for the considerable variation in the incidence of this type of carcinoma that has been reported by different workers. Leach (1950) classified six of his 39 cases of carcinoma of the pancreas as acinar; J.R. Miller et al. (1951) found 27 acinar types in their 202 cases; Cubilla and Fitzgerald (1975) found only three among their 406 cases; while Webb (1977), whose illustrations indicate that he accepted some quite poorly differentiated carcinomas as acinar, found 11 amongst 105 cases of pancreatic carcinoma, although four of the

11 were carcinomas of mixed ductal and acinar type. Of the 264 exocrine pancreatic tumours studied by Morohoshi et al. (1983), ten were classed as acinar carcinomas.

Macroscopically, there is little difference between the acinar type and the more common ductal carcinoma. According to J.R. Miller et al., the average diameter of their acinar carcinomas was 4.7 cm, compared with 4.3 cm for the mean diameter of ductal carcinomas and 8.9 cm for undifferentiated carcinomas of indeterminate origin. The association of marked fat necrosis or suppuration might, however, according to these authors, suggest that a carcinoma could be of the acinar type. Acinar cell carcinomas do not seem to occur in any special anatomical region of the pancreas.

Microscopically, relatively well-differentiated types, with a pattern that resembles normal pancreatic acinar tissue, have been illustrated by various authors (J.R. Miller et al. 1951; Ashley 1978), but acinar carcinomas are usually poorly differentiated and their recognition depends upon the identification of acinar cells (Figs 9.26–9.28). These are usually so packed together that their shape is round, columnar or triangular. They have regular round or oval nuclei that are frequently hyperchromatic and usually basal. There is little mitotic activity. The cytoplasm may be either purplish in haematoxylin and eosin preparations, or it may be quite eosinophilic. Microtubules that contain PAS-positive material can sometimes, according to Webb, be identified. Occasionally the cytoplasm of the tumour cells may contain eosinophilic granules. Because acinar cell carcinomas are often very anaplastic, some of the unusual types of carcinoma of the pancreas that have been reported are suspected to have been derived from acinar cells. Rosai (1968), for example, described two cases of carcinoma of the pancreas that were indistinguishable on light microscopy from giant cell tumours of bone, but which had ultrastructural features in both the giant cells and the stromal cells that suggested an acinar origin. Reports of similar carcinomas of the pancreas have been published by Jeffrey et al. (1983), and by Jalloh (1983) (Figs 9.29, 9.30). A carcinoma of this type has been found in the liver (Kuwano et al. 1984). Additional examples have since been reported; these include the case, described by Baniel et al. (1987), which suggested to the authors that the removal of an osteoclast-like giant cell tumour of the pancreas might justify an optimistic prognosis. Their patient was well, and free from recurrence or metastasis over 6 years after the removal of a tumour thought, at first, to be inoperable.

In the case described by Newbould et al. (1992), about half the neoplasm consisted of osteoclast-like

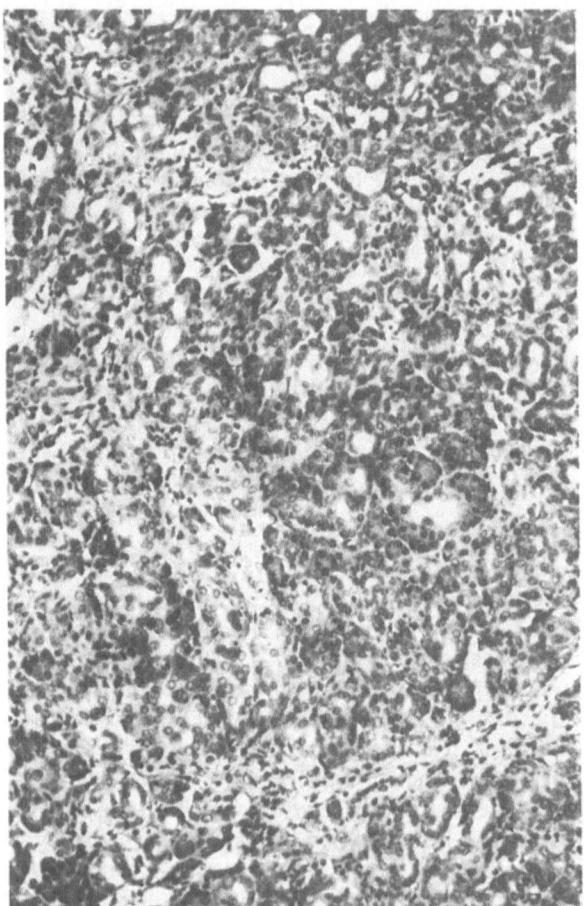

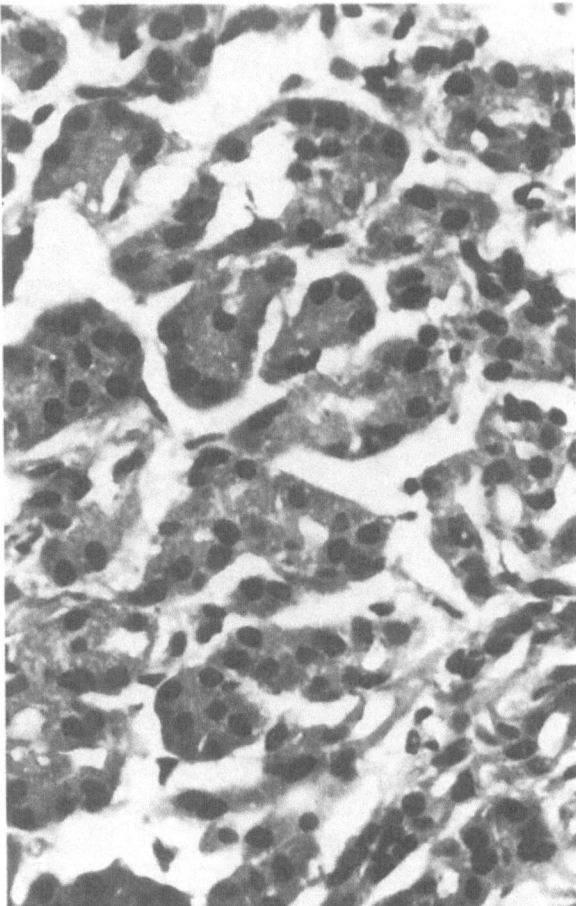

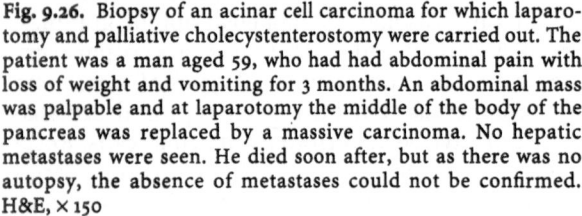

Fig. 9.26. Biopsy of an acinar cell carcinoma for which laparotomy and palliative cholecystenterostomy were carried out. The patient was a man aged 59, who had had abdominal pain with loss of weight and vomiting for 3 months. An abdominal mass was palpable and at laparotomy the middle of the body of the pancreas was replaced by a massive carcinoma. No hepatic metastases were seen. He died soon after, but as there was no autopsy, the absence of metastases could not be confirmed. H&E, × 150

Fig. 9.27. Higher-power view of the acinar carcinoma illustrated in Fig. 9.26. × 600

giant cell tumour with osteoid areas, while moderately differentiated adenocarcinoma accounted for the rest. The immunocytochemical studies carried out by the authors led them to conclude that the giant cells had had their origin in the bone marow and represented a non-neoplastic reaction against the carcinoma.

In acinar cell tumours the stroma is usually scanty, but may be plentiful.

It may be, as has been suggested by Willis (1967) and Ashley (1978), that it is neither useful nor possible to divide exocrine cancers of the pancreas accurately into ductal or acinar types, for mixed types undoubtedly occur, and Frantz (1959) stated that it

is generally accepted that acinar cells and islet cells can arise from duct epithelium. Ductal components certainly seem, as has been pointed out by Lafler and Hinderman (1961), to be able to differentiate into organoid structures that resemble both pancreatic acini and even islets, while the experimental work of Pour (1980) suggests that it is neoplasia of the ductules, rather than of the ductal epithelium, that is associated with organoid differentiation. Tanaka et al. (1988), however, have described atypical acinar lesions that they suggest are precursors of acinar cell carcinomas.

Whatever the origin of acinar cell carcinomas, they seem, as has been shown by the work of Hoorens et al. (1993), to have a capacity for differentiation in various directions. These authors believe, however, that they constitute an entity that is different from both ductal adenocarcinomas and endocrine tumours.

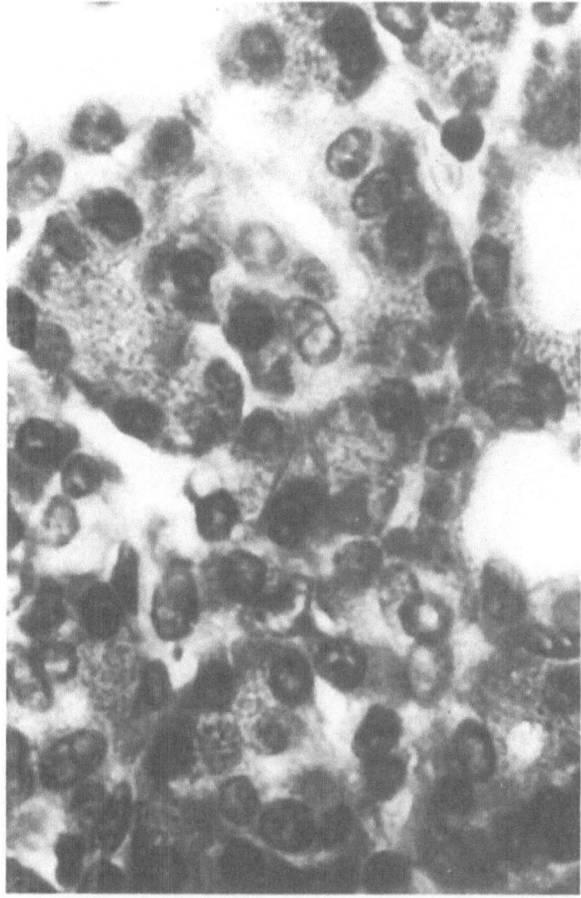

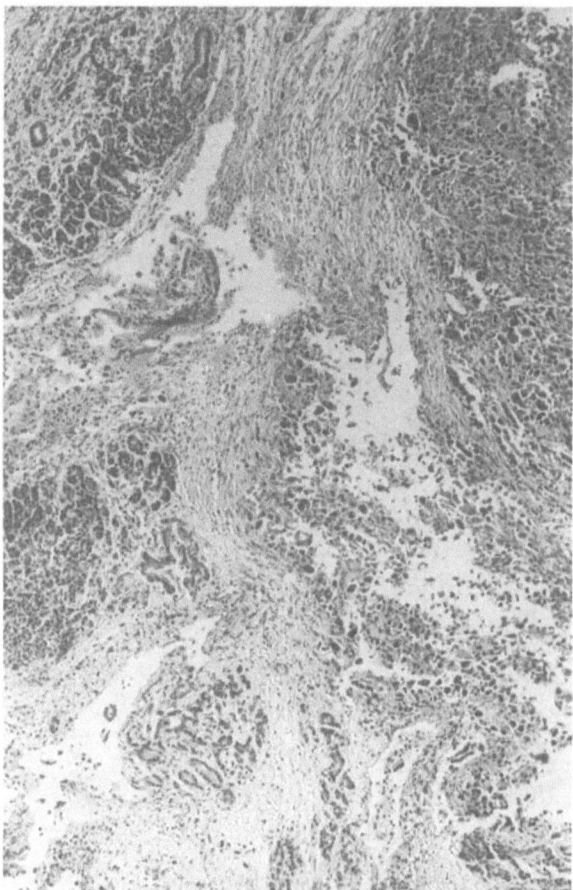

Fig. 9.28. Zymogen granules within the cells of the acinar carcinoma illustrated in Figs 9.26 and 9.27. × 1000

Fig. 9.29. The margin of an osteoclastoma-like carcinoma of the pancreas. (Courtesy of Dr Iona Jeffrey) H&E, × 60

Undifferentiated and Pleomorphic Carcinoma

The poorly differentiated or pleomorphic nature of the cells in many carcinomas of the pancreas makes it difficult to assign such tumours to either ductal or acinar types. Amongst the 202 cancers that were classified microscopically by J.R. Miller et al. (1951) there were ten that the authors considered to be of indeterminate origin. These they subdivided into a large cell type (six cases) and a small cell type (two cases). Sommers and Meissner (1954) were unable to assign an origin to 19 of the carcinomas in their series of 42 autopsied cases, while Cubilla and Fitzgerald (1975) were unable to classify 30 of their 406 cases and described another six as anaplastic. Morohoshi et al. (1983) were uncertain of the histogenesis of four of the 264 exocrine pancreatic tumours that they studied. All these workers record types that contain giant multinucleated cells, or

spindle cell forms that cause a sarcoma-like appearance; in the classification suggested by Frantz (1959), she includes a carcinosarcomatous type. More than one of the authors mention that, if enough material is available from these pleomorphic and bizarre tumours, areas of adenocarcinoma can sometimes be found peripherally. Most pleomorphic carcinomas include multinucleated giant cells, some of which may be phagocytic and have remnants of other carcinoma cells within their cytoplasm. Cubilla and Fitzgerald (1975) classified such tumours into a special group of giant cell carcinomas that made up 5% of their cases.

As Frantz (1959) has pointed out, it is tempting to subdivide the numerous microscopic variants of carcinoma of the pancreas but, until further information about their true nature is available, there seems to be little to be gained by doing so. It may well be that the poorly differentiated carcinomas,

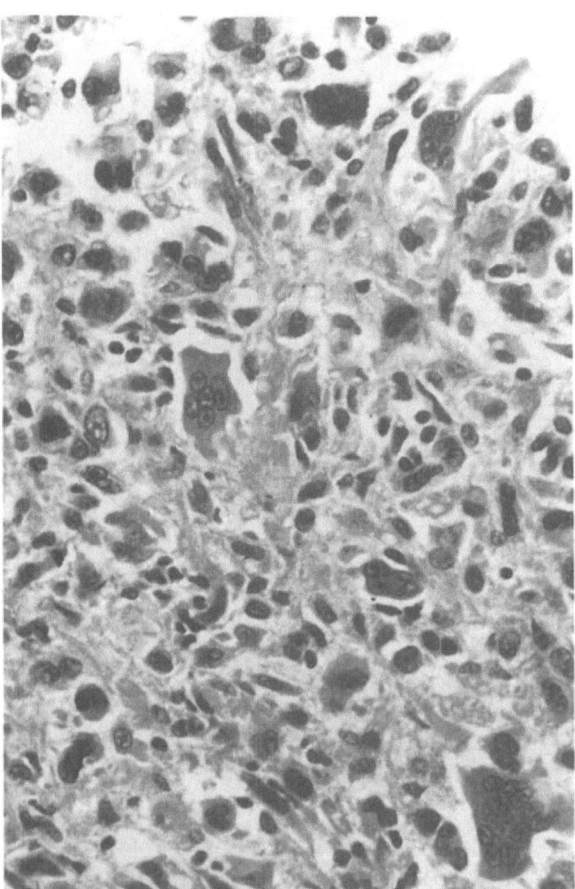

Fig. 9.30. A higher magnification of the tumour shown in Fig. 9.29. Osteoclast-like giant cells are present in a stroma of pleomorphic cells, some of which are spindle shaped. (Courtesy of Dr Iona Jeffrey) H&E, × 375

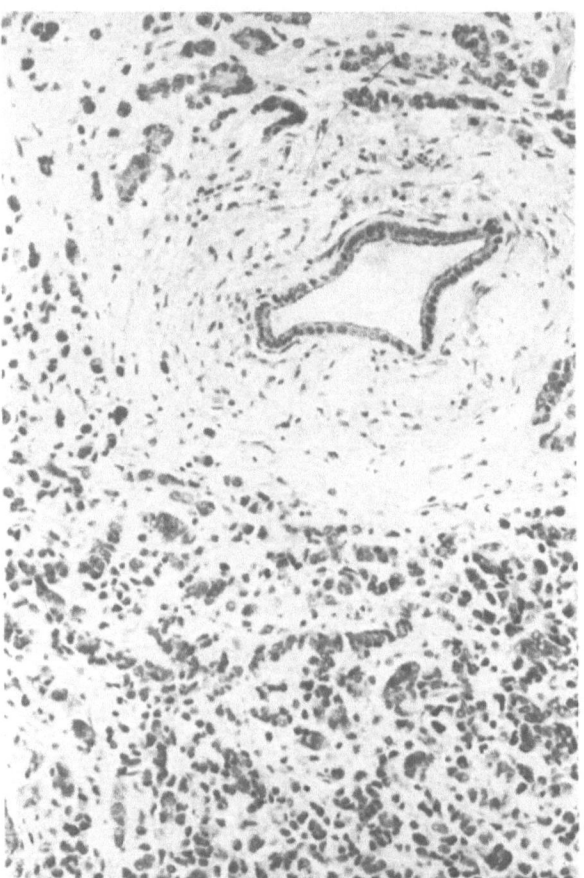

Fig. 9.31. Undifferentiated carcinoma of the pancreas surrounding the pancreatic duct, which is not, however, obstructed. This carcinoma, which measured 3 cm in diameter, was found in the head of the pancreas in a man aged 74, whose clinical history was of constipation for 18 weeks, and of left chest pain with cough and white sputum for 6 weeks before his admission. He was so cachectic that carcinoma of the oesophagus was suspected and oesophagoscopy was about to be undertaken when the patient died. At autopsy, there was secondary carcinoma in the liver, the adrenal glands and the spine. Lesions in the lung, thought with the naked eye to be secondary carcinoma, were found microscopically to be tuberculous. The carcinoma had not caused biliary obstruction. H&E, × 150

whose cell of origin is unrecognisable, include some non-functional islet cell carcinomas. The tumour whose microscopic appearance is illustrated in Figs 9.31 and 9.32 is an undifferentiated carcinoma of small cells to which an origin is difficult to assign. It contains, however, foci of calcification; such calcification is unusual in an exocrine carcinoma, but is sometimes a feature of islet cell carcinoma. Although there was no clinical or biochemical evidence of the secretion of insulin by this tumour, the calcification hints at an origin from islet cells.

Acinar–Endocrine Differentiation

Reports, such as that by Ulich et al. (1982), of an acinar–endocrine tumour of the pancreas, and of one with duct, endocrine and acinar differentiation (Schron and Mendelsohn 1984) have been published.

Tumours with such components, along with the experimental work of Pour (1980), and also his colleagues, suggest that ductular cells, including the centro-acinar cells, with their capacity to act as reserve cells for both endocrine and non-endocrine components of the pancreas, may be of previously unsuspected importance in the histogenesis of pancreatic malignancy.

In carcinomas in the region of the head of the pancreas there may, as has been mentioned in connection with the macroscopic appearances of carcinoma of the pancreas, be partial or complete obstruction of the main pancreatic duct and of the

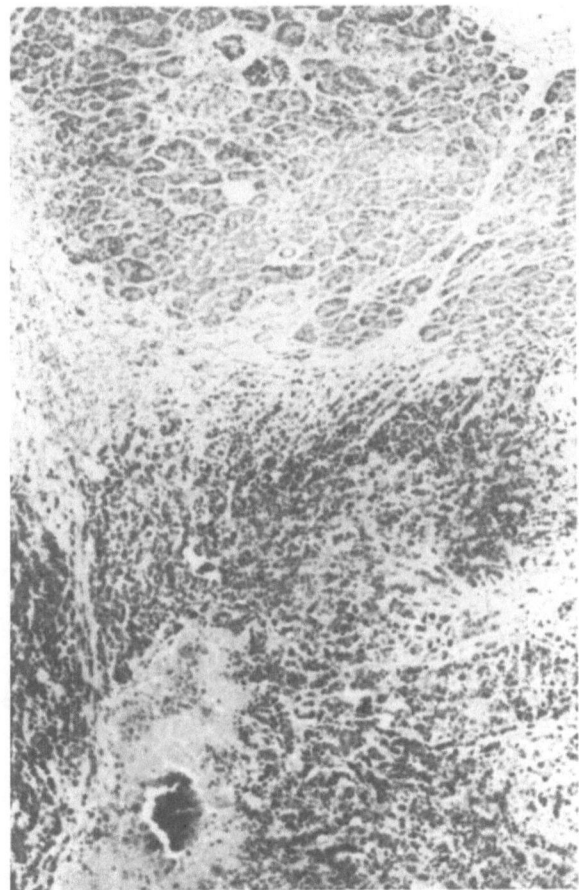

Fig. 9.32. A low-power view of the carcinoma illustrated in Fig. 9.22. The dark-staining material surrounded by a zone of pale-staining fibrous tissue was one of several foci of calcification in this tumour. H&E, × 60

accessory duct; this obstruction has secondary effects upon the ducts and the acinar tissues in the body and tail of the panceas. The changes were studied in detail by Haunz and Baggenstoss (1950). They found well-marked parenchymal atrophy that could be recognised only microscopically because the shape and size of the gland was often maintained by replacement of the glandular tissue by fat. Distension of the obstructed ducts was first associated with flattening of the epithelial lining, with subsequent desquamation of the cells. In the earlier stages they found dilatation and occasional rupture of acini that they considered to be responsible for focal areas of pancreatitis and fat necrosis. In the later stages nearly all the acinar tissue became replaced by fibrous tissue. Neither squamous metaplasia nor calcification occurred in the obstructed ducts and there were no signs of regeneration of ducts or acini. The average dilatation of the obstructed ducts was three and a half times the size of the normal duct and the amount of fatty replacement of the atrophic acinar tissue was more or less proportional to the degree of ductal dilatation. There was marked thinning of the walls of the main ducts but thinning was less noticeable or absent in the smaller tributaries. Fibrosis was the most conspicuous change and, in 11 of the 25 specimens studied, the entire pancreas, except for the carcinomatous portion, had become a mass of fibrous tissue, deteriorating ducts and persistent islets of Langerhans.

Effects upon the Pancreatic Islets

In many conditions associated with fibrosis and atrophy of the pancreas the persistence of the islets of Langerhans is striking; this is true also in the fibrosis associated with carcinoma of the pancreas, both in the areas of desmoplastic reaction to the carcinoma and in areas of fibrous replacement of atrophic glandular tissue. Willis (1952) was particularly impressed by the condition of the islets in both primary and secondary tumours (e.g. Fig. 9.33) of the pancreas and stated that: "At the advancing edges of the tumours the islets frequently appear to be increased in size and number, and in many cases the enlarged islets may be found intact within the substance of growths which have destroyed all other parenchymatous elements."

Carcinoid Tumours

Carcinoid tumours, both functional and non-functional, occur in the pancreas. Some may have their origin from Kulchitsky cells in the pancreatic ducts, but most appear to be derived from islet cells and will be discussed with the endocrine tumours of the pancreas.

Carcinoma of the Ampulla of Vater, Common Bile Duct and Duodenum

Such tumours are not pancreatic tumours and are thus outside the scope of this work, but their clinical effects may be so similar to carcinoma of the head of the pancreas that they are commonly discussed along with this condition. The carcinomas that arise from the common bile duct, the ampulla of Vater and the periampullary area of the duodenum are similar microscopically to the ductal type of carci-

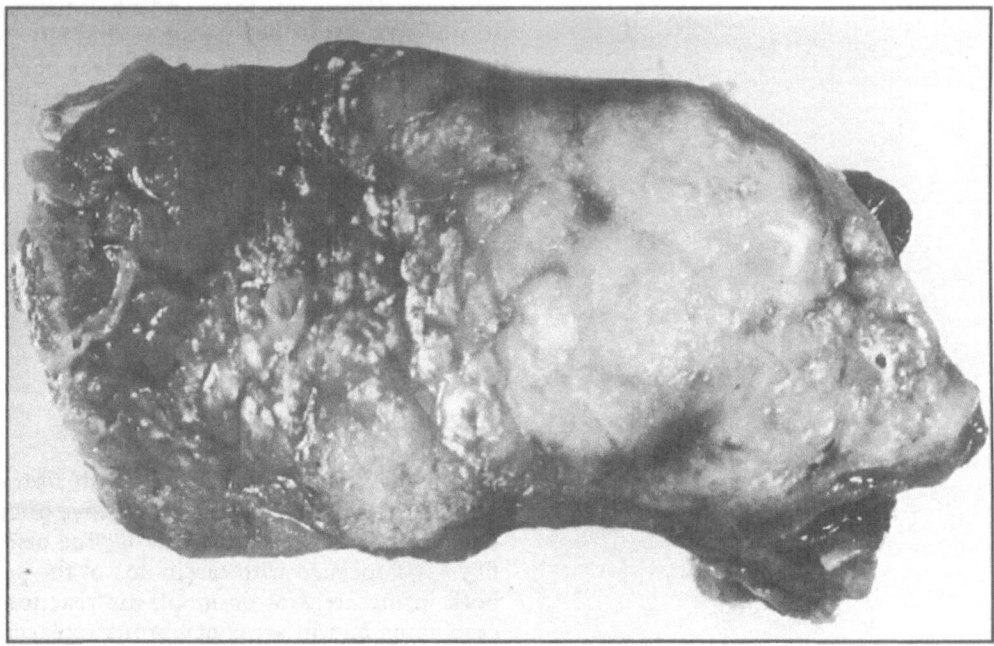

Fig. 9.33. Secondary carcinoma in the tail of the pancreas. The primary was an oat cell carcinoma of the lung and other secondary tumours were present in the body and head of the pancreas as well as in other organs. The macroscopic appearances of the tumour are indistinguishable from those of a primary carcinoma of the pancreas.

noma of the pancreas; the determination of the exact site of origin of an adenocarcinoma in the pancreatoduodenal region depends upon the macroscopic findings when a specimen is dissected. In certain, usually surgically removed, specimens, the site of origin of the tumour is self-evident, but when a large tumour in the head of the pancreas involves the common bile duct and ampulla as well as the pancreas, perhaps with ulceration also into the duodenum, it becomes impossible to ascertain its origin. This more advanced type of disease is the type likely to be found post-mortem and, since many of the figures for the incidence of carcinoma in different parts of the pancreas are the result of autopsy studies, the higher incidence of carcinoma in the head of the gland depends to some extent upon the inclusion of some carcinomas which are, in fact, biliary carcinomas or even duodenal carcinomas. Willis (1967) thought it probable that, if allowance were made for those cases in which carcinoma of the lower part of the bile duct had been erroneously included with carcinomas of the head of the pancreas, the frequency of cancers in the different parts of the pancreas would be found to be nearly proportional to the relative amounts of tissue in those parts. Allen-Mersh (1982), however, feels that the possible inclusion of a number of biliary carcinomas does not account for the higher inci-

dence of exocrine tumours in the head and neck regions of the pancreas. He carried out a quantitative study of 77 pancreases and found that the pancreatic head and neck constitute less than half of the whole pancreas and that, as there is no difference in the concentration of ductal epithelium in the head and body of the pancreas, a greater number of cells at risk is not the explanation for preponderance of cancers in the head of the pancreas. The findings by Pour et al. (1982) that pre-cancerous changes are most commonly situated in the head region also suggest that this region is specially vulnerable to neoplasia.

Microscopic Confirmation of a Diagnosis of Carcinoma of the Pancreas

Incisional Biopsy

In spite of the recent advances in imaging, it is often very desirable to confirm the clinical diagnosis of carcinoma of the pancreas by a biopsy of the part of the pancreas that looks or feels abnormal during a laparotomy, but the risks associated with an incisional biopsy include haemorrhage, pancreatitis, pseudocyst formation, abscess or fistula formation, and the possible liberation of carcinoma cells into the peritoneal cavity. Thus, if lymph nodes appear to be involved, or if metastatic nodules can be seen in the liver, most surgeons prefer to obtain a sample for microscopic examination from either a node or the liver. Certain groups, however, have found that, with appropriate safeguards, biopsy of the pancreas itself is justifiable, and relatively safe. George et al. (1975) reviewed 47 patients on whom open pancreatic biopsy had been carried out at the Royal Free Hospital in London, and concluded that the procedure was safe, valuable and accurate if it was carried out by the technique that they recommended. They considered it important to search for and, if necessary, deal with, any injury to the pancreatic duct that might have been caused by the removal of the sample. The samples they obtained measured 0.3 × 0.3 × 0.3 cm and allowed frozen sections to be examined with later confirmatory paraffin sections. The wound in the pancreas was repaired by a method similar to that used to seal a perforated peptic ulcer, and the area was drained.

In 1976, Lightwood et al. published the results of a retrospective analysis of 171 pancreatic biopsies carried out during laparotomies in hospitals in San Francisco between 1972 and 1976. The most common site to be sampled was the head of the pancreas but samples were also obtained from the body and tail regions. Most of the specimens were obtained by direct wedge biopsy but samples were also obtained transduodenally, sometimes in combination with a direct biopsy. Specimens were also obtained by the use of the Vim–Silverman needle. The pathologist's diagnosis was found to be correct in 86% of the 171 cases in which the subsequent course of the illness, the findings at autopsy or a later biopsy confirmed the diagnosis. Biopsy and diagnosis made from frozen sections yielded no false-positive diagnosis of cancer, but biopsy interpretation was falsely negative in 15 of 87 patients with cancer, the true diagnosis being made when metastases appeared, when a second operation was carried out, or at autopsy. The authors considered that wedge biopsy had a lower complication rate (3%) than biospy with the Vim–Silverman needle (14%), even when the two methods were used under comparable circumstances, for example when a lesion was situated deeply within the pancreas. They felt that the removal of a wedge of tissue allowed the depths of the wound to be scrutinised, with the ligation of blood vessels or the open ends of transected ducts, if necessary. Biopsy by direct needle puncture was also less accurate in their experience, with a

false-negative rate of 25%. Pancreatic biopsy in the total series of 171 patients gave rise to complications in 4.7% and caused one death, but Lightwood and his colleagues concluded that pancreatic biopsy with confirmation of malignancy should precede pancreaticoduodenectomy in most cases of suspected cancer.

The histological interpretation of the samples obtained by biopsy of the pancreas is notoriously difficult (Klöppel 1984). First, the sample may not contain any of the true lesion. Thus, even when a carcinoma is present, the pathologist may be given only the chronically inflamed pancreatic tissue that is commonly present in the vicinity of a carcinoma, and the surgeon should understand that a biopsy reported as showing chronic pancreatitis does not eliminate the possibility of an underlying carcinoma. Chronic pancreatitis may, of course, occur in the absence of a carcinoma and, because of atrophy and distortion of acini with proliferation of small ducts, it may lead to a false-positive diagnosis of carcinoma. However, a well-differentiated adenocarcinoma may provoke such a fibrous reaction that it may masquerade as chronic pancreatitis, unless something characteristic, such as a nerve whose sheath has been invaded by the carcinoma, should happen to have been included in the sample. It is important that the pathologist and the surgeon should both understand each other's problems and limitations. If samples are taken during an exploratory operation with one of the types of hollow needle, the diagnostic problems are not only more difficult for the pathologist but, as the core sample is only about 2 mm in diameter, it is not possible to cut frozen sections and then prepare confirmatory paraffin sections, as can usually be done with an incisional biopsy. As has already been mentioned, Lightwood et al. found that the needle biopsy was a less accurate diagnostic procedure and was more liable to produce complications, while Smith (1979) has stated that it is thoroughly unsafe to carry out a biopsy with a hollow needle on a suspected lesion in the head of the pancreas.

Nevertheless, a method by which carcinoma of the pancreas can be diagnosed with confidence, without a laparotomy, at a stage when a surgical cure may be attempted, has been the subject of much work by various groups. The recognition of malignant cells in aspirates from the duodenum (Lemon and Byrnes 1949; Wenger and Raskin 1958; Butler 1972) was followed by the study of cells obtained by the endoscopic cannulation of the pancreatic duct (Endo et al. 1974; Hatfield et al. 1976). The collection of samples for cytology is usually followed by the injection of a radiological opaque contrast medium to carry out endoscopic retrograde pancreatography and a description of the collection and examination of the cells in the pancreatic fluid has been given by Klöppel (1984). Following stimulation of the gland by the administration of secretin, fluid is collected from the cannulated duct by suction with a syringe, and is put into ice-cooled tubes. Up to 4 ml of fluid containing well-preserved cells may be obtained; the cells are stained by the Papanicolaou method. Normal duct cells have a round-to-oval nucleus with regular chromatin content and, usually, no visible nucleoli. They may be arranged in clusters or sheets and their cytoplasm is well defined and sometimes contains vacuoles of mucus. Degenerate cells have pyknotic nuclei. Malignant cells occur in clusters; they have abnormal nuclei and a high nucleocytoplasmic ratio. The nuclear abnormalities include irregular enlargement with indentation of the membrane, unevenly dispersed coarse chromatin and prominent nucleoli.

Klöppel tabulated the accuracy of the results of endoscopic aspiration cytology in carcinoma of the pancreas as obtained by six different groups, whose results had been published, and found that the average accuracy was between 60% and 70%. In a study in which he, himself, had participated (Klapdor et al. 1980) an accurate diagnosis of malignancy was achieved in 12 of 14 cases, but in the larger series of 44 cases of carcinoma of the pancreas studied by Kameya et al. (1981) positive results were obtained in only 23 (52.3%). When endoscopic aspiration cytology is combined with endoscopic retrograde pancreatography, much more accurate results are obtained in the diagnosis of pancreatic carcinoma.

The disadvantages of methods that involve the endoscopic cannulation of the pancreatic duct are that the procedure requires much time and experience. The cytological diagnosis also requires much time and experience (personal communication from Professor Moossa).

Percutaneous Cytology of Pancreatic Lesions

It is sometimes important to obtain confirmation of a diagnosis of carcinoma of the pancreas when neither endoscopy nor laparotomy can be undertaken. If the probable site of the lesion can be determined by one or other of the techniques used to obtain an image of the pancreas, a fine needle may be passed through the skin and through any intervening organ, into the selected part of the pancreas. The needle is directed under ultrasonic guidance, and the technique for the procedure has been described, amongst others, by Hovdenak et al. (1982). These workers carried out the procedure on

55 patients without complications. They were able to aspirate adequate material in 33 of the 41 patients with pancreatic malignancy and made a cytological diagnosis of cancer in 31, with no false-positive results. It is perhaps surprising that percutaneous fine-needle biopsy of the pancreas, in which the fine needle is likely to pass through the walls of the stomach, small intestine or colon and may pierce major blood vessels, rarely causes complications. In fact, no complications followed the procedure in the 55 patients reported by Hovdenak et al. from the Middlesex Hospital in London, or by Tatsuta et al. (1983) in Japan in their 26 patients. In one of the 28 patients subjected to fine-needle aspiration biopsy by McLoughlin et al. (1978) there was an exacerbation of pancreatitis after the puncture, and malignant seeding of the needle tract occurred in the single cases reported by Smith et al. (1980) and by Ferrucci et al. (1979). The apparent rarity of needle tract seeding by malignant cells in clinical practice is surprising, for such seeding is said to be common in experimental studies. This has been discussed by Bergenfeldt et al. (1988) in a paper in which they described two cases of cutaneous implantation of tumour in the needle tract after fine-needle biopsy of pancreatic carcinoma.

The cells obtained by percutaneous pancreatic aspiration may be acinar, ductal, endothelial, of connective tissue or inflammatory (Tao et al. 1978). Acinar cells are the most common; they have round nuclei with finely granular chromatin, in an abundant finely granular cytoplasm. Cells from ducts are columnar, while mesothelial or endothelial cells occur in sheets. Malignant cells have irregular enlarged nuclei with distinct nuclear membranes and prominent nucleoli; they occur in clumps. A poorly differentiated adenocarcinoma will yield cells with much pleomorphism and much necrotic debris. In the case of leiomyosarcoma of the pancreas diagnosed by percutaneous fine-needle biopsy by Tatsuta et al., the tumour cells were spindle shaped and had elongated nuclei that contained fine chromatin and several nucleoli of medium size.

Ultrasound Guided Core Biopsy of the Pancreas

The use of a specially adapted "Tru-cut" needle, fired by a spring-loaded device and inserted under ultrasonographic guidance was pioneered in England by workers at the Middlesex Hospital between 1986 and 1989. The instrument and its use to obtain samples for histological examination from various organs, including the pancreas, were described by Jennings et al. (1989). Also in 1989,

Rode et al. reported the value of these methods in the diagnosis of neuroendocrine tumours of the pancreas, followed, in 1990, by the results of 602 percutaneous biopsies on 241 consecutive patients (Rode and Lees 1990). Their tissue samples allowed 20 serial paraffin sections to be cut; histological diagnosis could be made in all the cases in which the tumours were sampled successfully. In 71, inflammatory cells without tumour were all that could be found; such cases were the most difficult and were diagnosed provisionally as having chronic pancreatitis. The follow-up studies were incomplete in 1990. In 24 of the 170 neoplasms diagnosed (14%), the lesion was potentially treatable.

Laparoscopic Biopsy of the Pancreas

Laparoscopic biopsy of the pancreas has been used by Hanafusa et al. (1990) in their study of the pancreas in diabetes, but this method does not seem to have been used yet in the diagnosis of pancreatic cancer.

Use of Tumour Markers in Diagnosis

Much research has been devoted to the recognition of a marker substance, or substances, whose presence in body fluids or in samples of tumour tissue would be of value in the laboratory diagnosis of pancreatic cancer. In 1981, Klavins reviewed the results available up to that time and concluded that there was no well-defined specific marker; there has been little advance since that time. Substances that have been investigated include carcinoembryonic antigen (CEA), tissue polypeptide antigen (TPA) and various artificially created antitumour antigens.

CEA is a glycoprotein with a substantial carbohydrate component that is secreted in small amounts by normal mucus-secreting epithelial cells. Carcinomas of the alimentary canal, especially colorectal tumours, often cause significant elevations of the level of CEA in the serum and a few carcinomas of the pancreas have also been found to have this effect. Horie et al. (1984), for example, in their study of the relationship of the plasma levels of CEA to the histological type of the tumour in 17 cases of pancreatic carcinoma, found that it was only in the two in which the cancer was of the acinar cell type, or had an acinar cell component, that there was a marked increase of the level of carcinoembryonic antigen in the plasma. In tissue sections, CEA can be demonstrated by immunohistochemistry; Allum

et al. (1986) used immunoperoxide staining with two anti-CEA monoclonal antibodies in normal, chronically inflamed and malignant pancreatic tissue. Positive staining was not found in the normal specimens but in the pancreatic cancers the expression of CEA was related to the degree of differentiation of the tumour. Positive staining was, however, also observed in the cases of chronic pancreatitis.

TPA is an unconjugated membrane protein without sugar, lipid or prosthetic groups. Antibodies raised against TPA react immunologically with various proteins with molecular weights between 20 000 and 45 000. High TPA values had been noted in the serum of patients with pancreatic cancer, and comparison of TPA and CEA serum levels in discriminating between pancreatic cancer and chronic pancreatitis was carried out by Panucci et al. (1986). They concluded that TPA was more sensitive than CEA in the diagnosis of pancreatic cancer, but could not discriminate between pancreatic cancer and certain non-pancreatic digestive diseases. Other possible marker substances that have been investigated include immunoreactive elastase (Hamano et al. 1987; Nakaizumi et al. 1992) and the androgen hormones (Tulassay et al. 1988).

Artificial markers that may have some value in the diagnosis of cancer have been created by making monoclonal antibodies against cell lines of human cancers maintained as xenografts in laboratory animals. By the use of such antibodies various high molecular weight glycoprotein antigens have been recognised in tumour tissue or serum from patients with pancreatic adenocarcinoma. These tumour-associated antigens have been given names such as CA 19-9, DU-PAN-2, CA 125 and TAG 72, and their value as tumour markers has been studied by workers such as Tempero et al. (1989). Heyderman et al. (1990), in their study of epithelial markers in pancreatic carcinoma, were able to state that absence of staining for DD9-E7, their antibody raised against a human pancreatic xenograft, made a diagnosis of adenocarcinoma of the pancreas very unlikely, while Tian et al. (1992) found serum levels of CA 19-9 of prognostic value in pancreatic adenocarcinoma. In the meantime, however, it seems that a single reliable marker for pancreatic adenocarcinoma remains to be discovered.

Spontaneous Carcinoma of the Exocrine Pancreas in Animals

Malignant tumours of the exocrine pancreas are uncommon in domestic animals, but they are more common in cats and dogs than in herbivores. They involve the surrounding abdominal organs and are not always easy to distinguish from biliary carcinomas. In wild animals, carcinoma of the pancreatic region appears to be particularly common in bears (Appleby 1981). A clinicopathological study in 14 dogs with pancreatic carcinoma was reported in 1967 by Anderson and Johnson. An ultrastructural study of four cases of adenocarcinoma of the pancreas in dogs was carried out by Banner et al. (1978), who found that the tumours were of the acinar type. An acinar cell carcinoma of the pancreas in a cat has also been studied by light and electron microscopy by Banner et al. (1979).

References

Adelstein AM (1977) Certifying cause of death. Health Trends 9:78-81

Alanen KA, Joensuu H, Klemi PJ, Nevalainen TJ (1990) Clinical significance of nuclear DNA content in pancreatic carcinoma. J Pathol 160:313-320

Alderson MR (1987) Occupational cancer. In: Hunter's diseases of occupations, 7th edn. Raffle PAB, Lee WR, McCallum RJ, Murray R (eds) Hodder and Stoughton, London, pp 837-849

Allen-Mersh TG (1982) Significance of the site of origin of pancreatic exocrine adenocarcinoma. J Clin Pathol 35:544-546

Allum WH, Stokes HJ, Macdonald F, Fielding JWL (1986) Demonstration of carcinoembryonic antigen (CEA) expression in normal, chronically inflamed, and malignant pancreatic tissue by immunohistochemistry. J Clin Pathol 39:610-614

Anderson NV, Johnson KH (1967) Pancreatic carcinoma in the dog. J Am Vet Med Assoc 150:286-295

Apalakis A, Dussault J, Knight M, Smith R (1977) Relief of pain from pancreatic carcinoma. Ann R Coll Surg Engl 59:401-403

Appleby EC (1981) Report of meeting of Section of Comparative Medicine. Exocrine pancreatic disease. J R Soc Med 74:315-316

Arlen M, Brockunier A (1967) Clinical manifestations of carcinoma of the tail of the pancreas. Cancer 20:1920-1923

Armstrong B, Lea AJ, Adelstein AM, Donovan JW, White CC, Ruttle S (1976) Cancer mortality and saccharin consumption in diabetics. Br J Prev Soc Med 30:151-157

Ashley DJB (ed) (1978) Carcinoma of the pancreas. Evans' histological appearances of tumours, 3rd edn. Churchill Livingstone, London, pp 612-617

Auger C (1947) Acinous cell carcinoma of the pancreas with extensive fat necrosis. Arch Pathol 43:400-405

Baniel J, Konichezky M, Wolloch Y (1987) Osteoclast-type giant cell tumor of the pancreas. Acta Chir Scand 153:67-69

Banner BF, Alroy J, Pauli BU, Carpenter JL (1978) An ultrastructural study of acinic cell carcinomas of the canine pancreas. Am J Pathol 93:165-173

Banner BF, Alroy J, Kipnis RM (1979) Acinar cell carcinoma of the pancreas in a cat. Vet Pathol 16:543-547

Barbosa JJ De C, Dockerty MB, Waugh JM (1946) Pancreatic heterotopia: review of the literature and report of 41 authenticated surgical cases of which 25 were clinically significant. Surg Gynecol Obstet 82:527-542

Barkin JS, Fayne SD (1986) Chronic pancreatitis: update. M Sinai J Med 53:404-408

Barsky D (1978) Unusual tumor of the iris: a rare initial clinical manifestation of metastatic adenocarcinoma of the tail of the pancreas. Ann Ophthalmol 10:1539-1543

Bartholomew LG, Gross JB, Comfort MW (1958) Carcinoma of the pancreas associated with chronic relapsing pancreatitis. Gastroenterology 35:473-477

Barton CM, Hall PA, Hughes CM, Gullick WJ, Lemoine NR (1991) Transforming growth factor alpha and epidermal growth factor in human pancreatic cancer. J Pathol 163:111-116

Bauerlein TC, de la Vega F (1963) A diagnostic sign of carcinoma of the body and tail of the pancreas (abstract). Gastroenterology 44:816

Benarde MA, Weiss W (1982) Coffee consumption and pancreatic cancer: temporal and spatial correlation. Br Med J i:400-402

Bender RA, Brennan MF (1978) The role of percutaneous liver biopsy in the pretreatment evaluation of pancreatic adenocarcinoma. Am J Surg 135:207-209

Benjamin E, Wright DH (1980) Adenocarcinoma of the pancreas of childhood: a report of two cases. Histopathology 4:87-104

Bergenfeldt M, Genell S, Lindholm K, Ekberg O, Aspelin P (1988) Needle-tract seeding after percutaneous fine needle biopsy of pancreatic carcinoma. Acta Chir Scand 154:77-79

Berk JE (1941) Diagnosis of carcinoma of the pancreas. Arch Intern Med 68:525-559

Bliss WR, Birch B, Martin MM, Zollinger RM (1950) Localization of referred pancreatic pain induced by electric stimulation. Gastroenterology 16:317-323

Blot WJ, Fraumeni JF, Stone BJ (1978) Geographic correlates of pancreas cancer in the United States. Cancer 42:373-380

Bourhis J, Lacaine F, August M, Huguier M (1987) Protective effect of oestrogen in pancreatic cancer [letter]. Lancet ii:977

Bowden L (1958) Pancreatic carcinoma: disparity in size of neoplasm as compared with size of gross tumefaction. Arch Surg 76:559-563

Boyd RV (1964) Pemphigoid and carcinoma of the pancreas. Br Med J i:1092

Branganza JM, Howat HT (1972) Cancer of the pancreas. Clin Gastroenterol 1:219-237

Braganza JM, Howat HT (1979) Carcinoma of the pancreas. In: Howat HT, Sarles H (eds) The exocrine pancreas. Saunders, London, pp 484-519

Brayko CM, Doll DC (1982) Squamous cell carcinoma of the pancreas associated with hypercalcemia. Gastroenterology 83:1297-1299

British Medical Journal (1976) Pancreatic pain. i:921-922

British Medical Journal (1978) Non-bacterial thrombotic endocarditis. i:197-198

Brown RK, Moseley V, Pratt TD, Pratt JH (1952) The early diagnosis of cancer of the pancreas based on the clinical and pathological study of one hundred autopsied cases. Am J Med Sci 223:349-363

Burch GE, Ansari A (1968) Chronic alcoholism and carcinoma of the pancreas: a correlative hypothesis. Arch Intern Med 122:273-275

Burns WA, Matthews MJ, Hamosh M, Weide GV, Blum R, Johnson FB (1974) Lipase-secreting acinar cell carcinoma of the pancreas with polyarthropathy. Cancer 33:1002-1009

Butler EB (1972) Pancreatic cytology. Clin Gastroenterol 1:53-60

Chaudhuri MR (1971) Non-bacterial thrombotic endocarditis in association with mucus-secreting adenocarcinomas. Br J Dis Chest 65:98-104

Chen J, Baithun SI (1985) Morphological study of 391 cases of exocrine pancreatic tumours with special reference to the classification of exocrine pancreatic carcinoma. J Pathol 146:17-29

Chen J, Baithun SI, Ramsay MA (1985) Histogenesis of pancreatic carcinomas: a study based on 248 cases. J Pathol 146:65-76

Chen KTK, Brittin G (1980) Peritoneal dissemination of pancreatic adenocarcinoma with granulomatous reaction. Arch Pathol Lab Med 104:163–164

Ching CK, Black R, Helliwell T, Savage A, Barr H, Rhodes JM (1988) Use of lectin histochemistry in pancreatic cancer. J Clin Pathol 41:324–328

Cibull ML, Seligson GR, Mouradian JA, Fialk MA, Pastmantier M (1978) Immunoblastic lymphadenopathy and adenocarcinoma of the pancreas. Cancer 42:1883–1885

Cihak RW, Kawashima T, Steer A (1972) Adenoacanthoma (adenosquamous carcinoma) of the pancreas. Cancer 29:1133–1140

Cliffton EE (1956) Carcinoma of the pancreas. Am J Med 21:760–780

Cochrane AL, Moore F (1981) Death certification from the epidemiological point of view. Lancet ii:742–743

Collure DWD, Burns GP, Schenk WG (1974) Clinical, pathologic, and therapeutic aspects of carcinoma of the pancreas. Am J Surg 128:683–689

Costa J (1977) Benign epithelial inclusions in pancreatic nerves. Am J Clin Pathol 67:306–307

Court-Brown WM, Doll R (1965) Mortality from cancer and other causes after radiotherapy for ankylosing spondylitis. Br Med J ii:1327–1332

Cubilla AL, Fitzgerald PJ (1975) Morphological patterns of primary nonendocrine human pancreas carcinoma. Cancer Res 35:2234–2248

Cubilla AL, Fitzgerald PJ (1980) In: Fitzgerald PJ, Morrison AB (eds) The pancreas. Williams and Wilkins, Baltimore, pp 82–110

Cubilla AL, Fortner J, Fitzgerald PJ (1978) Lymph node involvement in carcinoma of the head of the pancreas area. Cancer 41:880–887

Curth HO, Hilberg AW, Machacek GF (1962) The site and histology of the cancer associated with malignant acanthosis nigricans. Cancer 15:364–382

Cuzick J, Babiker AG (1989) Pancreatic cancer, alcohol, diabetes mellitus and gall bladder disease. Int J Cancer 43:415–421

Darwin E (1796) Zoonomia, vol 2. Printed for J Johnson, London, p 701

Davis DL, Hoel D, Fox J, Lopez A (1990) International trends in cancer mortality in France, West Germany, Italy, Japan, England and Wales, and the USA. Lancet ii:474–481

Davis JC, Hipkin LJ (1977) Clinical endocrine pathology. Blackwell, Oxford, pp 343–367

Devesa S, Silverman DT (1988) Protective effect of oestrogen in pancreatic cancer. Lancet ii:905–906

Doll R, Peto R (1977) Mortality amongst doctors in different occupations. Br Med J i:1433–1436

Drapiewski JF (1944) Carcinoma of the pancreas: a study of neoplastic invasion of nerves and its possible clinical significance. Am J Clin Pathol 14:549–556

Dreiling DA, Blum L, Saunders M (1955) Thrombophlebitis, blood coagulation, and pancreatic disease: a study of the pancreatic secretion in patients with thrombophlebitis. Arch Intern Med 96:490–495

Duff GL (1939) The clinical and pathological features of carcinoma of the body and tail of the pancreas. Bull Johns Hopkins Hosp 65:69–99

Ellis DL, Kaflea SP, Chow JC et al. (1987) Melanoma growth factors, acanthosis nigricans, the sign of Leser-Thélat, and multiple acrochordons. N Engl J Med 317:1582–1587

Elmer-Dewitt P (1992) Running against cancer. Time (March 9th): 40–41

Endo Y, Morii T, Tamura H, Okuda S (1974) Cytodiagnosis of pancreatic malignant tumours by aspiration under direct vision using a duodenal fiberscope. Gastroenterology 67:944–951

Fayemi AO, Deppisch LM (1977) Coronary embolism and myocardial infarction associated with nonbacterial thrombotic endocarditis. Am J Clin Pathol 68:393–396

Ferguson LJ, Watts JMcK (1980) Simultaneous cancer of the pancreas occurring in husband and wife. Gut 21:537–540

Ferrari BT, O'Halloran RL, Longmire WP, Lewin KJ (1979) Atypical papillary hyperplasia of the pancreatic duct mimicking obstructing pancreatic carcinoma. N Engl J Med 301:531–532

Ferrucci JT, Wittenberg J, Margolles MN, Carey RW (1979) Malignant seeding of the tract after thin-needle aspiration biopsy. Radiology 130:345–346

Foster GS (1972) Case records of the Massachusetts General Hospital. Case 25-1972. N Engl J Med 286:1353–1359

Foster JR, Idle JR, Hardwick JP, Bars R, Scott P, Braganza JM (1993) Induction of drug-metabolizing enzymes in human pancreatic cancer and chronic pancreatitis. J Pathol 169:457–463

Fontham ETH, Correa P (1989) Epidemiology of pancreatic cancer. Surg Clin North Am 69:551–567

Frantz VK (1959) Tumors of the pancreas. Armed Forces Institute of Pathology, Washington, DC (Atlas of tumor pathology, section 7, fascicles 27, 28)

Fras I, Litin EM, Pearson JS (1967) Comparison of psychiatric symptoms in carcinoma of the pancreas with those in some other intra-abdominal neoplasms. Am J Psychiatry 123:1553–1562

Fraser R (1963) A case of cachexia and vague abdominal pain. Br Med J i:245–248

Fraumeni JF (1975) Cancers of the pancreas and biliary tract: epidemiological considerations. Cancer Res 35:3437–3446

Gambill EE (1971) Pancreatitis associated with pancreatic carcinoma: a study of 26 cases. Mayo Clin Proc 46:174–177

George P, Brown C, Gilchrist J (1975) Operative biopsy of the pancreas. Br J Surg 62:280–283

Gillam PMS (1961) A case of thrombophlebitis migrans. Br Med J i:721–722.

Gold EB, Gordif L, Diener MD, Seltser R, Boitnott JK, Bynum TE, Hutcheon DF (1985) Diet and other risk factors for cancer of the pancreas. Cancer 55:460–467

Grauer FW (1939) Pancreatic carcinoma: a review of thirty-four autopsies. Arch Intern Med 63:884–898

Grieve DC (1973) Adenocarcinoma of the pancreas: a review of 100 cases. J R Coll Surg Edinb 18:221–226

Gross L, Friedberg GK (1936) Nonbacterial thrombotic endocarditis. Arch Intern Med 58:620–640

Gullick HD (1959) Carcinoma of the pancreas: a review and critical study of 100 cases. Medicine 38:47–84

Haenszel W, Kurihara M (1968) Studies of Japanese migrants: 1. Mortality from cancer and other diseases among Japanese in the United States. J Natl Cancer Inst 40:43–68

Hall RC, Krementz ET (1968) Diagnosis and treatment of pancreatic cancer. Br J Hosp Med 1:168–178

Hamano H, Hayakawa T, Kondo T (1987) Serum immunoreactive elastase in diagnosis of pancreatic disease: a sensitive marker for pancreatic cancer. Dig Dis Sci 32:50–56

Hanafusa T, Miyazaki A, Miyagawa J et al. (1990) Examination of islets in the pancreas biopsy specimens from newly diagnosed Type 1 (insulin dependent) diabetic patients. Diabetologia 33:105–111

Hartveit F, Maartmann-Moe H (1982) Pancreatic cancer: a hidden disease in the elderly? Clin Oncol 8:223–229

Hatfield ARW, Smithies A, Wilkins R, Levi AJ (1976) Assessment of endoscopic retrograde cholangio-pancreatography (ERCP) and pure pancreatic juice cytology in patients with pancreatic disease. Gut 17:14–21

Haunz EA, Baggenstoss AH (1950) Carcinoma of the head of the pancreas: the effects of obstruction on the ductal and acinar systems. Arch Pathol 49:367–386

Hayes RL, Pinson TJ, Leffall LD (1966) Adenocarcinoma of the pancreas metastatic to the mandible. Oral Surg 21:61–66

Herrera MF, van Heerden JA, Katzmann JA, Weiland LH, Nagorney DM, Ilstrup D (1992) Evaluation of DNA nuclear pattern as a prognostic determinant in resected pancreatic ductal adenocarcinoma. Ann Surg 215:120–124

Heuch I, Kvåle G, Jacobsen BK, Bjelke E (1983) Use of alcohol, tobacco and coffee, and risk of pancreatic cancer. Br J Cancer 48:637–643

Hewer TF (1961) The metastatic origin of alveolar-cell tumour of the lung. J Pathol Bacteriol 81:323–330

Heyderman E, Larkin SE, O'Donnell PJ et al. (1990) Epithelial markers in pancreatic carcinoma: immunoperoxidase localisation of DD9, CEA, EMA and CAM 5.2. J Clin Pathol 43:448–452

Higgins GA, Recant L, Fischman AB (1979) The glucagonoma syndrome: surgically curable diabetes. Am J Surg 137:142–148

Hobbs JR, Evans DJ, Wong OM (1974) Renal tubular obstruction by mucoproteins from adenocarcinoma of the pancreas. Br Med J ii:87–89

Hobbs RD, Stewart AF, Ravin ND, Carter D (1984) Hypercalcemia in small cell carcinoma of the pancreas. Cancer 53:1552–1554

Hoorens A, Lemoine NR, McLellan E et al. (1993) Pancreatic acinar cell carcinoma: an analysis of cell lineage markers, p53 expression, and Ki-*ras* mutation. Am J Pathol 143:685–698

Höpker W-W (1987) Epidemiologie der Pankreaserkrankungen. Verh Dtsch Ges Pathol 71:144–160

Horie A, Yano Y, Kotoo Y, Miwa A (1977) Morphogenesis of pancreatoblastoma, infantile carcinoma of the pancreas. Cancer 39:247–254

Horie Y, Gomyoda M, Kishimoto Y et al. (1984) Plasma carcinoembryonic antigen and acinar cell carcinoma of the pancreas. Cancer 53:1137–1142

Hovdenak N, Lees WR, Pereira J, Beilby JOW, Cotton PB (1982) Ultrasound-guided percutaneous fine-needle aspiration cytology in pancreatic cancer. Br Med J iv:1183–1184

Hubran RH, Molina JM, Reddy MN, Boitnott JK (1987) A neoplasm with pancreatic and hepatocellular differentiation presenting with subcutaneous fat necrosis. Am J Clin Pathol 88:639–645

Huntrakoon M (1983) Oncocytic carcinoma of the pancreas. Cancer 51:332–336

Igarashi M, Card GG, Johnson PE, Alford BR (1979) Bilateral sudden hearing loss and metastatic pancreatic adenocarcinoma. Arch Otolaryngol 105:196–199

Jalloh SS (1983) Giant cell tumour (osteoclastoma) of the pancreas – an epithelial tumour probably of pancreatic acinar origin. J Clin Pathol 36:1171–1175

Jeffrey I, Crow J, Ellis BW (1983) Osteoclast-type giant cell tumour of the pancreas. J Clin Pathol 36:1165–1170

Jennings PE, Donald JJ, Coral A, Rode J, Lees WR (1989) Ultrasound-guided core biopsy. Lancet i:1369–1371

Jick H, Dinan BJ (1981) Coffee and pancreatic cancer [letter]. Lancet ii:92

Johnson JR, Zintel HA (1963) Pancreatic calcification and cancer of the pancreas. Surg Gynecol Obstet 117:585–588

Kameya S, Kuno N, Kasugai T (1981) The diagnosis of pancreatic cancer by pancreatic juice cytology. Acta Cytologica 25:354–360

Kaplan N, Angrist A (1943) The mechanism of jaundice in cancer of the pancreas. Surg Gynecol Obstet 77:199–204

Karwinski B, Svendsen E, Hartveit F (1989) Changes in the cancer spectrum at autopsy: 1978–1984. J Pathol 157:117–125

Kay S, Harrison JM (1969) Unusual pleomorphic carcinoma of the pancreas featuring production of osteoid. Cancer 23:1158–1162

Keller RT, Logan GM (1977) Adenocarcinoma of the pancreas associated with neurofibromatosis. Cancer 39:1264–1266

Kepler EJ (1933) Symposium: Polyglandular dyscrasias involving abnormalities of sexual characteristics. Mayo Clin Proc 8:102–110

Kern HF, Röher HD, von Bülow M, Klöppel G (1987) Fine structure of three major grades of malignancy of human pancreatic adenocarcinoma. Pancreas 2:2–13

Kessler II (1970) Cancer mortality among diabetics. J Natl Cancer Inst 44:673–686

Kinlen L, Goldblatt P, Fox J, Yudkin J (1984) Coffee and pancreas cancer: controversy in part explained? Lancet i:282–283

Kircher T, Nelson J, Burdo M (1985) The autopsy as a measure of accuracy of the death certificate. N Engl J Med 313:1263–1269

Klapdor R, Soehendra N, Klöppel G, Steiner D (1980) Diagnosis of pancreatic carcinoma by means of endoscopic pancreatography and pancreatic cytology. Hepatogastroenterology 27:227–230

Klavins JV (1981) Tumor markers of pancreatic carcinoma. Cancer 47:1597–1601

Klöppel G (1984) Pancreatic biopsy. In: Klöppel G, Heitz PU (eds) Pancreatic pathology. Churchill Livingstone, Edinburgh, pp 114–122

Kozuka S, Sassa R, Taki T et al. (1979) Relation of pancreatic duct hyperplasia to carcinoma. Cancer 43:1418–1428

Krain LS (1970) The rising incidence of carcinoma of the pancreas – real or apparent? J Surg Oncol 2:115–124

Krain LS (1971) The rising incidence of carcinoma of the pancreas: further epidemiological studies. J Chronic Dis 23:685–690

Ku Y, Kawa Y, Fujiwara S et al. (1989) Hemodynamic study of occlusion of the splenic vein caused by carcinoma of the pancreas. Surg Gynecol Obstet 168:17–24

Kune GA, Cole R, Bell S (1975) Observations on the relief of pancreatic pain. Med J Aust 2:789–791

Kuwano H, Sonoda T, Hashimoto H, Enjoji N (1984) Heptocellular carcinoma with osteoclast-like giant cells. Cancer 54:837–842

Lafler CJ, Hinderman DL (1961) A morphological study of pancreatic carcinoma with reference to multiple thrombi. Cancer 14:944–951

Lancet (1829) State of the pancreas in smokers [letter]. ii:177

Lancet (1978) Cancer of the pancreas: the world scene. i:1109

Lancet (1990) Regulating *ras* [editorial]. Lancet 336:1291–1292

Leach WB (1950) Carcinoma of the pancreas: a clinical and pathological analysis of 39 autopsied cases. Am J Pathol 26:333–347

Lemoine NR, Hughes CM, Barton CM et al. (1992) The epidermal growth factor receptor in human pancreatic cancer. J Pathol 166:7–12

Lemon HM, Byrnes WW (1949) Cancer of the biliary tract and pancreas: diagnosis from cytology of duodenal aspirations. JAMA 141:254–257

Levin DL, Connelly RR (1973) Cancer of the pancreas: available epidemiologic information and its implications. Cancer 31:1231–1236

Levison DA (1979) Carcinoma of the pancreas. J Pathol 129:203–223

Libman E, Sacks B (1924) A hitherto undescribed form of valvular and mural endocarditis. Arch Intern Med 33:701–737

Lièvre J-A (1974) Les panniculites et les lésions ostéo-articulaires au cours des affections du pancréas. Ann Med Interne 125:45–49

Lightwood R, Reber HA, Way LW (1976) The risk and accuracy of pancreatic biopsy. Am J Surg 132:189–194

Lindelöf B, Sigurgeirsson B, Tegner E et al. (1991) PUVA and cancer: a large-scale eipdemiological study. Lancet ii:91–93

Lisa JR, Trinidad S, Rosenblatt MB (1964) Pulmonary manifestations of carcinoma of the pancreas. Cancer 17:395–401

Longnecker DS, Curphey TJ (1975) Adenocarcinoma of the pancreas in azaserine-treated rats. Cancer Res 35 : 2249–2258

Lorge RE, Richards P (1976) Carcinoma of the pancreas and acute renal failure. Br Med J i: 24

Lymboura M, Leathem AJ (1991) Helix pomatia lectin binding to various carcinomas and the possible relationship to prognosis [abstract]. J Pathol 163 : 180A

MacDermott RP, Kramer P (1973) Adenocarcinoma of the pancreas in four siblings. Gastroenterology 65 : 137–139

MacDonald RA, Robbins SL (1957) The significance of nonbacterial thrombotic endocarditis: an autopsy and clinical study of 78 cases. Ann Intern Med 46 : 255–273

MacMahon B, Yen S, Trichopoulos D, Warren K, Nardi G (1981) Coffee and cancer of the pancreas. N Engl J Med 304 : 630–633

Mancuso TF, Sterling TD (1974) Relations of place of birth and migration in cancer mortality in the US: a study of Ohio residents. J Chronic Dis 27 : 459–474

Marks LJ, Berde B, Klein LA et al. (1968) Inappropriate vasopressin secretion and carcinoma of the pancreas. Am J Med 45 : 967–974

Matsui Y, Aoki Y, Ishikawa O et al. (1979) Ductal carcinoma of the pancreas. Arch Surg 114 : 722–726

McLoughlin MJ, Ho C-S, Langer B, McHattie J, Tao L-C (1978) Fine needle aspiration biopsy of malignant lesions in and around the pancreas. Cancer 41 : 2413–2419

McWhirter WR, Stiller CA, Lennox EL (1989) Carcinomas in childhood: a registry-based study of incidence and survival. Cancer 63 : 2242–2246

Mellor H, Taylor I, Roath S, Francis JL (1989) Trousseau's syndrome: whole blood procoagulant in breast and colorectal cancer. J Clin Pathol 42 : 489–494

Mersey Regional Hospital Authority (1977) Analysis of malignant cases registered 1971, 1972, 1973. Mersey Regional Health Authority, Liverpool

Mikal S, Campbell AJA (1950) Carcinoma of the pancreas: diagnostic and operative criteria based on one hundred consecutive autopsies. Surgery 28 : 963–969

Miller EM, Dockerty MB, Wollaeger EF, Waugh JM (1951) Carcinoma of the region of the papilla of Vater: a study of cases in which resection was performed. Surg Gynecol Obstet 92 : 172–182

Miller JR, Baggenstoss AH, Comfort MW (1951) Carcinoma of the pancreas: effect of histological type and grade of malignancy on its behaviour. Cancer 4 : 233–241

Mills PK, Beeson WL, Abbey DE, Fraser GE, Phillips RL (1988) Dietary habits and past medical history as related to fatal pancreas cancer risk among Adventists. Cancer 61 : 2578–2585

Milner RDG, Mitchinson MJ (1965) Systemic Weber–Christian disease. J Clin Pathol 18 : 150–156

Mizumoto K, Inagaki T, Koizumi M et al. (1988) Early pancreatic duct adenocarcinoma. Hum Pathol 19 : 242–244

Morgan RGH, Wormsley KG (1977) Progress report: cancer of the pancreas. Gut 18 : 580–596

Morgan RGH, Levison DA, Hopwood D, Saunders JHB, Wormsley KG (1977) Potentiation of the action of azaserine on the rat pancreas by raw soya bean flour. Cancer Lett 3 : 87–90

Morohoshi T, Held G, Klöppel G (1983) Exocrine pancreatic tumours and their histological classifications: a study based on 167 autopsy and 97 surgical cases. Histopathology 7 : 645–661

Motojima K, Urano T, Nagata Y, Shiku H, Tsurifune T, Kanematsu T (1993) Detection of point mutations in the Kirsten-ras oncogene provides evidence for the multicentricity of pancreatic carcinoma. Ann Surg 217 : 138–143

Nagai H, Kuroda A, Morioka Y (1986) Lymphatic and local spread of T1 and T2 pancreatic cancer: a study of autopsy material. Ann Surg 204 : 65–71

Nagakawa T, Kayahara M, Ueno K et al. (1992) A clinicopathologic study on neural invasion in cancer of the pancreatic head. Cancer 69 : 930–935

Nakaizumi A, Tatsuta M, Uehara H et al. (1992) A prospective trial of early detection of pancreatic cancer by ultrasonographic examination combined with measurement of serum elastase 1. Cancer 69 : 936–940

Neil HAW, Fairer JG, Coleman MP, Thurston A, Vessey MP (1987) Mortality amongst male anaesthetists in the United Kingdom, 1957–83. Br Med J iii: 360–362

Newbould MJ, Benbow EW, Sene A, Young M, Taylor TV (1992) Adenocarcinoma of the pancreas with osteoclast-like giant cells: a case report with immunocytochemistry. Pancreas 7 : 611–615

Nix GAJJ, Dubbelman C, Wilson JHP, Schütte HE, Jeckel J, Postema RR (1991) Prognostic implication of tumor diameter in carcinoma of the head of the pancreas. Cancer 67 : 529–535

Nomura A, Stemmermann GN, Heilbrun LK (1981) Coffee and pancreatic cancer [letter]. Lancet ii: 415

Norell S, Ahlbon A, Olin R et al. (1986) Occupational factors and pancreatic cancer. Br J Indust Med 43 : 775–778

Oelbaum MH, Strich J (1953) Thrombophlebitis migrans and carcinoma of body and tail of pancreas. Br Med J ii: 907–909

Offerhaus GJA, Giardello FM, Moore GW, Teromette AC (1987) Partial gastrectomy: a risk factor for carcinoma of the pancreas? Hum Pathol 18 : 285–288

Osborne RR (1950) Functioning acinous cell carcinoma of the pancreas accompanied by widespread focal fat necrosis. Arch Intern Med 85 : 933–943

Panucci A, Fabris C, Del Favero G et al. (1986) Is tissue polypeptide antigen more accurate than serum CEA for diagnosing pancreatic cancer? J Clin Pathol 39 : 75–77

Paulino-Netto A, Dreiling DA, Baronofsky ID (1960) The relationship between pancreatic calcification and cancer of the pancreas. Ann Surg 151 : 530–537

Pour P (1980) Experimental pancreatic ductal (ductular) tumors. In: Fitzgerald PJ, Morrison AB(eds) The pancreas. Williams and Wilkins, Baltimore, pp 111–139

Pour P, Krüger FW, Althoff J, Cardesa A, Mohr U (1975) A new approach to induction of pancreatic neoplasms. Cancer Res 35 : 2259–2268

Pour PM, Sayed S, Sayed G (1982) Hyperplastic, preneoplastic and neoplastic lesions found in 83 human pancreases. Am J Clin Pathol 77 : 137–152

Rack FJ, Elkins CW (1950) Experiences with vagotomy and sympathectomy in the treatment of chronic recurrent pancreatitis. Arch Surg 61 : 937–943

Ray BS, Console AD (1949) The relief of pain in chronic (calcareous) pancreatitis by sympathectomy. Surg Gynecol Obstet 89 : 1–8

Reddy JK, Rao MS (1975) Pancreatic adenocarcinoma in inbred guinea pigs induced by N-methyl-N-nitrosourea. Cancer Res 35 : 2269–2277

Rich RH, Weber JL, Shandling B (1986) Adenocarcinoma of the pancreas in a neonate managed by pancreatoduodenectomy. J Pediatr Surg 21 : 806–808

Rickles FR, Edwards RL (1983) Activation of blood coagulation in cancer: Trousseau's syndrome revisited. Blood 62 : 14–31

Robertson JC, Eeles GH (1970) Syndrome associated with pancreatic acinar cell carcinoma. Br Med J ii: 708–709

Robinson A, Scott J, Rosenfeld DD (1970) The occurrence of carcinoma of the pancreas in chronic pancreatitis. Radiology 94 : 289–290

Rode J, Lees WR (1990) Pancreatic percutaneous biopsy in 241 consecutive patients [abstract]. J Pathol 161 : 357A

Rode J, Dowsett JF, Lees WR (1989) Pancreatic neuroendocrine tumours diagnosed by percutaneous core biopsy [abstract]. J Pathol 157 : 174A

Rohner RF, Prior JT, Sipple JH (1966) Mucinous malignancies, venous thrombosis and terminal endocarditis with emboli: a syndrome. Cancer 19 : 1805–1812

Rosai J (1968) Carcinoma of pancreas simulating giant cell tumor of bone: electron microscopic evidence of its acinar cell origin. Cancer 22:333–344

Sack GH, Levin J, Ball WR (1977) Trousseau's syndrome and other manifestations of chronic disseminated coagulopathy in patients with neoplasms: clinical, pathophysiologic, and therapeutic features. Medicine 56:1–32

Salm R (1960) Scirrhous adenocarcinoma arising in a lipomatous pseudohypertrophic pancreas. J Pathol Bacteriol 79:47–52

Salm R (1968) Carcinoma arising in a lipomatous pseudohypertrophic pancreas. Br Med J iii:293

Salmon PA (1966) Carcinoma of the pancreas and extra-hepatic biliary system. Surgery 60:554–565

Scarpelli DG (1956) Fat necrosis of bone marrow in acute pancreatitis. Am J Pathol 32:1077–1087

Schron DS, Mendelsohn G (1984) Pancreatic carcinoma with duct, endocrine, and acinar differentiation: a histologic, immunocytochemical, and ultrastructural study. Cancer 54:1766–1770

Segi M, Kurihara M, Matsuyama T (1969) Cancer mortality for selected sites in 24 countries, no. 5, 1964–1965. Department of Public Health, Tohoku University School of Medicine, Sendai, Japan

Serebro H (1965) A diagnostic sign of carcinoma of the pancreas. Lancet i:85–86

Silver GB, Lubliner RK (1948) Carcinoma of the pancreas: a clinicopathologic survey. Surg Gynecol Obstet 86:703–716

Smith FP, Macdonald JS, Schein PS, Ornitz RD (1980) Cutaneous seeding of pancreatic cancer by skinny-needle aspiration biopsy [letter]. Arch Intern Med 140:855

Smith JP, Yates PO (1955) The thrombotic syndrome associated with carcinoma. J Pathol Bacteriol 70:111–117

Smith, Lord of Marlow (1979) Surgery of cancer of the pancreas. In: Howat HT, Sarles H (eds) The exocrine pancreas. Saunders, London, pp 520–535

Smith R (1958) Malignant tumours of the pancreas. In: Raven RW (ed) Cancer, 2. Butterworths, London, pp 186–206

Sneddon IB (1963) The skin markers of malignancy. Br Med J ii:405–409

Sommers SC, Meissner WA (1954) Unusual carcinomas of the pancreas. Arch Pathol 58:101–111

Sproul EE (1938) Carcinoma and venous thrombosis: the frequency of association of carcinoma in the body or tail of the pancreas with multiple venous thrombosis. Am J Cancer 34:566–585

Stocks P (1970) Cancer mortality in relation to national consumption of cigarettes, solid fuel, tea and coffee. Br J Cancer 24:215–225

Tanaka T, Mori H, Williams GM (1988) Atypical and neoplastic acinar cell lesions of the pancreas in an autopsy study of Japanese patients. Cancer 61:2278–2285

Tao L-C, Ho C-S, McLoughlin MJ, McHattie J (1978) Percutaneous fine needle aspiration biopsy of the pancreas. Acta Cytologica 22:215–220

Tatsuta M, Yamamoto R, Yamamamura H, Okuda S, Tamura H (1983) Cytologic examination and CEA measurement in aspirated pancreatic material collected by percutaneous fine-needle aspiration biopsy under ultrasonic guidance for the diagnosis of pancreatic carcinoma. Cancer 52:693–698

Tavassoli FA, Lynch RG (1974) Occult carcinoma of the pancreas in a 17 year old patient with immunosuppressed leukemia. Gastroenterology 66:1054–1057

Tempero M, Takasaki H, Uchida E et al. (1989) Co-expression of CA19-9, DU-PAN-2, CA125, and TAG-72 in pancreatic adeno-

carcinoma. Am J Surg Pathol 13 (suppl 1):89–95

Thomas JP, Shields R (1970) Associated autonomic dysfunction and carcinoma of the pancreas. Br Med J iv:32

Thompson CM, Rodgers LR (1952) Analysis of the autopsy records of 157 cases of carcinoma of the pancreas with particular reference to the incidence of thrombo-embolism. Am J Med Sci 223:469–478

Tian F, Appert HE, Myles J, Howard JM (1992) Prognostic value of serum CA19-9 levels in pancreatic adenocarcinoma. Am Surg 215:350–355

Trousseau A (1865) Phlegmatia alba dolens. Clinique médicale de L'Hôtel-Dieu de Paris, tome troisième. Baillière, Paris, pp 660–662

Tulassay Z, Sándor Z, Bodrogi L, Papp J, Fehér T (1988) An endocrine marker for pancreatic cancer. Br Med J iv:1447–1448

Ulich T, Cheng L, Lewin KJ (1982) Acinar-endocrine cell tumor of the pancreas: report of a pancreatic tumor containing both zymogen and neuroendocrine granules. Cancer 50:2099–2105

Volk BW, Wellmann KF (1977) Cancer and diabetes. In: Volk BW, Wellmann KF (eds) The diabetic pancreas. Baillière Tindall, London, pp 311–316

Vorherr H, Massry SG, Utiger RD, Kleeman CR (1968) Antidiuretic principle in malignant tumor extracts from patients with inappropriate ADH syndrome. J Clin Endocrinol 28:162–168

Walker RJ (1970) The diagnosis of carcinoma of the pancreas. J R Coll Surg Edinb 15:185–190

Webb JN (1977) Acinar cell neoplasms of the exocrine pancreas. J Clin Pathol 30:103–112

Weger A-R, Graf A-H, Askensten U et al. (1987) Ploidy as prognostic determinant in pancreatic cancer [letter]. Lancet ii:1031

Weger A-R, Falkmer UG, Schwab G et al. (1990) Nuclear DNA distribution pattern of the parenchymal cells in adenocarcinomas of the pancreas and in chronic pancreatitis: a study of archival specimens using both image and flow cytometry. Gastroenterology 99:237–242

Wenger J, Raskin HF (1958) The diagnosis of cancer of the pancreas, biliary tract and duodenum by combined cytological and secretory methods: II. The secretin test. Gastroenterology 34:1009–1017

Whitfield AGW (1968) A case of pancreatic disease with peptic ulceration. Br Med J ii:494–498

Willett CG, Lewandrowski K, Warshaw AL, Efird J, Compton CC (1993) Resection margins in carcinoma of the head of the pancreas: implications for radiation therapy. Ann Surg 217:144–148

Williams RR, Horm JW (1977) Association of cancer sites with tobacco and alcohol consumption and socioeconomic status of patients: interview study from the third national cancer survey. J Natl Cancer Inst 58:525–547

Willis RA (1952) The spread of tumours in the human body. Butterworths, London, pp 135, 213, 309

Willis RA (1967) Pathology of tumours, 4th edn. Butterworths, London, pp 446–448

Wynder EL (1975) A epidemiological evaluation of the causes of cancer of the pancreas. Cancer Res 35:2228–2233

Wynder EL, Mabuchi K, Maruchi N, Fortner JG (1973) Epidemiology of cancer of the pancreas. J Natl Cancer Inst 50:645–667

Yoshioka H, Wakabayashi T (1958) Therapeutic neurotomy on head of pancreas for relief of pain due to chronic pancreatitis: a new technical procedure and its results. Arch Surg 76:546–554

Tumours and Hyperplasias of the Endocrine Pancreas

Although Neve, in 1891, described an adenoma that he had found by chance in the head of the pancreas, the microscopic appearances that he recorded do not allow the modern reader to identify that tumour as an adenoma of islet cells. The first recognition of an adenoma of islet cells is attributed to Nicholls in 1902. In 1903, Fabozzi described the pathological findings in five cases of carcinoma of the pancreas in each of which he found, and illustrated, microscopic appearances that seemed to show that the tumours had originated from islet cells, but his paper included no clinical information that might have distinguished his cases from carcinoma of the exocrine pancreas. Nicholls, who found a pea-sized nodule by accident on the anterior surface of the pancreas, attributed no clinical significance to the lesion, and, although similar tumours were soon found by others, it was not until insulin had been discovered that the possibility that tumours of islet tissue might be hormonally active was realised. In 1927, Wilder et al. described a case in which the patient, who was himself a doctor, suggested that his symptoms resembled the effects produced by excess of insulin. He was found to have a cystic tumour in the tail of the pancreas, with metastases in the liver and lymph nodes. Alcoholic extracts of the cancer tissue in the liver had an insulin-like action when they were injected into rabbits.

In the meantime, reports of adenomas of the islets of Langerhans had been accumulating and by 1926, Warren, by recording four of his own, brought the number of reported cases up to 20 and suggested that such tumours were not as rare as the small number of reports had suggested.

Special searches for such tumours proved him to be correct, for, as Spencer (1955) wrote: "The number of these tumours discovered varies directly with the care expended on the examination of the pancreas at every post-mortem." This was illustrated by the work of Lopez-Kruger and Dockerty (1947), who found that in 10 314 consecutive routine autopsies at the Mayo Clinic between 1926 and 1945, 44 pancreatic adenomas were discovered, an incidence of 0.4%, but that a carefully conducted study of 500 pancreases yielded eight tumours, an incidence of 1.6%. Spencer too, having become interested in islet cell adenomas, found five cases in 330 post-mortem examinations at St Thomas' Hospital, London, an incidence of 1.5%. Such findings have been confirmed, more or less, by later work and, in a review published in 1980, Creutzfeldt stated that the prevalence of islet cell tumours in unselected autopsy material was between 0.5% and 1.5%.

The interest aroused by the discovery that an islet cell tumour of the pancreas might produce effects similar to those of insulin resulted in numerous reports of insulin-like effects associated with both histologically benign and histologically malignant tumours of the islets, for example that by O'Leary and Womack (1934), who published an account of five operatively removed islet cell tumours each of which had been suspected clinically because of hypoglycaemia; only one of the five tumours had histological features that indicated malignancy. By 1942, Duff and Murray were able to review over 100 cases that had been recognised either clinically or at autopsy, and it became clear that there were two groups of islet cell tumours: those that produced the hypoglycaemic syndrome and those that did not. The authors considered that, in the absence of hyperinsulinism, an islet adenoma would remain unrecognised and unimportant until it became an incidental finding during an autopsy, and, also in the absence of hyperinsulinism, islet cell carcinomas would cause clinical effects similar to those of exocrine carcinomas of the pancreas. At that time neither anatomical nor histological criteria could distinguish between functioning and non-functioning tumours, but the pathologist was expected to differentiate between simple and malignant tumours, although it was recognised that adenoma-like tumours might have a low degree of malignancy.

The existence of truly non-functional tumours of islet cells, however, began to be questioned after Zollinger and Ellison (1955) described two patients with primary peptic ulcerations of the jejunum associated with non-specific islet cell tumours of the pancreas and were able to find previously published accounts of four similar cases. They postulated that a humoral factor, secreted by the non-beta islet cell tumours, caused hypersecretion of gastric acid that led to intractable ulcers of the upper gastrointestinal tract. The existence of such a hormone was later demonstrated by the work of Gregory et al. (1960), and shown to be the polypeptide substance gastrin (Gregory et al. 1967; McGuigan and Trudeau 1968). Gastrin is not secreted by any of the normal cells of the pancreatic islets; it is secreted normally by the G-cells of the mucosa of the pyloric antrum. The secretion of gastrin by a tumour of islet cells is an indication of functional metaplasia as well as of neoplastic change.

A second clinical syndrome associated with non-beta tumours of the pancreatic islets was recognised by Verner and Morrison in 1958. This syndrome consisted of intractable watery diarrhoea, hypokalaemia and either absent or much reduced secretion of gastric hydrochloric acid. A vasoactive peptide, originally obtained from intestines, and since shown to be secreted by the tumour cells, is the probable cause of the diarrhoea.

Descriptions of other clinical syndromes associated with non-beta tumours of islet cells followed; of these the glucagonoma syndrome is the most characteristic (Mallinson et al. 1974). The inappropriate secretion of glucagon is due to neoplasia of the alpha (A) cells of the islets. The full syndrome consists of a skin rash in which there is necrolytic migratory erythema with superficial destruction of the epidermis (tending to affect the lower abdomen, perineum and legs), diabetes or an abnormal glucose tolerance test, normocytic or normochromic anaemia, a sore red tongue, angular stomatitis, marked loss of weight, mental depression, vulnerability to infections, and a tendency to develop venous thromboses.

Tumours of delta (D) cells with excessive secretion of somatostatin have also been recognised (Larsson et al. 1977; Ganda et al. 1977; Krejs et al.

1979). The patients with such tumours suffer from abdominal pain, diarrhoea, steatorrhoea, achlorhydria and diabetes mellitus. In two patients a pancreatic tumour was discovered during operations for cholelithiasis. All the symptoms (including the cholelithiasis) have been attributed to the inhibitory effect of high concentrations of somatostatin upon the secretion of hormones by the pancreas, along with inhibition of the secretion and motility of the gastrointestinal tract, but the specificity of the inhibitory effects of somatostatin as the cause of a "somatostatinoma syndrome" have, however, been questioned by Klöppel and Heitz (1988).

The recognition of syndromes such as those that have just been mentioned suggests that, as the sensitivity of clinical diagnostic tests is improved and methods for the detection of hormonal activity in tumour cells become more refined, other syndromes may be discovered; functional activity may be found in islet cell tumours that have been regarded in the past as non-functioning. Already it has been found that hormones in addition to the dominant hormone responsible for the clinical syndrome may be produced by islet cell tumours. Thus a gastrinoma, causing the Zollinger–Ellison syndrome, may produce in addition to gastrin (its primary hormone), various secondary hormones such as insulin, glucagon, pancreatic polypeptide (PP), vasoactive intestinal peptide (VIP), secretin, ACTH and melanocyte-stimulating hormone. Likewise, secondary hormones may be produced in tumours that give rise to syndromes such as spontaneous attacks of hypoglycaemia, the Verner–Morrison syndrome and the glucagonoma syndrome. It has not been settled yet with certainty whether different types of endocrine cells within a pancreatic tumour that produces a multiplicity of hormones are responsible for the various hormones or whether a single type of neoplastically dedifferentiated cell produces several hormones, including those that are normally produced in significant amounts by pancreatic islet cells.

General Characteristics of Islet Cell Tumours

The general characteristics of islet cell tumours of the pancreas, functional or otherwise, have been assembled and discussed by Bloodworth and Greider (1982) and, more recently, by Klöppel and Heitz (1988). The review by the latter authors is based on their own collection of 365 examples of

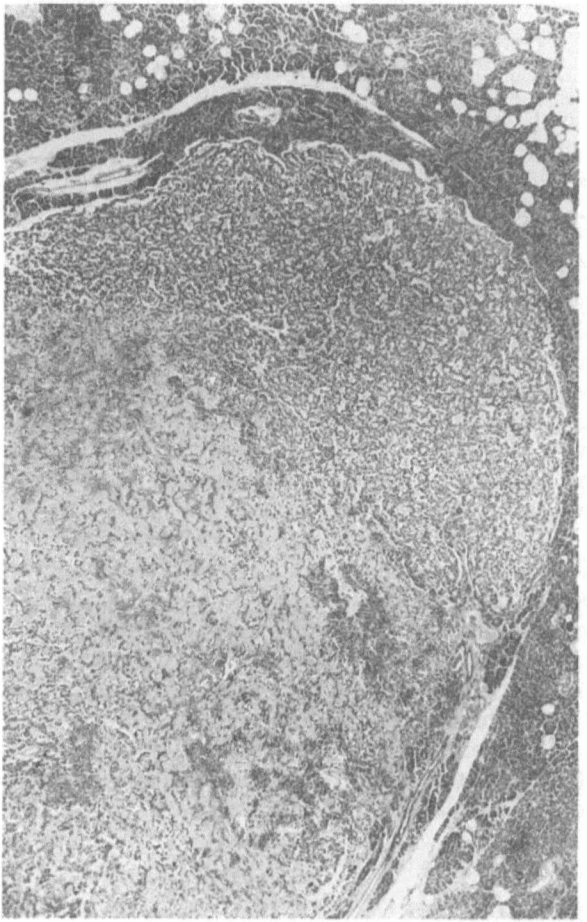

Fig. 10.1. Differing patterns within the same islet cell adenoma. One of many adenomas, without recognisable clinical effects, in a case of MEN 1. (Courtesy of Dr S. Banik) H&E, × 24

pancreatic endocrine tumours, supplemented by a study of the relevant literature. The size of such a collection is remarkable, for endocrine tumours of the pancreas are rare; for example, in 16 of the main surgical centres of what was then the Federal Republic of Germany, only 287 such tumours were removed between 1967 and 1976 (Kümmerle and Rückert 1978), an apparent incidence, according to Klöppel and Heitz, of about 30 tumours per year in a population of 62 million people. The latter authors attributed the abundance of the material available to them to the referral of many interesting specimens to their departments.

Most islet cell tumours occur in adults, but persistent hypoglycaemia due to an over-abundance of pancreatic islets (nesidioblastosis) may cause problems in neonatal infants. The localised tumours of adults may occur in any part of the pancreas and the

tumours that cause the Zollinger–Ellison syndrome may occur in the duodenum close to the pancreas.

The cut surface of islet cell tumours is usually grey but highly vascular tumours may resemble splenic tissue within the pancreas. The size ranges from 700 µm to several centimetres in diameter. Those less than 2 cm in diameter are usually benign and non-functional, but a small impalpable, but functioning, adenoma, may require intraoperative sonography for its recognition (Norton et al. 1988; London et al. 1988). Malignant tumours are usually over 6 cm in diameter when they are diagnosed. Islet cell tumours may be single or multiple; in multiple tumours each may differ histologically from its neighbours. The differentiation between benign and malignant tumours by routine histological methods is unreliable, but those causing the Zollinger–Ellison syndrome and the glucagonoma syndrome are usually malignant and cause metastases in lymph nodes and in the liver, while most tumours that cause the hypoglycaemic syndrome are benign. Any type of islet cell tumour may be one of the components of the multiple endocrine neoplasia syndrome, type 1 (MEN 1).

In routinely stained sections, certain histological patterns have been described but the pattern is liable to vary in different parts of the same tumour (Fig. 10.1) and there are often morphologically different cell types, some with clear cytoplasm, and others with an eosinophilic or basophilic cytoplasm with round, polygonal or ovoid outlines. The nuclei are usually only slightly hyperchromatic; abnormal or multiple nuclei are usually, though not invariably, rare. A fibrous stroma, in which there may be hyaline change, is common, and there is sometimes amyloid change or calcification in the stroma, especially in insulinomas.

The arrangement of the tumour cells has been described as being of three main types. There is a gyriform or whirling pattern in which cords of cells form loops and festoons. This is the pattern that is most easily recognised as resembling the structure of normal islets. Another pattern is the solid or medullary arrangement, with the cells in large clumps with little intervening stroma, while a glandular or alveolar arrangement of the cells may also be found, along with occasional duct-like structures, and, very rarely, with psammoma bodies. Although all the patterns may occur in the same tumour, one of the types usually predominates. There is no definite association between the predominant pattern and the predominant hormone produced by the tumour, nor is there any association between any of the patterns and the benign or malignant behaviour of the tumour. The cellular characteristics of malignant tumours rarely differ from those

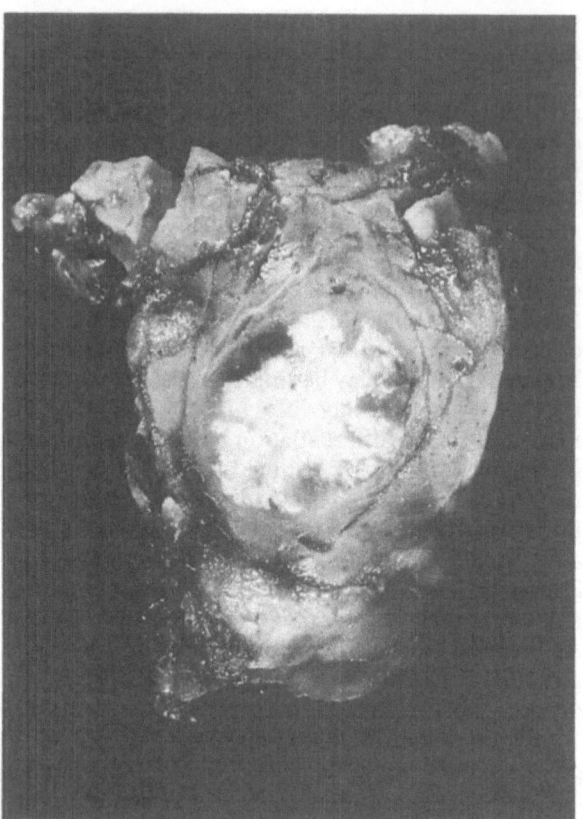

Fig. 10.2. An islet cell tumour, 1.8 cm in diameter, removed from a man aged 49, who had suffered from hypoglycaemic attacks for the previous year. Calcification was sufficiently marked to give the cut surface of the tumour a white colour.

of adenomas. The presence or absence of a capsule does not help in differentiating between simple and malignant tumours; when a capsule is present it is usually incomplete. The presence of tumour thrombi within veins is said (Ackerman and Rosai 1974) to be useful in the recognition of malignancy, as is the invasion of nerves (Bloodworth and Greider 1982), but in the majority of cases malignancy cannot be diagnosed histologically, even in cases in which metastases in the liver or lymph nodes have been seen during an operation.

Morphometric methods (Kenny et al. 1988) and nuclear DNA cytometric methods involving automatic or semi-automatic image analyses (Stipa et al. 1987; Rode et al. 1990), have shown promise in the recognition of islet tumours with malignant potential. Other methods depend upon the identification of marker substances by immunocytochemisty. Heitz et al. (1983), for example, in their study of tumours from 155 patients, found that the presence of the alpha-chain of human chorionic gonadotropin

indicated malignancy in functioning pancreatic endocrine tumours.

Immunocytochemistry is essential for the investigation of pancreatic endocrine tumours; this can usually be done on paraffin-embedded sections. Commercial kits are available for the immunoperoxidase staining of the hormones normally secreted by the cells of the pancreatic islets, and for many of the abnormal hormones secreted by endocrine tumours of the pancreas, as well as for the substances secreted by other tumours of the neuroendocrine system (Cohen and Budgeon 1982). In endocrine tumours that are not associated with any recognised clinical syndrome (i.e. apparently non-functioning tumours), the diagnosis is made according to the main product detected by immunocytochemistry (e.g. pancreatic polypeptide tumours (PPomas), neurotensinomas or calcitoninomas).

Ultrastructurally there are membrane-bound electron-dense secretory granules within the cells of well-differentiated functioning tumours, but atypical granules are common in poorly differentiated tumours and, even in a clinically functioning tumour, granules may be almost unrecognisable (Creutzfeldt 1980).

The general aspects of the progression and effects of malignant endocrine tumours of the pancreas will be discussed later.

Insulinomas

The information currently available about insulinomas has been reviewed by Heitz (1984) and by Klöppel and Heitz (1988). They are the commonest type of functioning pancreatic endocrine tumour. This may be because they are the type that has longest been recognised. By 1974, Stefanini et al. were able to review 1067 cases in which pancreatic tumours had caused clinical hypoglycaemia. There are, of course, many causes of hypoglycaemia other than pancreatic insulinomas, such as various types of non-pancreatic tumours. The hypoglycaemia accompanying such tumours is not usually associated with any significant increase in the level of insulin in the plasma; the cause of the hypoglycaemia in such cases is not understood (Bloodworth and Greider 1982).

Insulinomas represent 70%–75% of functioning pancreatic endocrine tumours. They affect both sexes equally and most of the patients are between 30 and 60 years of age, although some have been much older. They are rare in children, but in infants they may be associated with nesidioblastosis or focal adenomatosis (Heitz 1984).

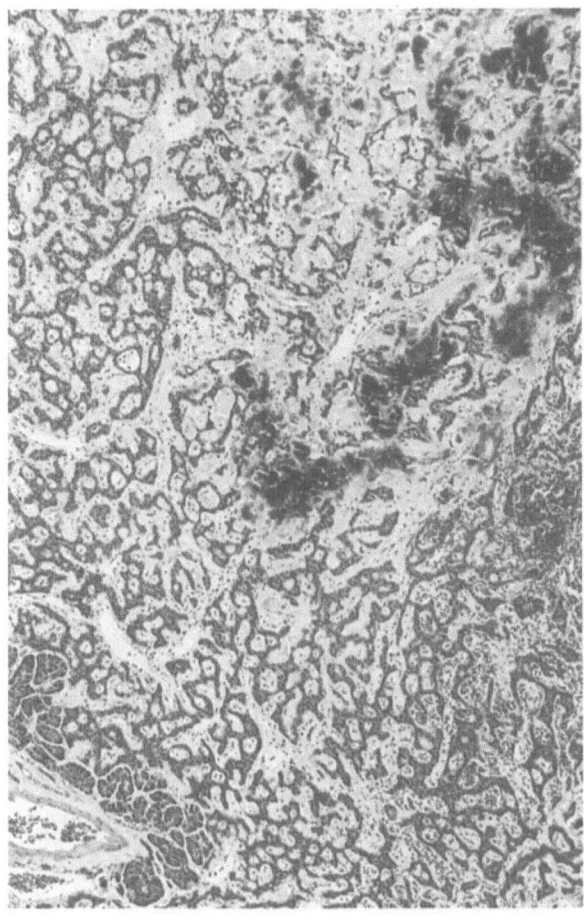

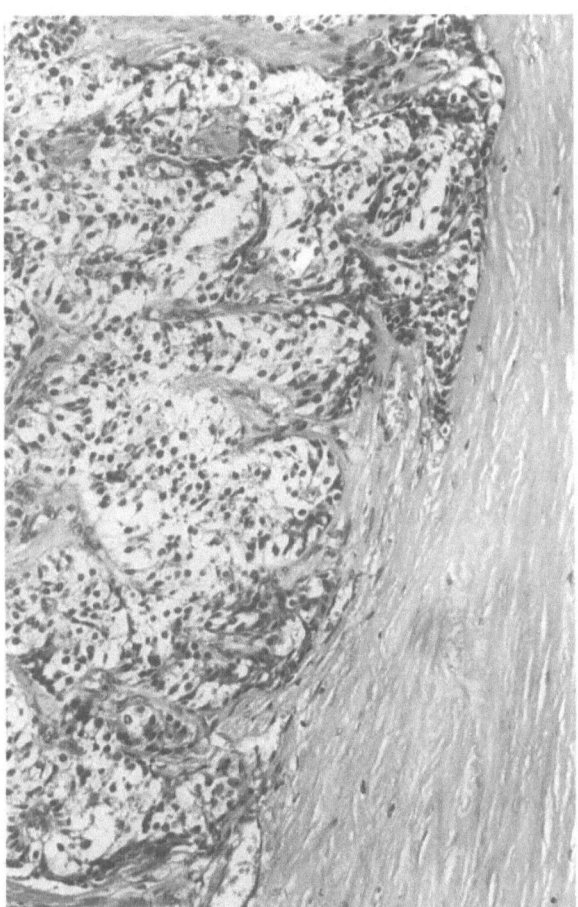

Fig. 10.3. The microscopic appearance of the tumour illustrated macroscopically in Fig. 10.2. No capsule separates the tumour cells from the small group of pancreatic acini included in the picture. H&E, × 60

Fig. 10.4. An insulinoma with a marked fibrous capsule. The tumour cells are of the type in which the cytoplasm is clear and empty-looking. H&E, × 150

Nearly all insulinomas are situated in the pancreas. They may occur in any part of the pancreas, and are usually solitary except in MEN 1. As a rule the tumours are less than 3 cm in diameter and weigh less than 10 g; the size is, however, unrelated to the severity of the symptoms (Figs 10.2–10.6). About half the insulinomas studied immunocytochemically by Heitz et al. (1982) contained cells that stained for hormones other than insulin as well as the cells that stained for insulin. Most insulinomas are benign but a relatively small number are malignant. In the papers referred to by Heitz, the percentage of insulinomas that behaved malignantly varied between 4% and 16% but, as has already been mentioned, the recognition of malignancy may be difficult and unreliable if metastatic spread has not occurred. In the better differentiated insulinomas, beta granules can usually be stained by methods

such as Gomori's aldehyde fuchsin technique. It is said that the less well-differentiated insulinomas contain less insulin than the well-differentiated types, but that the poorly differentiated tumours contain more proinsulin. In almost all insulinomas, however, the concentration of insulin is lower than in normal beta cells (Fig. 10.7) and there seems to be a defect in the production of insulin due to inadequate conversion of proinsulin to insulin. It has been proposed by Berger et al. (1983) that functioning insulinomas should be divided into two groups: A and B. In group A, the tumours contain many well-granulated typical beta cells, arranged in trabeculae; the cells give a uniform immunofluorescent reaction for insulin. Such tumours are associated clinically with a moderate elevation of proinsulin-like component and with almost complete suppressibility of serum insulin by somatostatin and

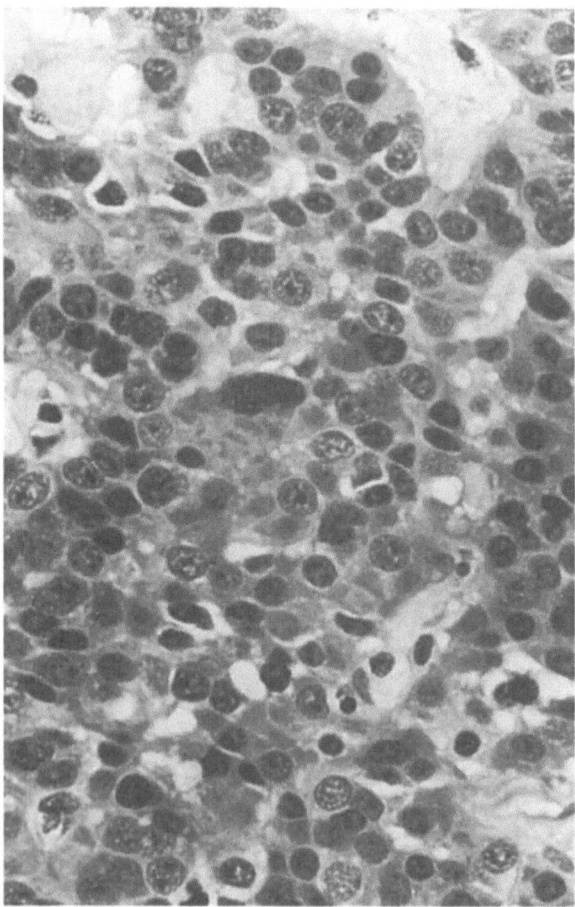

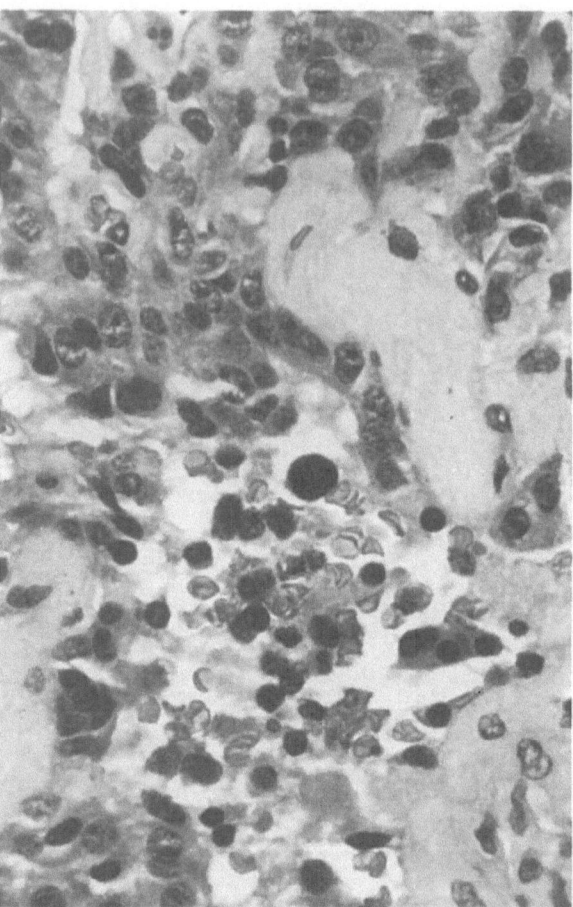

Fig. 10.5. An insulinoma in which the cytoplasm is more dense than in the cells in Fig. 10.3. Most nuclei contain a nucleolus and have a loose network of chromatin. A multinucleated cell is present near the centre of the field. H&E, × 600

Fig. 10.6. Another field in the sections from the tumour in Fig. 10.5. Some of the nuclei are hyperchromatic and there is a certain amount of hyaline stroma. H&E, × 500

diazoxide. In contrast, tumours in group B have few well-granulated typical B cells, and a medullary arrangement of the cells, while the immunofluorescent reaction for insulin is irregular. These tumours are associated with elevated levels of proinsulin-like component in the circulation and a marked resistance of insulin secretion to somatostatin and diazoxide inhibition. This proposed classification did not, however, help the authors to assess the clinical malignancy of the tumours.

The beta granules in the cells of an insulinoma can be seen in the electron micrographs shown in Figs 10.8 and 10.9. The microscopic appearances of the tumours in a case with multiple insulinomas in the pancreas, but without the features of MEN 1, are shown in Figs 10.10 and 10.11, while Figs 10.12 and 10.13 illustrate the macroscopic appearances of a malignant insulinoma.

Although extrapancreatic gastrinomas are well known, extrapancreatic insulinomas are very unusual (Holman et al. 1943) but a relatively recent case has been reported by Miyazaki et al. (1986). Their patient was a 47-year-old housewife who had had hyperglycaemic symptoms associated with an increase of immunoreactive insulin in her venous plasma. She was cured by the removal of an aberrant insulinoma from the distal duodenum, which measured 2.1 × 1.8 × 1.3 cm. Microscopically it consisted of islet cells without ducts or acini. Many of the cells reacted with anti-insulin serum and beta granules were seen on electron microscopy. A few cells reacted immunocytochemically for somatostatin and glucagon.

Some carcinoid tumours of the ileum have been found to secrete insulin (Adamson et al. 1971; Pelletier et al. 1984) in addition to serotonin, and

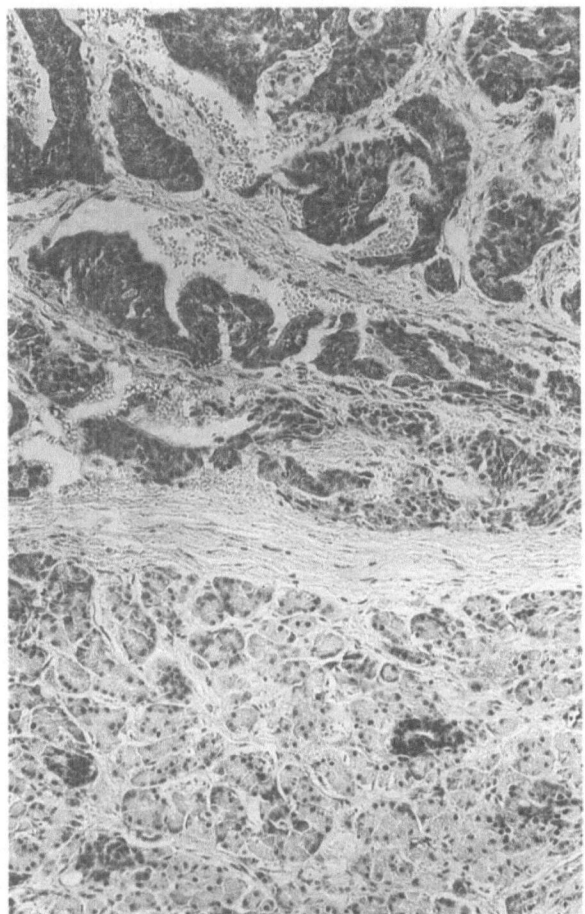

Fig. 10.7. The margin of an islet cell adenoma that caused hypoglycaemic attacks. The dark staining of the cells in the normal islets in the pancreas outside the capsule of the tumour indicates a positive immunoperoxidase reaction for insulin; a similar positive reaction can be recognised in the tumour cells. (Courtesy of Dr Anne Clark) PAP, × 120

diabetes mellitus. There is no such explanation for the calcification that occurs in some insulinomas. An insulinoma with areas of calcification is illustrated in Figs 10.2 and 10.3.

Psammoma bodies may be found in pancreatic endocrine tumours but they are not associated with any particular hormone. They are unusual in insulinomas but were present in one of the cases of insulinoma described by Yamashita et al. (1985).

Congenital Insulinomas

It has already been mentioned that insulinomas are rare in children, but, in the neonatal period, hyperinsulinaemia with dangerous hypoglycaemia is a well-known disorder of metabolism. The diffuse or focal hypertrophy and hyperplasia of islet tissue that is the usual cause of the condition is to be discussed later (pp. 212–213), but hyperinsulinaemia in the neonate may also be caused by a congenital insulinoma. Such a case has been described by Carney (1976) who described the clinical features and pathological findings, and was able to refer to 12 previously published examples of congenital insulinomas. Carney examined the tumour by electron microscopy and concluded that it had developed from the foetal ductal epithelium.

Cerebral Damage Due to Undiagnosed Insulinoma

Irreversible changes in the central nervous system due to severe or prolonged hypoglycaemia have been well known since the description in 1942 of the lesions in the brain in six fatal cases of hypoglycaemia by Lawrence et al. In one, the hypoglycaemia was found at autopsy to have been caused by an undiagnosed adenoma of pancreatic islet cells. A more recent report is that of Snook et al. (1986), of a woman who had had progressive neurological deterioration for 30 years before her death at the age of 48. Inappropriate insulin secretion was recognised before her death but she developed a fatal infection before the investigation of her metabolic abnormality had been completed. At autopsy, a well-differentiated islet cell tumour, 15 mm in diameter, was found in her pancreas. Her brain was atrophic and, on microscopic examination, there were infarct-like lesions of variable size in the cerebral and cerebellar hemispheres and basal ganglia, with relative sparing of the temporal lobes and hippocampus. In the cerebellum there was widespread loss of Purkinje cells.

Shames et al. (1968) described an insulin-secreting bronchial carcinoid. In these patients, the secretion of insulin was sufficient to cause hypoglycaemic symptoms in addition to the carcinoid syndrome, but the insulin-secreting cells were carcinoid tumour cells and not heterotopic pancreatic islet cells. To support this observation, Pelletier et al. showed that the tumour cells from their case were capable of forming both insulin and serotonin in tissue culture.

The deposition of amyloid material in the stroma of insulinomas is not unusual. This is not surprising, for the amyloid is of a type that appears to be associated with the production of insulin. This has been discussed in relation to the amyloid change that may occur in the islets of Langerhans in type II

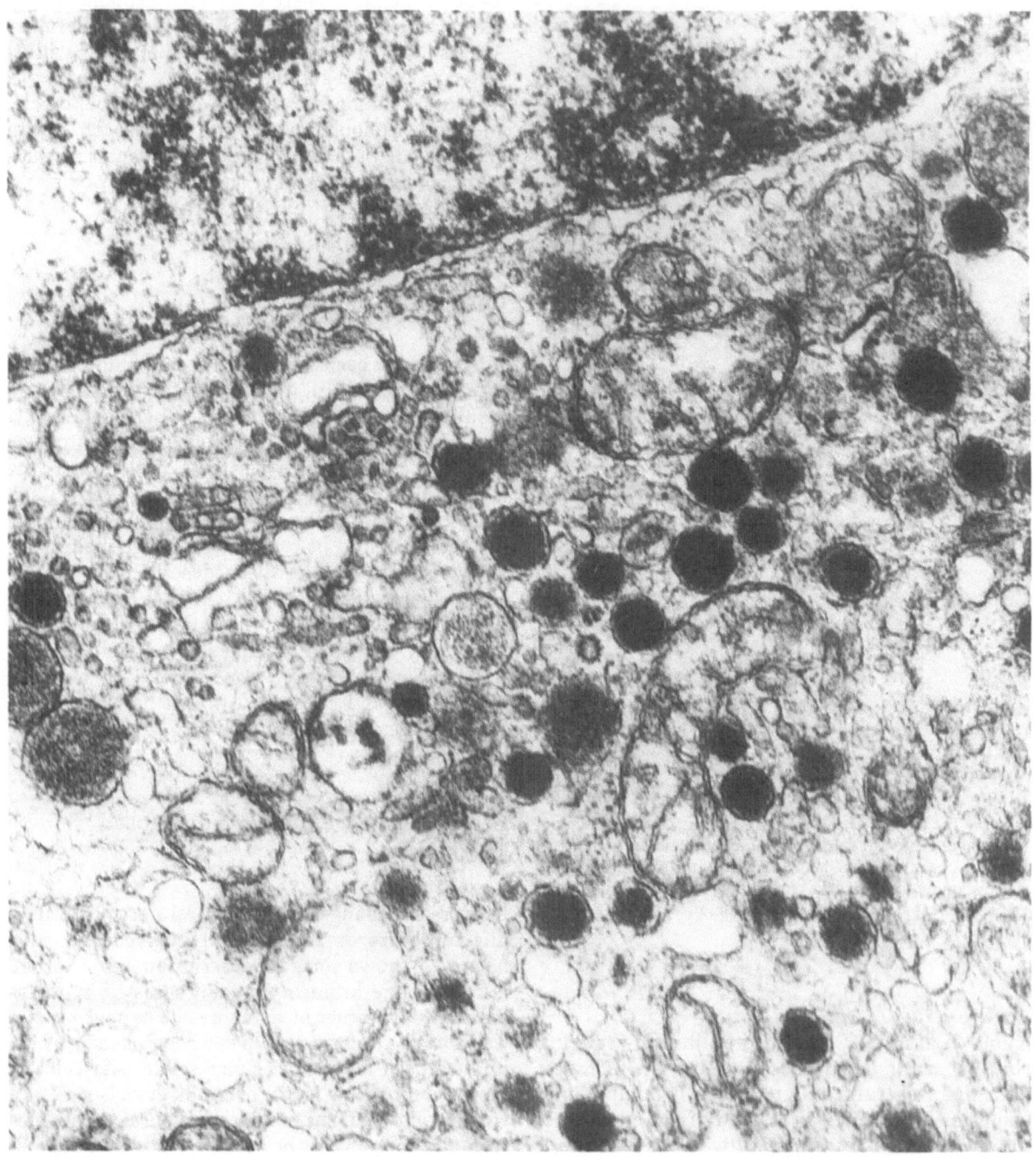

Fig. 10.8. Polymorphous, membrane-limited granules with electron-dense cores within clear halos in the cytoplasm of a cell in an islet cell tumour that caused hypoglycaemic attacks in a man aged 35. The upper area of the field is occupied by part of the nucleus. × 70 000

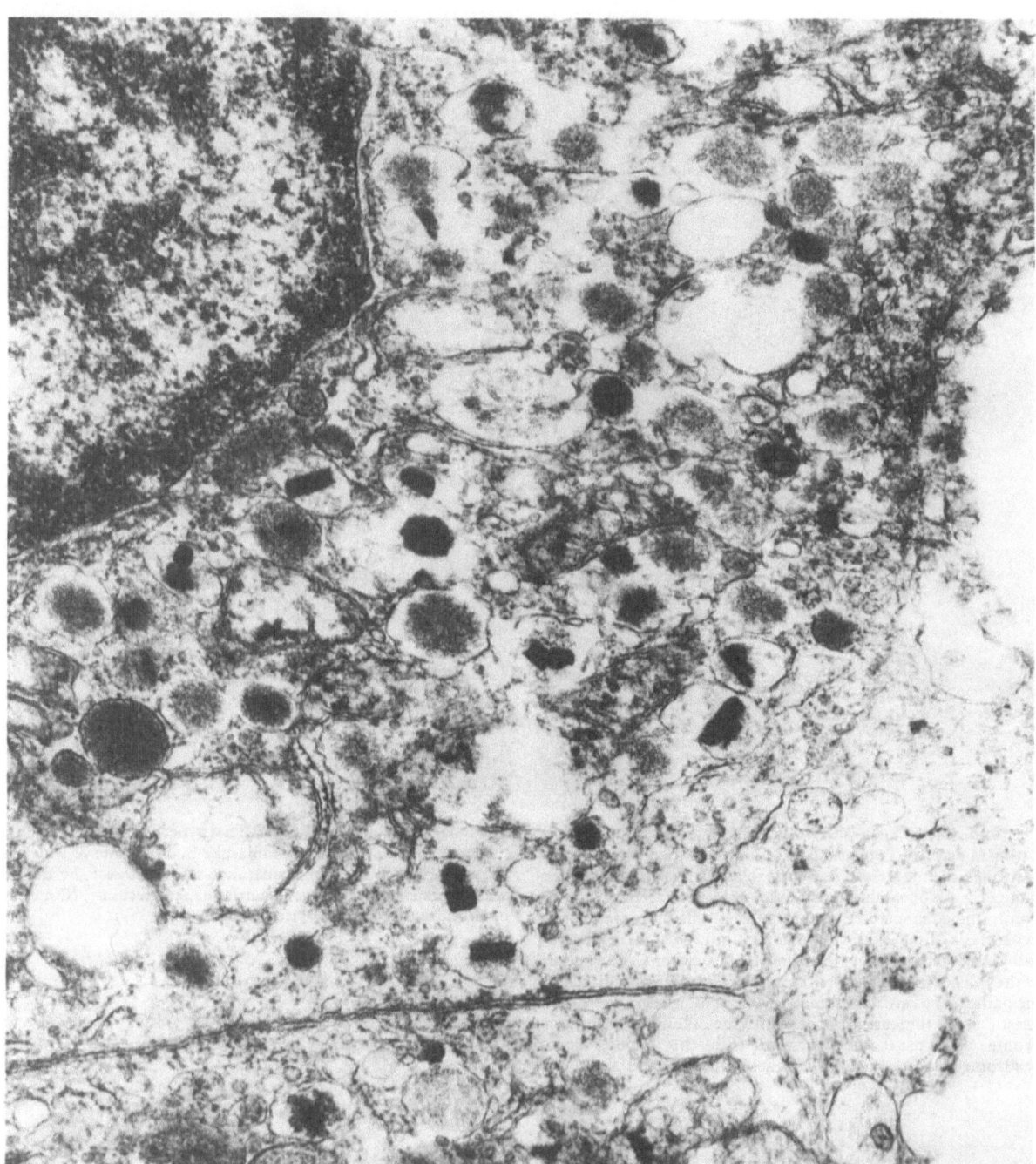

Fig. 10.9. Another cell in the islet cell tumour shown in Fig. 10.8. The cytoplasm contains secretory granules that include several of the crystalloid type. The crystalloid structure is characteristic of beta granules. × 42 000

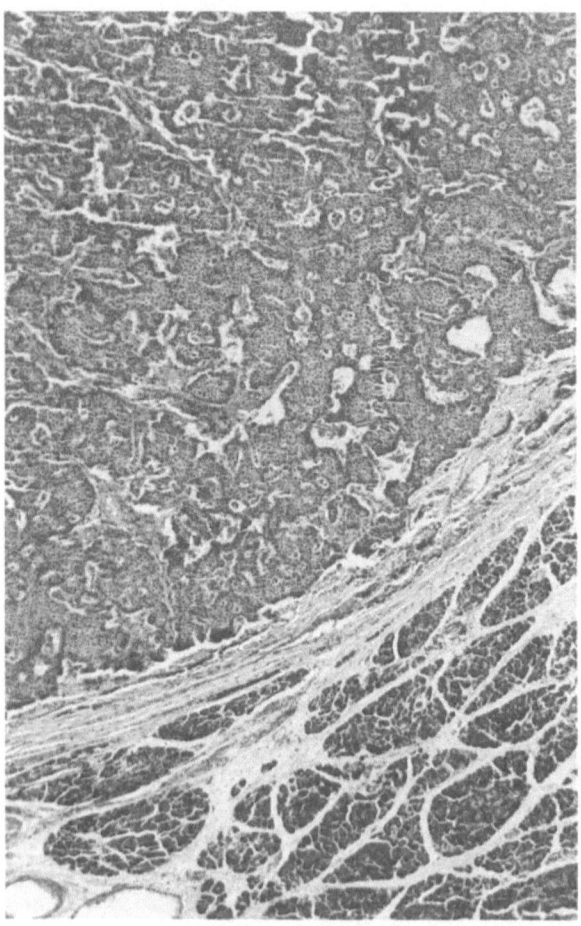

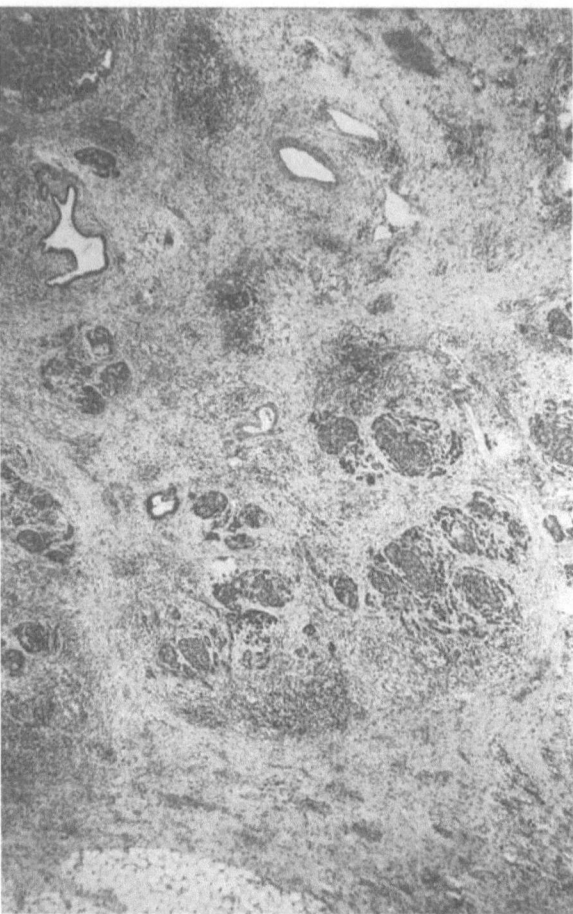

Fig. 10.10. One of many adenoma-like nodules in the pancreas of a woman aged 25. Two partial excisions of the pancreas, because of hypoglycaemic attacks, had to be followed by total pancreatectomy because of continuing episodes of hypoglycaemia. In addition to the adenoma-like nodules of islet cells there was diffuse hyperplasia of the islets, shown in Fig. 10.11. The patient was not recognised to be suffering from the MEN 1 syndrome. The pattern of the cells in the partially encapsulated nodule is reminiscent of the pattern of a carcinoid tumour. Such a pattern is more characteristic of the tumours associated with the Zollinger-Ellison syndrome than of those associated with the hypoglycaemic syndrome. (Courtesy of Dr Alexander Kennedy) H&E, × 60

Fig. 10.11. What appears to be diffuse hyperplasia of islets in the pancreas that contained adenoma-like nodules, one of which is shown in Fig. 10.10. The appearance may, however, be due to scarring caused by a previous partial pancreatectomy. (Courtesy of Dr Alexander Kennedy) H&E, × 24

Insulinomas in Animals

In the dog, a species in which insulinomas are now well recognised, most of the tumours are malignant (Feldman 1983). They tend to be multihormonal; Hawkins et al. (1987), in their series of 20 endocrine pancreatic tumours in dogs, found that insulin alone could be demonstrated in only three. O'Brien et al. (1987) produced results that were very similar; they studied 31 canine islet cell tumours and found that only three of these contained insulin as the only

identifiable hormone. As far as other species are concerned, spontaneous beta cell tumours have been found in the rat (Kovacs et al. 1976), in a polar bear (Alroy et al. 1980) and in ferrets (Luttgen et al. 1986).

Gastrinomas

Gastrinomas account for between 20% and 25% of pancreatic endocrine tumours and most are found in patients between 30 and 50 years of age, but, according to Heitz (1984), there is an age range of 7–92 years. They are the usual cause of the syndrome first recognised by Zollinger and Ellison in 1955. The

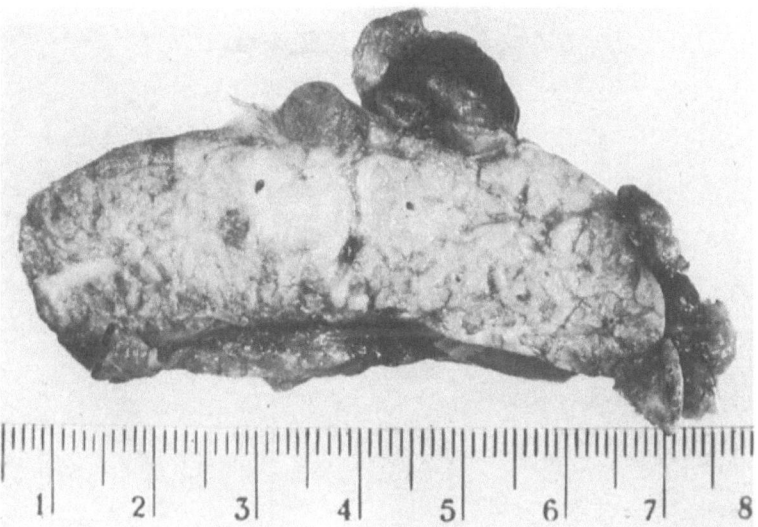

Fig. 10.12. The area of diffuse pallor in the middle region of the excised and bisected pancreas is a malignant insulinoma. The patient was a woman aged 38, whose history was that during the 10 months before her partial pancreatectomy she had been unable to move when she wakened in the morning, but became able to get up when she had been given a cup of sweet tea. Lymph nodes that contained secondary tumour are attached to the upper border of the specimen. The scale is in centimetres.

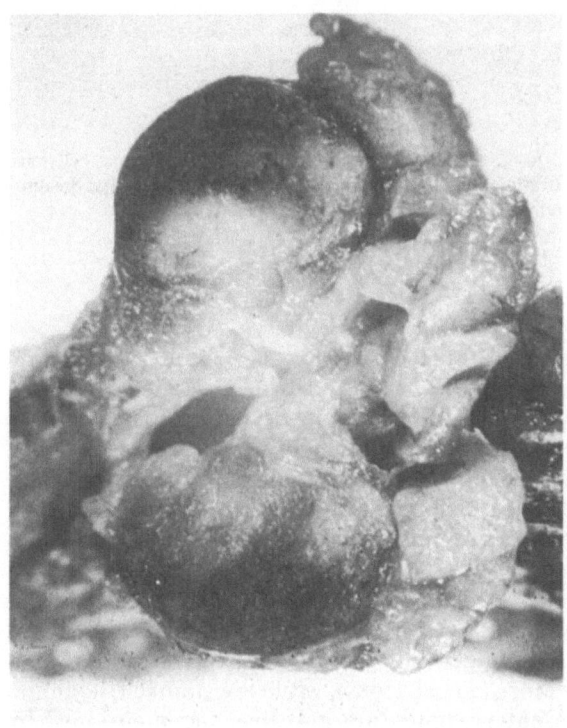

Fig. 10.13. One of the lymph nodes attached to the pancreas shown in Fig. 10.12. It has been bisected to show the pallor caused by replacement of the normal node by secondary malignant insulinoma. × 2

tumours are slightly more common in men. In 60% of the 260 cases of the Zollinger–Ellison syndrome reviewed by Ellison and Wilson in 1964 the tumours were malignant, 44% of the total cases having had metastatic lesions at the time of diagnosis. More recent studies (Creutzfeldt 1980), however, suggest that the true incidence of malignancy is at least 90%. Malignant tumours infiltrate locally, and metastatic spread is to the lymph nodes nearest to the tumour and to the liver. Involvement of the peritoneal cavity may occur but spread to organs outside the peritoneal cavity is unusual. Secondary deposits have, however, been recorded in the lungs (Ellison and Wilson 1964), the mediastinum and a supraclavicular lymph node (Friesen 1967), the skin (Colin-Jones et al. 1969) and the skeleton (Barton et al. 1986). The skeletal metastases described by Barton et al. developed in four women and two men; they were osteolytic as well as osteoblastic, affected the central skeleton and caused symptoms. In two patients the lesions were associated with hypercalcaemia with normal serum parathormone levels.

Most pancreatic gastrinomas are solitary and occur in either the head or tail of the pancreas, but Ellison and Wilson found that in 29% of the 260 cases they reviewed there were two separate tumours in different parts of the pancreas, while in 19% the whole gland was involved. Gastrinomas

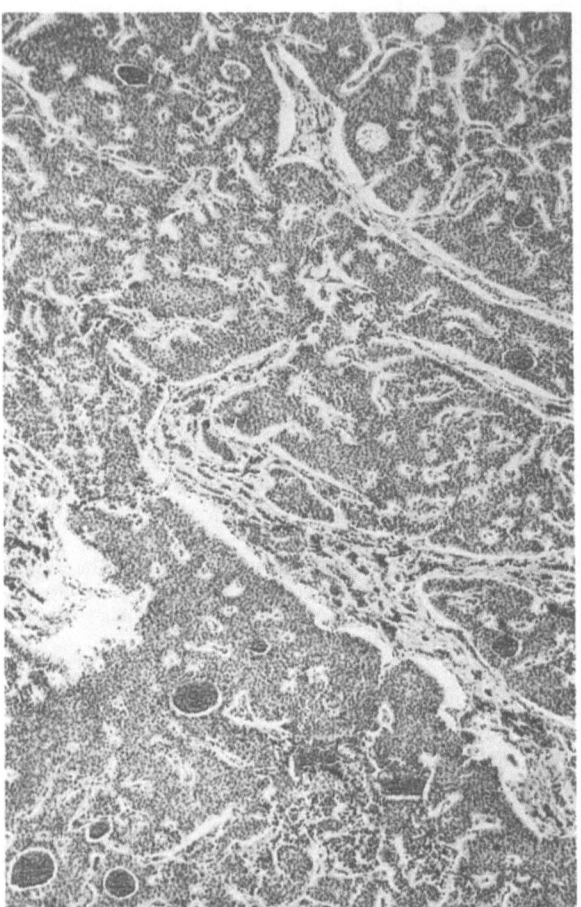

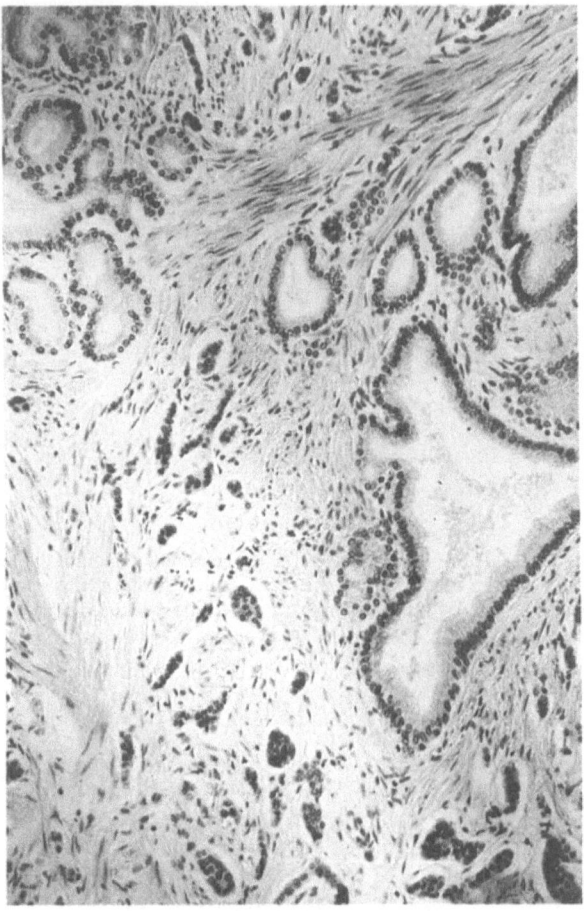

Fig. 10.14. An islet cell tumour of the head of the pancreas that caused the Zollinger–Ellison syndrome. The tumour was malignant, with infiltration of the wall of the duodenum and metastases in lymph nodes. (Courtesy of Dr J.M. Vetters) H&E, × 60

Fig. 10.15. Dark clumps of malignant gastrinoma cells are infiltrating the muscle and glandular tissue of the wall of the duodenum. (Courtesy of Dr J.M. Vetters) H&E, × 150

may also arise in sites other than the pancreas, the commonest site being the duodenum. In the 53 cases of the Zollinger–Ellison syndrome reported by Malagelada et al. (1983), there were five in which the tumour was in the wall of the duodenum; these were not examples of MEN 1. The series, however, included two other patients in which the Zollinger–Ellison syndrome was a manifestation of MEN 1; in these, gastrinomas were found in the duodenum. Surgical exploration was undertaken in 44 of the 53 patients studied by Malagelada et al., and in 13 of these no tumour could be found. In such cases the syndrome may be due to hyperplasia of gastrin-secreting cells in the antral mucosa of the stomach (Polak et al. 1972).

Friesen (1990) has discussed whether gastrinomas that appear to be primary tumours in lymph nodes near the pancreas are truly primary in heterotopic

pancreas tissue, or whether they are metastatic from an undetected primary neuroendocrine gastrinoma in, for example, the duodenal submucosa. Friesen's own experience, combined with his study of publications on the subject, convinced him that most nodal gastrinomas are really metastatic, but that a primary aberrant nodal gastrinoma must remain a rare possibility. Other rare sites for gastrinomas include a Meckel's diverticulum (Zollinger 1987). A gastrin-secreting ovarian cystadenoma that caused the Zollinger–Ellison syndrome has been reported by Morgan et al. (1985), while the stomach, jejunum, mesentery, omentum and liver are mentioned by Klöppel and Heitz (1988) as unusual and rare sites for primary gastrinomas.

Histologically, gastrinomas may resemble intestinal carcinoid tumours very closely (Figs 10.14 and 10.15), but they do not usually give a positive

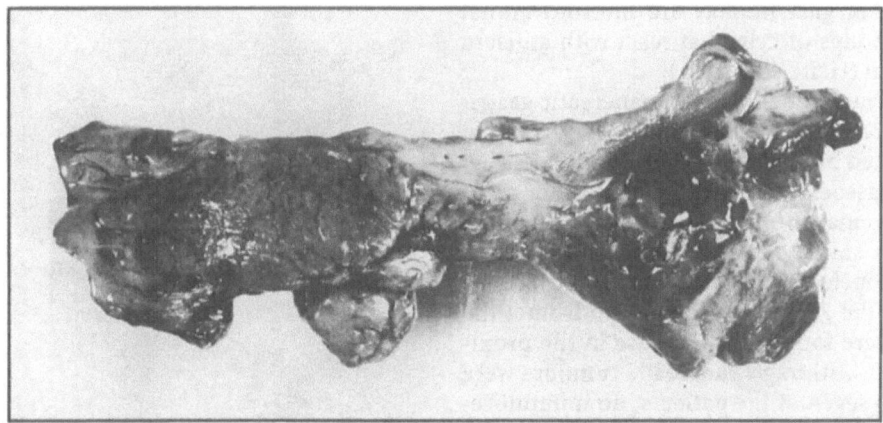

Fig. 10.16. An encapsulated pancreatic nodule (2 cm diameter), without recognisable infiltration or metastasis, found post-mortem in a woman aged 54, who had suffered from the Zollinger–Ellison syndrome for the 12 years that preceded her death. Various operations had been carried out because of the severe peptic ulceration and its complications. She became cachectic after total gastrectomy had been carried out in 1973 and died 3 months after the operation. During the final stages of her illness the gastrin level in her blood (as assessed by the late Prof R.A. Gregory) was 100 times in excess of normal. When the tumour was bisected it was found to be traversed by some fibrous septa in which there was a little calcification.

argentaffin reaction, neither can a positive alkaline diazo reaction be obtained. Many of their cells, however, give a positive reaction with Grimelius's silver stain. The histological features of gastrinomas on routine examination are not diagnostic, and their ultrastructural characters do not justify their identification, but immunocytochemistry will usually identify many cells that stain positively with antisera to gastrin. In occasional cases of the Zollinger–Ellison syndrome, however, in which hypergastrinaemia has been present, too little gastrin may remain in the tumour to react immuno-cytochemically. The naked eye and microscopic appearances of such a gastrinoma are shown in Figs 10.16 and 10.17.

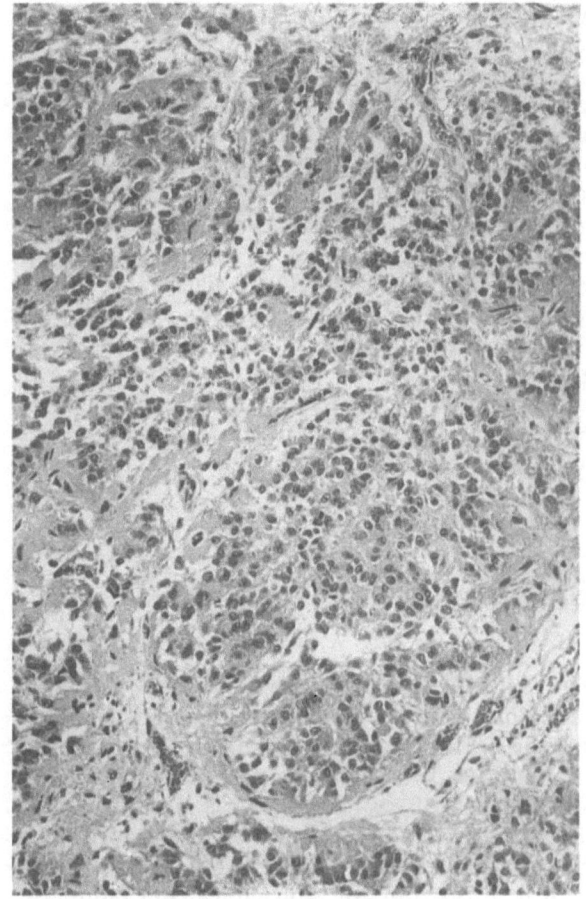

Fig. 10.17. This is the microscopic appearance of the tumour illustrated in Fig. 10.16. It consists of spheroidal cells in a background of hyaline tissue. No granules could be demonstrated by Gomori's aldehyde fuchsin method. Some rather indefinite, membrane-bound secretion vesicles with osmiophilic contents were seen on electron microscopy. Unfortunately the autopsy could not be carried out until 6 h after death and the ultrastructural details are unsatisfactory as a result. Although there had been hypergastrinaemia, attempts to demonstrate gastrin-positive cells using a antigastrin immunoperoxidase kit were unsuccessful. In this case the tumour is atypical in that its macroscopic and microscopic features are those of a benign adenoma. H&E, ×150

About 50% of gastrinomas are multihormonal and contain groups of cells that react with antisera to somatostatin (Heitz et al. 1982).

As has been mentioned already, pancreatic gastrinomas may occur as a component of MEN 1, as in the case reported by Vella et al. (1988), but, like gastrinomas unassociated with other endocrine tumours, they may be extra-pancreatic. In eight patients with MEN 1 and hypergastrinaemia described by Pipeleers-Marichal et al. (1990), seven of whom had the Zollinger–Ellison syndrome, the gastrinomas were found in every case in the proximal duodenum. Although pancreatic tumours were also present in seven of the patients, no immunoreactivity for gastrin was present in these tumours, except for a few scattered gastrin-positive cells in one. The authors pointed out, however, that the duodenal gastrinomas may be so small that they are liable to be missed; in five of their cases the duodenal tumours were multiple and were between 2 mm and 6 mm in diameter.

In animals, the Zollinger–Ellison syndrome has been reported in association with islet cell tumours in the pancreas in dogs (Jones et al. 1976; Straus et al. 1977; Happé et al. 1980; Rousseaux 1987), while Boosinger et al. (1988) described a dog with multihormonal pancreatic tumours. The tumours contained cells that reacted immunochemically for the presence of insulin, and others that contained pancreatic polypeptide, but were negative for gastrin as well as for various other peptide hormones. There were, however, multiple duodenal ulcers and hypertrophic gastric mucosal nodules; this is reminiscent of the human gastrinoma syndrome reported by Wynick (1990). In that patient, hypergastrinaemia and hyperglucagonaemia in a man with MEN 1 were relieved by the removal of a pancreatic adenoma that contained abundant glucagon but failed to stain for gastrin. When in situ hybridisation to detect gastrin messenger RNA was carried out, however, there was weak specific hybridisation in the tumour cells.

Glucagonomas

The clinical features associated with glucagon-secreting tumours of the pancreatic islets have already been mentioned in the earlier part of this chapter, but, with the exception of diabetes or an abnormal glucose tolerance test, it is difficult to fit together the components of the glucagonoma syndrome and the known physiological and pharmacological properties of glucagon. Glucagon was

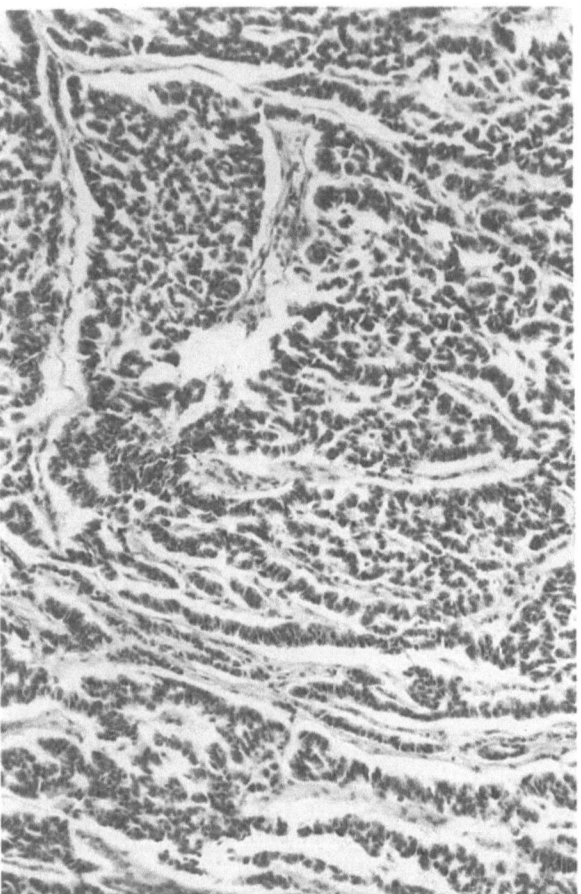

Fig. 10.18. The microscopic appearance of a malignant tumour of islet cells in the head of the pancreas in a man aged 59, who died with widespread replacement of his liver by multiple metastatic deposits that were microscopically similar to the pancreatic tumour. He had suffered from necrolytic migratory erythema for about 18 months before his death. The clinical and dermatological aspects of this case have been published by Verbov (1981). (Courtesy of Dr William Kenyon) H&E, × 150

discovered and named soon after the discovery of insulin (Kimball and Murlin 1923–1924) in the days when the relatively crude preparations of insulin contained a substance that caused a preliminary rise in the level of glucose in the blood before the insulin in the extracts had its hypoglycaemic effect. The substance was given the name glucagon. Glucagon received much attention because of its possible role in the aetiology of diabetes mellitus and it became established that glucagon is a polypeptide hormone; it has been synthesised completely in the laboratory. Its known functions were reviewed by Bloom in 1975, and, in spite of its many effects, such as the mobilisation of hepatic stores of glycogen to raise the blood glucose, and its effect

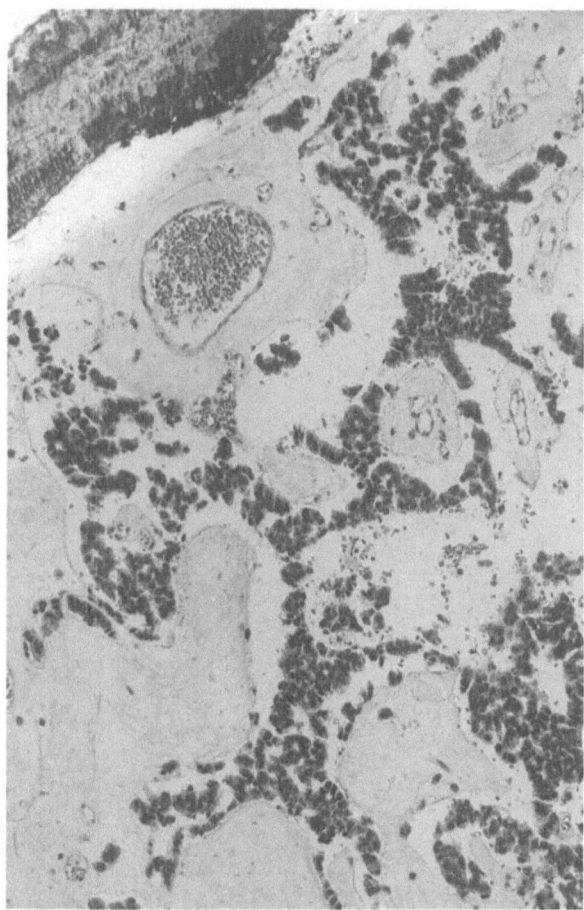

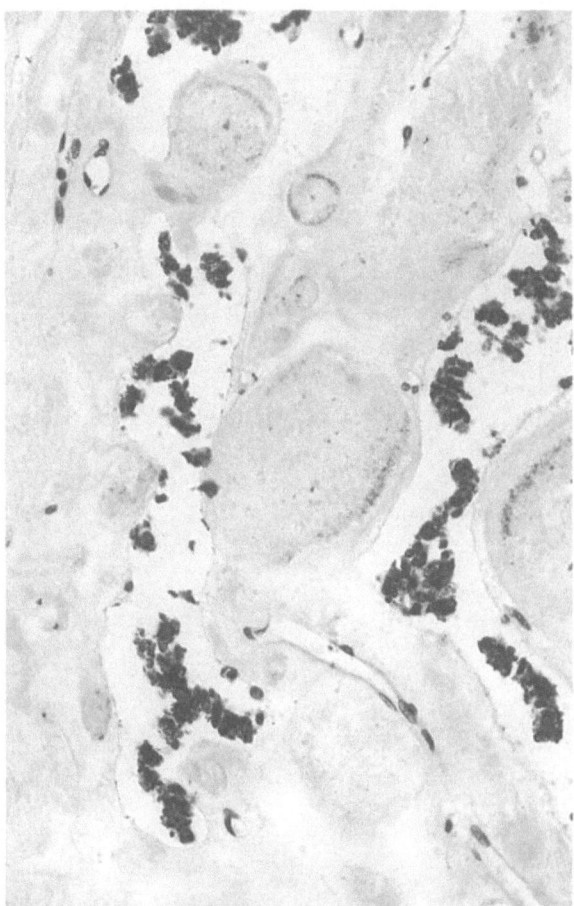

Fig. 10.19. Another part of the tumour shown in Fig. 10.18. This part of the tumour was separated from the more uniformly cellular region by a band of dense fibrous tissue, parts of which were heavily calcified, as can be seen in one corner of the illustration. (Courtesy of Dr William Kenyon) H&E, × 150

Fig. 10.20. Groups of cells that gave a positive reaction for glucagon by the immunoperoxidase method. Only relatively few glucagon-positive cells were present, although the skin lesions were of the type associated with the glucagonoma syndrome. Cells that reacted positively for pancreatic polypeptide were more abundant than glucagon-positive cells. (Courtesy of Dr William Kenyon) PAP, × 375

upon the heart and the pituitary and adrenal glands, as well as upon the functions of the pancreas and upon almost all parts of the alimentary canal, the features of the syndrome produced by a glucagon-secreting tumour of the alpha cells of the pancreas could scarcely have been predicted from the known effects of glucagon. In particular, the necrolytic migratory erythema, which is such a marked feature of the syndrome, is difficult to relate to the effects of hyperglucagonaemia; a number of morphologically characteristic glucogonomas are not actually associated with inappropriate secretion of glucagon (Heitz 1984). There is also some evidence that the necrolytic migratory erythema may be, at least partly, due to zinc deficiency, and the serum concentrations of amino

acids, which are depressed when the syndrome is present, rise to normal following the successful removal of a glucagonoma. Figs 10.18–10.22 illustrate a tumour associated with the glucagonoma syndrome.

In his review of the reports of glucagonomas, Heitz states that approximately 1% of pancreatic endocrine tumours are glucagonomas, and, according to Boden in 1987, about 100 cases had been reported up to that time. The syndrome tends to occur in subjects between 40 and 70 years of age, and the incidence is probably equal in the sexes, although it seemed at first that there was a slight female preponderance; it has not yet been reported in children. Tumours associated with the syndrome are usually malignant (60%–80%) and are large (up

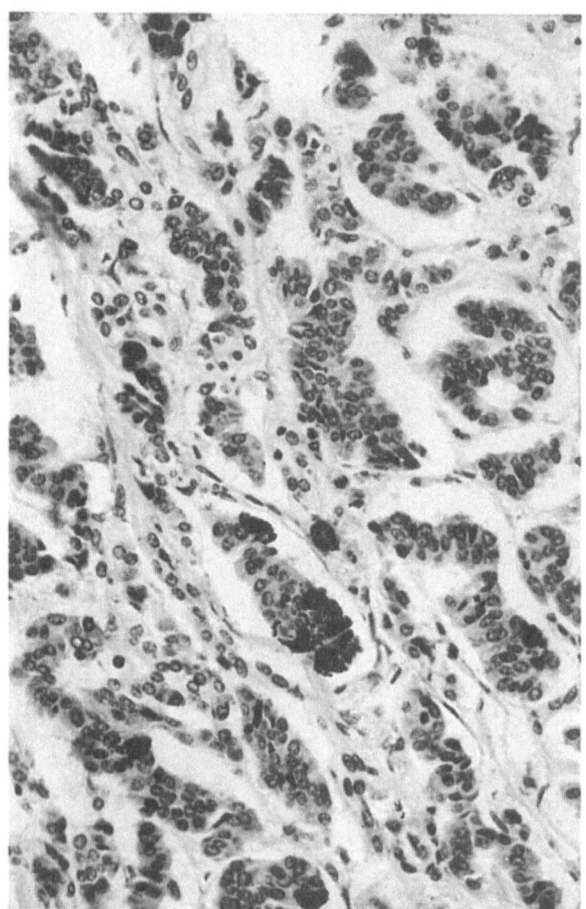

Fig. 10.21. Insulin-positive cells in the tumour shown in Figs 10.18–10.20. Insulin-positive cells were not originally found in the sections examined, but a few groups that reacted positively to the immunoperoxidase method for insulin were present in later sections. (Courtesy of Dr William Kenyon) PAP, × 375

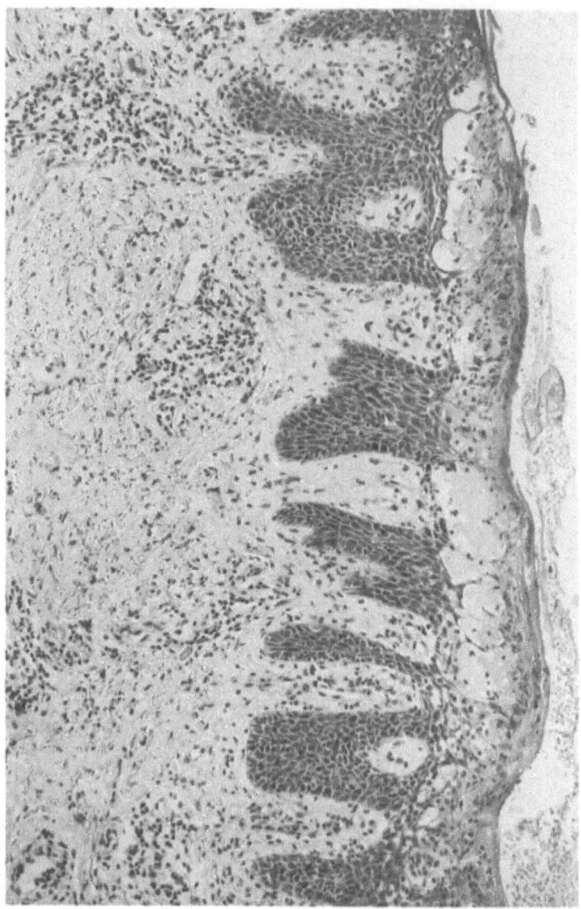

Fig. 10.22. A section of the skin from the patient whose pancreatic tumour is shown in Figs 10.18–10.21. A multilocular intraepidermal vesicle in which there are a few leucocytes is associated with marked spongiosis and some patches of infiltration by round cells in the underlying dermis. Clinically the skin condition was not of necrolytic migratory erythema. (Courtesy of Dr T. Steward and Dr Julian Verbov) H&E, × 150

to 300 g), while those unassociated with the syndrome are small (0.4–3 cm in diameter) and are benign. Such small tumours have usually been found incidentally during post-mortem examinations. A positive immunoperoxidase reaction for the presence of glucagon in such a case is illustrated in Fig. 10.23.

Microscopically, in sections stained with haematoxylin and eosin, glucagonomas have a trabecular or tubular arrangement of the tumour cells or, elsewhere, there may be solid masses of tumour cells separated by fibrovascular bands that may be partially calcified or have a hyaline appearance due to amyloid change. There may be large vascular spaces in hepatic metastatic deposits. The tumour cells are rounded or cuboidal, with dense nuclei and eosinophilic cytoplasm. Mitotic figures are rare even in tumours that have caused secondary deposits; they are also rare in the metastases.

The immunostaining of the glucagon in glucagonomas is sometimes straightforward, but the tumours may secrete proglucagon, a larger molecular precursor of glucagon. The larger molecule contains the amino acid sequence of glucagon with, in addition, at least four other peptides, each of which may function as separate entities. These peptides are: glycentin, a glycentin-related pancreatic peptide and two different glucagon-like peptides. Hamid et al. (1986) used antibodies against each of these substances in a study of ten pancreatic tumours that had been associated with the glucagonoma syndrome in patients with high levels

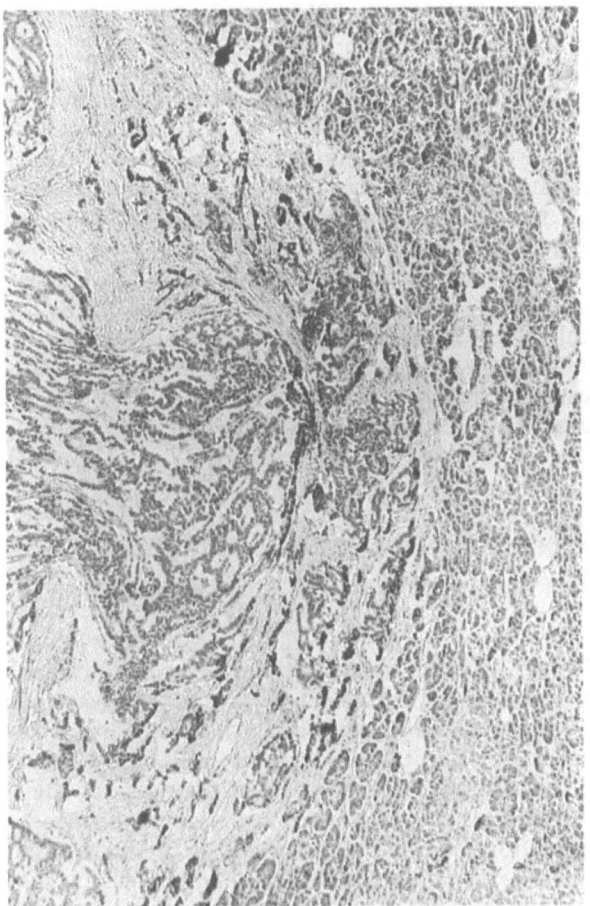

Fig. 10.23. A microscopic tumour of islet cells found post-mortem in a pancreas. Groups of cells that react positively for glucagon by the immunoperoxidase method are present at the periphery of the tumour. The patient had been diabetic but no other features of the glucogonoma syndrome had been present and it is probable that the tiny tumour was of no clinical significance. (Courtesy of Dr Anne Clark) PAP, × 60

of circulating glucagon. Nine of the tumours were obtained surgically and one at autopsy. Five of the ten were malignant, as shown by the presence of metastases. The tumours were investigated by histology, histochemistry, immunocytochemistry and electron microscopy. All showed immunoreactivity to one or other of the peptides derived from proglucagon, although only seven were found to contain immunoreactive pancreatic glucagon. The presence of secretory granules in eight of the tumours was demonstrated by electron microscopy, argyrophilia or chromogranin immunoreactivity. Neuron specific enolase was present in all the tumours by immunostaining, thereby indicating their neuroendocrine nature. Moreover, the intensity of the immunostain was higher in four of the

five malignant tumours than in the other six tumours. Pancreatic polypeptide was present in non-glucagon cells in six of the ten tumours.

According to Bordi et al. (1979), in their electron microscopic study of eight glucagonomas, the tumours unassociated with the syndrome contained easily recognised alpha granules, whereas the tumours associated with the syndrome contained granules that were mainly atypical. Using immuno-fluorescent staining for glucagon and glycentin, the same authors found that, in all tumours but one, a number of cells were positive with both types of antisera, a finding closely similar to that made with non-neoplastic alpha cells by Ravazzola and Orci (1980).

As already noted, asymptomatic tumours are usually benign but, in general, neither morphology nor hormone assay can distinguish between functional and non-functional tumours, for it seems that glucagonomas may form glucagon without discharging it as secretion. Morphology and assay of hormones cannot differentiate between benign and malignant tumours (Bloodworth and Greider 1982).

Glucagonomas have occurred as a component of the MEN 1 syndrome (Croughs et al. 1972). Four of nine relatives of a patient with a glucagonoma and the glucagonoma syndrome were found by Boden and Owen (1977) to have familial hyperglucago-naemia as an autosomal dominant trait. A renal tumour that secreted enteroglucagon, a form of glucagon that can be distinguished from pancreatic glucagon, and whose effects were upon the structure and function of the small intestine, was reported by Bloom (1972). A metastasis in the liver from an undifferentiated carcinoma of the lung was found by Unger and Bochner (1964) to contain both glucagon and insulin.

A malignant endocrine tumour of the pancreas that originally had the typical effects of an insulinoma, but which later caused the glucagonoma syndrome, was reported in 1979 by Ohneda et al. A similar mixed endocrine pancreatic tumour has been reported by D'Arcangues et al. (1984); the patient suffered from hyperinsulinism and hypoglycaemia during the earlier stages of his illness, but gradually became normoglycaemic with hyperglucagonaemia, and developed many of the features of the glucagonoma syndrome. The patient, who was still alive at the time of the report, had survived for 17 years after an islet cell carcinoma with hepatic metastases had been recognised at laparotomy. Immunoperoxidase studies with antisera to insulin, glucagon and somatostatin upon the pancreatic tumour and upon the metastatic deposits in his liver were strongly positive for insulin and glucagon as well as weakly positive for somatostatin.

Somatostatinomas

The recognition of a syndrome associated with islet cell tumours that secrete the inhibitory hormone somatostatin, a peptide normally secreted by the anterior pituitary gland, has already been mentioned. In most of the reported cases, the pancreatic tumours were solitary and, although the patient reported by Ganda et al. (1977) appeared to be cured 20 months after an apparently circumscribed tumour in the head of the pancreas had been removed by a radical operation, most somatostatinomas are malignant. Hepatic metastases were already present when most of the reported patients underwent laparotomy. Either the head or the tail of the pancreas may be the site of the tumour; tumours in the head may infiltrate the wall of the duodenum. The pancreatic tumours have been between 3 cm and 8 cm in diameter. Microscopically, first impressions often suggest a carcinoid tumour, but, ultramicroscropically, secretory granules said to be typical of D cells can be found. The confirmation of the diagnosis depends upon the recognition of a greatly increased level of somatostatin immunoreactivity in the plasma – there was a 40-fold elevation in the case reported by Pipeleers et al. (1979) – and the presence of many cells that react immunocytochemically when sections are tested for the presence of somatostatin. In addition to somatostatin, hormones such as calcitonin may be present (Galmiche et al. 1978; Krejs et al. 1979), or ACTH, which, in the patient reported by Kovacs et al. in 1977, was sufficient to cause clinical symptoms. Somatostatinomas have been reported in the duodenum (Kaneko et al. 1979; Somers et al. 1983; Jensen et al. 1984) and in the cystic duct (Goodman et al. 1984). Between 1980 and 1986 there were reports of 27 cases of pancreatic somatostatinoma and 21 of intestinal somatostatinoma (Vinik et al. 1987). It is of interest that 21 of the 27 patients with pancreatic somatostatinoma had diabetes mellitus, while only three of the 21 with intestinal somatostatinoma had diabetes.

Microscopically, some of the reported cases of duodenal somatostatinoma have contained psammoma bodies and, having reviewed the literature, Taccagni et al. (1986) stated that somatostatinomas with psammoma bodies are found only in the duodenum and do not produce significant amounts of peptides other than somatostatin. X-ray dispersive microanalysis in the duodenal somatostatinoma reported by Albrecht et al. (1989) showed that the psammoma bodies contained calcium apatite cystals.

Somatostatinomas may be a component of the MEN syndromes and, as reported by Cantor et al. (1982) and Stamm et al. (1986), von Recklinghausen's neurofibromatosis may also be associated. By 1988, Swinburn et al. found that 18 cases with duodenal carcinoid tumours associated with neurofibromatosis had been reported and that, in seven of these, the duodenal carcinoids had been identified as somatostatinomas.

In pancreatic islet cell tumours in dogs, somatostatin may be secreted as one of the components in multihormonal tumours, but no pure somatostatinomas were found in the 20 canine islet cell tumours studied by Hawkins et al. (1987), or in the 31 tumours studied by O'Brien et al. (1987).

Islet Cell Tumours Associated with the Verner–Morrison Syndrome

The Verner–Morrison syndrome, as it was described by Verner and Morrison (1958), consisted of severe, refractory, watery diarrhoea accompanied by striking hypokalaemia, in association with non-beta islet cell tumours of the pancreas. In their report, they postulated the existence of some, as yet unrecognised, hormone that was secreted by the tumour of islet cells, to cause excessive secretion by the intestinal mucosa with consequent watery diarrhoea and loss of potassium from the body. The developments in the understanding of the syndrome that took place between 1958 and 1980 have been reviewed by Morrison (1980), in which he tabulated the main features of every published example of the syndrome up to 1978, and included two cases reports that had appeared before the syndrome was recognised in 1958. In these early cases (Brown et al. 1950; Moldawer et al. 1954), non-beta adenomas of islet cells had been found, but the authors had regarded these tumours as non-functioning. The case reports, however, included information that convinced Verner and Morrison that they were, in fact, examples of the Verner– Morrison syndrome. In addition to the components of the syndrome as described originally, it became recognised that gastric achlorhydria, or at least hypochlorhydria, was often an additional component, and this was useful in distinguishing the syndrome from the Zollinger-Ellison syndrome, in which watery diarrhoea sometimes occurs . Thus "pancreatic cholera", a name that has been used for the syndrome, is less appropriate than other suggested names such as those made up of the initial letters of the features of the syndrome: WDHA for watery diarrhoea, hypokalaemia and achlorhydria, or WDHH for patients with gastric hypochlorhydria rather than complete achlorhydria. With the development of radioimmunoassay, the estimation of the level of gastrin in the serum became the most reliable way of differentiating between cases of the Zollinger–Ellison syndrome with diarrhoea, and true cases of the Verner–Morrison syndrome; the serum gastrin is greatly increased in the former, but is normal in the latter.

In addition to the essential components of the Verner–Morrison syndrome, less constant features may be present, such as abnormal glucose tolerance, and, during the diarrhoeal attacks, mild hypercalcaemia. Flushing of the face and skin eruptions have also been recorded.

As a result of his review of over 100 published examples of the syndrome, Morrison (1980) concluded that it affected men and women in equal numbers, although it had previously been thought to occur more commonly in women.

The hormone, or hormones, produced by the non-beta islet cell tumours, and responsible for the syndrome, have not been established to the complete satisfaction of all the investigators, but the vasoactive intestinal polypeptide (usually referred to by the initial letters VIP), is believed by many to be responsible and the pancreatic tumours have become known as VIPomas.

VIP received its name because it was isolated from the intestine of pigs, but its true origin has now been recognised to have been the nerves in the intestine. It is present in nerves throughout the central and peripheral nervous systems and there are high concentrations in the gastrointestinal tract. Its biological actions include the stimulation of intestinal secretion, vasodilatation, inhibition of secretion of gastric acid, stimulation of glycogenolsis and the production of hypercalcaemia.

In 1973, Bloom et al. found raised plasma and tumour concentrations of VIP in patients with the Verner–Morrison syndrome and in a patient with a retroperitoneal tumour, identified as a ganglioneuroblastoma, who had severe secretory diarrhoea. By 1981, Long et al. were able to report the results of their study of 52 patients with pancreatic tumours, and ten with ganglioneuroblastomas, who had raised VIP concentrations. All the patients had severe secretory diarrhoea, weight loss, dehydration, hypokalaemic acidosis and a raised plasma urea concentration. Reduced gastric acid secretion was present in 72%. There was no elevation of the level of plasma VIP in patients with diarrhoea due to other types of tumour or non-neoplastic disease, nor in hormone-secreting tumours not associated with diarrhoea. In the meantime it was shown experimentally (Modlin et al. 1978; Krejs et al. 1980; Krejs 1980; Kane et al. 1983) that VIP caused diarrhoea in animals and in human volunteers. Biochemical abnormalities of the Verner–Morrison syndrome, such as hypokalaemic acidosis, prerenal uraemia and hypophosphataemia, are usually attributed to the effects of the diarrhoea. In 65% of the patients studied by Long et al. (1981), the plasma concentration of pancreatic polypeptide was increased, but excess of pancreatic polypeptide is not considered to be a cause of diarrhoea; a tumour that secreted pancreatic polypeptide alone was found not to be associated with diarrhoea (Bordi et al. 1978). Also in a number of the reported cases of the Verner–Morrison syndrome immunocytochemistry has shown that hormones other than VIP, or in addition to VIP, were being formed in the tumours, and various peptides and prostaglandins have been associated with the syndrome (Sandler et al. 1968; Gutniak et al. 1980). Relatively recently, peptide histidine isoleucine has been found to be abnormally high in the plasma of patients with VIPomas in whom plasma VIP was also elevated (Bloom et al. 1983).

VIPomas represent 3%–5% of all pancreatic endocrine tumours and Heitz (1984) has discussed their main characteristics. He states that 50%–75% are malignant, and that their size is between 2 cm and 7 cm in diameter. Microscopically, they have a solid or trabecular structure and occasional mitotic figures may be present. Many of the cells give a positive reaction to the silver impregnation method of Grimelius, and VIP can usually, but not always, be demonstrated by immunocytochemical methods. Electron microscopy is unhelpful in that only some of the tumour cells contain secretory granules and these are difficult to identify.

The histological, histochemical, ultrastructural and biochemical aspects of 32 VIP-producing tumours have been reported by Capella et al. (1983). In 31 of these, the tumours were situated in the pancreas; in the remaining one, the tumour was in the jejunum.

The Verner–Morrison syndrome may occur in the absence of any localised endocrine tumour in the pancreas, but in association with diffuse hyperplasia of the islets, and with islet cells scattered singly or in small groups in the exocrine tissue (Morrison 1980). Removal of the pancreas has been shown to cure this syndrome. In such a case, it is difficult to reconcile the apparent cure with the pathological findings for, as was mentioned earlier, VIP is not produced in normal pancreatic islet cells, and VIP secretion in the hyperplastic islets would have had to be demonstrated to prove that they had been responsible for the syndrome.

It has already been stated that the Verner–Morrison syndrome may be caused by ganglioneuroblastomas, but other non-pancreatic tumours have occasionally been associated with the syndrome. A list of such tumours, with their main symptoms, has been tabulated by Morrison; it includes a bronchial carcinoid tumour, a bronchial adenoma and phaeochromocytomas. A pancreatic tumour, other than an islet cell tumour, has also been reported to have caused the syndrome (Rood et al. 1988); the pancreatic tumour was a mucinous adenocarcinoma that was found by immunohistological staining to be secreting both VIP and PP, as well as the mucin that had been demonstrated by histochemistry. It is of interest that this patient had been found by Gibbard et al. (1988) to have increased secretion of tears as well as secretory diarrhoea. These observers considered the increased lacrimation to be a newly recognised feature of the VIP syndrome. Electron microscopy demonstrated two populations of granules whose significance was not clear to the authors. Another example of the VIP syndrome in association with a mucin-secreting carcinoma of the pancreas has been reported by Ordóñez et al. (1988), who described the tumour as an amphicrene carcinoma of islet cells, based on the histochemical and ultrastructural demonstration of mucin secretion and the immunohistochemical finding of chromogranin and PP reactivity in the same tumour cells. Although there had been a marked elevation of the serum VIP, this hormone could not be demonstrated immunohistochemically in a biopsy from one of the hepatic metastases.

Watery diarrhoea caused by oversecretion of VIP by a pancreatic tumour may occur in the MEN 1 syndrome, as has been reported by Hutcheon et al. (1979). In the family these authors studied, a son had the VIPoma syndrome, associated with an islet cell tumour and a parathyroid adenoma, while his father had the Zollinger–Ellison syndrome associated with multiple pancreatic islet cell adenomas.

The report of a combination of the VIPoma syndrome with the glucagonoma syndrome by Cavallo-Perin (1988) will be discussed later in relation to combined endocrine syndromes.

Tumours Producing Pancreatic Polypeptide (PPomas)

Pancreatic polypeptide (PP) was first found incidentally during the extraction of insulin from chicken pancreas in 1968, and was found later to be present in the pancreas of many species of animal including dogs and man (Gersell et al. 1979). The human product is sometimes referred to as HPP to distinguish it from PP obtained from other animals. In 1976, it was found by Polak et al. to be present in more than half of 33 endocrine tumours whose effects had been those of either insulinoma, gastrinoma, vipoma or glucagonoma; its presence did not seem to influence the effects of the dominant hormone secreted by these tumours. Somewhat similar results were those of Larsson et al. (1976), who found that more than half the 18 endocrine pancreatic tumours they examined contained more than one type of hormone-producing cell, but that clinical symptoms were attributable to only one of the hormones produced by the mixed tumours. Their series contained four tumours associated with the watery diarrhoea syndrome; in three of these the tumours contained both VIP and human pancreatic polypeptide. In the fourth tumour in this group, however, there was a preponderance of HPP cells and there was a 1000-fold elevation of the serum HPP levels, while the VIP levels were within the normal range; they felt that this provided evidence that HPP might be a possible cause of the watery diarrhoea syndrome. Another clinical finding in association with a PP-producing pancreatic tumour is the skin rash reported by Choksi et al. (1988). The rash was erythematous, scaly, pruritic and papular; it affected the face, chest, hands, abdomen and perineum in a 56-year-old white woman; the pancreatic tumour responded well to chemotherapy and the rash disappeared.

Examples of pure PPomas have been found by Bordi et al. (1978) and Heitz et al. (1982), but such pancreatic tumours were non-functioning, and Heitz (1984) concluded that it was not possible to attribute symptoms to the effects of circulating pancreatic polypeptide in patients with PPomas. This opinion has been repeated more recently by Klöppel and Heitz (1988) as a result of their additional experience of many pancreatic endocrine tumours.

Although pancreatic polypeptide may be secreted in association with other hormones by malignant endocrine tumours of the pancreas, as in the cases reported by Tomita et al. (1983) and by Norbin et al. (1984), pure PPomas are usually benign (Heitz et al. 1982). One of the ten PPomas studied by Heitz and his colleagues was situated in the duodenal mucosa. The illustration of the microscopic appearance of the latter tumour, when stained by haematoxylin and eosin, is of clumps of cells with small nuclei and clear cytoplasm lying beside a duodenal gland. There is no definite alveolar arrangement and no significant amount of stroma. An adjacent illustration shows that, by an immunological unlabelled antibody enzyme method, many of the cells give a positive reaction for the presence of PP within their cytoplasm.

An infiltrating endocrine tumour of the papilla of Vater, with unusual morphological appearances, has been reported by Ljungberg et al. (1981) as having immunoreactivity to HPP. A malignant gastric tumour in a woman aged 64 was reported by Solt et al. (1984) to be made up of cells, most of which were immunoreactive to PP antiserum. This patient had suffered from flushing, tachycardia, headache and lacrimation when her plasma PP level was 700 times in excess of normal. These symptoms lessened and the levels of PP in the plasma fell after embolisation of the hepatic artery had been carried out to reduce the effects of secretion by hepatic metastases. The authors claim that their case is the first reported example of a gastric PP-producing endocrine tumour. An earlier example of an extrapancreatic polypeptide-producing tumour is that reported in the liver by Warner et al. (1980). The cells in that tumour contained electron-dense granules that were taken to indicate the formation of various peptides, but immunofluorescence studies with antibodies to several polypeptide hormones detected PP-containing tumour cells only. It was suggested that the tumour might have originated from intrahepatic bile ducts. Other extra-pancreatic tumours that have been reported to secrete PP include gangliocytic paragangliomas of the duodenum, in which PP was found by Perrone et al. (1985) along with various other hormones, and in 21 of the 25 carcinoid tumours of the rectum examined by Alumets et al. (1981), a condition also quite often found to be in association with other peptide hormones.

Ectopic Hormones Produced by Functioning Pancreatic Tumours

Gastrin is, of course, the best known of the ectopic hormones produced by pancreatic islet cell tumours; the Zollinger–Ellison syndrome due to gastrinomas has already been discussed. Occasionally, endocrine secretions produced by pancreatic islet cell tumours may cause well-recognised syndromes, usually resulting from non-pancreatic endocrine secretions. Thus Cushing's syndrome due to islet cell carcinoma of the pancreas was reported by O'Riordan et al. (1966) and, more recently, by others such as Clark and Carney (1984) and by Melmed et al. (1987), who demonstrated that a case of Cushing's syndrome was due to ectopic

proopiomelanocortin gene expression by an islet cell carcinoma of the pancreas. Acromegaly, due to the production of ectopic growth hormone by a pancreatic islet cell tumour has been reported (Melmed et al. 1985) and to the secretion of growth-hormone-releasing factor by pancreatic endocrine tumours (Thorner et al. 1982; Rivier et al. 1982; Bostwick et al. 1984; Saeger et al. 1986).

Hypercalcaemia due to the secretion of parathormone by a pancreatic endocrine carcinoma has been reported by Arps et al. (1986) and to the secretion of parathormone and its related protein by another pancreatic endocrine carcinoma (Wynick et al. 1990). The carcinoid syndrome caused by carcinoid tumours of the pancreas is discussed later (see p. 206).

Pancreatic Neuroendocrine Tumours with Combined Hormonal Syndromes

Pancreatic endocrine tumours commonly produce multiple hormones, but, in the well recognised syndromes, the clinical effects are attributable to a single dominant hormone, an excess of which can be detected in the patient's serum and in the tumour. Mixed syndromes may, however, occur occasionally, when effects due to hormones that are not secreted by normal islet cells may be produced. An example of such a mixed syndrome was published by Lokich et al. (1987). Their patient with metastatic islet cell carcinoma had Cushing's syndrome and the Zollinger–Ellison syndrome simultaneously. The authors were able to refer to eight previously published examples of this syndrome, in one of which the pancreatic tumour developed in a pancreas already damaged by calcifying chronic pancreatitis (Allison et al. 1985).

A malignant pancreatic endocrine tumour with hepatic metastases causing a combination of the glucagonoma syndrome and the VIPoma syndrome has been reported by Cavallo-Perin et al. (1988). The authors believed this to be the first reported case in which there was both immunocytochemical and clinical evidence of the secretion of both glucagon and VIP by a pancreatic endocrine tumour.

Carcinoid Tumours of the Pancreas

The appearances of carcinoid tumours of the small intestine and appendix are so similar to certain tumours of islet cells, especially those associated with the Zollinger–Ellison syndrome, that the term carcinoid–islet tumour was suggested by Weichert et al. (1967). Carcinoid tumours are known to secrete serotonin (5-hydroxytryptamine) and, when they have produced secondary deposits in the liver, sufficient serotonin may be secreted to cause the clinical and anatomical effects of the carcinoid syndrome, which has been the subject of reviews by Campbell (1959), Grahame-Smith (1972) and Marks (1979). The main features of the syndrome are episodes of flushing of the skin and endocardial fibrosis, most marked upon the walls and valves of the right side of the heart, with eventual cardiac failure. The staining reactions by which carcinoid tumours are recognised are those that demonstrate argyrophilia in the tumour cells, for example the Grimelius method, and the presence of argentaffin granules within the tumour cells, as can be shown for example by the Masson–Fontana technique. Dense core granules can also be found within the tumour cells by electron microscopy. The carcinoid tumours that stain most characteristically by the methods used for light microscopy are those found in the ileum and appendix, that is, in structures derived from the embryonic mid-gut. Tumours that may cause the carcinoid syndrome have also been found in organs derived from the primitive foregut, for example the bronchi, proximal duodenum and pancreas. Though these may be argyrophilic, they often do not contain argentaffin granules. Carcinoids in hindgut-derived structures usually do not stain typically and seldom cause the carcinoid syndrome (Williams and Sandler 1963).

A monoclonal antibody that reacts against serotonin immunoreactive sites has been used by Wells et al. (1985), who found it to be more sensitive and more specific than either the Grimelius or Masson–Fontana techniques in the diagnosis of foregut and hindgut carcinoid tumours. Wells et al. applied their antibody technique to a number of islet cell tumours, a malignant one of which had caused the carcinoid syndrome as well as having secreted adrenocorticotrophic hormone. A positive reaction for the presence of serotonin in the tumour associated with the carcinoid syndrome was obtained. A similar reaction was obtained with another malignant islet cell tumour, but two islet cell adenomas reacted negatively. The presence of serotinin in the two positively reacting pancreatic islet cell tumours would justify their acceptance as true carcinoids of the pancreas according to the criterion suggested by Bloodworth and Greider (1982), namely that only tumours producing serotonin, or its precursor substance 5-hydroxytryptophan, should be regarded as true pancreatic carcinoids. That pancreatic tumours may form many types of polypeptide hormone has been shown by Pearse et al. (1974), who carried out a cytochemical analysis of 46

carcinoid–islet cell tumours. Of these, ten were found to contain gastrin, six insulin, five calcitonin, four adrenocorticotrophin, and one VIP, while four contained mixtures of hormones. A carcinoid–islet tumour of the pancreas has also been shown to contain prostaglandins (Sandler et al. 1968).

It is unusual for carcinoid–islet cell tumours of the pancreas to cause the carcinoid syndrome but, as these tumours are of the foregut type, in which the secretion of 5-hydroxytryptophan is common, it seems likely that the more sensitive methods that are becoming available will detect small amounts of 5-hydroxytryptophan or serotonin in the secretions of such tumours, along with the more dominant hormones that such tumours may be producing.

Examples of carcinoid tumours of the pancreas associated with the carcinoid syndrome have been reported by Peart et al. (1963), and by van der Sluys Veer et al. (1964). Peart and his colleagues believed that the carcinoid tumour in their case had arisen from the epithelium of the pancreatic ducts. In that reported by van der Sluys Veer et al., the chief effect of the tumour and its hepatic metastases was to cause hypoglycaemia, but, as the illness progressed, the carcinoid syndrome, as indicated by flushing of the skin, diarrhoea and bronchial asthma, developed, along with the excretion of 5-hydroxyindole acetic acid in amounts sufficient to indicate that the tumours were secreting either serotonin or its precursor 5-hydroxytryptophan. Somewhat similar changes in the hormonal effects of functioning islet cell tumours, with replacement of the original hypoglycaemic syndrome by the effects of another hormone, have already been mentioned (Ohneda et al. 1979; D'Arcangues et al. 1984). Additional examples of pancreatic carcinoid tumours are those reported by Wilander et al. (1981) and Ordóñez et al. (1985), while the collection of 84 cases of pancreatic islet cell tumour accumulated during 35 years at the Cleveland Clinic included two cases of carcinoid tumour (Broughan et al. 1986). Such reports indicate that the malignancy of carcinoid–islet cell tumours tends to be high, with metastatic spread to lymph nodes, the liver and elsewhere.

Mixed Endocrine–Exocrine Tumours

Reports of such tumours in the pancreas are still infrequent, but is becoming recognised that, if carcinomas in other organs, especially adenocarcinomas of the alimentary canal, are stained appropriately and examined carefully, endocrine cells will be found. Such searches are, however, not normally undertaken unless clinical and biochemical evidence had indicated that the endocrine cells were causing a significant functional effect. When searches have been carried out, cells with the features of both exocrine and endocrine cells have been found (Reid et al. 1982; Chejfec et al. 1985; Bosman 1989). The cells with such features have been called "amphicrene" cells. Their exact origin and fundamental biological significance is debatable but, in large bowel carcinomas, it has been suggested by Arends et al. (1986) that the presence of cells with immunoreactivity for serotonin identifies a subpopulation of colorectal carcinomas with a relatively poor prognosis.

As far as the pancreas in concerned, cells immunoreactive to pancreatic endocrine hormones have been reported by Eusebi et al. (1981), Reid et al. (1982), Chejfec et al. (1985), Kniffin et al. (1988) and Ordóñez et al. (1988), in mucinous adenocarcinomas of the pancreas. In the case reported by Ordóñez et al., as was mentioned on p. 204, the watery diarrhoea, hypokalaemia syndrome was associated with an amphicrene carcinoma. Numerous cells that stained immunocytochemically for pancreatic polypeptide were present and there was also diffuse positive reactivity for chromogranin and neuron specific enolase. There was no staining for any of the other hormonal polypeptides investigated. The latter included insulin, glucagon, somatostatin and serotonin. In the case reported by Kniffin et al., immunohistochemical staining demonstrated neuron specific enolase, and positive reactions for serotonin, glucagon, gastrin and bombesin in a hepatic metastasis. Negative reactions for insulin and somatostatin were obtained. Simultaneous immunostaining and mucin staining demonstrated tumour cells that contained both peptide hormones and mucin vacuoles. The pancreatic cancer and its hepatic metastases were associated with a nodular skin rash in which esoinophil leucocytes were abundant, together with lymphocytes and histiocytes in the upper dermis.

What is, to the authors' knowledge, the first malignant islet cell tumour with rhabdomyosarcomatous differentiation, has been reported by Ferreiro et al. (1989). This was a widely metastatic tumour of the pancreas in which there were focal areas with a rhabdomyosarcomatous appearance. In such areas, desmin was identified by immunohistochemistry. Cross-striations were not seen by light microscopy but z-lines and thick filaments were seen on electron microscopy. In other immunohistochemical studies, positive staining was obtained for chromogranin, somatostatin, and, focally, for gastrin-releasing peptide (bombesin). Parathormone was positive in 70% of the cells and hypercalcaemia had been an important clinical feature of the patient's illness.

The Malignant Behaviour of Pancreatic Endocrine Carcinomas

The capacity that neuroendocrine cells have for reproduction is suspected to be much less than the reproductive capacity of the adjacent exocrine cells, at least in the intestine, and, although the turnover times for pancreatic endocrine cells is not known, their ability to divide is probably limited (Pearse 1984). This limited capacity is in keeping with the difficulty in differentiating histologically between simple and malignant endocrine tumours of the pancreas, and in keeping also with the relatively slow progress of the disease associated with some of the malignant endocrine tumours, even when mestastatic disease has developed: the patient described by D'Arcangues et al. (1984) was still alive 17 years after hepatic metastases had been proved by biopsy to be present. Such long survival, however, cannot be taken for granted, for, in the 30 patients with islet cell carcinoma reported by Cubilla and Hajdu in 1975, the average survival was only 3.9 years, with a range of survival time from 3 months to 14 years. Survival tended to be poor in the patients with hypoglycaemia. They found that liver, regional lymph nodes, bones and peritoneum were common sites for metastases. Most of the tumours were found in the body or tail of the pancreas and the primary tumour was more than 6 cm in diameter in 25 of the 30 patients; in 26 there was metastatic disease at the time of diagnosis.

The results of a study of the DNA profiles and nuclear parameters in the pancreatic endocrine tumours from 39 patients diagnosed between 1969 and 1989 by Lee et al. (1993), using computerised video image analysis, led the authors to conclude that ploidy studies may be useful in predicting malignant potential.

Survival tends to be better in functioning pancreatic endocrine malignant tumours than in the non-functioning tumours (Thompson et al. 1988). In the 365 tumours analysed by Klöppel and Heitz (1988), 64% of non-functioning tumours were malignant. The reason may be that non-functioning tumours are slow in causing symptoms and are thus large and advanced before they are recognised. It is confidently stated by Eckhauser et al. (1986) that non-functioning neuroendocrine tumours of the pancreas are locally aggressive, have a propensity to metastasise early, and are rarely curable by surgery.

Malignant pancreatic endocrine tumours may occasionally become cystic and resemble pseudocysts; three cystic pancreatic endocrine tumours have been described by Thompson et al. (1984). Two of these tumours, both of which were gastrinomas, were treated by drainage into the intestine before the true nature of the lesion was recognised. In the third patient, two pancreatic endocrine tumours, one of which was cystic, together with microadenomatosis and nesidioblastosis in the adjacent pancreas, were part of MEN 1.

Cystic Change in Pancreatic Endocrine Tumours

Cystic change in malignant pancreatic endocrine tumours has just been mentioned, but such a change is not invariably a sign of malignancy. Two of the cystic pancreatic cancers described by Thompson et al. (1984) were gastrinomas, which are usually malignant. The endocrine nature of the large cystic carcinoma of the pancreas reported by Kamisawa et al. (1987) was diagnosed by immunohistochemistry and not by functional endocrine effects of the tumour. Following total pancreatectomy, the patient survived for five and a half years, although hepatic metastases, some of which were cystic, were known to be present. The collection of 67 cystic tumours of the pancreas studied by Warshaw et al. (1990) included two examples of cystic islet cell tumours, but few details of these two tumours are included in the report. One of the cystic endocrine pancreatic tumours described by Thompson et al. was in a patient with MEN 1. A cystic tumour of the pancreas in an unusual example of the MEN 1 syndrome in a 29-year-old man has been reported briefly by Scheimberg et al. (1991). Cystic change has not, however, been a feature of the numerous other examples of the syndrome that have been published. The clinical importance of the change is that, unless careful biopsies are carried out during surgery, the cystic tumours may be mistaken for pseudocysts and be treated by drainage instead of by excision.

Portal Hypertension Due to Islet Cell Tumours

Portal hypertension with haemorrhage from the resulting oesophageal varices was caused by an islet cell carcinoma in a case reported by Ponsky et al. (1979). An apparently non-functioning tumour that extended from the head of the pancreas to within 1 cm of the tail had caused an arteriovenous fistula that increased the portal venous flow sufficiently to cause portal hypertension. In the case recorded by Chellappa et al. (1986) too, a non-functioning malignant islet cell tumour presented with left-sided portal hypertension due to non-occlusive obstruction of the splenic vien.

Response of Islet Cell Tumours to Chemotherapy

Unlike pancreatic exocrine carcinomas, malignant endocrine tumours of the pancreas may respond well to chemotherapy as described by Hansen et al. (1988), but the results are somewhat variable, and Thompson et al. (1988), who used chemotherapy only to relieve symptoms in patients who had received palliative, but non-curative, surgery, found that the survival time of such patients was disappointing.

Pancreatic Islet Cell Tumours in Multiple Endocrine Adenopathy

Several syndromes that may be familial, or may occur sporadically, involve neoplasia of two or more endocrine glands. The syndromes may sometimes be the result of hyperplasia of the affected glands without true neoplasia and, for that reason, Montgomery and Welbourn (1975) have suggested that the syndromes be referred to as multiple endocrine adenopathy syndromes, but the multiple endocrine neoplasia syndrome is undoubtedly the more commonly used term, with MEN as the accepted contraction. The neoplasms may be benign or malignant.

There are two main types but, as there are several variants of each type, the features of the two sometimes overlap. In type 1 (MEN 1) the neoplasia or hyperplasia usually affects the anterior pituitary, the pancreatic islets and the parathyroids. Occasionally the adrenal cortex and the thyroid gland may be involved. In type 2 (MEN 2), medullary carcinoma of the thyroid is associated with phaeochromocytoma and with parathyroid hyperplasia or neoplasia. Both types also have eponyms, type 1 being known as Wermer's syndrome (Wermer 1954, 1963), and type 2 as Sipple's syndrome (Sipple 1961). When they are familial the syndromes are inherited as an autosomal dominant trait with high penetration and variable expression (Steiner et al. 1968). The sexes are affected equally and the disease may become manifest at any age; a woman aged 81 with MEN 1 was reported by Gelston et al. (1982). Sporadic cases are more common than familial cases (Croisier et al. 1971).

Pancreatic lesions are found in between 50% and 80% of the patients with MEN 1 (Heitz 1984). The abnormalities consist of localised or widespread ducto-insular proliferation of endocrine cells, hyperplastic islets and one or more islet cell tumours. The tumours are usually less than 1 cm in diameter and their microscopic appearance in routinely stained sections is said by Wermer (1974) to be so characteristic as to be diagnostic of MEN 1, and to indicate that a search for other tumours should be carried out. The characteristic appearances consist of a ribbon-like pattern in which the tumour cells form long parallel or interlacing rows that contrast with the irregular or alveolar structure of islet cell tumours of the non-genetic type. The ribbon pattern does not, however, indicate the cell type or functional activity of the tumours, which require ultrastructural and immunocytochemical studies for their detailed analysis, and which may be either monohormonal or multihormonal.

The hormonal effects of these tumours may be those of gastrinoma (50% of patients), insulinoma (30%) or VIPomas (12%). The glucagonoma syndrome is rare. The secretion of multiple hormones is common. In gastrinomas that cause the Zollinger–Ellison syndrome, malignancy is common, but in insulinomas, though they are often multiple, the tumours are usually benign. The successful removal of an insulinoma has been known, however, to be followed years later by the endocrine effects of other types of functioning pancreatic endocrine tumours (Heitz 1984), as has been described by Sardi and Singer (1987).

Neural abnormalities, including tumours of nerve tissues, and multiple lipomas have been associated with pancreatic endocrine tumours or hyperplasias. The association of lipomas and adenomas of the pituitary, parathyroid and pancreatic islets was noted by Marshall and Sloper (1954). An association between von Hippel–Lindau disease and pancreatic islet cell tumours has been reported by Probst et al. (1978), whose case also had syringomyelia, and by Hull et al. (1979), while the study by Lamiell et al. (1989) of 43 cases of von Hippel–Lindau disease has shown increased risk of pancreatic malignancy as well as of renal cancer, phaeochromocytoma and

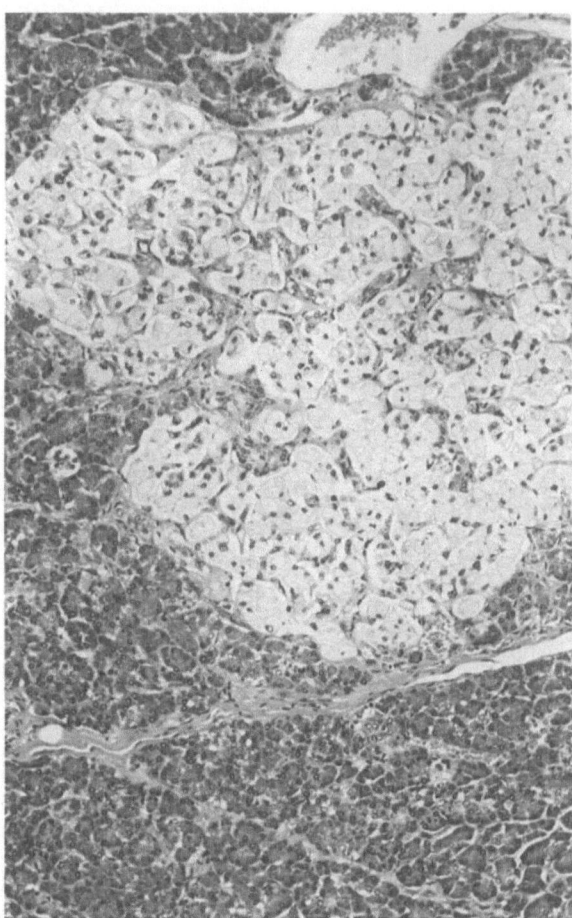

Fig. 10.24. One of several adenomas of islet cells, only one of which was recognisable macroscopically, in the pancreas of a man aged 35, who died of haemorrhage from a cerebellar haemangioblastoma. A similar adenoma was present in heterotopic pancreatic tissue in the duodenum, and there was also a clear cell carcinoma of one kidney. Bilateral adrenal phaeochromocytomas were also present. H&E, × 150

malignancy of the central nervous system. The pancreatic lesions of von Hippel–Lindau disease are discussed in Chap. 3 and also in Chap. 8. Figs 10.24 and 10.25 illustrate one of the pancreatic islet cell tumours and part of a cerebellar haemangioblastoma in a 35-year-old man. His death was caused by haemorrhage from the haemangioblastoma. At autopsy he was found to have a clear cell carcinoma of one kidney, bilateral adrenal phaeochromocytomas and islet cell tumours in the head and body of the pancreas, with an additional islet cell tumour in heterotopic pancreatic tissue in the duodenum. No intestinal carcinoid tumour was found and there was no neurofibromatosis. No family history was available.

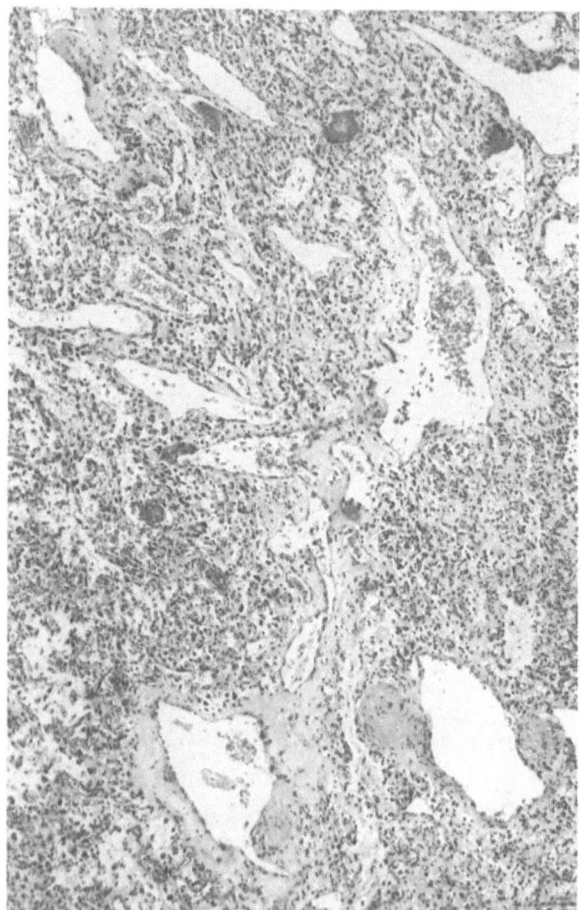

Fig. 10.25. Part of a cerebellar haemangioblastoma associated with multiple endocrine tumours. One of the adenomas of the pancreatic islets is shown in Fig. 10.24. H&E, ×70

Nesidioblastosis has been found in association with a congenital neuroblastoma by Grotting et al. (1979) and insulinoma in association with an adrenal medullary ganglioneuroma by Hale et al. (1987). In 1987 also, Griffiths et al. published the results of a study they undertook to clarify the syndromes in which endocrine lesions and neural abnormalities were associated. Their material consisted of nine cases of their own, in which von Recklinghausen's neurofibromatosis was present concurrently with carcinoid tumours in the duodenum; to these they added 20 published cases. In 18, a duodenal carcinoid was associated with neurofibromatosis, with in some cases, phaeochromocytomas in addition. When these were compared with six published cases of von Hippel–Lindau disease, in which single or bilateral phaeochromocytomas were present, it was found that all six had had pancreatic

islet cell tumours and that none had had a carcinoid tumour. None of the cases with neurofibromatosis and duodenal carcinoid tumours had an islet cell tumour of the pancreas. The authors concluded that the association of neurofibromatosis, duodenal carcinoid tumour and phaeochromocytoma formed a distinctive neuroendocrine syndrome that should be sharply separated from the association of von Hippel–Lindau complex with islet cell tumour and phaeochromocytoma. Such a conclusion certainly seems justified from the material available to these authors, but such associations are probably not invariable, for occasional cases in which neurofibromatosis and von-Hippel–Lindau disease were associated have been reported (Tishler 1975).

It may be mentioned in passing that in the duodenal carcinoids in the cases reviewed by Griffiths et al. (1987), psammoma bodies were often present, along with diffuse somatostatin reactivity in the carcinoid tumours.

The association of multiple islet cell adenomas with secondary haemochromatosis is discussed in the chapter on diabetes and haemochromatosis (Chap. 6).

A potentially useful screening test for the recognition of MEN 1 has been described by Friesen et al. (1983), who found significant elevation of the basal fasting levels of HPP in all of six patients with MEN 1 and in only three of 15 non-familial patients with sporadic islet cell tumours.

Nesidioblastosis and Adenomatosis in the Adult

Nesidioblastoma was the name, derived from the Greek word for an island, used by Laidlaw (1938) for a tumour of islet cells. He also suggested the word nesidioblastosis to describe the ductulo-insular structures that appeared to be forming new islet tissues near the nesidioblastomas that he described. A real, or at least apparent, increase of islet tissue is common in cases of chronic pancreatitis and in congenital cystic fibrosis of the pancreas. Such apparent neo-formation may not however, represent a true increase of islet tissue, and in chronic pancreatitis and cystic fibrosis a proportion of the cases eventually develop diabetes mellitus (see Chaps 4 and 11). Proliferation of ductules with differentiation towards islets is common in the pancreas of adults with intrapancreatic endocrine tumours (Laidlaw

1938; Creutzfeldt 1977) and is usually well marked in MEN 1 (Vance et al. 1972). In the latter condition it seems likely that the adenomas are formed by the conversion of hyperplastic islet tissue into microscopically or macroscopically recognisable neoplasms. Vance and his colleagues put forward the suggestion that in the MEN 1 syndrome the basic inherited abnormality is the abnormal proliferation of islet cells and of adenomatosis, whose secretion of an abnormal hormone, such as gastrin, or a normal pancreatic hormone in excess, leads to the other components of the syndrome.

Adenomatosis of the pancreas without tumours that could be seen or felt, and without any recognised components of MEN 1 has been described by Bickerstaff et al. (1955) and by Garland (1957). In both of these patients there were hypoglycaemic episodes that were relieved by partial pancreatectomy, and in each case the resected pancreas looked normal. In the case described by Bickerstaff et al., two areas that felt firm and were thought to be adenomas did not correspond to the microscopic adenomas that were discovered later. These adenomas, which were discovered in transverse sections taken at 1 cm intervals along the 11 cm length of resected distal pancreas, varied in diameter from 0.2 mm to 7 mm. In addition to the collections of islet cell tissue that were regarded as tumours, there were hyperplastic and normal islets throughout the specimen. The largest tumours tended to lie on the surface of the gland. The microscopic appearances of the tumours were very similar to those of normal islets. They were, however, much larger and were distributed irregularly. In Garland's case, the largest adenomas were 4 mm in diameter and could be seen with the naked eye when the resected distal pancreas had been sectioned at 0.5 cm intervals. Familial adenomatosis of islet cells, without other components of the MEN 1 syndrome but with diabetes in other members of the family, was reported by Tragl and Mayr in 1977.

More recently, Carlson et al. (1987) described the case of a 21-year-old black man with hypoglycaemia and hyperinsulinism, which were taken to indicate the effects of an insulinoma. No adenoma could be recognised, however, when the pancreas was explored, but hyperplasia of the islets was found in frozen sections and a 70%–75% resection of the pancreas was carried out. Further studies confirmed the presence of nesidioblastosis in macroscopically normal pancreatic tissue, which also contained a few microscopic foci of adenomatosis. When the patient was discharged from hospital his symptoms had been relieved and his blood chemistry was normal. There was no family history or other evidence to suggest that the case might be an example of the MEN 1 syndrome. In 1987 also, Jerkins et al. reported a 63-year-old man in whom nesidioblastosis with microadenomatosis associated with hypersecretion of pancreatic polypeptide coexisted with medullary carcinoma of the thyroid. The authors interpreted this as an example of the overlapping of the MEN syndrome types 1 and 2. Further studies of nesidioblastosis were undertaken by Wotherspoon and Rode in 1989. Their 11 cases of nesidioblastosis included two adults, one of whom had MEN 1 syndrome. They found that nesidioblastosis represented a spectrum that ranged from a diffuse increase in cell clusters budding from ductular epithelium, as in embryological development, to multinodular islet cell hyperplasia which, in adults, might form part of a multiple endocrine neoplasia syndrome.

Nesidioblastosis Due to Therapy

Hypertrophy and hyperplasia of the islets of Langerhans has been attributed to various types of therapy. Novak et al. (1979) observed nesidioblastosis in three children with Fanconi's pancytopenia, who had been treated with androgen anabolic steroids for many months before their deaths, during which time the steroids had caused intolerance of glucose. The pancreatic lesions were associated with benign liver cell tumours. Another patient with anaemia due to pure red cell aplasia, who developed multiple islet cell adenomas, has been described by Sidi et al. (1984). This patient had developed secondary haemochromatosis because of the many blood transfusions he had received during the 15 years that preceded his death and the authors attributed the pancreatic adenomas to the advanced chronic pancreatitis with fibrous replacement of almost all the exocrine tissue of the pancreas that had been produced by the deposition of haemosiderin.

Nesidioblastosis attributable to the effects of secretly self-administered chlorpropamide has been reported by Rayman et al. (1984) in a 25-year-old woman who was thought to be suffering from an insulinoma because of recurrent attacks of hypoglycaemia associated with inappropriately high plasma insulin levels. Partial pancreatectomy was carried out and nesidioblastosis, without an insulinoma, was found in the excised pancreas. After her discharge from hospital the woman had another episode of hypoglycaemia, during which a high concentration of chlorpropamide was found in her blood. Similarly high concentrations of chlorpropamide were also found in stored pre-operative samples of her blood, and were taken to indicate that the case was one of self-poisoning.

sudden unexpected death in the neonatal period (Polak and Wigglesworth 1976).

Hyperplasia of Pancreatic Islets Associated with Extrapancreatic Lymphoma and Sarcoma

Quite unexplained but, in the opinion of the authors, significant, hyperplasia of the pancreatic islets was found by Hart and Hinerman (1965) in patients who had died with extrapancreatic lymphoma or sarcoma. Their conclusion was based on measurements of the diameters of the pancreatic islets in 10 cases of lymphoma and 12 of sarcoma, with similar measurements of the islets in 20 cases of accidental death for comparison. Somewhat similar results were obtained by Ghosh et al. (1973) when they qualitatively and quantitatively compared the islets in 15 cases of chondrosarcoma with those of 12 controls. They suggest that the alteration of carbohydrate metabolism that may be associated with neoplastic conditions might have been responsible.

The existence of nesidioblastosis is now accepted by most workers but, because of the difficulty of making accurate assessment of the amount of islet tissue, as has been discussed in an earlier chapter, there is still some scepticism about its existence. Thus, in an examination of the pancreases, obtained at autopsy, from 207 adults, and without either clinical or autopsy evidence of insular overactivity, Karnauchow (1982) found ductulo-insular complexes, together with insular cells among the acini, in 10.6% of the specimens, the nesidioblastosis being somewhat more common in the male subjects. Goudswaard et al. (1984) also concluded from a study of the normal pancreas in 49 cases in age groups from foetal to adult life that nesidioblastosis is a normal feature of development and that there is wide variation in all age groups. Its incidence tends to diminish with advancing age. In three of five cases originally thought to be true examples of nesidioblastosis, they found small insulinomas when a more careful search was carried out; this led them to conclude that, if true hyperplasia is present, it points to the presence of an islet tumour.

The difficulties that exist in the identification of true nesidioblastosis exist also in the interpretation of the pancreatic lesions associated with the syndrome of hyperinsulinaemic hypoglycaemia in infancy, a condition which, if persistent, will lead to permanent damage to the nervous system (Lucas et al. 1988). It has also been blamed for having caused

The Pancreas in Persistent Hyperinsulinaemic Hypoglycaemia in Infancy

In 1941, Potter et al., from a study of the pancreas in the foetus and the newborn infant, found that an increased amount of islet tissue may be found in the foetal pancreas in the presence or absence of abnormal sugar metabolism in the mother or infant. There are many abnormalities of metabolism that may cause hypoglycaemia in the neonate or in the young baby; the main causes have been tabulated and discussed by Pagliara et al. (1973); the list included hyperinsulinism. Such hyperinsulinism may be transient, as in the babies of diabetic mothers, but there are other cases in which the hyperinsulinism and hypoglycaemia are persistent. Such cases justify the surgical exploration of the pancreas. A small insulinoma may be found – an illustration of a nodule of compact endocrine cells on the surface of the pancreas of a 4-month-old infant with hyperinsulinaemic hypoglycaemia is shown by Klöppel and Heitz (1984) – but insulinomas are rare in infancy. More commonly, the pancreas seems normal at laparotomy. In such patients, however, it is considered justifiable to carry out a subtotal pancreatectomy, a procedure that has been found to relieve the hyperinsulinism and hypoglycaemia, though it may not always prevent persistent cerebral impairment (Gampa et al. 1976), while the results of Dunger et al. (1988) suggest that even after 95% pancreatectomy, pancreatic function is not usually seriously impaired 1–2 years later. Similar results were obtained by Warden et al. (1988). Heitz et al. (1977) carried out a morphological and quantitative analysis of seven specimens of pancreatic tissue removed for the relief of persistent hyperinsulinaemic hypoglycaemia in infants. The results were based on specific immunostaining and electron microscopy with quantification, for which a television image conversion analyser branched on-line to a calculator was used. In five of the cases there were multiple foci of ducto-insular proliferation, in one there was focal adenomatosis and in one there was a solitary encapsulated adenoma. An almost five-fold increase in the mean total area occupied by endocrine tissue, as compared with age-matched controls, was found. The ratio of B cells per total endocrine area in the hypoglycaemic cases was very similar (62%) to that per islet of the controls (59%). Similar findings in their study of the pancreas removed from a case of hyperinsulinaemic hypoglycaemia in a neonate were reported by Shermeta et al. (1980), who postulated that the state of the pancreas represented an abnormal continuation of the prenatal proliferation of pancreatic endocrine cells. They suggested, moreover, that hyperplasia might be a specific overproduction of the secondary islets, said by Liu and Potter (1962) to be formed in the developing pancreas, while adenomatosis represented an abnormal continuation of the primary islets that are normally replaced by the secondary islets.

The significance of nesidioblastosis as the cause of hyperinsulinaemic hypoglycaemia has been questioned by Gould et al. (1983). They obtained subtotal pancreatectomy specimens from seven infants with persistent hyperinsulinaemic hypoglycaemia and studied them by electron and conventional light microscopy, and by immunocytochemistry, for the presence of insulin, glucagon, somatostatin and HPP. Their findings, quantitated morphometrically in four of the cases, were compared with the findings in the pancreases, obtained at autopsy, of four infants that had died of other causes. Like Heitz et al. (1977), they found an increase in the total endocrine cell volume in the hyperinsulinaemic infants. They found, however, that one of the control pancreases had a total endocrine cell mass comparable with that of the hypoglycaemic cases, and, if they used the anatomical definition of nesidioblastosis as being the presence of abundant endocrine cells intermingled with exocrine acini and ducts, in addition to the endocrine cells that were organised into islets, then nesidioblastosis might be observed in neonates and infants, regardless of the presence or absence of an associated endocrine syndrome. They concluded that nesidioblastosis, as defined anatomically, could not be considered to be the cause of hyperinsulinaemic hypoglycaemia. In reaching this conclusion they may have been influenced by the fact that one of the hypoglycaemic infants remained hypoglycaemic after two operations, the first of which was an almost total pancreatectomy, and the second of which was to remove the stump of the pancreas and to cauterise its base. Subtotal pancreatectomy was apparently successful in producing a cure in two of the cases, and possibly in a third who could not be followed up. In one, and possibly in two others, the hypoglycaemia had caused neurological damage.

As more material had accumulated, Goossens et al. (1989) were able to review the anatomical findings in the pancreases of 24 cases of persistent hyperinsulinaemic hypoglycaemia. Like earlier workers (Heitz et al. 1977; Klöppel and Heitz 1984) they found that nesidioblastosis occurred in two main forms – one focal and one diffuse – and that in their material the two types were equally frequent. In the focal type there was nodular hyperplasia of islet-like cell clusters, including ducto-insular complexes and hypertrophied insulin-positive cells with giant nuclei. In nine of their cases, such foci were solitary, while in three, two or more foci were present. The diffuse type involved the entire pancreas and consisted of islets of varying size and ducto-insular complexes, both of which contained hypertrophic insulin cells. In nine of the 12 specimens with the diffuse type of nesidioblastosis, the abnormalities were easily recognisable using routine histological methods, but in three the appearances were normal when conventional histological staining alone was used, the abnormalities being recognisable only by immunostaining. The authors admitted that there were diagnostic difficulties in such cases. They made the important observation in the two of the patients in whom second operations were necessary, after six and eight years respectively, that the lesions were still present and that the pancreases had not matured into normality as the children grew up.

The Pancreas in Temporary Hyperinsulinaemia Due to Maternal Diabetes Mellitus

In spite of the variability in the amount of islet tissue in the pancreas of the newborn infant, which makes assessment so difficult, it has usually been found that the islet tissue is increased in the pancreases of infants of diabetic mothers, or even of pre-diabetic mothers. Moreover the accumulation of eosinophil granulocytes around the enlarged islets, first noted by Cardell (1953), is now thought to be an important diagnostic characteristic of the effects of maternal diabetes upon the neonatal pancreas. Such abnormalities are presumed to regress in infants that survive the neonatal period.

Lesions of the Nervous System Caused by Neonatal Hypoglycaemia

The injuries to nerve cells caused in the adult brain by severe, prolonged or repeated episodes of hypoglycaemia have already been mentioned, thus it is not surprising that similar damage has been found in the central nervous system of fatal cases of neonatal hypoglycaemia. The case histories and necropsy findings of six infants who suffered from prolonged hypogylcaemia in the first week of life have been described by Anderson et al. (1967). In three, the hypoglycaemia had not been treated; in these there was extensive degeneration of nerve cells throughout the central nervous system, with, in two, damage also to glial cells. The spinal cord was affected as well as the brain. In the three cases in which the hypoglycaemia had been corrected and in which the babies had died later from other causes, the abnormalities were only slight. This was attributed to successful treatment of the hypoglycaemia.

References

Ackerman LV, Rosai J (1974) Surgical pathology, 5th edn. Mosby, St Louis, p 575

Adamson AR, Grahame-Smith DG, Bogomoletz V, Maw DSJ, Rothnie NG (1971) Malignant argentaffinoma with carcinoid syndrome and hypoglycaemia. Br Med J iii: 93–94

Albrecht S, Gardiner GW, Kovacs K, Isle G, Kaiser U (1989) Duodenal somatostatinoma with psammoma bodies. Arch Pathol Lab Med 113: 517–520

Allison MC, Renfrew CC, Webb WJS, Chappell ME, Pounder RE (1985) Neuroendocrine islet cell tumour producing gastrin and ACTH in a patient with calcifying chronic pancreatitis. Gut 26: 426–428

Alroy J, Baldwin D, Maschgan ER (1980) Multiple beta cell neoplasms in a polar bear. Vet Pathol 17: 331–337

Alumets J, Alm P, Falkmer S et al. (1981) Immunohistochemical evidence of peptide hormone in endocrine tumors of the rectum. Cancer 48: 2409–2415

Anderson JM, Milner RDG, Strich SJ (1967) Effects of neonatal hypoglycaemia on the nervous system: a pathological study. J Neurol Neurosurg Psychiatry 30: 295–310

Arends JW, Wiggers T, Vestijnen K, Bosman FT (1986) The occurrence and clinicopathological significance of serotonin immunoreactive cells in large bowel carcinoma. J Pathol 149: 97–102

Arps H, Dietel M, Schulz A, Janzarik H, Klöppel G (1986) Pancreatic endocrine carcinoma with ectopic PTH production and paraneoplastic hypercalcaemia. Vichows Arch [A] 408: 497–503

Barton JC, Hirschowitz BI, Maton PM, Jensen RT (1986) Bone metastases in malignant gastrinoma. Gastroenterology 91: 1179–1181

Berger M, Bordi C, Cüppers H-J et al. (1983) Functional and morphologic characterization of human insulinomas. Diabetes 32: 921–931

Bickerstaff ER, Dodge OG, Gourevitch A, Hearn GW (1955) Adenomatosis of the islets of Langerhans. Br Med J ii: 997–1000

Bloodworth JMB, Greider MH (1982) The endocrine pancreas and diabetes mellitus. In: Bloodworth JMB (ed) Endocrine pathology, 2nd edn. Williams and Wilkins, Baltimore, pp 556–721

Bloom SR (1972) An enteroglucagon tumour. Gut 13: 520–523

Bloom SR (1975) Glucagon. Br J Hosp Med 13: 150–158

Bloom SR, Polak JM, Pearse AGE (1973) Vasoactive intestinal peptide and watery-diarrhoea syndrome. Lancet ii: 14–16

Bloom SR, Christofides ND, Delamarter J, Buell G, Kawashima E, Polak JM (1983) Diarrhoea in VIPoma patients associated with cosecretion of a second active peptide (peptide histidine isoleucine) explained by single coding gene. Lancet ii: 1163–1165

Boden G (1987) Insulinoma and glucagonoma. Semin Oncol 14: 253–262

Boden G, Owen OE (1977) Familial hyperglucagonemia – an autosomal dominant disorder. N Engl J Med 296: 534–538

Boosinger TR, Zerbe CA, Grabau JH, Pletcher JM (1988) Multihormonal pancreatic endocrine tumor in a dog with duodenal ulcers and hypertrophic gastropathy. Vet Pathol 25: 237–239

Bordi C, Togni R, Baetens D, Ravazzola D, Malaisse-Lagae F, Orci L (1978) Human islet cell tumor storing pancreatic polypeptide: a light and electron microscopic study. J Clin Endocrinol Metab 46: 215–219

Bordi C, Ravazzola M, Baetens D, Gorden P, Unger RH, Orci L (1979) A study of glucagonomas by light and electron microscopy and immunofluorescence. Diabetes 28: 925–936

Bosman FT (1989) Endocrine cells in non-endocrine tumours. J Pathol 159: 181–182

Bostwick DG, Quan R, Hoffman AR, Webber RJ, Chang J-K, Benesch KG (1984) Growth-hormone-releasing factor immunoreactivity in human endocrine tumors. Am J Pathol 117: 167–170

Broughan TA, Leslie JD, Soto JM, Hermann RE (1986) Pancreatic islet cell tumors. Surgery 99: 671–678

Brown CH, Neville WE, Hazard JB (1950) Islet cell adenoma without hypoglycaemia causing duodenal obstruction. Surgery 27: 616–620

Campbell ACP (1959) The pathological relationships of 5-hydroxytryptamine. In: Collins DH (ed) Modern trends in pathology. Butterworths, London, pp 231–247

Cantor AM, Rigby CC, Beck PR, Mangion D (1982) Neurofibromatosis, phaeochromocytoma, and somatostatinoma. Br Med J iv: 1618–1619

Capella C, Polak JM, Buffa R et al. (1983) Morphologic patterns and diagnostic criteria of VIP-producing endocrine tumors. Cancer 52: 1860–1874

Cardell BS (1953) Hypertrophy and hyperplasia of the pancreatic islets in new-born infants. J Pathol Bacteriol 66: 335–346

Carlson T, Eckhauser ML, DeBaz B, Khiyami A, Park CH (1987) Nesidioblastosis in an adult: an illustrative case and collective review. Am J Gastroenterol 82: 566–571

Carney CN (1976) Congenital insulinoma (nesidioblastoma): ultrastructural evidence for histogenesis from pancreatic ductal epithelium. Arch Pathol Lab Med 100: 352–356

Cavallo-Perin P, DePaoli M, Guiso G et al. (1988) A combined glucagonoma and VIPoma syndrome. Cancer 62: 2576–2579

Chejfec G, Capella C, Solcia E, Jao W, Gould VE (1985) Amphicrine cells, dysplasias, and neoplasias. Cancer 56: 2683–2690

Chellappa M, Chan Kit Yee, Gill DS (1986) Left-sided portal hypertension from malignant islet cell tumour of the pancreas: review with a case report. J R Coll Surg Edinb 31: 251–252

Choksi UA, Sellin RV, Hickey RC, Samaan NA (1988) An unusual skin rash associated with a pancreatic polypeptide-producing tumor of the pancreas. Ann Intern Med 108: 64–65

Clark ES, Carney JA (1984) Pancreatic islet cell tumor associated with Cushing's syndrome. Am J Surg Pathol 8: 917–924

Cohen C, Budgeon LR (1982) Commercial immunoperoxidase kits in the study of 13 pancreatic islet cell tumors. Am J Clin Pathol 78: 364–366

Colin-Jones DG, Copping RML, Gibbs DD, Sharr MM (1969) Malignant Zollinger–Ellison syndrome with gastrin-containing skin metastases. Lancet i: 492–494

Creutzfeldt W (1977) Endocrine tumors of the pancreas. In: Volk BW, Wellmann KF (eds) The diabetic pancreas. Baillière Tindall, London, pp 551–590

Creutzfeldt W (1980) Endocrine tumors of the pancreas: clinical, chemical and morphological findings. In: Fitzgerald PJ, Morrison AB (eds) The pancreas. Williams and Wilkins, Baltimore, pp 208–230

Croisier J-C, Azerad E, Lubetzki J (1971) L'adénomatose polyendocrinienne (syndrome de Wermer). A propos d'une observation personnelle. Revue de la litérature. Semaine Hôpitaux Paris 47:494–525

Croughs RJM, Hulsmans HAM, Israël DE, Hackeng WHL, Schopman W (1972) Glucagonoma as part of the polyglandular adenoma syndrome. Am J Med 52:690–698

Cubilla AL, Hajdu S I (1975) Islet cell carcinoma of the pancreas. Arch Pathol 99:204–207

D'Arcangues CM, Awoke S, Lawrence GD (1984) Metastatic insulinoma with long survival and glucagonoma syndrome. Ann Intern Med 100:233–235

Duff GL, Murray EGD (1942) The pathology of islet cell tumors of the pancreas. Am J Med Sci 203:437–451

Dunger DB, Burns C, Ghale GK, Muller DPR, Spitz L, Grant DB (1988) Pancreatic exocrine and endocrine function after subtotal pancreatectomy for nesidioblastosis. J Pediatr Surg 23:112–115

Eckhauser FE, Cheung PS, Vinik AI, Strodel WE, Lloyd RV, Thompson NW (1986) Non-functioning malignant neuroendocrine tumors of the pancreas. Surgery 100:978–988

Ellison EW, Wilson SD (1964) The Zollinger–Ellison syndrome: reappraisal and evaluation of 260 registered cases. Ann Surg 160:512–528

Eusebi V, Capella C, Boudi A, Sess F, Bezzadini P, Mancini AM (1981) Endocrine-paracrine cells in pancreatic exocrine carcinomas. Histopathology 5:599–613

Fabozzi S (1903) Ueber die Histogenese des primären Krebses des Pankreas. Beitr Path Anat Allg Path 34:199–214

Feldman EC (1983) Diseases of the endocrine pancreas. In: Ettinger SJ (ed) Textbook of veterinary internal medicine. Diseases of the dog and cat, 2nd edn. Saunders, Philadelphia, pp 1644–1645

Ferreiro J, Lewin K, Herron RM, Bhuta S (1989) Malignant islet cell tumor with rhabdomyosarcomatous differentiation. Am J Surg Pathol 13:422–427

Friesen SR (1967) Effect of total gastrectomy on the Zollinger–Ellison tumor: observations by second-look procedures. Surgery 62:609–613

Friesen SR (1990) Are "aberrant nodal gastrinomas" pathogenetically similar to "lateral aberrant thyroid" nodules? Surgery 107:236–238

Friesen SR, Tomita T, Kimmel JR (1983) Pancreatic polypeptide update: its roles in detection of the trait for multiple endocrine adenopathy syndrome, type 1 and pancreatic polypeptide-secreting tumors. Surgery 94:1028–1037

Galmiche JP, Colin R, Dubois PM et al. (1978) Calcitonin secretion by a pancreatic somatostatinoma [letter]. N Engl J Med 299:1252

Gampa G, Gargantini L, Grigolato PG, Chiumello G (1976) Hypoglycemia of infancy caused by beta cell nesidioblastosis. Am J Dis Child 128:226–231

Ganda OP, Weir GC, Soeldner JS et al. (1977) "Somatostatinoma": a somatostatin-containing tumor of the endocrine pancreas. N Engl J Med 296:963–967

Garland H (1957) Pancreatic islet adenomatosis with hypoglycaemic episodes. Br Med J ii:969–971

Gelston AL, Delisle M-B, Patel YC (1982) Multiple endocrine adenomatosis type 1: occurrence in an octogenarian with high levels of circulating pancreatic polypeptide. JAMA 247:665–666

Gersell DJ, Gingerich RL, Greider MH (1979) Regional distribution and concentration of pancreatic polypeptide in the human and canine pancreas. Diabetes 28:11–15

Ghosh L, Huvos AG, Miké V (1973) The pancreatic islets in chondrosarcoma. Am J Pathol 71:23–32

Gibbard JP, Dartt DA, Rood RP, Rossi SR, Gray KL, Donowitz M (1988) Increased tear secretion in pancreatic cholera: a newly recognised symptom in an experiment of nature. Am J Med 85:552–554

Goodman ZD, Albores-Saavedra J, Lundblad DM (1984) Somatostatinoma of the cystic duct. Cancer 53:498–502

Goossens A, Gepts W, Saudubray J-M et al. (1989) Diffuse and focal nesidioblastosis: a clinicopathological study of 24 patients with persistent neonatal hyperinsulinemic hypoglycemia. Am J Surg Pathol 13:766–775

Goudswaard WB, Houthoff HJ, Koudstaal J, Bosman FT, Zwierstra RP (1984) Nesidioblastosis and islet cell hyperplasia of the pancreas – a secondary phenomenon – not a disease entity [abstract]. J Pathol 143:301A

Gould VE, Memoli VA, Dardi LE, Gould NS (1983) Nesidiodysplasia and nesidioblastosis of infancy: structural and functional correlations with the syndrome of hyperinsulinemic hypoglycemia. Pediatr Pathol 1:7–31

Grahame-Smith DG (1972) The carcinoid syndrome. Heinemann, London

Gregory RA, Tracy HJ, French JM, Sircus W (1960) Extraction of a gastrin-like substance from a pancreatic tumour in a case of Zollinger–Ellisin syndrome. Lancet i:1045–1048

Gregory RA, Grossmann MI, Tracy HJ, Bentley PH (1967) Nature of the secretagogue in Zollinger–Ellison tumours. Lancet ii:543–544

Griffiths DFR, Williliams GT, Williams ED (1987) Duodenal carcinoid tumours, phaeochromocytoma and neurofibromatosis: islet cell tumour, phaeochromocytoma and the von Hippel–Lindau complex: two distinctive neuroendocrine syndromes. Q J Med (New Series) 64:769–782

Grotting JC, Kassel S, Dehner LP (1979) Nesidioblastosis and congenital neuroblastoma: a histologic and immunocytochemical study of a new complex neurocrystopathy. Arch Pathol Lab Med 103:642–646

Gutniak M, Rosenquist U, Grimelius L et al. (1980) Report on a patient with watery diarrhoea syndrome caused by a pancreatic tumour containing neurotensin, enkephalin, and calcitonin. Acta Med Scand 208:95–100

Hale PJ, Suarez V, Williams A, Baddeley RM, Nattrass M (1987) Insulinoma and ganglioneuroma. Br J Surg 74:1183

Hamid QA, Bishop AE, Sikri KL, Varndell IM, Bloom SR, Polak JM (1986) Immunocytochemical characterization of ten pancreatic tumours, associated with the glucagonoma syndrome, using antibodies to separate regions of the pro-glucagon molecule and other neuroendocrine markers. Histopathology 10:119–133

Hansen R, Helm J, Wilson JF, Wilson S (1988) Non functioning islet cell carcinoma of the pancreas: complete response to continuous 5-fluorouracil infusion. Cancer 62:15–17

Happé RP, van der Gaag I, Lamens CBHW, van Toorenburg J, Rehfeld JF, Larsson L-I (1980) Zollinger–Ellison syndrome in three dogs. Vet Pathol 17:178–186

Hart WR, Hinerman DL (1965) Hyperplasia of pancreatic islets associated with extrapancreatic lymphoma and sarcoma. Metabolism 14:1158–1168

Hawkins KL, Summers BA, Kuhajda FP, Smith CA (1987) Immunocytochemistry of normal pancreatic islets and spontaneous islet cell tumors in dogs. Vet Pathol 24:170–179

Heitz PU (1984) Pancreatic endocrine tumours. In: Klöppel G, Heitz PU (eds) Pancreatic pathology. Churchill Livingstone, Edinburgh, pp 206–232

Heitz PU, Klöppel G, Häckl WH, Polak JM, Pearse AGE (1977) The pathologic basis of persistent hyperinsulinemic hypoglycemia in infants. Diabetes 26:632–642

Heitz PU, Kasper M, Polak JM, Klöppel G (1982) Pancreatic endocrine tumors: immunocytochemical analysis of 125 tumors. Hum Pathol 13 : 263–271

Heitz PU, Kasper M, Klöppel G, Polak JM, Vaitukaitis JL (1983) Glycoprotein-hormone alpha-chain production by pancreatic endocrine tumors: a specific marker for malignancy. Cancer 51 : 277–282

Holman CE, Wood DA, Stockton AB (1943) Unusual cases of hyperinsulinism and hypoglycemia. Arch Surg 47 : 165–177

Hull MT, Warfel KA, Muller J, Higgins JH (1979) Familial islet cell tumors in von Hippel-Lindau's disease. Cancer 44 : 1523–1526

Hutcheon DF, Bayless TM, Cameron JL, Baylin SB (1979) Hormone-mediated watery diarrhea in a family with multiple endocrine neoplasms. Ann Intern Med 90 : 932–934

Jensen SL, Christiansen LA, Oxholm A-M, Holst JJ (1984) Duodenal somatostatinoma. Br J Surg 71 : 159

Jerkins TW, Sacks HS, O'Dorisio TM, Tuttle S, Solomon SS (1987) Medullary carcinoma of the thyroid, pancreatic nesidioblastosis and microadenosis, and pancreatic polypeptide hypersecretion: a new association and clinical and hormonal responses to long-acting somatostatin analog SMS 201–995. J Clin Endocrinol Metab 64 : 1313–1319

Jones BR, Nicholls MR, Badman R (1976) Peptic ulceration in a dog associated with an islet cell carcinoma of the pancreas and an elevated plasma gastrin level. J Small Animal Pract 17 : 593–598

Kamisawa T, Fukayama M, Koike M, Tabuta I, Okamoto A (1987) A case of malignant cystic endocrine tumor of the pancreas. Am J Gastroenterol 82 : 86–89

Kane MG, O'Dorisio TM, Krejs GJ (1983) Production of secretory diarrhea by intravenous infusion of vasoactive intestinal polypeptide. N Engl J Med 309 : 1482–1485

Kaneko H, Yanaihara N, Ito S et al. (1979) Somatostatinoma of the duodenum. Cancer 44 : 2273–2279

Karnauchow PN (1982) Nesidioblastosis in adults without insular hyperfunction. Am J Clin Pathol 78 : 511–513

Kenny BD, Hamilton PW, Sloan JM, Buchanan KD, Johnston C (1988) The use of morphometry in the histological assessment of pancreatic islet cell tumours [abstract]. J Pathol 154 : 90A–91A

Kimball CP, Murlin JR (1923–1924) Aqueous extracts of pancreas: some precipitation reactions of insulin. J Biol Chem 58 : 337–346

Klöppel G, Heitz PU (1984) Persistent hyperinsulinaemic hypoglycaemia in infancy. In: Klöppel G, Heitz PU (eds) Pancreatic pathology. Churchill Livingstone, Edinburgh, pp 193–205

Klöppel G, Heitz PU (1988) Pancreatic endocrine tumors. Pathol Res Pract 183 : 155–168

Kniffin WD, Spencer SV, Memoli VA, LeMarbre PJ (1988) Metastatic islet cell amphicrine carcinoma of the pancreas: association with an eosinophilic infiltration of the skin. Cancer 62 : 1999–2004

Kovacs K, Horvath E, Ilse RG, Ilse D (1976) Spontaneous pancreatic beta cell tumor in the rat. Vet Pathol 13 : 286–294

Kovacs K, Horvath E, Ezrin C, Sepp H, Elkan I (1977) Immunoreactive somatostatin in pancreatic islet-cell carcinoma accompanied by ectopic ACTH syndrome. Lancet i : 1365–1366

Krejs GJ (1980) Effect of VIP infusion on water and ion transport in the human large intestine [letter]. Gastroenterology 78 : 1200

Krejs GJ, Òrci L, Conlon JM et al. (1979) Somatostatinoma syndrome: biochemical morphologic and clinical features. N Engl J Med 301 : 285–292

Krejs GJ, Fordtran JS, Bloom SR et al. (1980) Effect of VIP infusion on the water and ion transport in the human jejunum. Gastroenterology 78 : 722–727

Kümmerle F, Rückert K (1978) Chirurgie des endokrinen Pankreas in der Bundesrepublik. Engebnisse einer Umfrage.

Dtsch Med Wochenschr 103 : 729–732

Laidlaw GF (1938) Nesidioblastoma, the islet cell tumor of the pancreas. Am J Pathol 14 : 125–134

Lamiell JM, Salazar FG, Hsia YE (1989) von Hippel–Lindau disease affecting 43 members of a single kindred. Medicine 68 : 1–29

Larsson L-I, Schwartz T, Lundquist G et al. (1976) Occurrence of human pancreatic polypeptide in pancreatic endocrine tumors. Possible implication in the watery diarrhea syndrome. Am J Pathol 85 : 675–684

Larsson L-I, Hirsch MA, Holst JJ et al. (1977) Pancreatic somatostatinoma: clinical features and physiological implications. Lancet i : 666–668

Lawrence RD, Meyer A, Nevin S (1942) The pathological changes in the brain in fatal hypoglycaemia. Q J Med (New Series) 11 : 181–201

Lee CS, Charlton IG, Williams RA, Dhillon AP, Rhode J (1993) Malignant potential of aneuploid pancreatic endocrine tumours. J Pathol 169 : 451–456

Liu HM, Potter EL (1962) Development of the human pancreas. Arch Pathol 74 : 439–442

Ljungberg O, Järnerot G, Rolny P, Wickbom G (1981) Human pancreatic polypeptide (HPP) immunoreactivity in an infiltrating endocrine tumour of the papilla of Vater with unusual morphology. Virchows Arch [A] 392 : 119–126

Lokich J, Bothe A, O'Hara C, Federman M (1987) Metastatic islet cell tumor with ACTH, gastrin, and glucagon secretion. Cancer 59 : 2053–2058

London NJM, Bolia A, Millac P, James RFL, Bell PRF (1988) Localization of an occult impalpable insulinoma by intraoperative ultrasonography. J R Soc Med 81 : 663–664

Long RG, Bryant MG, Mitchell SJ, Adrian TE, Polak JM, Bloom SR (1981) Clinicopathological study of pancreatic and ganglioneuroblastoma tumours secreting vasoactive intestinal polypeptide (VIPomas). Br Med J ii : 1767–1771

Lopez-Kruger R, Dockerty MB (1947) Tumors of the islets of Langerhans. Surg Gynecol Obstet 85 : 495–511

Lucas A, Morley R, Cole TJ (1988) Adverse neurodevelopmental outcome of moderate neonatal hypoglycaemia. Br Med J 297 : 1304–1308

Luttgen PP, Storts RW, Rogers KS, Morton LD (1986) Insulinoma in a ferret. J Am Vet Med Assoc 189 : 920–921

Malagelada JR, Edis AJ, Adson MA, van Heerden JA, Go VLW (1983) Medical and surgical options in the management of patients with gastrinoma. Gastroenterology 84 : 1524–1532

Mallinson CN, Bloom SR, Warin AP, Salmon PR, Cox B (1974) A glucagonoma syndrome. Lancet ii : 1–5

Marks C (1979) Carcinoid tumors: a clinicopathologic study. GK Halland, Boston, MA

Marshall AHE, Sloper JC (1954) Pluriglandular adenomatosis of the pituitary, parathyroid and pancreatic islet cells associated with lipomatosis. J Pathol Bacteriol 68 : 225–229

McGuigan JE, Trudeau WL (1968) Immunochemical measurement of elevated levels of gastrin in the serum of patients with pancreatic tumors of the Zollinger-Ellison variety. N Engl J Med 278 : 1308–1313

Melmed S, Ezrin C, Kovacs K, Goodman RS, Frohman LA (1985) Acromegaly due to secretion of growth hormone by an ectopic pancreatic islet cell tumor. N Engl J Med 312 : 9–17

Melmed S, Yamashita S, Kovacs K, Ong J, Rosenblatt S, Braunstein G (1987) Cushing's syndrome due to ectopic pro-opiomelanocortin gene expression by islet cell carcinoma of the pancreas. Cancer 59 : 772–778

Miyazaki K, Funakoshi A, Nishihara S, Wasada T, Koga A, Ibayashi H (1986) Aberrant insulinoma in the duodenum. Gastroenterology 90 : 1280–1285

Modlin JM, Bloom SR, Mitchell SJ (1978) Experimental evidence of vasoactive intestinal peptide as the cause of the watery diarrhea syndrome. Gastroenterology 75:1051:1054

Moldawer PM, Nardi GL, Raker JW (1954) Concomitance of multiple adenomas of the parathyroids and pancreatic islets with tumor of the pituitary: a syndrome with familial incidence. Am J Med Sci 228:190–206

Morgan DR, Wells M, MacDonald RC, Johnston D (1985) Zollinger–Ellison syndrome due to gastrin-secreting ovarian mucinous cystadenoma. Br J Obstet Gynaecol 92:867–869

Montgomery DAD, Welbourn RB (1975) Medical and surgical endocrinology. Edward Arnold, London, pp 487–500

Morrison AB (1980) Islet cell tumors and the diarrheogenic syndrome. In: Fitzgerald PJ, Morrison AB (eds) The pancreas. Williams and Wilkins, Baltimore, pp 185–207

Neve ET (1891) On the morbid anatomy of the pancreas. Lancet ii:659–661

Nicholls AG (1902) Simple adenoma of the pancreas arising from an island of Langerhans. J Med Res 8:385–395

Norbin A, Berg M, Ericsson M, Ingemansson S, Olsson E, Sundler F (1984) Pancreatic polpeptide-producing tumors. Report on two cases. Cancer 53:2688–2691

Norton JA, Cromack DT, Shawker TH et al. (1988) Intraoperative ultrasonographic localization of islet cell tumors: a prospective comparison to palpation. Ann Surg 207:160–168

Novak R, Willmas J, Johnson W (1979) Hypertrophy and hyperplasia of islets of Langerhans associated with androgen therapy. Arch Pathol Lab Med 103:483–485

O'Brien TD, Hayden DW, O'Leary TP, Caywood DD, Johnson KH (1987) Canine pancreatic endocrine tumors: immunohistochemical analysis of hormone content and amyloid. Vet Pathol 24:308–314

Ohneda A, Otsuki M, Fugiya H, Yaginuma N, Kokubo T, Ohtani H (1979) A malignant insulinoma transformed into a glucagonoma syndrome. Diabetes 28:962–969

O'Leary JL, Womack N (1934) Histology of adenoma of the islets of Langerhans. Arch Pathol 17:291–310

Ordóñez NG, Manning JT, Raymond AK (1985) Argentaffin endocrine carcinoma (carcinoid) of the pancreas with concomitant breast metastases: an immunohistochemical and electron microscopic study. Hum Pathol 16:746–751

Ordóñez NG, Balsaver, AM, Mackay B (1988) Mucinous islet cell (amphicrine) carcinoma of the pancreas associated with watery diarrhea and hypokalemia syndrome. Hum Pathol 19:1458–1461

O'Riordan JLH, Blanshard GP, Maxham A, Nabarro JDN (1966) Corticotrophin-secreting carcinomas. Q J Med (New Series) 35:137–147

Pagliara AS, Karl IE, Haymond M, Kipnis DM (1973) Hypoglycemia in infancy and childhood. Part I. J Pediatr 82:365–379

Pearse AGE (1984) Islet development and the APUD concept. In: Klöppel G, Heitz PU (eds) Pancreatic pathology. Churchill Livingstone, Edinburgh, p 127

Pearse AGE, Polak JM, Heath CM (1974) Polypeptide hormone production by "carcinoid" apudomas and their relevant cytochemistry. Virchows Arch [B] 16:95–109

Peart WS, Porter KA, Robertson JIS, Sandler M, Baldock E (1963) Carcinoid syndrome due to pancreatic-duct neoplasm secreting 5-hydroxytryptophan and 5-hydroxytryptamine. Lancet i:239–242

Pelletier G, Cortot A, Launay J-M et al. (1984) Serotonin-secreting and insulin-secreting ileal carcinoid tumor and the use of in vitro culture of tumoral cells. Cancer 54:319–322

Perrone T, Sibley RK, Rosai J (1985) Duodenal gangliocytic paraganglioma: an immunohistochemical and ultrastructural study and a hypothesis concerning its origin. Am J Surg Pathol 9:31–41

Pipeleers D, Somers G, Gepts W, de Nutte N, de Vroede M (1979) Plasma pancreatic hormone levels in a case of somatostatin-

oma: diagnostic and therapeutic implications. J Clin Endocrinol Metab 49:572–579

Pipeleers-Marichal M, Somers G, Willems G et al. (1990) Duodenal gastrinomas as a source of hypergastrinemia and Zollinger–Ellison syndrome in patients with multiple endocrine neoplasia type 1. N Engl J Med 322:723–727

Polak JM, Wigglesworth JS (1976) Islet-cell hyperplasia and sudden infant death. Lancet ii:570–571

Polak JM, Stagg B, Pearse AGE (1972) Two types of Zollinger–Ellison syndrome: immunofluorescent, cytochemical and ultrastructural studies of the antral and pancreatic gastrin cells in different clinical states. Gut 13:501–512

Polak JM, Bloom SR, Adrian TE, Heitz PU, Bryant MG, Pearse AGE (1976) Pancreatic polypeptide in insulinomas, gastrinomas, VIPomas, and glucagonomas. Lancet i:328–330

Ponsky JL, Hoffman M, Rhodes RS (1979) Arteriovenous fistula and portal hypertension secondary to islet cell tumor of the pancreas. Surgery 85:408–411

Potter EL, Seckel HPG, Stryker WA (1941) Hypertrophy and hyperplasia of the islets of Langerhans of the fetus and the newborn infant. Arch Pathol 31:467–482

Probst A, Lotz M, Heitz P (1978) von Hippel-Lindau's disease, syringomyelia and multiple endocrine tumors: a complex neuroendocrinopathy. Virchows Arch [A] 378:265–272

Ravazzola M, Orci L (1980) Glucagon and glicentin immunoreactivity are topologically segregated in the alpha granule of the human pancreatic A cell. Nature 284:66–67

Rayman G, Santo M, Salomon F et al. (1984) Hyperinsulinaemic hypoglycaemia due to chlorpropamide-induced nesidioblastosis. J Clin Pathol 37:651–654

Reid JD, Song-Lim Y, Pretrelli M, Jaffe R (1982) Ductoinsular tumors of the pancreas: a light, electron microscopic and immunohistochemical study. Cancer 49:908–915

Rivier J, Spiess J, Thorner M, Vale W (1982) Chracterization of a growth hormone releasing factor from a human pancreatic islet tumour. Nature 300:276–278

Rode J, Williams RA, Charlton IG, Dhillon AP, Moss E (1990) Nuclear DNA analysis in benign and malignant islet cell tumours [abstract]. J Pathol 160:154A

Rood RP, De Lellis RA, Dayal Y, Donowitz M (1988) Pancreatic cholera syndrome due to a vasoactive intestinal polypeptide-producing tumor: further insights into the pathophysiology. Gastroenterology 94:813–818

Rousseaux CG (1987) Ultrastructure of a canine gastrinoma. J Comp Pathol 97:605–607

Saeger W, Schulte HM, Klöppel G (1986) Morphology of a GHRH producing pancreatic islet cell tumor causing acromegaly. Virchows Arch [A] 409:547–554

Sandler M, Karim SMM, Williams ED (1968) Prostaglandins in amine-peptide-secreting tumours. Lancet ii:1053–1055

Sardi A, Singer JA (1987) Insulinoma and gastrinoma in Werner's disease (MENI). Arch Surg 122:835–836

Scheimberg IB, Bishop AE, Colfour AM, Williamson RCN, Polak JM (1991) A new pattern of neuroendocrine tumours in MEN 1 [abstract]. J Pathol 163:165A

Shames JM, Dhurandhar NR, Blackard WG (1968) Insulin-secreting bronchial carcinoid tumor with widespread metastases. Am J Med 44:632–637

Shermeta DW, Mendelsohn G, Haller JA (1980) Hyperinsulinemic hypoglycemia of the neonate associated with persistent fetal histology and function of the pancreas. Ann Surg 191:182–186

Sidi Y, Liban E, Solomon F, Pinkhas J (1984) Multiple islet cell adenomas in a patient with secondary hemochromatosis. Arch Pathol Lab Med 108:690–692

Sipple JH (1961) The association of pheochromocytoma with carcinoma of the thyroid gland. Am J Med 31:163–166

Snook JA, van der Star R, Weller RO (1986) Insulinoma producing progressive neurological deterioration over 30 years.

Br Med J 293:241-242

Solt J, Kádas I, Polak JM et al. (1984) A pancreatic-polypeptide-producing tumor of the stomach. Cancer 54:1101-1104

Somers G, Pipeleers-Marichal M, Gepts W, Pipeleers D (1983) A case of duodenal somatostatinoma: diagnostic usefulness of calcium-pentagastrin test. Gastroenterology 85:1192-1198

Spencer H (1955) Pancreatic islet-cell adenomata. J Pathol Bacteriol 69:259-267

Stamm B, Hedinger CE, Saremaslani P (1986) Duodenal and ampullary carcinoid tumors. Virchows Arch [A] 408:475-489

Stefanini P, Carboni M, Patrassi N, Basoli A (1974) Beta-islet cell tumors of the pancreas: results of a study on 1067 cases. Surgery 75:597-609

Steiner AL, Goodman AD, Powers SR (1968) A study of a kindred with pheochromocytoma, medullary thyroid carcinoma, hyperparathyroidism and Cushing's disease: multiple endocrine neoplasia type 2. Medicine 47:371-409

Stipa F, Arganini M, Bibbo M et al. (1987) Nuclear DNA analysis of insulinomas and gastrinomas. Surgery 102:988-998

Straus E, Johnson GF, Yallow RS (1977) Canine Zollinger-Ellison syndrome. Gastroenterology 72:380-381

Swinburn BA, Mee Ling Y, Lane MR, Nicholson GI, Holdaway IM (1988) Neurofibromatosis associated with somatostatinoma: a report of two patients. Clin Endocrinol 28:353-359

Taccagni GL, Carlucci M, Sironi M, Cantabone A, de Carlo V (1986) Duodenal somatostatinoma with psammoma bodies: an immunohistochemical and ultrastructural study. Am J Gastroenterol 81:33-37

Thompson GB, van Heerden JA, Grant CS, Carney JA, Ilstrup DM (1988) Islet cell carcinomas of the pancreas: a twenty-year experience. Surgery 104:1011-1017

Thompson NW, Ekhauser FE, Vinik AI, Lloyd RV, Fiddian-Green RG, Strodel WE (1984) Cystic neuroendocrine neoplasms of the pancreas and liver. Ann Surg 199:158-164

Thorner MO, Perryman RL, Cronin MJ et al. (1982) Successful treatment of acromegaly by removal of a pancreatic islet tumor secreting a growth hormone-releasing factor. J Clin Invest 70:965-977

Tishler PV (1975) A family with coexistent von Recklinghausen's neurofibromatosis and von Hippel–Lindau's disease: diseases possibly derived from a common gene. Neurology 25:840-844

Tomita T, Friesen SR, Kimmel JR, Doull V, Pollock HG (1983) Pancreatic polypeptide-secreting islet cell tumors. A study of three cases. Am J Pathol 113:134-142

Tragl K-H, Mayr WR (1977) Familial islet-cell adenomatosis. Lancet ii:426-428

Unger RH, Bochner J (1964) Identification of insulin and glucagon in a bronchogenic metastasis. J Clin Endocrinol Metab 24:823-831

Vance JE, Stoll RW, Kitabchi AE, Buchanan KD, Hollander D, Williams RH (1972) Familial nesidioblastosis as the predominant manifestation of multiple endocrine adenomatosis. Am J Med 52:211-227

van der Sluys Veer J, Choufoer JC, Querido A, van der Heul RO, Hollander CF, van Rÿssel TG (1964) Metastasising islet-cell tumour of the pancreas associated with hypoglycaemia and carcinoid syndrome. Lancet i:1416-1419

Vella MA, Cowie AGA, Gorsuch AN, Watson LCA (1988) Giant gastrinoma in a patient with multiple endocrine adenopathy (type 1). J R Soc Med 81:359-360

Verbov J (1981) Necrolytic migratory erythema associated with an islet cell tumour of the pancreas. Dermatologica 163:189-194

Verner JV, Morrison AB (1958) Islet cell tumor and a syndrome of refractory watery diarrhea and hypokalemia. Am J Med 25:374-380

Vinick AI, Strodel WE, Eckhauser FE, Moattari AR, Lloyd R (1987) Somatostatinomas, PPomas, neurotensinomas. Semin Oncol 14:263-281

Warden MJ, German JC, Buckingham BA (1988) The surgical management of hyperinsulinism in infancy due to nesidioblastosis. J Pediatr Surg 23:462-465

Warner TFCS, Seo IS, Madura JA, Polak JM, Pearse AGE (1980) Pancreatic-polypeptide-producing apudoma of the liver. Cancer 46:1146-1151

Warren S (1926) Adenomas of the islands of Langerhans. Am J Pathol 2:335-340

Warshaw AL, Compton CC, Lewandrowski K, Cardenosa G, Mueller PR (1990) Cystic tumors of the pancreas: new clinical, radiologic and pathologic observations in 67 patients. Ann Surg 212:432-445

Weichert R, Reed R, Creech O (1967) Carcinoid-islet tumors of the duodenum. Ann Surg 165:660-669

Wells CA, Taylor SM, Cuello CA (1985) Argentaffin and argyrophil reactions and serotonin content of endocrine tumours. J Clin Pathol 38:49-53

Wermer P (1954) Genetic aspects of adenomatosis of endocrine glands. Am J Med 16:363-371

Wermer P (1963) Endocrine adenomatosis and peptic ulcer in a large kindred. Inherited multiple hormone-producing tumors and mosaic pleiotropism in man. Am J Med 35:205-212

Wermer P (1974) Multiple endocrine adenomatosis: multiple hormone-producing tumours, a familial syndrome. Clin Gastroenterol 3:671-684

Wilander E, El-Salhy M, Willén R, Grimelius L (1981) Immunocytochemistry and electron microscopy of an argentaffin endocrine tumour of the pancreas. Virchows Arch [A] 392:263-269

Wilder RM, Allan FN, Power MH, Robertson HE (1927) Carcinoma of the islands of the pancreas: hyperinsulinism and hypoglycemia. JAMA 89:348-355

Williams ED, Sandler M (1963) The classification of carcinoid tumours. Lancet ii:238-239

Wotherspoon AC, Rode J (1989) Nesidioblastosis: a histological and immunocytochemical study of 11 cases [abstract]. J Pathol 157:170A

Wynick D (1990) Gastrinoma syndrome in multiple endocrine neoplasia. Br Med J 301:489-490

Wynick D, Ratcliffe WA, Heath DA, Ball S, Barnard M, Bloom SR (1990) Treatment of a malignant endocrine tumour secreting parathyroid hormone related protein. Br Med J 300:1314-1315

Yamashita Y, Okuzono Y, Yokota T et al. (1985) Morphologic study of three cases of insulinoma: histochemical and ultra-structural studies. Cancer 55:841-847

Zollinger RM (1987) Gastrinoma: the Zollinger-Ellison syndrome. Semin Oncol 14:247-252

Zollinger RM, Ellison EH (1955) Primary peptic ulcerations of the jejunum associated with islet cell tumors of the pancreas. Ann Surg 142:709-728

11 Secondary Tumours, Lymphomas and Rare Tumours

Secondary Tumours

Secondary tumours of the pancreas are common but, as they seldom produce clinical symptoms or recognisable disturbances of pancreatic function, they have been considered in the past to be of little practical importance. The modern methods of producing images of the pancreas, and of its ducts and vessels, may, however, have made information about secondary tumours of the organ more than purely academic.

Secondary tumours of the pancreas may be the result of the spread of malignant tumours by any of the usual routes; direct invasion by the extension of cancers of neighbouring organs is relatively common, especially in carcinoma of the stomach (Fig. 11.1) or the transverse colon. The lymph nodes in the vicinity of the pancreas may also be the site of primary or secondary tumours that may infiltrate the pancreas. Willis (1973), for example, in his series of 500 necropsies found that direct invasion was the commonest way in which secondary tumours reached the pancreas, with 18 examples of this type of spread, 13 of these having primary carcinoma of the stomach. Cubilla and Fitzgerald (1980), however, found only 16 cases of invasion of the pancreas from cancer of contiguous organs amongst 2587 consecutive autopsies carried out between 1973 and 1978 at Memorial Hospital in New York; but, like Willis, they found that the stomach was the commonest site for the primary tumour, with the colon as the next most common site. In Cubilla and Fitzgerald's series, metastatic spread by the blood stream was the most common cause of secondary tumours in the pancreas. They found that metastatic tumour was present in the pancreas in 273 cases, with carcinoma of the breast as the commonest type of primary tumour. Carcinoma of the lung, however (Figs 11.2, 11.3), was the primary cancer in almost the same number of cases, the figures being 51 primary carcinomas of the breast, and 49 primary carcinomas of the lung. The next most common type of cancer in their series to cause blood-borne secondary tumours in the pancreas was malignant melanoma (23 cases). This condition was noted to have caused secondary cancer of the pancreas over a century ago by Cruveilhier (1830) in his *Anatomie Pathologique du Corps Humain*, an atlas that was published in instalments between 1829 and 1835. Willis, in a series of 127 cases with haemic metastatic tumours of the pancreas, found that the primary tumours responsible were carcinoma of the lung in 34, malignant melanoma in 31, carcinoma of the kidney in 12, and carcinoma of the breast in 12. Although these findings differ slightly from those of Cubilla and Fitzgerald in relation to carcinoma of the breast, they confirm the importance of carcinoma of the lung and of malignant melanoma as the primary causes of secondary tumours of the pancreas. Of course, any type of malignancy that disseminates itself by the blood stream may involve the pancreas, which seems, unlike the spleen, to have no special resistance against metastatic cancer.

Secondary blood-borne tumours of the pancreas are almost invariably associated with multiple metastases in other organs, and in the pancreas itself, secondary tumours tend to be multiple rather

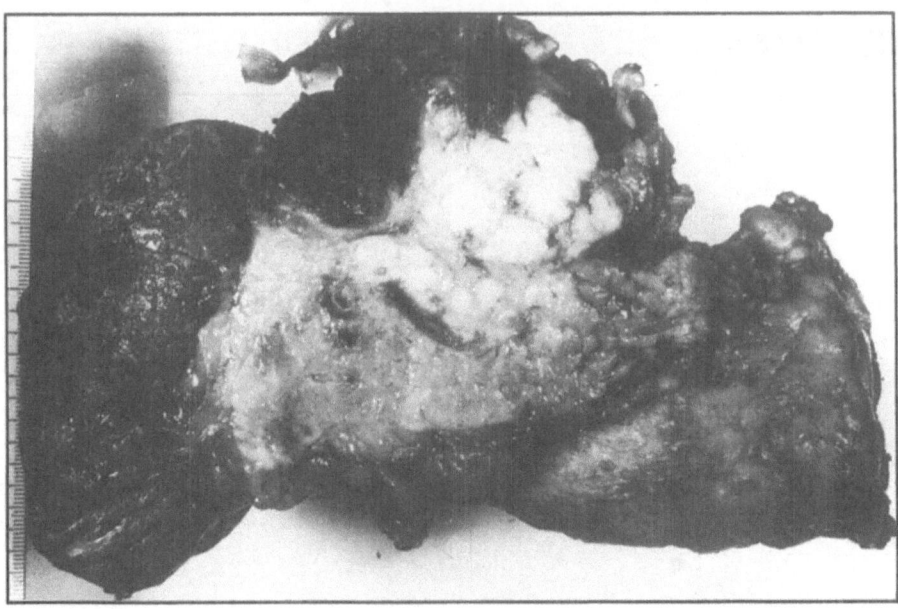

Fig. 11.1. Direct invasion of the pancreas by carcinoma. The specimen has been photographed from its posterior aspect. The patient had carcinoma of the stomach with spread to lymph nodes, from which invasion of the pancreas can be seen to be taking place.

than single. In cases studied by Willis, the pancreatic metastases were multiple in 40 and single in 19. They are usually well defined, seldom become large enough to be palpable clinically, and may cause surprisingly little disruption of the pattern of the duct system when radio-opaque material is injected postmortem. Willis could find only one reference to secondary carcinoma in the head of the pancreas that caused obstructive jaundice. It was a case which, at autopsy, was found to have a latent primary carcinoma of the prostate. He also referred to a publication that recorded fat necrosis in the omentum and perirenal fat in association with haemorrhagic metastases in the pancreas from a primary carcinoma of the lung. If diabetes is associated with secondary carcinoma, it is likely to be coincidental for,

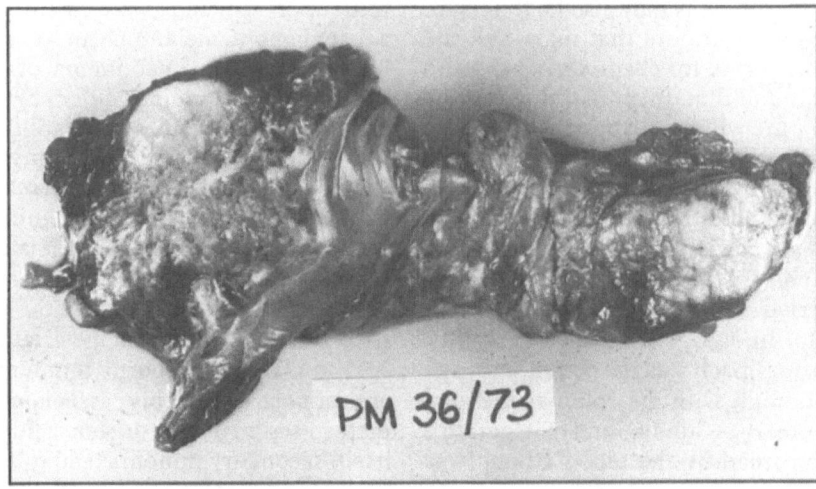

Fig. 11.2. Blood-borne secondary carcinoma of the pancreas. Deposits of secondary carcinoma are present in both the head and the tail.

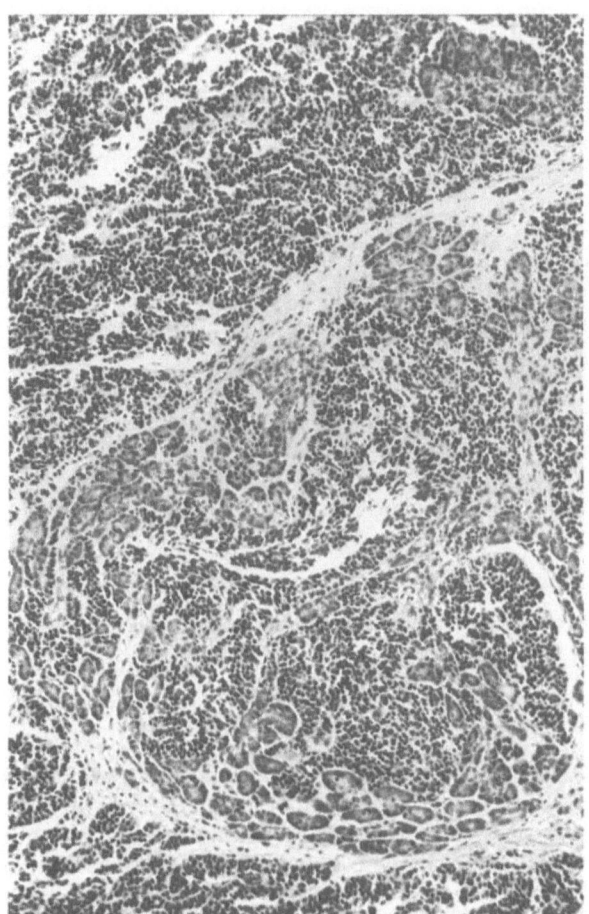

Fig. 11.3. Blood-borne secondary carcinoma of the pancreas. Pancreatic acini are embedded in secondary carcinoma of the anaplastic small cell (oat cell) type of carcinoma from a primary carcinoma of the lung. H&E, × 105

as with primary cancer of the pancreas, the islets of Langerhans often seem more conspicuous microscopically, being larger and more numerous at the advancing edges of secondary tumours. Willis also referred to published examples of lymphatic permeation of the pancreas from carcinoma of the stomach without gross tumour formation, although he had no personal experience of this type of secondary involvement of the pancreas.

An example of an unusual metastatic tumour of the pancreas was included by Fermelia et al. (1988) in their collection of unusual pancreatic lesions. The tumour presented as a large epigastric mass in a 60-year-old white woman, whose right breast had been removed by local excision 3 years previously because of a cystosarcoma phyllodes that weighed 2.5 kg. At laparotomy, a mass 16 × 16 × 9 cm replaced the body and tail of the pancreas. It had a

well-defined pseudocapsule, but the pancreatic duct was infiltrated and deformed by the tumour, whose microscopic appearances were similar to those of the previously removed breast tumour. The authors could find no previously reported example of cystosarcoma phyllodes with a pancreatic metastasis. The patient died within a year of surgery.

Pancreatic Involvement in Lymphoma

Lymphoma predominantly involving the pancreas is rare, but in their report of such a case, Cappell et al. (1989) were able to refer to 11 previously reported cases. They found that the condition comprised less than 0.2% of pancreatic malignancies and that it was almost never suspected clinically; it was usually found during surgery for suspected adenocarcinoma. All the reported cases were non-Hodgkin's lymphomas. Chylous ascites may be an associated feature (Fischer and Kabakow 1987). If the diagnosis is suspected, guided percutaneous needle biopsy is recommended. A good response to chemotherapy or radiotherapy would support a positive diagnosis.

Because there are peripancreatic lymph nodes, and because the coeliac and perigastric lymph nodes are nearby, lymphomatous diasease affecting any of these sites may lead to direct invasion of the pancreas. In a review of 323 patients with lymphoma who came to autopsy at the Memorial and James Ewing Hospitals in New York during the 5-year period 1960 to 1964, Ehrlich et al. (1968) found that the pancreas was the gastrointestinal organ most commonly invaded by tumour. There was invasion of the pancreas in 86 patients, of whom 53 had reticulum cell sarcoma, 18 lymphosarcoma (Figs 11.4, 11.5) and 15 Hodgkin's disease. Many of the patients with pancreatic involvement had suffered from pain that was attributed to the retroperitoneal tumours invading the pancreas. In four patients, secondary lymphoma in the head of the pancreas had caused obstructive jaundice.

In a later analysis of the autopsies carried out at Memorial Hospital from 1973 to the end of 1978, Cubilla and Fitzgerald (1980) found that, among the 2587 consecutive autopsies carried out during that time, there were 40 in which the pancreas was involved by malignant lymphoma and 19 in which there was leukaemic infiltration of the pancreas, seven showed involvement by Hodgkin's disease (Figs 11.6–11.10), and myelomatosis had involved the pancreas in one.

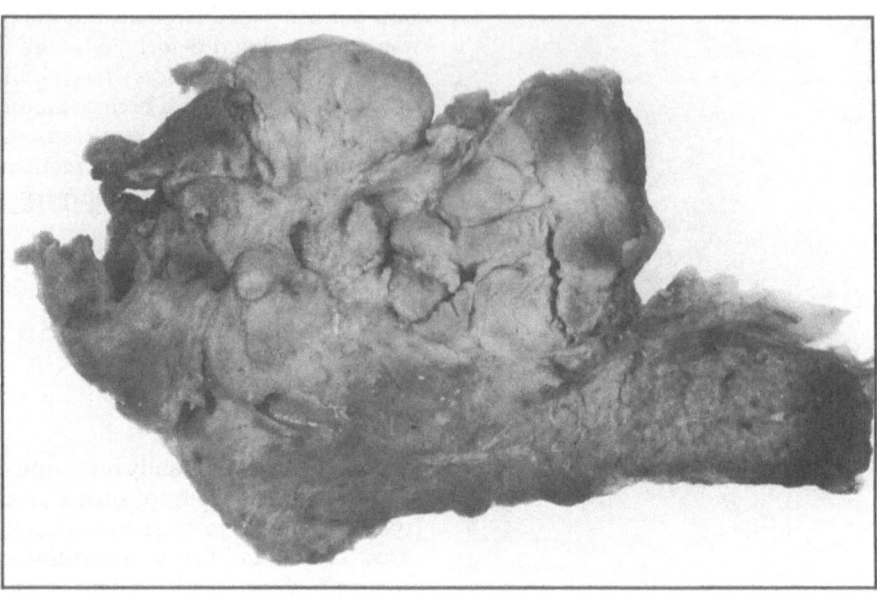

Fig. 11.4. Direct invasion of the pancreas by lymphosarcoma that has extended from adjacent lymph nodes affected by the disease.

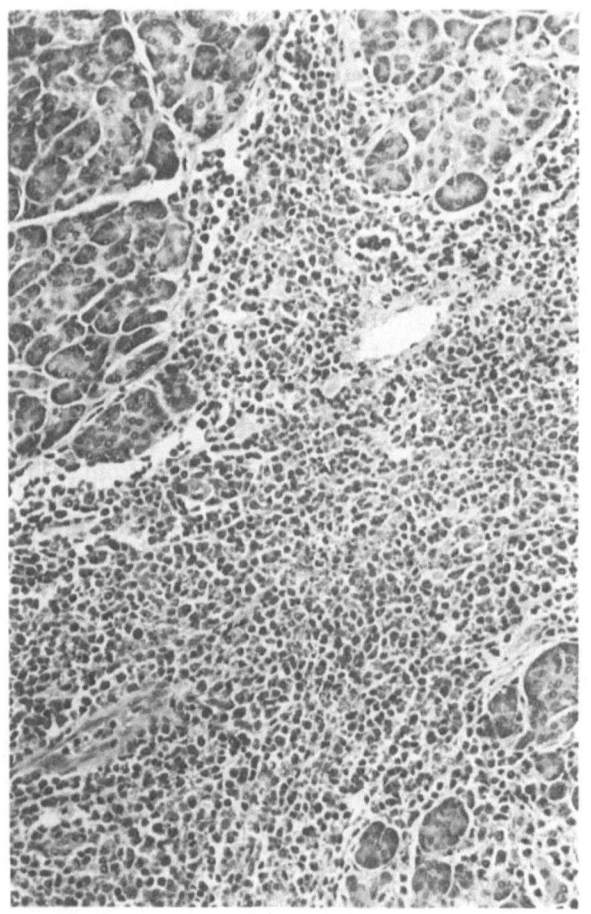

Such figures make it clear that the pancreas is considerably less likely to be involved by Hodgkin's disease than by the non-Hodgkin's lymphomas, but Gowing (1973), who reported the findings in 130 necropsies on patients who had been treated for Hodgkin's disease at the Royal Marsden Hospital in London, found that the pancreas was involved in 14, an incidence of 11%. Gowing's cases included ten examples of extranodal Hodgkin's disease; one of these had Hodgkin's disease in the liver, lungs, bones, kidneys and pancreas. When pancreatic involvement is present in Hodgkin's disease, it is seldom of clinical importance. Levitan et al. (1961), who made an analysis of 116 patients with Hodgkin's disease who became jaundiced, did not attribute the jaundice in any of these cases to Hodgkin's disease of the pancreas.

Burkitt's lymphoma seems to have a special tendency to involve extranodal sites and such sites include the pancreas (Wright 1970), but secondary invasion of the pancreas from retroperitoneal tumour masses is also very common in the advanced stages of the disease. In his post-mortem study of 50 cases of Burkitt's tumour, Wright (1964)

Fig. 11.5. The microscopic appearance of the pancreas illustrated in Fig. 11.4. Lymphosarcoma is infiltrating the interlobular septa and is beginning to infiltrate the lobules. H&E, × 150

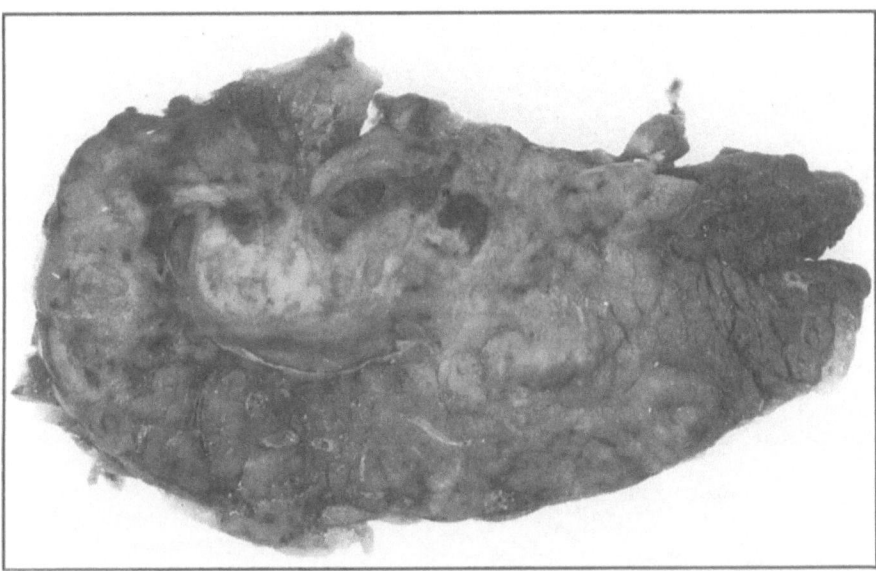

Fig. 11.6. Direct invasion of the pancreas by Hodgkin's disease that has extended from adjacent lymph nodes.

found that the pancreas was involved in 27. In 15 of these there were massive retroperitoneal tumours that made it impossible to determine whether the tumour had arisen within the pancreas or whether the gland had been invaded from outside; in some cases the pancreas could not be recognised at all in the retroperitoneal mass. The pancreatic tumour was described as diffuse, except in one, in which it was said to be nodular. The 50 cases of Burkitt's tumour included 35 children and 15 adults. The pancreas contained tumour in 20 of the children and seven of the adults, so that in the whole series the pancreas was involved in 54%. In a series of 45 cases of non-Hodgkin's, non-Burkitt's lymphoma that came to post-mortem in Uganda during the period when the cases of Burkitt's tumour were being col-

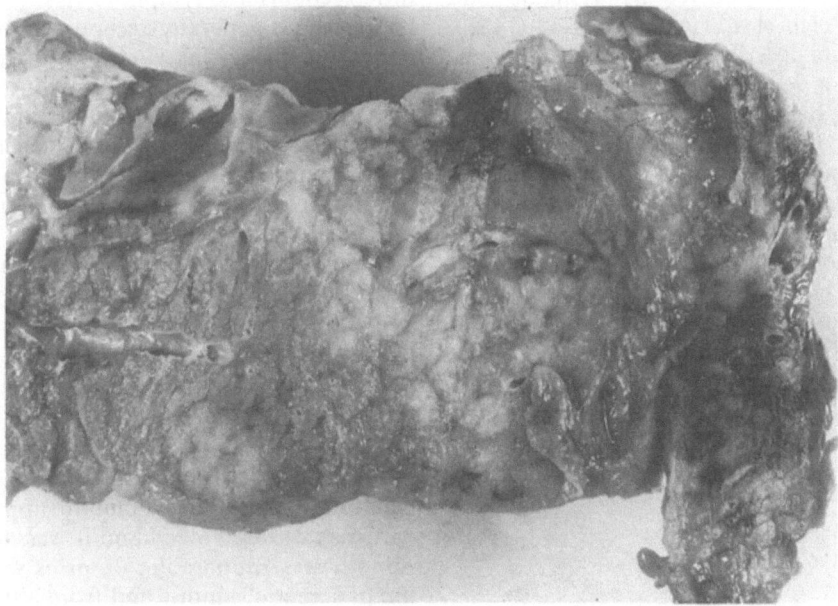

Fig. 11.7. Infiltration of the pancreas by neoplastic tissue in Hodgkin's disease. In this case it is not obvious whether the pancreatic involvement was the result of extension from adjacent nodes or not.

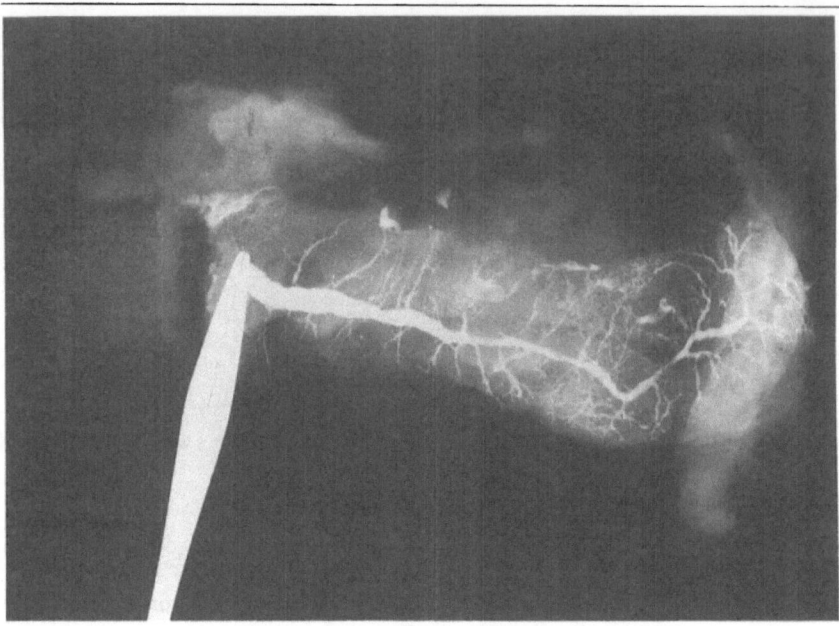

Fig. 11.8. A radiograph of the pancreas shown in Fig. 11.7, after the ducts had been injected with barium. Very little deformity of the duct system has been caused by the infiltration of the gland by the Hodgkin's tissue.

lected, the pancreas was involved in 12, an incidence of 27%.

Metastatic disease of the pancreas, as distinct from direct involvement, in malignant lymphomatous disease appears to be rare, but the pancreas may be the site of blood-borne secondary deposits in some cases of malignant lymphoma of the thyroid, as has been reported by Winship and Greene (1955), Welch et al. (1958) and Cox (1964). One of the patients described by Cox became jaundiced because of a deposit of secondary malignant lymphoma in the head of the pancreas, along with other secondary deposits in the cervical lymph nodes, duodenum, jejunum and kidneys. This distribution of secondary tumours is in keeping with the suggestion, made by Brewer and Orr (1953), that malignant lymphomas of the thyroid have a special tendency to metastasise to the gastrointestinal organs. Pancreatitis due to metastatic involvement of the pancreas from a primary lymphoma of the testis has been reported by Ade et al. (1991).

Rare Tumours

Sarcomas

When Ewing discussed sarcoma of the pancreas in 1941, he wrote that very few satisfactory reports of pancreatic sarcoma were available. Frantz, in 1959, also found the diagnosis questionable in many of the older reports of sarcoma of the pancreas. Ewing, however, having studied the publications that were available up to 1940, thought it probable that spindle cell sarcoma and lymphosarcoma might arise in the pancreas. The normal pancreas contains little recognisable lymphoid tissue, but extranodal lymphoma is generally accepted as being capable of appearing in organs such as the testes, in which lymphoid tissue is not usually present; thus, primary lymphosarcoma of the pancreas cannot be dismissed as impossible. There has, however, except for the studies of Burkitt's lymphoma, been only one relatively recent report of a malignant lymphoma of the pancreas. That tumour was diagnosed as a reticulosarcoma of the pancreas and the case was published by Ziarek et al. in 1975. The patient was a boy aged 12, who was found a laparotomy to have a solid yellowish-white tumour in the head of the pancreas. The tumour, which was adherent to the duodenum, had not caused obstructive jaundice but had encroached upon the portal vein and inferior vena cava sufficiently to cause a collateral circulation. Lynph nodes along the upper aspect of the pancreas were involved and it was decided that the tumour was inoperable. Biopsies were taken from the pancreatic tumour and from a lymph node. On microscopic examination, the normal appearances of both the pancreas and of the lymph node were

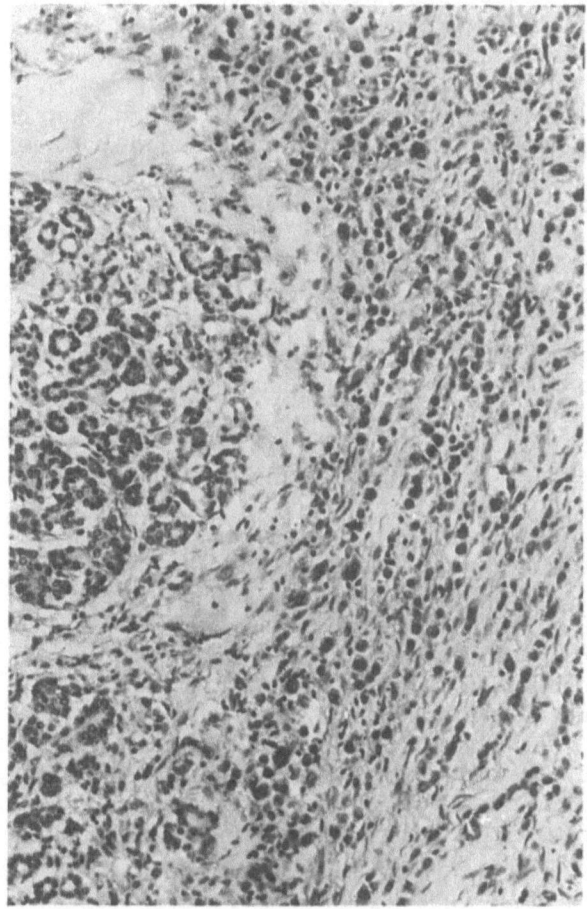

Fig. 11.9. A low-power view of the pancreas whose macroscopic appearance is shown in Fig. 11.6. As is usual when Hodgkin's disease has been fatal, almost all the reacting cells have disappeared and few cells other than the neoplastic cells are present. H&E, × 150

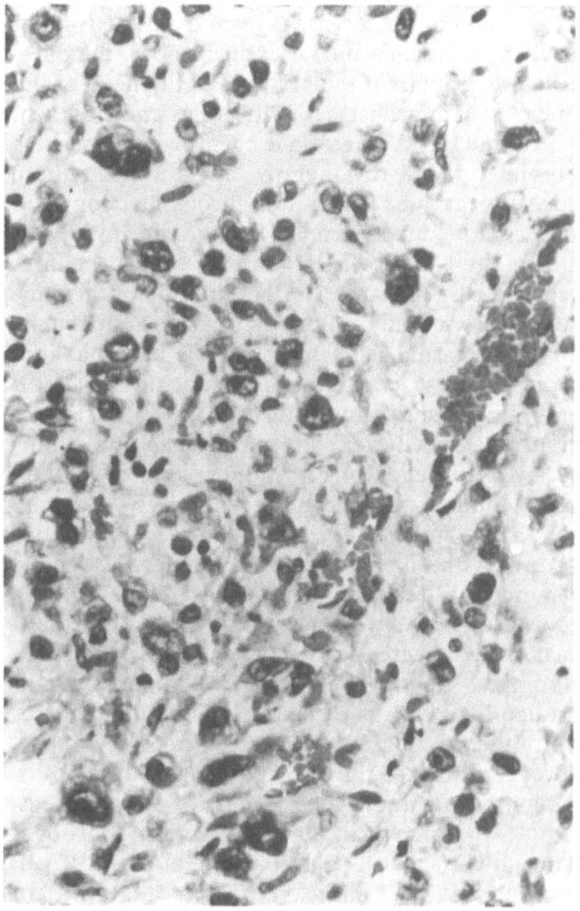

Fig. 11.10. A higher magnification of the Hodgkin's tissue shown in the previous figure. H&E, × 375

completely replaced by a homogeneous proliferation of reticulum cells and lymphocytes. There were many mitotic figures and a diagnosis of reticulosarcoma of the pancreas with invasion of lymph nodes was made. In spite of chemotherapy the patient died 3 months later in a cachectic state after a severe haematemesis. There was no autopsy.

From earlier reports, however, it seems that reticulum cell sarcomas and lymphomas are not invariably inoperable. Feather and Kuhn, for example, in 1951 carried out a total pancreatectomy in a man aged 29 for a pancreatic tumour that was diagnosed microscopically as a reticulum cell sarcoma. Although the tumour involved the duodenum and peripancreatic lymph nodes, the patient was alive and able to carry on his activities 1 year after the removal of his tumour. In childhood too, a lymphoid tumour is sometimes amenable to surgery;

there is a very short report, in an addendum to a paper by Becker (1957), of the successful removal by Robert E. Gross of a lymphoma of the head of the pancreas in a 2-year-old boy.

Extraskeletal plasma cell tumours have also been recorded as presenting as pancreatic tumours, and, at least in the case reported by Richards et al. (1958), there was a relatively long survival after a purely palliative procedure. The tumour, 9.5 cm in diameter, was situated in the head of the pancreas and the original biopsy was interpreted as Hodgkin's disease. The tumour was causing obstructive jaundice, and palliative cholecystjejunostomy was carried out. The patient, a woman 77 years old, then survived for 5 years before metastatic tumour in the neck was found microscopically to consist of extramedullary plasmacytoma and, after a review of the sections of the pancreatic tumour, it too was diagnosed as an extraskeletal plasmacytoma. The patient died of the disease 6 years from the time of her first attendance and, after an autopsy, the diagnosis was primary plasmacytoma of the head of the pancreas, with metastases in the lungs and stomach. The tumour in the neck had been made to regress completely by X-ray therapy, and the immediate cause of death was perforation through a neoplastic nodule in the duodenum just beyond the ampulla of Vater. The authors believed this to be the first recorded case of primary plasmacytoma of the pancreas. More recently, a tumour, diagnosed histologically as a plasma cell sarcoma of the pancreas in a woman aged 37, was fatal, with subcutaneous and cerebral metastases, in a little over a month after the tumour had been excised from the head of the pancreas (Doutre et al. 1976). In the case of metastatic extramedullary plasmacytoma reported by Akiyama and Krigel (1988), an 80-year-old woman, whose nasopharyngeal plasmacytoma appeared to have responded well to radiotherapy, developed multiple metastases, one of which was in the head of the pancreas. The pancreatic deposit caused a palpable abdominal tumour with biliary obstruction and simulated a primary carcinoma of the pancreas. A computed tomography-directed needle biopsy, however, indicated the true nature of the mass.

Reports of spindle cell sarcoma of the pancreas, and of leiomyosarcoma, include those of Brunschwig (1949), who treated a spindle cell sarcoma of the pancreas causing a secondary tumour in the left lung, by radical pancreatectomy, splenectomy and left total pneumonectomy at one operation, and also the case of leiomyosarcoma of the pancreas published by Ross (1951–1952). In the latter case, the sarcoma had caused complete replacement of the pancreas in a man aged 80. There were metastases in many organs, apparently by blood-spread, for there was no involvement of lymph nodes. The patient had had diabetes mellitus. Other published reports are those of Berman and Levene (1956), and of Brooke and Maxwell (1966). Berman and Levene treated a sarcoma of the pancreas, probably of smooth muscle origin, by pancreaticoduodenectomy. The tumour had invaded the ampullary region and the common bile duct, but the patient was well, except for postoperative diabetes, 1 year and 7 months after the operation. The patient that Brooke and Maxwell treated by pancreaticoduodenectomy was still alive after 8 years. The microscopic findings in the tumour they removed were that it was composed of pleomorphic spindle cells and stellate fibroblast-like cells mingled in a fine network. It also had large collagenous areas and was diagnosed as

a mesenchymal sarcoma, most likely a fibrosarcoma. It was in the head of the pancreas and had obstructed the common bile duct. The nearby lymph nodes were uninvolved.

What the authors believed to be the first report of a granulocytic sarcoma of the head of the pancreas was published by King et al. (1987). The tumour caused obstructive jaundice. Such tumours are usually precursors of myeloproliferative disease and in this patient acute myeloid leukaemia developed 6 months after the onset of the illness.

Malignant tumours of nerve sheaths may, of course, arise wherever there are nerves, but they are rare in viscera. A malignant tumour of spindle cells that was successfully removed from the head of the pancreas by Pack et al. (1958) was, however, diagnosed by these authors as a malignant neurilemmoma.

An "osteogenic" sarcoma of the pancreas is mentioned by Cubilla and Fitzgerald (1980) as having been encountered in the autopsy material of Memorial Hospital, New York, while the surgical files of that hospital contained one leiomyosarcoma, one malignant haemangiopericytoma and a malignant histiocytoma.

A leiomyosarcoma of the pancreas was diagnosed by Tatsuta et al. (1983) by percutaneous fine-needle aspiration cytology, the needle being directed towards the suspected site of the tumour with the assistance of ultrasonic imaging.

Sarcomatous degeneration in the remnant of an incompletely removed cystadenoma of the pancreas in a baby girl has been described by Grosfeld et al. (1970). The child was 18 months old when two cystic tumours, the larger 20 cm and the smaller 6 cm in diameter, were removed from the body and tail of the pancreas. The excision was down to the pancreatic tissue but no glandular tissue was actually removed. The resected tissue was diagnosed pathologically as benign cystadenoma of the pancreas. An abdominal mass was found 11 months later. At laparotomy its origin was in the pancreas and it involved the stomach and mesenteric vessels. Only partial removal was possible. The histological diagnosis on the excised tissue was that the tumour was a rhabdomyosarcoma that had originated in the wall of a recurrent pancreatic cystadenoma. The patient died 2 months later with metastatic disease in the brain, liver and retroperitoneum. There was no autopsy.

A tumour, diagnosed histologically as a myosarcoma, was reported by Fermelia et al. in 1988. A lobulated retroperitoneal mass was found to have replaced about 90% of the pancreas, sparing only part of the head, in an 86-year-old white woman.

After excision, the tumour measured 20 × 12 × 3 cm and consisted microscopically of "gigantocellular spindle cells and a fibre-forming sarcoma with areas of hyalinization and necrosis". Post-operatively the patient regained her normal weight and was asymptomatic for 7 months, but was then found to have hepatic metastases. She was treated by radiotherapy and died 16 months after surgery.

Primary Choriocarcinoma of the Pancreas

A case of primary pancreatic choriocarcinoma was reported by Childs et al. (1985). These authors believed this to be the first recorded example of choriocarcinoma as a primary pancreatic tumour. Their patient was a black male aged 42 years. The original diagnosis was one of inflammatory pseudocyst of the pancreas and drainage into the stomach was carried out. A specimen obtained for microscopy at the original operation was reported as consisting of necrotic carcinoma. During the 6 months that followed there were several episodes of gastrointestinal bleeding and gynaecomastia developed. A marked elevation of the serum chorionic gonadotrophin level was found and biopsy specimens from metastases in the skin and axillary lymph nodes had the microscopic appearances of choriocarcinoma; chorionic gonadotrophin was demonstrated in the cancer cells by immunocytochemistry. Chemotherapy reduced the level of the serum gonadotrophin quite dramatically but the patient died of *Klebsiella* sepsis during his fourth course of chemotherapy 1 year after the diagnosis of choriocarcinoma had been established. At autopsy the gross appearances were of a primary pancreatic cancer with metastases. Subsequently, 2 mm serial sections of both testes excluded the possibility of an occult primary testicular choriocarcinoma. In discussing the origin of the tumour, the authors suggested that cells of the choriocarcinoma had been produced by metaplasia of cells in a pancreatic carcinoma. Earlier writers, Sommers and Meissner (1954) for example, while studying unusual carcinomas of the pancreas, had noted cells that resembled those of choriocarcinoma but it was the availability of immunocytochemistry, combined with clinical and biochemical evidence, that convinced Childs and his colleagues that their case was one of true choriocarcinoma of the pancreas.

Pancreatic Tumours of Vascular Tissue

Benign vascular malformations similar to the cavernous haemangiomas that are commonplace in the liver seem to be very rare in the pancreas. The publication by Dixon and Whitlock (1934) arouses the suspicion that, if a haemangioma occurs in the pancreas, it may be less stable than the usual hepatic haemangioma. In the case described by Dixon and Whitlock a recurrent tumour that weighed 2400 g was removed from the body of the pancreas of a 28-year-old woman. The specimen was sufficiently encapsulated to be excisable and was a single, large, degenerating, multilocular, cystic haemangioendothelioma. Microscopically there were parts of the tumour that were highly cellular and undifferentiated, but there were also areas of typical haemangioma, and areas of partial differentiation. One lymph node attached to the tumour was secondarily involved. In the tumour described by Chappell (1973) as a benign haemangioendothelioma, however, there was no evidence of a pre-existing hamartomatous angioma. That tumour was situated in the head of the pancreas of an 11-year-old boy. Although it was only an inch in diameter it had caused jaundice by obstructing the lower end of the common bile duct, and had to be treated by pancreaticoduodenectomy. In another example of haemangioendothelioma of the head of the pancreas (Tunell 1976) there was also obstruction of the common bile duct together with the duodenum, and a by-pass operation was carried out in the hope that involution of the tumour could be induced by radiotherapy.

Angiosarcomas of the pancreas are mentioned among the older reports of sarcoma of the pancreas that were reviewed by Ewing (1941), and a surgical specimen of a malignant haemangiopericytoma of the pancreas was found by Cubilla and Fitzgerald in the files of Memorial Hospital, New York.

The following case history is an example of a malignant tumour of vascular tissue that appeared to have arisen in the pancreas. An elderly woman, whose exact age is not available, sustained a fracture of the neck of her femur and, during an operation to fix the fracture, sarcoma-like material was found in the bone. When a skeletal survey was carried out there were multiple osteolytic lesions similar to those of myelomatosis. The patient died, and in addition to the lesions in the bones, it was found, post-mortem, that there was a spherical mass, 5 cm in diameter, in the body of the pancreas, associated

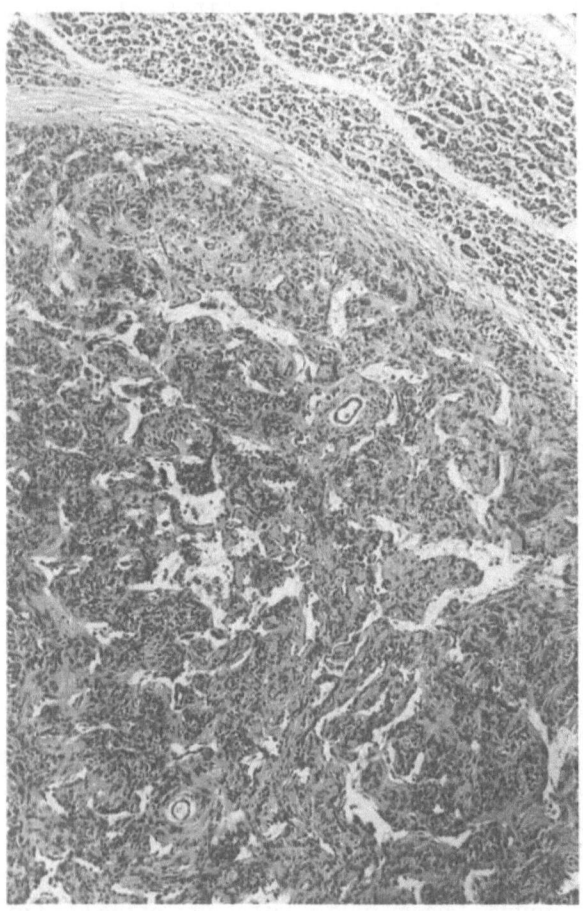

Fig. 11.11. The margin of a vascular tumour of the pancreas, thought to be a malignant haemangiopericytoma. (Courtesy of Dr D.G. Miller) H&E, × 60

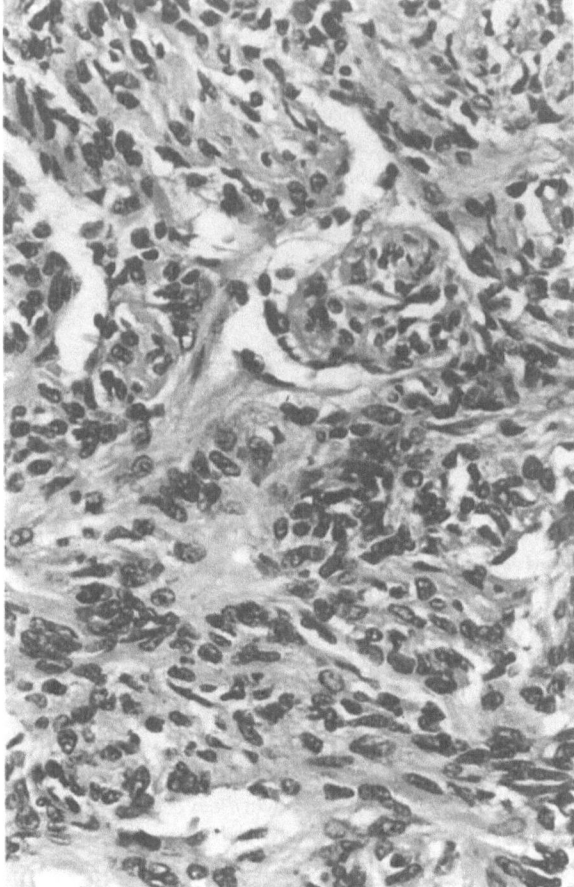

Fig. 11.12. A higher magnification of the tumour shown in Fig. 11.11. (Courtesy of Dr D.G. Miller) H&E, × 375

with enlargement of the adjacent lymph nodes and a few small lesions in the liver. Dr D.G. Miller, of Warrington General Hospital, who carried out the autopsy, made a diagnosis of malignant haemangiopericytoma of the pancreas, with metastatic deposits in the skeleton, lymph nodes and liver. The microscopic appearance of the tumour, in sections provided by Dr Miller and reproduced with his permission, are shown in Figs 11.11–11.13.

Lymphangioma of the Pancreas

Lymphangioma of the pancreas is rare, but a number of reports have been published. These are

discussed in the chapter on cystic tumours of the pancreas, pp. 139–140.

Tumours of the Exocrine Pancreas in Infancy and Childhood

Several of the rare tumours that have been referred to in the earlier parts of this chapter were in children; any tumour of the pancreas in a child is a rarity. Congenital tumours may occur, for example the tumour described as a lymphosarcoma by L'Huillier in 1904. That tumour was in the head of the pancreas of a female neonate who died of umbilical sepsis. It measured 32 × 21 mm and was com-

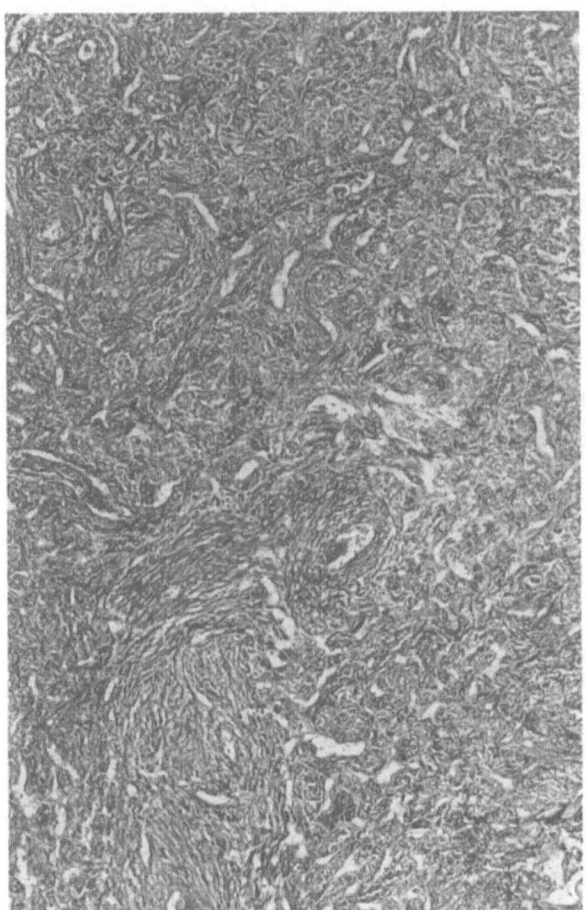

Fig. 11.13. A reticulin preparation of the tumour illustrated in Fig. 11.12. (Courtesy of Dr W. Taylor) Gordon and Sweet, × 60

posed of lymphocytes and giant cells. An apparently congenital adenoma of the pancreas was noted by Potter (1952). That tumour was 1 cm in diameter and was sharply circumscribed. It was said to lie in the pancreas "immediately distal to the duodenum". Microscopically, it was composed of wide interlacing bands of cells, with plump oval nuclei and poorly demarcated cell boundaries. It was thought to be derived from acinar epithelium.

Functioning tumours of islet cells have also been recognised in neonatal infants as well as in older children (Rickham 1975); such tumours have already been discussed (Chap. 10).

Young children, of 2 years old or less, have been found to have cystadenomas of the pancreas (Gundersen and Janis 1969; Grosfeld et al. 1970; Gille et al. 1972) and carcinoma of the pancreas was reported in a child of 15 months by Becker in 1957.

In 1964, Moynan et al. reported a case of carcinoma of the pancreas with metastases in a female child aged five and a half years, and reviewed reports of the 15 earlier cases of non-functioning carcinoma of the pancreas in childhood that had appeared in the world literature. The carcinoma they described had arisen in the head of the pancreas and had caused secondary nodules in the liver, retroperitoneum, tracheo-bronchial region and pelvis of the left kidney. Microscopically there was much variation in the appearances in different places. There were glandular structures as well as sheets of spindle cells and acanthomatous areas. There was some secretion of mucin and perineural lymphatics were invaded. A somewhat similar carcinoma of the pancreas in a 4-year-old girl was described by Frable et al. in 1971. In 1973, Tsukimoto et al., having reported the occurence of adenocarcinoma of the head of the pancreas in a 4-year-old Japanese girl, were able to review 11 additional cases of pancreatic carcinoma in children under 15 years old, most having been published in the Japanese literature. The name pancreaticoblastoma was used by Cubilla and Fitzgerald (1980) for their own report of a highly malignant tumour in the pancreas of a 4-year-old boy. The tumour was resected by the Whipple's procedure but the boy died with pulmonary metastases 1 year after the operation. The microscopic appearances of the pancreaticoblastoma included areas of small cell adenocarcinoma, non-keratinising squamous cell elements, malignant spindle cells and benign areas of mesenchymal tissue, in which there were areas of chondroid and osteoid tissue as well as mature bone. In discussing earlier reports of this type of tumour, Cubilla and Fitzgerald referred to the case published by Taxy (1976) and suggested that the tumour in that case was also a pancreaticoblastoma. One of the two tumours described by Benjamin and Wright (1980) appears also to have been a pancreaticoblastoma. Ultrastructural studies of such tumours have demonstrated zymogen granule-like structures that suggest acinar cell differentiation.

Solid and Papillary, Papillary and Cystic Epithelial Neoplasms of the Pancreas

Recent reports show that this tumour of girls and young women is no longer a rarity. It is discussed in the chapter on cystic pancreatic tumours, pp. 135–138.

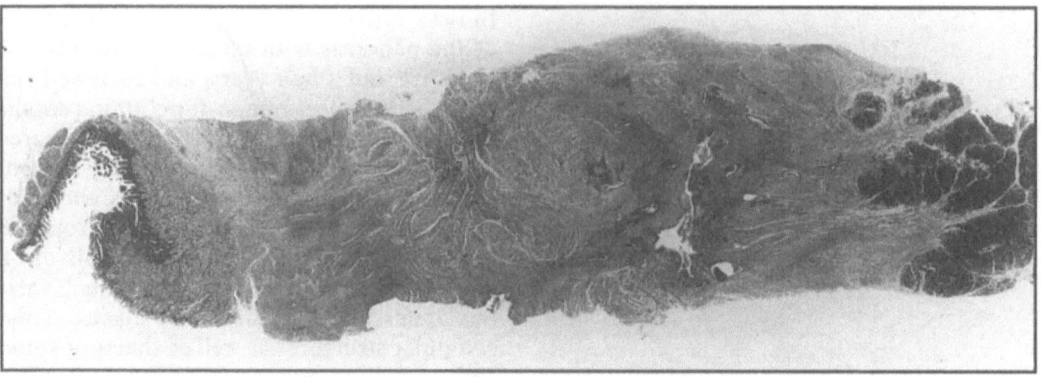

Fig. 11.14. A section through a tumour-like lesion between the head of the pancreas and the duodenum. The lesion consisted mainly of smooth muscle. The wall of the duodenum is on the left and the head of the pancreas on the right. (Courtesy of Dr W. Taylor) H&E, × 2.5

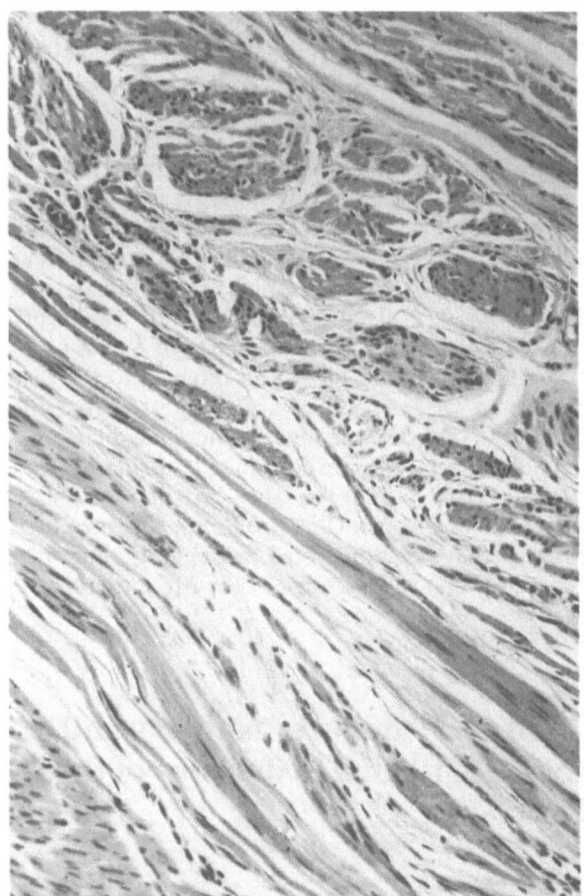

Fig. 11.15. The smooth muscle fibres that were the main constituent of the lesion illustrated in Fig. 11.14. (Courtesy of Dr W. Taylor) H&E, × 150

Tumour-like Lesions

From time to time tumour-like lesions that are probably not true neoplasms may be found in the pancreas; they may or may not be associated with clinical effects. Dr William Taylor, of Fazakerley Hospital, Liverpool has kindly provided information about, and material from, a case of this type.

The patient was a man aged 31, who was referred to the Royal Liverpool Hospital in October 1980 because he had had pain in the right side of the upper abdomen for the previous 15 months. The pain radiated to the epigastrium and to the back. The patient had anorexia and had lost 15 kg in weight. On pancreatic scintiscanning there was decreased uptake in the head of the pancreas, ultrasound scanning demonstrated an area of decreased echogenicity and displacement of the superior mesenteric artery, while computerised tomography indicated that a mass, 5 × 4 cm, in the head of the pancreas was distorting the duodenal loop. At laparotomy a mass was present in the head of the pancreas and pancreaticoduodenectomy was carried out.

The mass turned out to consist, for the most part, of smooth muscle fibres that formed a tumour-like lesion, with poorly defined margins, between the duodenum and the head of the pancreas. Fig. 11.14 illustrates the appearances of a section through the lesion, with the adjacent duodenum and pancreas. The muscle fibres were well differentiated and there were no abnormalities of the nuclei, and no mitotic activity to suggest malignancy. In the head of the

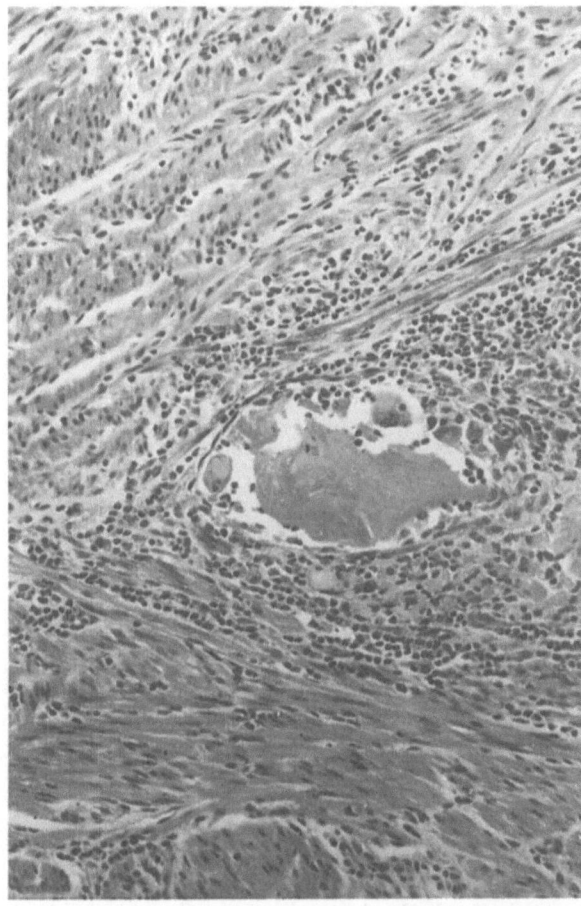

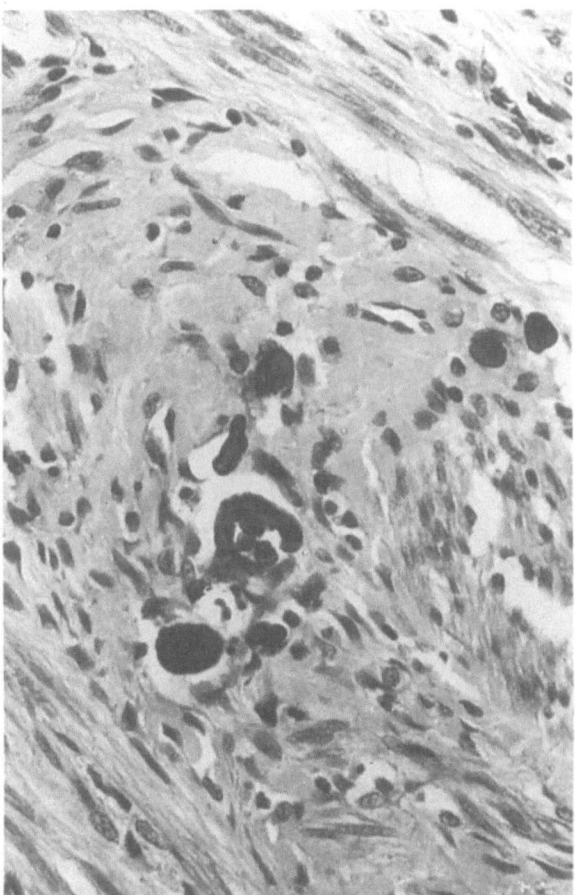

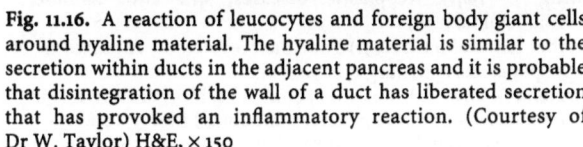

Fig. 11.16. A reaction of leucocytes and foreign body giant cells around hyaline material. The hyaline material is similar to the secretion within ducts in the adjacent pancreas and it is probable that disintegration of the wall of a duct has liberated secretion that has provoked an inflammatory reaction. (Courtesy of Dr W. Taylor) H&E, × 150

Fig. 11.17. Small foci of calcification among the muscle fibres illustrated in Fig. 11.15. (Courtesy of Dr W. Taylor) H&E, × 375

pancreas some relatively large ducts contained laminated eosinophilic material and in places the epithelium in contact with the inspissated secretion had broken down, with resulting inflammatory changes around the duct. In some places it seemed that smaller ducts had disintegrated completely to leave eosinophilic material surrounded by a reaction that included foreign body giant cells. There were occasional small foci of calcification that might have been the result of calcification of retained secretion, or might have been due to degenerative changes in the muscle fibres. Some of the microscopic appearances are illustrated in Figs 11.14–11.17. The true nature of the lesion is obscure, but Dr Taylor's suggestion is that the "tumour" may be a hamartomatous malformation of smooth muscle with superimposed inflammation.

If true lipomas of the pancreas, as distinct from the diffuse lipomatosis that may accompany pancreatic hypoplasia, occur at all, they must be very rare, and have received little attention. Fig. 11.18 illustrates a collection of fat in the head of the pancreas that simulated a true neoplasm. The patient, a man aged 71, died of bronchopneumonia and hypertensive heart disease; there was nothing in the clinical history that suggested any pancreatic disease, but the fatty area of the head of the pancreas was mistaken for an unsuspected carcinoma until microscopic examination was carried out.

A traumatic neuroma of the tail of the pancreas following splenectomy for injury 26 years previously has been reported by Geddy and Venables (1991).

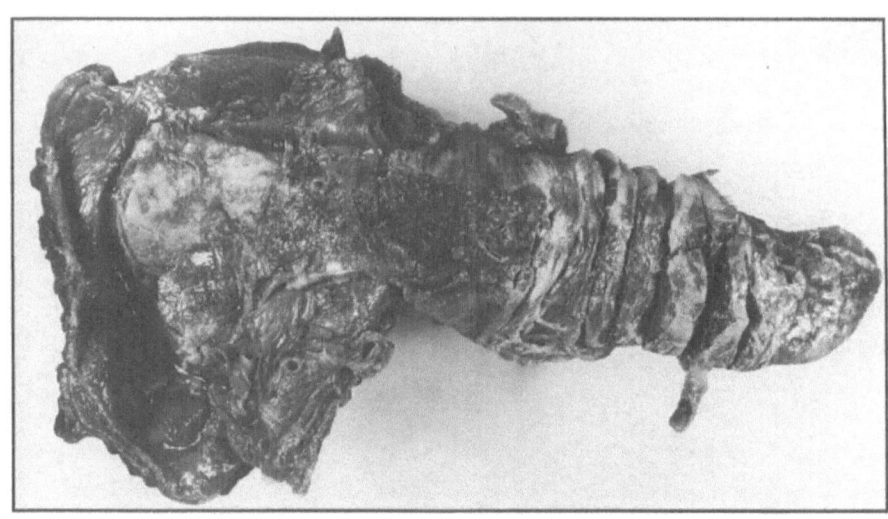

Fig. 11.18. An accumulation of fat in the upper part of the head of the pancreas that was mistaken for a tumour on examination with the naked eye.

References

Ade C, Hatton M, Hamilton Stewart P, Naylor B, Parker D (1991) Testicular lymphoma with pancreatitis. J R Soc Med 84:309–310

Akiyama H, Krigel RL (1988) Metastatic extramedullary plasmacytoma: a case report and review of the literature of a rare pseudocarcinoma. Am J Hematol 27:115–117

Becker WF (1957) Pancreaticoduodenectomy for carcinoma of the pancreas in an infant: report of a case. Ann Surg 145:864–872

Benjamin E, Wright DH (1980) Adenocarcinoma of the pancreas of childhood: a report of two cases. Histopathology 4:87–104

Berman JK, Levene N (1956) Sarcoma of the pancreas. Arch Surg 73:894–896

Brewer DB, Orr JW (1953) Struma reticulosa: a reconsideration of the undifferentiated tumours of the thyroid. J Pathol Bacteriol 65:193–208

Brooke WS, Maxwell JG (1966) Primary sarcoma of the pancreas: eight-year survival after pancreaticoduodenectomy. Am J Surg 112:657–661

Brunschwig A (1949) Radical pancreatectomy and splenectomy with left total pneumonectomy at one sitting for sarcoma of the pancreas and pulmonary metastases. Cancer 2:576–580

Cappell MS, Yao F, Cho KC, Axiotis CA (1989) Lymphoma predominantly involving the pancreas. Dig Dis Sci 34:942–947

Chappell JS (1973) Benign hemangioendothelioma of the pancreas treated by pancreaticoduodenectomy. J Pediatr Surg 8:431–432

Childs CC, Korsten MA, Choi H-SH, Schwarz R, Fisse RD (1985) Pancreatic choriocarcinoma presenting as inflammatory pseudocyst. Gastroenterology 89:426–431

Cox MT (1964) Malignant lymphoma of thyroid. J Clin Pathol 17:591–601

Cruveilhier J (1830) Anatomie pathologique du corps humain, 19e livraison. Baillière, Paris, p 2

Cubilla AL, Fitzgerald PJ (1980) Cancer (non-endocrine) of the pancreas: a suggested classification. In: Fitzgerald PJ, Morrison AB (eds) The pancreas. Williams and Wilkins, Baltimore, pp 82–110

Dixon CF, Whitlock ME (1934) Hemangio-endothelioma of pancreas probably originating in hemangioma: report of a case. Surg Clin North Am 14:701–703

Doutre L-P, Leger H, Bobois JP, Diard F (1976) Sarcome plasmocytaire extra-squeletique à localisation pancréatique. Chirurgie 102:130–135

Ehrlich AN, Stadler G, Geller W, Sherlock P (1968) Gastrointestinal manifestations of malignant lymphoma. Gastroenterology 54:1115–1121

Ewing J (1941) Neoplastic diseases, 4th edn. Saunders, Philadelphia, p 767

Feather HE, Kuhn CL (1951) Total pancreatectomy for sarcoma of the pancreas. Ann Surg 134:904–912

Fermelia D, Ozeran L, Sostrin S, Shabot M, Morgenstern L (1988) Unusual lesions of the pancreas. Mt Sinai J Med 55:132–137

Fischer MG, Kabakow B (1987) Lymphoma of the pancreas. Mt Sinai J Med 54:423–426

Frable WJ, Still WJS, Kay S (1971) Carcinoma of the pancreas, infantile type: a light and electron microscopic study. Cancer 27:667–673

Frantz VK (1959) Tumours of the pancreas. Armed Forces Institute of Pathology, Washington, DC, pp 7–28 (Atlas of tumour pathology, section 7, fascicles 27, 28)

Geddy PM, Venables CW (1991) Traumatic neuroma of the tail of the pancreas following splenectomy. Postgrad Med J 67:90–91

Gille P, Barbier G, Leclerc D, Bauer J (1972) Cystadenome pancréatique chez un enfant de 2 ans. Ann Chirurg Infant 13:437–442

Gowing NFC (1973) Modes of death and post-mortem studies. In: Smithers, Sir D (ed) Hodgkin's disease. Churchill Livingstone, Edinburgh, p 165

Grosfeld JL, Claworthy HW, Hamoudi AB (1970) Pancreatic malignancy in children. Arch Surg 101:370–375

Gundersen AE, Janis JF (1969) Pancreatic cystadenoma in childhood: report of a case. J Pediatr Surg 4:478–481

King DJ, Ewan SWB, Sewell HF, Dawson AA (1987) Obstructive jaundice: an unusual presentation of granulocytic sarcoma. Cancer 60:114–117

Levitan R, Diamond HD, Carver LF (1961) Jaundice in Hodgkin's disease. Am J Med 30:99–111

L'Huillier A (1904) Uber ein Fall von kongenitalen Lymphosarkom des Pankreas. Virchows Arch 178 : 507–509

Moynan RW, Neerhout RC, Johnson TS (1964) Pancreatic carcinoma in childhood. J Pediatr 65 : 711–720

Pack GT, Trinidad SS, Lisa JR (1958) Rare primary somatic tumors of the pancreas. Arch Surg 77 : 1000–1003

Potter EL (1952) Pathology of the fetus and the newborn. Year Book, Chicago, pp 162–163

Richards WG, Katzmann FS, Coleman FC (1958) Extramedullary plasmacytoma arising in the head of the pancreas. Cancer 11 : 649–652

Rickham PP (1975) Islet cell tumors in childhood. J Pediatr Surg 10 : 83–86

Ross CF (1951–1952) Leiomyosarcoma of the pancreas. Br J Surg 39 : 53–56

Sommers SC, Meissner WA (1954) Unusual carcinomas of the pancreas. Arch Pathol 58 : 101–111

Tatsuta M, Yamamoto R, Yamamura H, Okuda S, Tamura H (1983) Cytologic examination and CEA measurement in aspirated pancreatic material collected by percutaneous fine-needle aspiration biopsy under ultrasonic guidance for the diagnosis of pancreatic carcinoma. Cancer 52 : 693–698

Taxy JB (1976) Adenocarcinoma of the pancreas in childhood: report of a case and a review of the English language literature. Cancer 37 : 1508–1518

Tsukimoto I, Wataknabe K, Lin J-B, Nakajima T (1973) Pancreatic carcinoma in children in Japan. Cancer 31 : 1203–1207

Tunell WP (1976) Hemangioendothelioma of the pancreas obstructing the common bile duct and duodenum. J Pediatr Surg 11 : 827–830

Welch JW, Chesky VE, Hellwig CA (1958) Malignant lymphoma of thyroid. Surg Gynecol Obstet 106 : 70–76

Willis RA (1973) The spread of tumours in the human body, 3rd edn. Butterworths, London, pp 216–217

Winship T, Greene R (1955) Reticulum cell sarcoma of the thyroid gland. Br J Cancer 9 : 401–408

Wright DH (1964) Burkitt's tumour: a post-mortem study of 50 cases. Br J Surg 51 : 245–251

Wright DH (1970) Gross distribution and haematology. In: Burkitt DP, Wright DH (eds) Burkitt's lymphoma. Livingstone, Edinburgh p 248

Ziarek S, Deddouche M, Nekkache M, Taleb M (1975) Réticulosarcome du pancréas. A propos d'un cas cheq l'enfant. Med Chir Dig 4 : 195–196

Although both acute and chronic pancreatitis are very familiar entities, the definition and classification of each has provided a surprising degree of difficulty. Many authors have classified pancreatitis, each with a different emphasis on clinical findings, pathogenesis and pathology, but no single effort has gained universal approval. Several consensus conferences have addressed the problem (Sarles 1965; Sarner and Cotton 1984a, 1984b; Singer et al. 1985; Sarles et al. 1989), but their conclusions have generally served to fuel debate (Banks et al. 1985; Nordback et al. 1986; Glazer 1988) rather than illuminate clinical practice.

There has been no significant difficulty in distinguishing acute pancreatitis from chronic pancreatitis, but subdivision within these major categories has been more controversial. For instance, the first consensus conference, which was held in Marseilles in 1963, made a distinction between acute pancreatitis and relapsing acute pancreatitis, defining both as conditions likely to resolve when the primary cause was removed (Sarles 1965). The next conferences, held in Cambridge in 1983 (Sarner and Cotton 1984a, 1984b) and in Marseilles in 1984 (Singer et al. 1985), did not address the question of relapse, but were at pains to divide acute pancreatitis into mild and severe. The Cambridge conference achieved this by using the presence of multisystem failure, local complications and systemic complications, all diagnosed on clinical grounds, to define severe disease (Sarner and Cotton 1984a, b). In contrast, the Marseilles conference also proposed criteria that included morphological observations unlikely

to be available to the clinician (Singer et al. 1985). A proposed modification by Banks et al. (1985) is also unsuitable for simple clinical categorisation. Failure to achieve a conclusion satisfactory to all is illustrated by the fact that yet another consensus conference was held in Rome in 1988 (Sarles et al. 1989). Add to this the observation by Czernobilsky and Mikat (1964) that estimates of the incidence of pancreatitis in autopsy studies range from 0.13% to 66%, and it can readily be appreciated that the condition is less well defined than is generally realised.

A note of caution must be sounded about terminology. The title of this chapter reflects the general belief that the condition generally known as acute pancreatitis is aseptic in origin, and is used in particular to distinguish this condition from pancreatic inflammation caused by specific microorganisms. However, the implication that the process is sterile is misleading (Keynes 1980, 1988), for there is both clinical and experimental evidence that bacteria have a significant role, at least in determining the severity of inflammation even if they do not initiate it. Pancreatitis caused by particular organisms will be discussed in Chap. 14.

Research into the causes of acute pancreatitis has followed two main pathways. Some workers have enumerated associated conditions: Gambill (1973), Dürr (1979) and Gyr et al. (1984) have accumulated a wide range of references to the results of such labours. Others have studied pathogenesis, and a number of intermediary mechanisms have been defined, particularly by experimental studies. However, in many circumstances, clear correlations between the initiating lesions and the mechanisms of progression remain to be established.

Aetiology and Mechanism

Biliary Disease

There is a close developmental and anatomical association between the biliary and pancreatic ducts, and so it is not surprising that biliary lesions are occasionally complicated by pancreatic disease. Certainly, gallstones are seen much more frequently in patients presenting with acute pancreatitis than they are in controls. Howard's (1960a) compilation of published results includes reports that the incidence of gallstones in patients with acute pancreatitis is anything between 16% and 96%; a more recent study (Dürr 1979) revealed a range of 5% to 63%, with an average of 41% for the accumulated total of 3836 cases.

Opie, in 1901, noted that a gallstone could obstruct the common channel found distal to the anastomosis between the common bile duct and the pancreatic duct, and that this could lead to reflux of bile into the pancreas. From this observation, he developed a concept of obstructive biliary pancreatitis which has remained influential ever since. Support for this concept can be derived from studies such as that of Acosta et al. (1980), who found impacted gallstones at the ampulla of Vater in 49 of 78 patients with acute pancreatitis who were operated on early in the course of the disease, or who were subjected to autopsy after dying in the acute phase. Where there was no demonstrable obstruction of the ampulla, they suggested that the stone might have passed on into the duodenum. They support this contention by quoting their own earlier studies (Acosta and Ledesma 1974; Acosta et al. 1977), in which gallstones were found in the stools of 34 of 36 patients with acute pancreatitis, compared with three of 36 cases with uncomplicated cholelithiasis. Further interesting evidence has been produced by physicians who have investigated acute pancreatitis by endoscopic retrograde cholangiopancreatography. When the duodenal papilla is visualised early during an acute attack, stones can be seen in the common duct in a significant number of patients, whereas visualisation after the clinical symptoms have settled detects stones in very few (Neoptolemos et al. 1988).

Observations have been made during cholecystectomy carried out to prevent recurrences of pancre-

atitis, and compared with the findings in patients undergoing cholecystectomy with no history of pancreatitis. Kelly (1984) noted that patients with acute pancreatitis are more likely to have small gallstones (below 5 mm in diameter) in the gall bladder, and more likely to have impacted stones in the common bile duct. Where there were stones impacted in the ampulla of Vater, they were less than half the size in patients with acute pancreatitis than in those who did not have pancreatitis. The cystic duct in such individuals had a larger internal diameter, and there was more likely to be reflux of radiological contrast medium from the biliary tree into the pancreatic duct. Amstrong et al. (1985) and Amstrong and Taylor (1986) produced similar findings, and in addition noted that patients with acute pancreatitis had a greater number of gallstones in the gall bladder and in the common bile duct, together with a larger common channel. A complementary approach was reported by Houssin et al. (1983), who categorised patients according to the size of their gallstones and then demonstrated an inverse relation between stone diameter and the prevalence of pancreatitis. The ultimate expression of this finding, that small stones are more likely than larger ones to be associated with acute pancreatitis, was the recent observation that many patients with apparently idiopathic acute pancreatitis had biliary microlithiasis or biliary sludge (Lee et al. 1992; Steinberg 1992). Biliary sludge is defined on ultrasonographic grounds as an echogenic material found in the dependent part of the gall bladder; a disparate group of conditions predispose to the formation of biliary sludge, including total parenteral nutrition, pregnancy, bone marrow transplantation and the acquired immune deficiency syndrome (Lancet 1992). Further, disruption of gallstones by extracorporeal lithotripsy may reduce their size to a level where their passage down the bile ducts is able to cause acute pancreatitis (Dion et al. 1992).

Although this mass of evidence confirms that cholelithiasis and acute pancreatitis are associated, it has done little to clarify the pathogenetic mechanisms involved, both in terms of disruption of major duct plumbing and biochemistry of ductal and acinar cells.

Three possible mechanisms of ductal change exist, including the concept of bile reflux already described. The second possibility, that of complete obstruction of the pancreatic duct, can readily be discarded: experimental ligation of the duct and ductal obstruction by tumour give chronic inflammation and scarring rather than acute change. Further, this model cannot explain the association with biliary microlithiasis, and the observation that the common channel tends to be longer in patients with acute pancreatitis. Although Opie's (1901) ideas have been extraordinarily influential, they no longer exactly reflect current thinking.

The third mechanism, which postulates a primary role for duodenal contents, is less readily discarded because Opie's concept has not been supported by experimental results. In particular, it was noted that introduction of bile into the pancreatic duct under physiological pressures did not cause a significant degree of inflammatory change. Even when injection was at elevated pressures, changes were limited to interstitial pancreatitis, and it is only when other conditions were also changed that a severe necrotising lesion could be produced. One of the conditions that can produce a necrotising form of the disease is the presence of infection, a finding that prompted the suggestion that the role of gallstones is to make the ampulla of Vater sufficiently patulous as they pass through it to permit reflux of duodenal contents into the pancreatic duct. This model also overcame what was once thought to be a fundamental difficulty with the bile reflux hypothesis: the exocrine secretions of the pancreas are produced as proenzymes, which are only activated within the duodenum. If the reflux is of duodenal contents rather than bile, then activated pancreatic enzymes would be present in the pancreatic duct. Modern ideas about functional changes within the ducts and acini, discussed later in this chapter, also need to be taken into account.

Ethanol

Pancreatitis is clearly linked to alcohol abuse, though the association is particularly with chronic pancreatitis. When acute pancreatitis develops in an alcoholic, it typically does so after a drinking binge or a heavy meal (Keddie and Corson 1966), but there is almost certainly pre-existing damage to the organ as a response to years of hard drinking. Machado et al. (1984) provided pathological evidence of progression from a chronic to an acute lesion when they noted that focal necrosis was present in 12 of 117 pancreatectomy specimens removed for chronic alcoholic pancreatitis. Although there may also be a group of individuals whose pancreases have a particular susceptibility to alcohol and who may develop pancreatitis after only a very small amount (Sarles et al. 1976), a bout of heavy drinking in an individual without previous persistent heavy exposure is believed to be very unlikely to cause pancreatitis.

Dürr (1979) collected reports on the incidence of clinically recognisable acute pancreatitis in chronic alcoholics, and found the quoted prevalence to range from 0.9% to 9.5%. Further, he reported that the incidence of pancreatic damage at autopsy appeared to range from 17% to 45%, though these figures are difficult to interpret because the lesions included would appear to be impossible to distinguish from others, especially those sometimes referred to as terminal pancreatitis (Whipple 1907; Stein and Powers 1958). It is, of course, possible that alcohol is a factor in the development of these focal areas of necrosis and inflammation; Czernobilsky and Mikat (1964) found a history of alcohol abuse in 16.3% of their cases. More recently, Seligson et al. (1982) demonstrated minimal histological alterations in the pancreas in apparent cases of acute alcoholic pancreatitis. Such findings will remain difficult to interpret until a satisfactory definition of alcoholism can be obtained, and until some index of consumption can be devised which is more reliable than the patients' self-reported intake.

Malagelada (1986) reviewed the pathophysiology of alcoholic pancreatitis and delineated three main hypotheses by which damage might occur. The first of these is that there is direct injury of acinar cells by ethanol, or its metabolic product acetaldehyde, both carried to the pancreas by the blood stream. Experimental studies have shown evidence of persistent acinar cell damage in rats fed on an ethanol diet, comparable with changes in chronic pancreatitis in human alcoholics, but there is no evidence that this mechanism is responsible for acute pancreatic damage. Similarly, the second hypothesis, which was that the proteinaceous plugs found in pancreatic ducts in alcohol abusers can lead to inflammation, is more easily used to explain chronic alcoholic pancreatitis. The third hypothesis is more readily adapted to explain acute pancreatitis, and has similarities with the duodenal reflux theory of biliary pancreatitis. In particular, Malagelada (1986) found the experimental studies of Jalovaara and Apaja (1978) to be significant. They found that bile from rats on a routine diet was no more harmful than normal saline when injected retrogradely into the pancreatic duct, whereas bile from ethanol-fed rats caused severe damage. However, when rats on routine and high-ethanol diets are treated with the same kind of bile, they demonstrate similar susceptibility to damage. This implies that alcohol modifies the characteristics of the bile, rather than the susceptibility of the pancreas, at least in relation to the development of acute pancreatitis. In addition to evidence that alcohol intake changes the composition of bile, there is considerable evidence that it changes the pressure within the pancreatic duct. For example, intragastric infusion of alcohol raises pancreatic duct pressure, and intraduodenal infusion lowers it.

Therapeutic Agents

A wide range of commonly used drugs have been reported to cause acute pancreatitis. The evidence against many of these agents consists only of a handful of case reports, and, because many of the drugs are prescribed frequently and widely, many of the supposed associations are probably simple coincidences. Some of the relationships are supported by deliberate rechallenges carried out after clinical recovery, and others by accidental second exposures. For instance, one young woman attended four different venereal disease clinics without revealing her previous drug history at each successive attendance, and so was given metronidazole for four consecutive bouts of pelvic inflammatory disease; she developed acute pancreatitis each time (Sanford et al. 1988).

Bourke et al. (1978) attempted to overcome this problem of separating coincidence from causation by taking careful drug histories from 100 patients recovering from their first attack of acute pancreatitis; each individual was matched with a control of the same sex and similar age. The investigators were able to show a statistically significant excess exposure amongst the study group to only two drugs: cyclopenthiazide and frusemide. Other differences were also found, but the disproportions were not statistically significant.

Mallory and Kern (1980) resorted to a literature review, and concluded that azathioprine, thiazides, sulphonamides, frusemide, oestrogens and tetracycline did "seem to cause pancreatitis". They also thought that there was suggestive, but less convincing, evidence, to incriminate asparagine, chlorthalidone, corticosteroids, ethacrynic acid, phenformin and procainamide; evidence against other drugs was, in their view, dubious and contradictory. A more recent review by Banerjee et al. (1989) classified associations in a similar way, though some drugs have been promoted or demoted between categories; they agreed that there is a definite association with azathioprine, thiazides, sulphonamides, frusemide and tetracycline. They saw the association with oestrogen as only probable, but thought the association with cisplatin and L-asparaginase to be definite.

The difficulty with reaching a sensible consensus is illustrated by the discussion of frusemide in the major reviews already quoted (Mallory and Kern 1980; Banerjee et al. 1989). Both discussed a case report by Jones and Oelbaum (1975), but, whereas Mallory and Kern implied that symptoms recurred after a second challenge, Banerjee et al. thought that they did not. Despite the fact that both reviews included frusemide as a definite cause of pancreatitis, the authors were able to accumulate very few reasonably convincing reports from the literature. Jones and Oelbaum's (1975) report was of a 64-year-old woman who had mild left ventricular failure following a myocardial infarct; she developed acute pancreatitis after 4 weeks' treatment with frusemide. The drug was withdrawn, but symptoms recurred when it was reintroduced at low doses. Stenvinkel and Alvestrand (1988) described acute pancreatitis beginning about 24 hours after the start of a regimen that included high-dose frusemide, together with a similar drug called bumetanide. Symptoms recurred following rechallenge with frusemide, but not bumetanide. Circumstantial evidence came from Bourke et al.'s (1978) statistical study, and from observations that elevated serum and urine amylase levels commonly accompany frusemide exposure (Kristensen et al. 1980). It has been suggested that this increased enzyme secretion may be sufficient to cause pancreatitis; alternatively, frusemide might lower plasma volume sufficiently to cause pancreatic ischaemia. An alternative interpretation is that the serum amylase is raised because frusemide reduces renal excretion, and that this has nothing to do with pancreatitis (Kristensen et al. 1980).

There is more compelling evidence against the thiazides; Johnston and Cornish (1959) described four cases in patients on chlorothiazide. Several other cases can be found in the literature where rechallenge was avoided, for instance, because the patient was pregnant (Mallory and Kern, 1980). Apart from clinical observations of acute pancreatitis, many patients develop an asymptomatic elevation of serum amylase shortly after starting a course of thiazides (Cornish et al. 1965). Mice given chlorothiazide may develop acute pancreatitis after 1–6 months (Cornish et al. 1965). The mechanism of acute pancreatitis associated with thiazides is not understood; Banerjee et al. (1989) suggested direct toxicity.

A putative association with tetracycline is complicated by the fact that acute fatty change of the liver is often associated with acute pancreatitis. Acute fatty change of the liver is, of course, a rare but potentially fatal complication of tetracycline therapy; acute renal failure may also occur in these patients (Whalley et al. 1964). In such cases, it is not clear whether pancreatitis was a complication of the administration of the drug itself, or whether it merely followed the fatty change. For example, Kunelis et al. (1965) describe autopsies on 12 subjects who had developed acute fatty change of liver; of eight who had been given tetracycline, six had acute pancreatitis, and of four who had not been given tetracycline, three had acute pancreatitis. However, Elmore and Roggs (1981) describe a single patient where acute fatty change followed tetracycline administration without liver disease. This was a 13-year-old girl, who had been prescribed tetracycline by a dermatologist for severe cystic acne. Three months after withdrawal of the drug and recovery from the acute pancreatitis, the same dermatologist prescribed a different proprietary preparation of tetracycline, and acute pancreatitis recurred.

Sulphonamides are definitely associated with acute pancreatitis; case reports of symptom recrudescence on rechallenge were provided by Barrett and Thier (1963), Block et al. (1970) and Brazer and Medoff (1988). Brazer and Medoff's case was of a young woman who was being treated with sulphasalazine for ulcerative colitis, and who developed fever, rash, abdominal pain and leucocytosis 10 weeks after treatment was started. Two years later, she was given sulphamethoxazole for urinary tract infection, and developed abdominal pain and hyperamylasaemia within hours. It was found that her lymphocytes were capable of stimulation with sulphasalazine, sulphamethoxazole and sulphapyridine, which led Brazer and Medoff (1988) to suggest that the mechanism of acute pancreatitis was an allergic one.

Early investigations of the possible risks of azathioprine were complicated by the practice of using it only as a part of potent immunosuppressive cocktails with various other drugs during anticancer therapy. In such circumstances, acute pancreatitis might be caused by the direct toxic actions of the other drugs, or by opportunistic infections. More recently, it has been found that azathioprine can be used in Crohn's disease, in association with other drugs far less toxic than those used by oncologists, thus allowing better evidence to be accumulated (Singleton et al. 1979). Even so, clarification is limited by the fact that it is possible that Crohn's disease itself can cause acute pancreatitis (Matsumoto et al. 1989). Acceptance of a positive association between azathioprine and acute pancreatitis (Mallory and Kern 1980; Banerjee et al. 1989) seems to be based on two case reports. Nogueria and Freedman (1972) described a woman who had been treated with steroids for a number of years, and who then developed acute pancreatitis 3 weeks after azathioprine was added to her treatment; symptoms disappeared when azathioprine

was withdrawn, but recurred hours after its reintroduction. Kawanishi et al.'s (1973) patient was on azathioprine, sulphapyridine and diphenoxylate, but had recrudescence of pancreatitis only when rechallenged with azathioprine; sulphapyridine rechallenge produced no symptoms. However, Frick et al. (1991) could find no excess of acute pancreatitis in patients given azathioprine to induce immunosuppression following renal transplantation.

The position is unusual for another chemotherapeutic agent, L-asparaginase. This drug is thought to be associated with a substantial and predictable dose-related incidence of acute pancreatitis, as opposed to the sporadic and apparently idiosyncratic cases linked with other drugs. Since it is never used on its own, absolute proof of a causative role remains lacking (Mallory and Kern 1980; Banerjee et al. 1989), though Mallory and Kern were able to review ten large studies. Pancreatitis was observed in all but one of these, with an average incidence of 7%. However, they could find no rechallenge studies, and felt that the only controlled trial was marred by poor case matching. The mechanism of toxicity is unknown, though a direct toxic effect is likely (McLean et al. 1982).

Cisplatin, another potent cytotoxic drug, was accepted as a definite cause of pancreatitis by Banerjee et al. (1989), despite the fact that the only evidence they can quote is a single case report (Bunin et al. 1985). Two further cases occurred in young men treated for germ cell tumours with cisplatin, bleomycin and vinblastine.

The position with the oestrogen contraceptive pill is analogous to the difficulties with implicating tetracycline as a cause of acute pancreatitis; it is difficult to determine whether the effect is direct, or whether it is mediated by some complication of oestrogen therapy. It is clear that acute pancreatitis occurs disproportionately frequently in women taking the contraceptive pill (Davidoff et al. 1973; Parker 1983), but almost all those who develop acute pancreatitis have had hyperlipidaemia. Hyperlipidaemia is a known complication of taking oestrogen, and is itself a cause of acute pancreatitis; other drugs causing hyperlipidaemia have also been implicated in this kind of mechanism (Durrington and Cairns 1982). Foster and Powell (1975) described acute pancreatitis associated with the contraceptive pill in a woman shown not to have hyperlipidaemia.

Corticosteroid therapy is particularly difficult to evaluate. Although Mallory and Kern (1980) were able to find over 40 cases suggesting a link between steroids and acute pancreatitis, they remained unsure about their significance. Many were patients with serious pre-existing diseases that might have caused acute pancreatitis independently, and most were also on other drugs. In addition, they could find no evidence of a rechallenge test, and concluded that a causative link was only probable. Nine years later, Banerjee et al. (1989) thought the link unlikely, though some evidence exists in favour of a true association. Some of the patients were children, who otherwise rarely suffer from acute pancreatitis; a few carefully studied adult patients had no other demonstrable cause. Carone and Liebow (1957) described acute pancreatic lesions in 28.5% of autopsy subjects who had received oral steroids or ACTH. Steroids have been shown to induce pancreatitis in experimental animals (Bencosme and Lazarus 1956). The mechanism remains obscure.

A further drug that has recently emerged as a probable cause of acute pancreatitis is pentamidine. This is frequently used as an aerosolised preparation in the treatment of *Pneumocystis carinii* pneumonia, a condition that is an extremely common complication of the acquired immune deficiency syndrome. As with steroids, interpretation is difficult because the patients are often on multiple preparations, and are susceptible to other possible causes of acute pancreatitis (Hart 1989; Kumar et al. 1989; Schwartz and Cappell 1989). Murphey and Josephs (1981) were able to demonstrate recrudescent symptoms on rechallenge, but Schwartz and Cappell (1989) were not. The role of pentamidine as a cause of diabetes mellitus is discussed on p. 103.

Another drug recently accepted to be a cause of acute pancreatitis is valproic acid, which is particularly used for the treatment of petit mal and other less common forms of epilepsy (Camfield et al. 1979; Batalden et al. 1979). In one example, where acute pancreatitis occurred soon after long-term treatment with clonazepam was abandoned in favour of valproic acid, it recurred 2 days after rechallenge.

In addition to difficulties about determining whether or not any particular drug is really a cause of acute pancreatitis, there are also problems with establishing mechanisms. Older papers quote disparate mechanisms for different drugs, few with anything other than speculation to support them. More recently, Braganza (1991a) pointed out that all the drugs that she accepts as definite causes of acute pancreatitis are known to generate reactive chemical intermediates when processed via the cytochrome P450 system, and that the pancreas has definite and inducible cytochrome P450 enzymes of its own. This hypothesis replaces a previous one developed at a time when it was thought that cytochrome P450 systems were found in hepatocytes but not in the pancreas, whereby it was necessary to speculate that reactive intermediates could be generated in hepatocytes and be introduced into the pancreas by retrograde flow of bile into the pancreatic duct at the ampulla of Vater.

Hereditary Factors

The inherited condition of cystic fibrosis of the pancreas (mucoviscidosis) is a disease that affects the secretions in many organs; the pancreatic component is relatively unimportant as far as survival of the patients is concerned. Moreover, although there are important changes in the pancreas in mucoviscidosis, the inflammatory component of the commoner pancreatic lesions is trivial. The pancreatic effects of cystic fibrosis have been discussed in Chap. 4. There are, however, a number of reports of families in which certain members were unusually vulnerable to attacks of pancreatitis. In these families, the tendency to pancreatitis is inherited as a dominant mechanism, but penetrance is not complete, and the disease may skip a generation. Males and females are affected with equal frequency. The earlier reports of affected families have been reviewed by McConnell (1966), and in 1975 Sibert tabulated the families that had been reported up to that time, when he gave an account of a British family with hereditary pancreatitis. The clinical picture of hereditary pancreatitis has been described by Gross (1973); it closely resembles that of nonhereditary pancreatitis. The sequels and complications, too, are similar. Although most of the affected families have been American, they have had Anglo-Saxon Caucasian roots, and it has been suggested by Sibert that the condition may be underdiagnosed in Britain. Affected families living in Ireland, France and New Zealand are mentioned by Gross, who also refers to reports of the disease among the natives of the Kerala state of India. Attacks of the disease tend to begin in childhood, with irregular recurrences and a tendency to cease, at least in the family described by Sibert, at about the age of 40 years. There seems to be a special tendency for calculi to form in the main pancreatic ducts (Rohrmann et al. 1981), and there is perhaps some risk of eventual malignancy (Kattwinkel et al. 1973) i.e. (see p. 303).

Aminoaciduria is an associated metabolic abnormality in some, but not all, of the affected families; there was no aminoaciduria in the British family studied by Sibert (1975). A recent observation quoted by Braganza (1991a) is that those patients who have acute pancreatitis associated with inherited disorders of the metabolism of branched-chain amino acids generate a toxic intermediate, isovaleric acid. This is interesting, because isovaleric acid is very similar to valproic acid, which is thought by some to be a definite cause of acute pancreatitis.

Inherited Metabolic Abnormalities

Hyperlipidaemia and Hyperlipoproteinaemia

Although the importance of hyperlipidaemia in the aetiology of acute and relapsing pancreatitis is unclear (Dürr 1979), there are various reports that implicate hyperlipidaemia as a cause of pancreatitis. It is true that patients with pancreatitis may develop hyperlipidaemia, but in familial hyperlipidaemia with xanthomatosis, as in a patient reported by Klatskin and Gordon (1952), the abormality of lipid metabolism antedated the attacks of abdominal pain, and, when dietary adjustments reduced the hyperlipidaemia, the attacks of abdominal pain improved. Since that time, the hyperlipidaemias and hyperlipoproteinaemias have been classified more precisely, and Fredrickson et al. (1967) state that it is the patients with type IV or type V hyperlipidaemia, according to their classification, that are particularly liable to develop acute pancreatitis. In such patients, pancreatitis is strongly associated with alcohol abuse (Dickson et al. 1984), and it may be that the hyperlipidaemia is not primary, but secondary to alcohol abuse. However, Dickson et al. described acute pancreatitis in a pregnant woman with Fredrickson type I hyperlipidaemia.

Guzmán et al. (1985) studied a Chilean population where cholelithiasis is the predominant cause of acute pancreatitis. He found, in subjects with pancreatitis, that lipid clearance was abnormal following a dose of 100 g of sunflower oil in those both with and without gallstones, when compared with controls who had not had pancreatitis. This metabolic abnormality persisted for at least 6 months after their first attack of acute pancreatitis, leading the authors to suggest that it was independent of the metabolic derangements that accompany the acute phase, and may have preceded it. An alcoholic aetiology can also be excluded in children with acute pancreatitis with a background of hyperlipidaemia (Poulsen 1950).

Acute Intermittent Porphyria

Acute intermittent porphyria may cause severe abdominal symptoms that resemble those of acute pancreatitis but, according to Gambill (1973), if there is a family history of porphyria and if porphyrins can be demonstrated in the urine, porphyria should be the diagnosis. He states, moreover, that pancreatic enzyme levels will not, usually, be elevated in acute porphyria. In 1954, however, there was a report by Saint et al. that, in two of the three patients with acute porphyria that they studied,

there was evidence of mild pancreatitis and they suggested this to be the cause of the abdominal pain. One of the patients died and, at necropsy, the pancreas was atrophic and contained areas of recent necrosis. Because, as has been pointed out earlier, "terminal pancreatitis" is not uncommonly found after death from many types of illness, this seems less than satisfactory proof that pancreatitis was the cause of the abdominal pain. In their other patient, who did not die, the diagnosis of pancreatitis depended on the finding of raised serum amylase several times during the acute stage of the illness. Though serum amylase estimation is important in the diagnosis of pancreatic disease, it is not an entirely infallible guide (Salt and Schenker 1976). Thus, the statement by Saint (1954), in a paper published later in the same year, that there was unequivocal evidence of mild pancreatitis must be accepted with reservations. In the paper by Kobza et al. (1976), however, there is an account of a 36-year-old woman, who, during her first attack of acute intermittent porphyria, had simultaneously increased levels of serum amylase and lipase, as well as an increased amylase clearance to creatine clearance ratio; these findings justified a diagnosis of pancreatitis. Sonotomography showed a homogeneously enlarged pancreas. The patient suffered an identical attack of abdominal pain 40 weeks after the first episode. The authors did not attempt to explain the pathogenesis of the pancreatitis, but Saint (1954) has suggested that ischaemia due to spasm of the smooth muscle of blood vessels may cause the damage, while the possibility of some locally acting vasoconstrictor substance was discussed by Denny-Brown and Sciarra (1945) in relation to the pathogenesis of the visceral disorders of porphyria.

Suicidal or Accidental Poisoning

Pancreatitis has been reported by Gaultier et al. (1964) as a complication of the illness that followed a suicidal attempt with coal gas, and by Cooper and Macaulay (1982) in a joiner who was poisoned accidentally with a wood preservative that had zinc naphthanate and pentachlorophenol as its active ingredients. Various other aliphatic or hydrogenated hydrocarbons are amongst the xenobiotics that may cause acute pancreatitis following exposure in the workplace (Braganza et al. 1986).

Hypercalcaemic States

The suggestion that pancreatitis might be a complication of hyperparathyroidism, and might serve as a diagnostic signpost to overactivity of the parathyroid glands, was made by Cope et al. in 1957. In their paper they referred to previously published cases in which pancreatitis or pancreatic calcification had coincided with hyperparathyroidism. Further work (Mixter et al. 1962) more or less established that pancreatitis was a complication of hyperparathyroidism, and it is now known that both primary hyperparathyroidism and hyperparathyroidism secondary to renal failure are associated with acute pancreatitis (Sitges-Serra et al. 1988). Patients with familial primary hyperparathyroidism are also at risk (Peters et al. 1966). In 1969, Banks and Janowitz stated that between 7% and 19% of hyperparathyroid subjects had had documented pancreatitis. However, another American study, carried out at the Mayo Clinic by Herskovic et al. (1967), found only 15 cases of pancreatitis in 400 examples of hyperparathyroidism. Bess et al. (1980) found an even lower rate of association, not significantly different from the rate of acute pancreatitis in other hospital patients, suggesting a coincidental rather than a causal relationship. In Europe, Schmidt and Creutzfeldt (1970) estimated that the incidence of pancreatitis in hyperparathyroidism was 6.5%. In hyperparathyroid crisis, the incidence of pancreatitis may be as high as between 25.5% and 34% (Dürr 1979). When acute pancreatitis is associated with hyperparathyroid crisis, the patient may present as one of diabetic ketoacidosis (Payne and Tanenberg 1980).

It is now clear that the factor that predisposes to pancreatitis is hypercalcaemia. Frick et al. (1990) showed that acute hypercalcaemia can induce acinar cell necrosis and intraductal protein precipitates in the pancreases of both rats and guinea pigs. Acute pancreatitis has been associated with diseases, other than hyperparathyroidism, where marked hypercalcaemia is a feature; medically induced hypercalcaemia may also be associated. One patient on home haemodialysis for renal failure caused by chronic pyelonephritis became hypercalcaemic, and subsequently developed acute pancreatitis, when the deionizer that softened the water in her dialysis system failed (Evans and Slapak 1975). Acute pancreatitis complicated a calcium infusion test in a man with end-stage renal disease (Hochgelerent and David 1974), and may follow the hypercalcaemia that can occur during total parenteral nutrition (Manson 1974; Izsak et al. 1980).

Leeson and Fourman (1966) described a patient with hypoparathyroidism in whom hypercalcaemia was induced by toxic doses of vitamin D, who then developed acute pancreatitis. De Waele et al. (1989) described a man who presented on four occasions with acute pancreatitis, with a very high serum calcium on each occasion; eventually, it was found that he was taking excess doses of vitamin D as self-medication. Gafter et al. (1976) observed acute pancreatitis in a patient with hypercalcaemia following bone destruction by secondary breast carcinoma. Dazai et al. (1991) described two examples of acute pancreatitis following hypercalcaemia induced by T-cell leukaemia; Senba et al. (1991) have seen four similar patients.

In the condition of familial hypocalciuric hypercalcaemia, which is inherited by an autosomal dominant mechanism, and which differs from primary hyperparathyroidism in that the renal excretion of calcium is reduced, pancreatitis tends to occur and may be severe (Davies et al. 1981; Marx et al. 1981). The pathogenetic mechanism is obscure, though Baer and Neu (1966) suggested high serum ionised calcium is sufficiently thrombogenic to cause multiple microthrombi within the pancreas. Alternatively, the role of calcium as a co-factor in the autocatalytic activation of trypsin may be important (Longnecker 1991).

Structural and Functional Abnormalities

There is much clinical and experimental evidence that structural or functional narrowing of the bile duct is harmful to the pancreas, leading to chronic pancreatitis or acute oedematous pancreatitis, but progression to acute necrotising pancreatitis is less well understood. The importance of migrating gallstones, or gallstones impacted at or near the ampulla of Vater, as causes of obstruction, has already been discussed, while congenital variations in the arrangement of the ducts, for example pancreas divisum, in which it is suspected that there may be inadequate drainage of parts of the pancreas, have also been covered in Chap. 1. Other causes of obstruction of the ducts include epithelial metaplasia (Rich and Duff 1936) and tumours of the pancreas or duodenum. Gambill (1971), for example, found that attacks of abdominal pain that suggested acute pancreatitis occurred in 31% of 26 patients that were found later to have carcinoma of the pancreas, while microscopic signs of pancreatitis were present in 26 of 255 patients with pancreatic or ampullary carcinoma. More recently, Wilson and Imrie (1986) have described a patient in whom recurrent acute pancreatitis was found eventually to have been due to a carcinoma of the body of the pancreas. Parasitic worms in the pancreatic ducts have been associated with acute pancreatitis (Novis 1923; Duncan 1948), and duodenal diverticula were thought by Ogilvie (1941) and Caos (1989) to have promoted acute pancreatitis by their obstructive effect upon the pancreatic duct. Willemer et al. (1992) discussed recurrent acute pancreatitis in a young man with an intraluminal duodenal diverticulum.

Earlier studies suggested that normal bile alone, at the pressures generated within the pancreatic duct, is not capable of direct induction of experimental acute pancreatitis, but more recent observations and hypotheses have re-established a possible role. Pancreatic enzymes can be activated without exposure to the duodenal milieu, even while still in the acinar cell (Steer et al. 1984). Under conditions of persistent intraductal hypertension, the secretory vacuoles of the acinar cells fail to release their contents into the acinar lumens, and eventually fuse with the lysosomes of the same cells. Following this process, which is known as crinophagy, the pancreatic proenzymes are activated by the lysosomal enzymes and might, at least in theory, go on to damage the pancreatic substance (Steer and Meldolesi 1988).

Another possible role for bile has gained recent prominence. In particular circumstances, bile can be shown to contain highly reactive free radicals. These are not present in significant quantities in normal bile, but they can be generated by the activity of hepatocytic enzymes, the cytochrome P450 systems (Braganza 1991b). The hypothesis is that "toxic" bile can be produced by the liver and causes acute pancreatitis if it refluxes into the pancreatic duct. This model not only provides a possible explanation for biliary pancreatitis, but might also explain drug-induced pancreatitis; hepatic microsomal enzymes are capable of converting certain drugs into highly reactive intermediates excreted via the bile. In addition, it has been suggested that comparable reactive intermediates might be formed from xenobiotics accidentally introduced into the body in the work place. Some of these compounds are capable of participating in a sequence of oxidation–reduction cycles, with potential damage to tissue at each cycle. These ideas have recently had to be reformulated, following the discovery of cytochrome P450 systems in the pancreas itself, whereby the role of bile has been downgraded.

Other sources of highly reactive toxic intermediates exist, including the activated neutrophil polymorph. One of the important mechanisms of bacterial killing in the phagocyte is the production of oxygen-derived free radicals. These are generated from molecular oxygen during the respiratory burst that follows phagocytosis. Although bacterial killing occurs primarily within the phagolysosome formed from the phagosome and one or more lysosomes after phagocytosis, there is a short phase during which lysosomal and specific granule contents may be spilled into the environment around the poly-

morph. This occurs because fusion with the cell membrane in the phagosome can happen before it has fully enclosed its prey, leading to the phenomenon picturesquely referred to as "regurgitation during feeding". Some recent research has therefore investigated the possibility that the oxidative capacity of toxic bile can be derived from the neutrophil polymorph.

The initial consequence of this oxidative stress, whatever its source, is believed to be failure of the normal polarised secretion from the apex of the cell (Sanfey et al. 1986), for which the term "pancreastasis" has been coined (Braganza 1991b). This inevitably leads to a build-up of pancreatic enzymes within the cytoplasm of pancreatic acinar cells, which then causes an increase of enzyme flow along a pathway of non-polarised secretion through the base of the cell into the interstitium (Musa and Case 1991). This pathway carries small quantities of enzymes in healthy pancreases, accounting for the presence of pancreatic enzymes in small amounts in the plasma of healthy individuals. Under normal circumstances, the enzymes are carried from the pancreatic interstitium to the blood stream by the lymphatics, but when the majority of the acinar cell secretions drains to the interstitium rather than the acinar lumen, the lymphatics rapidly become overloaded (Hollender et al. 1983).

If the oxidative stress is reduced or reversed, then normal secretory polarity may be restored; experimental studies suggest that this is the situation in those cases of acute oedematous pancreatitis which resolve without the more severe sequelae of haemorrhage and necrosis. In other patients, the lesion progresses to acute necrotising pancreatitis. Ohlsson and Genell (1991) put forward a complex, but compelling, hypothesis to explain this disastrous progression, suggesting that the activation of trypsin is important. In large enough doses, trypsin alone causes severe haemorrhage (Beck et al. 1964), although the full-blown picture of necrotising pancreatitis is not produced (Creutzfeldt and Schmidt 1970). Ohlsson and Genell (1991) believe that when the concentration of trypsin increases to a level where it overwhelms the protective inhibitory effects of alpha$_1$-antitrypsin (alpha$_1$-proteinase inhibitor) and alpha$_2$-macroglobulin, then a number of physiological cascades are set in motion and various pancreatic proenzymes may be activated. These cascades include complement activation, plasma coagulation and fibrinolysis, together with the activation of kallikrein and, subsequently, bradykinin, and lead to pancreatic necrosis. This in turn leads to the recruitment of neutrophil polymorphs and macrophages. The validity of the latter component of this sequence is supported by the presence of leucocytic products within the pancreatic tissue and within ascitic fluid (Balldin et al. 1989; Axelsson et al. 1990), and by the early appearance of neutrophil polymorphs in experimental acute pancreatitis (Uden et al. 1989).

Recent developments have modified the idea, probably first propounded by Klebs in 1868 (cited in Ohlsson and Genell 1991) and raised to the status of formal hypothesis by Chiari in 1896, that "pancreatic ferments" are responsible for pancreatic autodigestion. However, in addition to the central role of trypsin already mentioned, the activity of other enzymes still remains crucial. Both chymotrypsin and elastase, when instilled alone, produce oedema and haemorrhage, and, like trypsin, a limited degree of necrosis (Anderson and Schiller 1968; Geokas 1968). In contrast, lipolytic enzymes cause the full-blown picture of extensive necrosis of the pancreas and damage to adjacent structures. Phospholipase A readily damages cellular membranes (Schmidt and Creutzfeldt 1969), releasing metabolic products, such as lysolecithin, which are themselves cytotoxic, and does so without the intervention of inhibitors such as those that control the proteolytic enzymes (Lankisch 1988). Lipase is generally held to be responsible for the fat necrosis that characteristically surrounds the pancreas, and, although lipase has no direct effect on acinar cells, detergents released by fat necrosis may be less innocuous (Nagai et al. 1989).

Abnormalities of Perfusion

Emboli and Infarcts

Healthy living epithelial cells, such as those that line the small intestine and almost certainly those that line the ducts and form the acini of the pancreas, are not digested by the enzymes secreted by the pancreas. It is when the pancreas has become devitalised in some way that it becomes vulnerable to autodigestion; most observers agree that vascular lesions are important in the pathogenesis of some cases of acute pancreatitis. The experimental work up to 1968 was reviewed by McCutcheon (1968) who pointed out that infarcts of the pancreas could occur as distinct lesions unassociated with acute pancreatitis and concluded that the diffuse vascular lesions of acute pancreatitis were secondary to the action of active enzymes.

It is true that infarcts of the pancreas can occur as a separate entity (this is discussed in Chap. 5), but the dividing line between haemorrhagic infarction of the pancreas and haemorrhagic pancreatitis are

quite indefinite and, indeed, the two conditions may coincide (Gambill et al. 1948). The importance of vascular lesions in the pathogenesis of acute pancreatitis has been based mainly upon the results of experiments in animals. Rich and Duff (1936) stated that in human and experimental haemorrhagic pancreatitis there was a constant and specific vascular lesion characterised by rapid necrosis of the walls of arteries and veins, with haemorrhage due to rupture of the necrotic vessels. They attributed the lesion to the effects of trypsin. Other investigators, however, concluded that vascular lesions might actually initiate acute haemorrhagic pancreatitis. Thus Thal and Brackney (1954), who induced fulminating haemorrhagic pancreatitis by provoking a Schwartzman reaction in the pancreases of rabbits and goats, expressed their opinion that this condition might develop entirely on a vascular basis. In their experiments, they introduced endotoxin into the pancreatic duct at pressures well below those required to produce ductal rupture, followed 24 hours later by the intravenous injection of toxin. In experimental controls, in which the intravenous provocative dose was omitted, pancreatic necrosis never occurred. In the pancreases of the animals with haemorrhagic pancreatitis, hyaline thrombi were seen microscopically in the capillaries and venules. Further experiments (Thal and Molestina 1955; Thal and Brackney 1954) also impressed Thal and his colleagues with the importance of extensive thrombosis of small vessels as a cause of pancreatic necrosis. Later studies of the Schwartzman type of reaction in causing experimental haemorrhagic pancreatitis in dogs (Bliss and Sibley 1969) indicated that there is marked variation in the sensitivity of individuals to reactions of this type and the authors suggested that variations in individual sensitivity might explain the infrequency of acute haemorrhagic pancreatitis in man.

A number of researchers have attempted to cause acute pancreatitis in animals by the expedient of ligating the pancreatic arteries or veins, but with negative results (Menguy et al. 1957; Popper et al. 1978), though others were able to produce acute pancreatitis in a proportion of subjects by simple vascular ligation alone (Block et al. 1954). However, when additional insults, such as ligation of the pancreatic duct with the administration of secretin, are introduced, haemorrhagic necrosis can be predictably induced (Popper et al. 1978).

A wide range of relatively inert substances have been injected into the arterial supply of the pancreas in an attempt to unravel this problem, including wax, lycopodium powder, air, oil, metallic mercury and polythene microspheres of graded sizes (Prinz 1991). Early experiments with mercury injections produced infarct-like lesions of acute pancreatic necrosis (Smyth 1940), leading to the conclusion that the vascular lesions identified by Rich and Duff (1936) were the results of pancreatitis, rather than a cause. Further attempts to produce acute pancreatitis by the injection of substances into the vascular tree have, however, produced variable results, and it is likely that the precise size of the vessels that are occluded is crucial. This appears to have been demonstrated by the experiments of Pfeffer et al. (1962). These workers were able to produce all gradations of pancreatitis in dogs by controlled injections of sterile polythene microspheres that varied in size from 8 μm to 400 μm in diameter into the pancreatic blood vessels. They found that the severity of the lesion was inversely proportional to the size of the micropheres, the larger microspheres inducing the less severe lesions, and that haemorrhagic pancreatitis resulted within 11 hours in every case when microspheres with diameters between 8 μm and 20 μm were injected. This is interpreted to indicate that collateral blood flow is important in preventing the evolution of infarction and consequent acute pancreatitis. Waldner (1992) reviews a wide range of experimental methods whereby pancreatic blood flow is artificially disrupted, and discusses the practical problems associated with these methods.

Experimental embolic pancreatitis in animals has clinically important correlates in man, and it has been suggested that an example of acute haemorrhagic pancreatitis that followed incompatible blood transfusion occurred because of microthrombi within the circulation (Ackerman 1942; Hardaway and McKay 1959). Baer and Neu (1966) investigated an elderly woman with primary hyperparathyroidism, who died of acute pancreatitis; they found microthrombi in renal glomeruli and pancreatic vessels, and speculated that these were precipitated because the high levels of ionised calcium in the blood stream promoted thrombogenesis. Probstein et al. (1957) investigated 23 patients with atheromatous emboli, and found pancreatic involvement in 12. Mild acute pancreatitis was present in five, and severe acute pancreatitis in another five. Pellegrini et al. (1977) described a man in whom thromboembolism of the coeliac axis apparently led to acute pancreatitis.

Thrombotic thrombocytopenic purpura (TTP), a rare and poorly understood condition characterised by microthrombi in the arterioles and capillaries of many organs, is sometimes associated with acute pancreatitis (Amorosi and Ultmann 1966; Olsen 1973), and is therefore said to cause acute pancreatitis. Jackson et al. (1989) challenged this received wisdom, describing a middle-aged woman who was recovering from an acute attack of pancreatitis, when a sudden drop in the haematocrit and in the numbers of platelets heralded the onset of TPP. They argue that TTP is a syndrome that not only causes acute pancreatitis, but can itself be the consequence of acute pancreatitis.

A clinical paradigm even more closely similar to the experimental models occurs when transcatheter arterial embolisation is used for the treatment of conditions such as gastrointestinal haemorrhage, hypersplenism and advanced carcinoma (Miller et al. 1985). Kishimoto et al. (1989) monitored serum amylase levels in a study of patients undergoing transcatheter arterial embolisation, as well as chemotherapy, for hepatocellular carcinoma. They found little or no elevation of amylase in patients receiving chemotherapy alone, or those receiving chemotherapy with lipiodol embolisation; there was slight hyperamylasaemia in patients receiving chemotherapy with gelatin sponge embolisation, and marked hyperamylasaemia in those subjected to chemotherapy with gelfoam powder embolisation. Acute pancreatitis developed in one patient who had gelfoam embolisation.

A recent study by Kusterer et al. (1991) readdressed, in a novel manner, the problem first discussed in respect of Rich and Duff's studies, wherein there was controversy about whether vascular lesions provoked or followed acute pancreatitis. In this study, acute pancreatitis was induced by the intraductal injection of sodium taurocholate. Vascular changes were observed by in vivo microscopy, showing permeability changes and blood stasis that clearly reflect the changes in blood vessels associated with early acute inflammation elsewhere in other organs. This is taken to mean that vascular changes are generally secondary.

Shock and Ischaemia

It seems probable that in most cases of acute haemorrhagic pancreatitis in man the vascular factor in the pathogenesis of the lesion is only one of several, but in certain types of pancreatitis the vascular factor may the most important, or even the only, cause of the lesions. In shock, pancreatic lesions not only occur but may be of clinical importance for, as has been pointed out by McGovern (1971), acute necrotising pancreatitis, as well as causing shock, may be a complication of shock and be the direct cause of death. Acute pancreatitis was found in six of the 100 autopsies on those dying of shock studied by McGovern. The importance of intravascular coagulation in shock has been emphasised by Hardaway (1962) and Hardaway et al. (1962).

Further demonstrations of the susceptibility of the pancreas to ischaemic injury in shock were those of Warshaw and O'Hara (1978) and Gmaz-Nikulin et al. (1981). Warshaw and O'Hara combined a retrospective study of autopsy material from patients who had died after either oligaemic or non-oligaemic shock, with a prospective study of 13 selected patients who had been in shock. In the prospective study they looked for hyperamylasaemia, hyperlipidaemia, elevation of the amylase/creatine clearance ratio, and elevation of the circulating isoamylases that are specifically derived from the pancreas. Their findings in the autopsy study were that there was an incidence of major pancreatic injury in 9% of cases of oligaemic shock if there was not concomitant acute renal tubular necrosis, but an incidence of 50% in those with renal tubular necrosis. Among patients who had died after non-oligaemic shock, there was an incidence of pancreatic injury of 12% in subjects without renal tubular necrosis, and an incidence of 35% in those with acute renal tubular necrosis. In the prospective study, four of the 13 patients had clinical evidence of pancreatitis, with one fatality from fulminating pancreatitis, while the remaining nine had hyperamylasaemia, the amylase being of the pancreatic type, without evidence of pancreatitis.

Many cases of acute pancreatitis following shock are not identified by the attending clinicians during life. Tilney et al. (1973) studied 18 patients who had required dialysis for acute renal failure following surgical repair of ruptured atheromatous aneurysms of the abdominal aorta. Only one patient survived, and two others had clinically identified pancreatitis. Of the remaining 15, nine were found to have severe acute pancreatitis at autopsy.

Surgery in general is associated with post-operative acute pancreatitis, though most cases are limited and localised, and presumed to be related to direct handling. White et al. (1970) studied 70 cases of post-operative acute pancreatitis, and ascribed 54 of them to surgical trauma. Some of the remaining 16 followed abdominal surgical procedures in which the pancreas should not be handled, and several were associated with extra-abdominal surgery, such as transurethral resection of the prostate, hip replacement, parathyroidectomy for parathyroid carcinoma, and radical mastectomy. The authors thought that the common factor when direct trauma could be excluded was intraoperative hypotension.

Cardiac surgery requiring cardiopulmonary bypass is particularly prone to be associated with post-operative acute pancreatitis. Feiner (1976) described 182 complete autopsies in adult patients who had died within 10 weeks of cardiac surgery, and found pancreatic inflammation in 34. She felt that five of these owed more to coincidental factors,

such as unsuspected retroperitoneal lymphoma invading the pancreas, abscess caused by disseminated candidiasis, or perforated duodenal ulcer; the other 29 cases had no such factor. She reported that, in some cases, pancreatic necrosis was limited to the peripheries of lobules, a pattern more recently shown to be particularly associated with vascular insufficiency (Foulis 1980). As with acute pancreatitis associated with other kinds of surgery, clinical acumen identifies only a minority. Haas et al. (1985) describe a series in which 12 examples of acute pancreatitis after cardiopulmonary bypass (of which nine were severe) were detected clinically, over a period during which 35 examples were found at autopsy, including 27 with pancreatic or peripancreatic necrosis. They found that prolonged intraoperative hypotension had been recorded in all nine cases of severe acute pancreatitis that were clinically diagnosed, and indicate that they believe the association to reflect the high sensitivity of the pancreas to hypoperfusion. They went on to study prospectively a small cohort of cardiac surgery patients, and found hyperamylasaemia in over one-quarter. Rattner et al. (1989) confirmed their observation, performing a prospective study of 300 patients undergoing cardiopulmonary bypass, of whom 96 developed hyperamylasaemia; 56 of these had isolated, asymptomatic hyperamylasaemia, but 32 also had elevations of serum lipase or pancreatic isoamylase, often with mild upper gastrointestinal symptoms, defined by the authors as subclinical pancreatitis. Eight patients developed overt pancreatitis. The authors made the unexpected and unexplained observation that mortality was much greater in the patients with isolated hyperamylasaemia than in those without hyperamylasaemia.

In Rattner et al.'s study, those patients who developed overt pancreatitis were, in general, also those who developed renal tubular damage ascribed to hypoperfusion, this supporting the previous contention that the cause of acute pancreatitis in such patients is ischaemia.

A further prospective study of another 300 patients was carried out by the same group (Fernandez-del Castillo et al. 1991). On multivariate analysis, they found significant associations between pancreatic damage and pre-operative renal insufficiency, valve surgery (rather than coronary artery bypass grafts), post-operative hypotension, and perioperative administration of calcium chloride. Calcium chloride is given because it is believed to be beneficial to myocardial contractility, but, once the dose exceeds 800 mg m^{-2} of body surface, the risk of pancreatic damage increases rapidly. The authors pointed out that hypercalcaemia causes vasoconstriction, though they did not make it clear

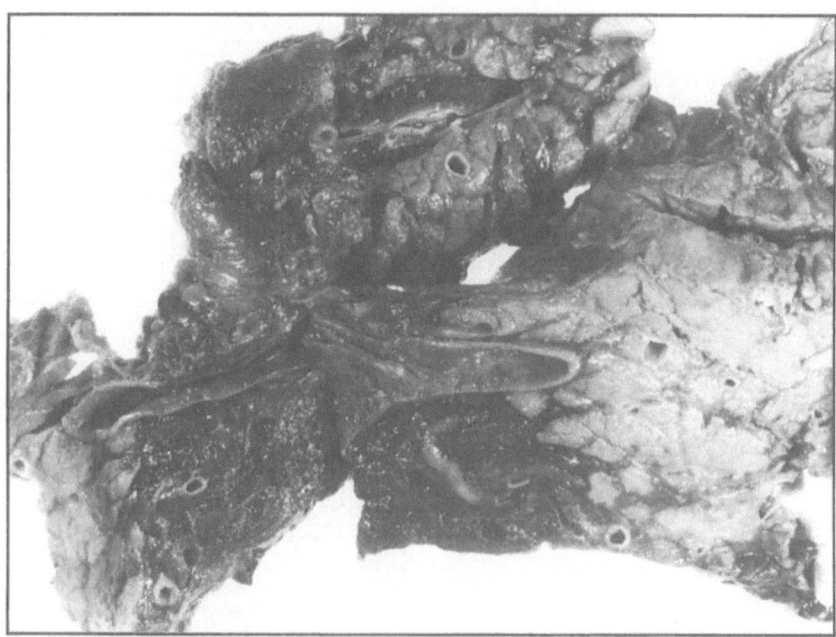

Fig. 12.1. A macroscopic view of a section through the region of the head of the pancreas from a woman aged 89, who became hypothermic while suffering from hypothyroidism. The common bile duct, which has been opened by the section, is surrounded by a haematoma. The woman was found dead and the duration of the pancreatitis is not known.

whether they think this to be the direct cause of pancreatic injury.

Hypothermia

Accidental hypothermia remains common in so-called developed countries (Rango 1984; Randall et al. 1985). Hypothermia was the certified cause of death in 152 individuals in England and Wales in 1990 (Office of Population Censuses and Surveys 1991), a figure that is inevitably an underestimate (Randall 1986).

A substantial proportion of patients found to be hypothermic before death prove to have evidence of pancreatic damage after death (Duguid et al. 1961; Mant 1969; Maclean and Emslie-Smith 1977; Moss 1986). The lesions may be focal or diffuse, with evidence of damage on naked eye examination in up to 80% of patients (Maclean and Emslie-Smith 1977); additional patients may have foci of fat necrosis identifiable only on microscopy (Mant 1969). Similar lesions are seen in deliberate iatrogenic hypothermia, which once enjoyed a short-lived vogue as therapy for advanced cancer (Sano and Smith 1940; Smith 1940).

It has long been suspected that acute pancreatitis is associated with hypothermia because the latter disease makes the circulation sluggish, causing hypoperfusion of the pancreas. Foulis (1980, 1982, 1984) provided the most cogent support for this hypothesis, showing that pancreatic necrosis in such cases is perilobular, where blood supply is most vulnerable. He goes on to demonstrate that other patterns of damage can be seen when a hypothermic patients dies with pancreatic lesions; he supports the previous contention that hypothermia may cause "microcirculatory shock" within the pancreas in some patients, but also points out that the two conditions may be coincidental complications of alcohol abuse, or that acute pancreatitis could lead to hypothermia in a socially isolated patient unable to get medical help. Drug-induced pancreatitis may have led to hypothermia in a case seen by one of the current authors (Benbow 1988). Some of the pancreatic lesions associated with hypothermia are illustrated in Figs 12.1–12.10.

The Role of Bacteria

Whilst it is generally accepted that acute pancreatitis is not primarily a bacterial infection, Keynes (1980, 1981, 1988) has persistently supported the viewpoint that bacterial infection may convert interstitial pancreatitis into necrotising pancreatitis, while noting that severe pancreatitis can be induced by bile reflux in germ-free dogs (Nance and Cain

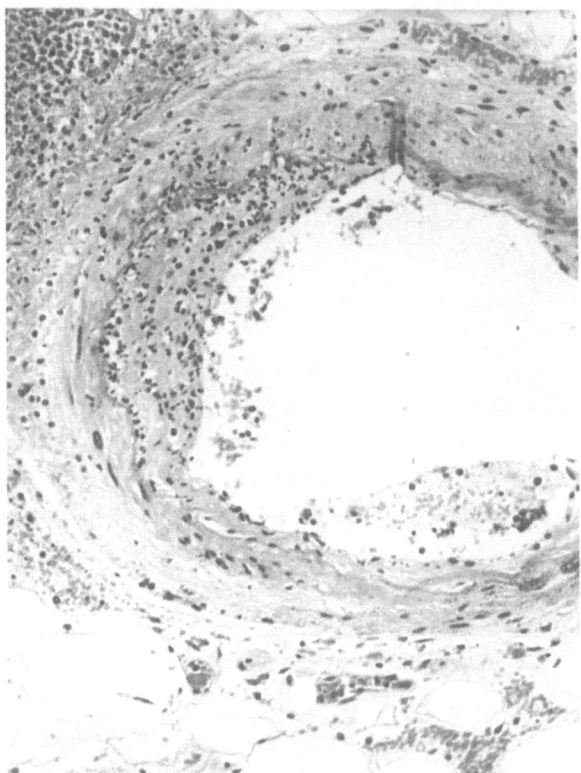

Fig. 12.2. A necrotic segment in the wall of a medium-sized artery in the pancreas illustrated in Fig. 12.1. H&E, × 150

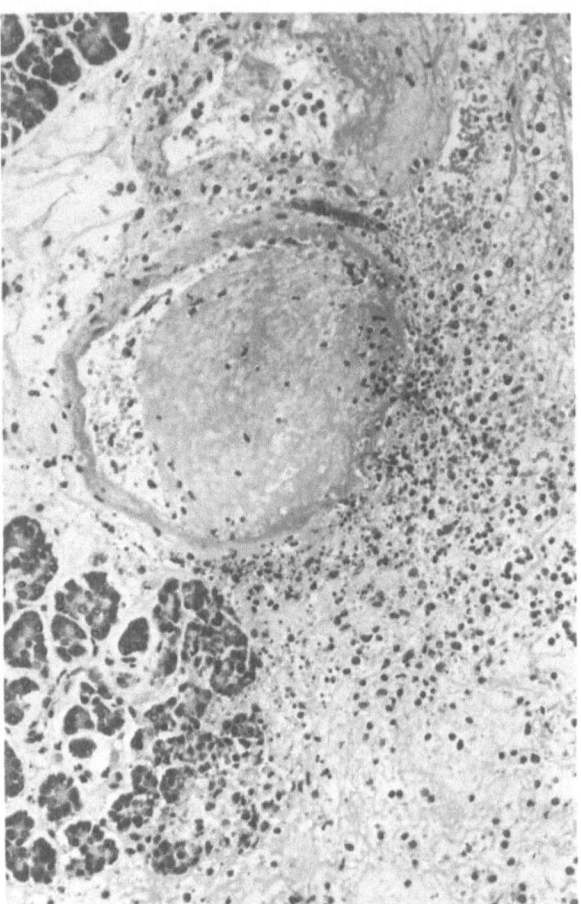

Fig. 12.3. Necrosis, mainly of the interstitial tissue, of the pancreas illustrated in Fig. 12.2. The walls of a small vein are necrotic and the lumen is almost filled by thrombus. H&E, × 150

1967). He was able to quote a number of studies, spread over most of the twentieth century, to support his views (Flexner 1901; Archbald 1919; Ivy and Gibbs 1952; Armstrong et al. 1984), together with his own experimental work (Keynes 1980). For instance, Armstrong et al. (1984) were able to induce haemorrhagic pancreatitis in rats by injecting bile infected with *Escherichia coli* into the pancreatic ducts, but not if they injected sterile bile or infected bile that had been filtered. However, other studies show that bacteria are not an essential prerequisite for lethal pancreatitis: Rattner et al. (1989) induced necrotising pancreatitis in mice, and found a similar rate of infection in those killed by the disease as in those that survived.

There is also plentiful information in the literature to suggest a possible mechanism by which bacteria might become important. Only those bacteria capable of producing membrane-damaging cytotoxins are able to convert acute interstitial pancreatitis into acute necrotising pancreatitis in experimental animals (Keynes 1988). In addition to producing their own toxins, these bacteria are able to promote the release of further toxic compounds from the host tissues, such as lysolethicin. When acutely inflamed pancreas is surgically resected and bacteriological cultures taken, then all positive cultures show toxin producers (Warshaw and Jin 1985; Malangoni et al. 1986; Beger et al. 1986). Gregg (1977) used endoscopic retrograde cholecystopancreatography to sample pancreatic duct juice; in patients with acute pancreatitis whose cultures were positive, the pancreatitis was more severe. Similarly, bacterial contamination of the pancreas can be demonstrated during the surgical removal of necrotic pancreatic tissue, and is associated with a higher mortality (Beger et al. 1986; Bittner et al. 1987).

Other Possible Causes

Even after extensive investigation, a substantial minority of cases of acute pancreatitis have no demonstrable underlying cause, and single case

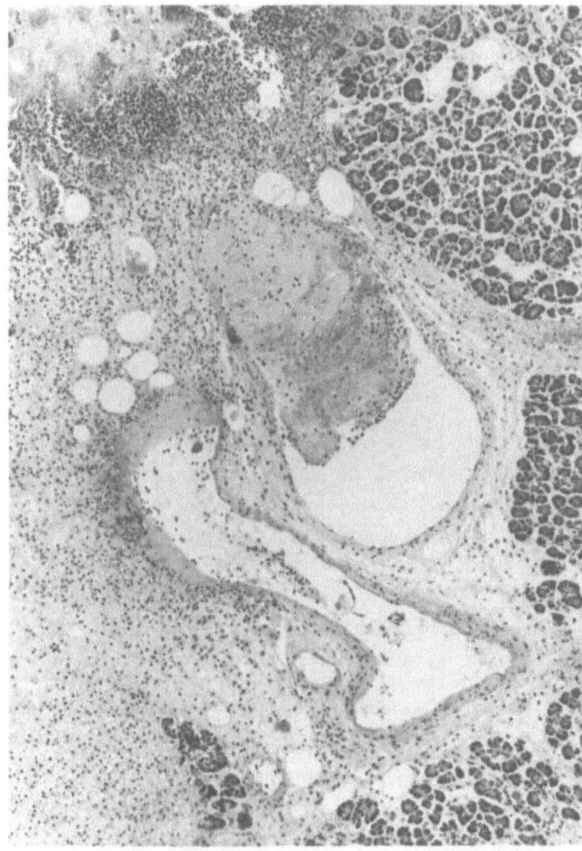

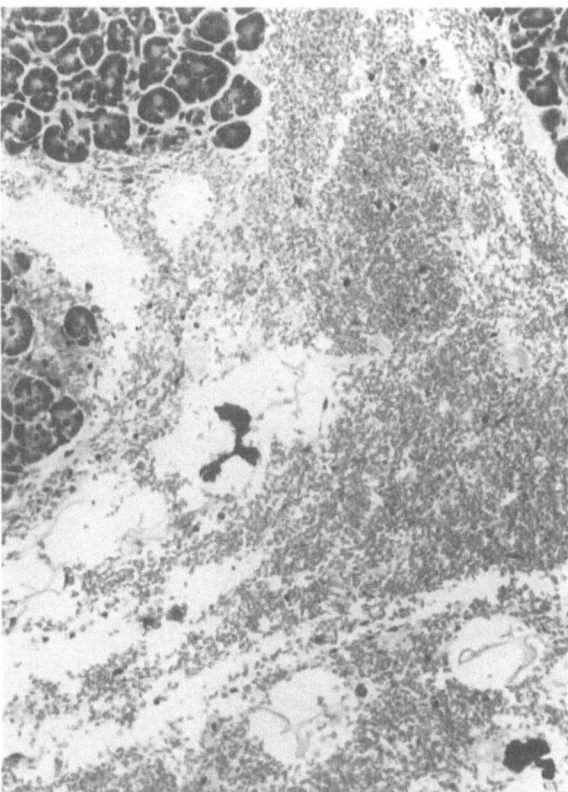

Fig. 12.4. Fat necrosis with adjacent oedema and leucocytic infiltration in the interstitial tissue of the pancreas illustrated in Fig. 12.3. There is partial occlusion of the lumen by thrombus in two segments of vein. H&E, × 60

Fig. 12.5. Haemorrhage and fat necrosis in the interstitial tissue of the pancreas illustrated in Figs 12.1–12.4. Deposits of brown pigment appear to be derived from damaged fat. In this case the pancreatitis was mainly interstitial but, unlike the characteristic picture of acute interstitial pancreatitis, haemorrhage was well marked. H&E, × 150

reports and descriptions of possible minor associations abound in the literature. Many of these associations are probably coincidental, but a few are sufficiently well-established to represent probable cause and effect.

DiVittorio et al. (1983) studied 168 patients with systemic lupus erythematosus (SLE), and found that seven had suffered from acute pancreatitis. In four of these seven, the clinical symptoms improved without the patients' steroid doses being reduced, which tends to exclude steroids as a cause of their pancreatitis. Reynolds et al. (1982) reported 20 examples of patients with SLE who had also suffered from acute pancreatitis, and found no possible cause other than the SLE in four of them; in one patient, acute pancreatitis appeared to be the first manifestation of SLE. In a more recent review, Eaker and Toskes (1989) described 66 patients with acute pancreatitis associated with SLE: ten were on drug-free regimens when acute pancreatitis became

symptomatic, and acute pancreatitis was the mode of presentation in four.

Matsumoto et al. (1989) described two examples of acute pancreatitis in patients with Crohn's ileo-colitis, in neither of whom could they find any of the usual causes of acute pancreatitis. By searching the literature, they found reports of 40 other patients in whom the two diseases coincided, with no other potential cause for the acute pancreatitis in about one-third.

A recently reported association is of interest, and is difficult to dismiss because of the large numbers of case histories studied. Parrilla Paricio et al. (1990) reviewed the case histories of 434 individuals who had been shown to have cholesterolosis of the gall bladder, and found that 98 (25.8%) of the 379 patients who had also had gallstones had a history of acute pancreatitis. Even more curiously, 27 (49.0%) of the 55 individuals with cholesterolosis, but no gallstones, had a history of pancreatitis.

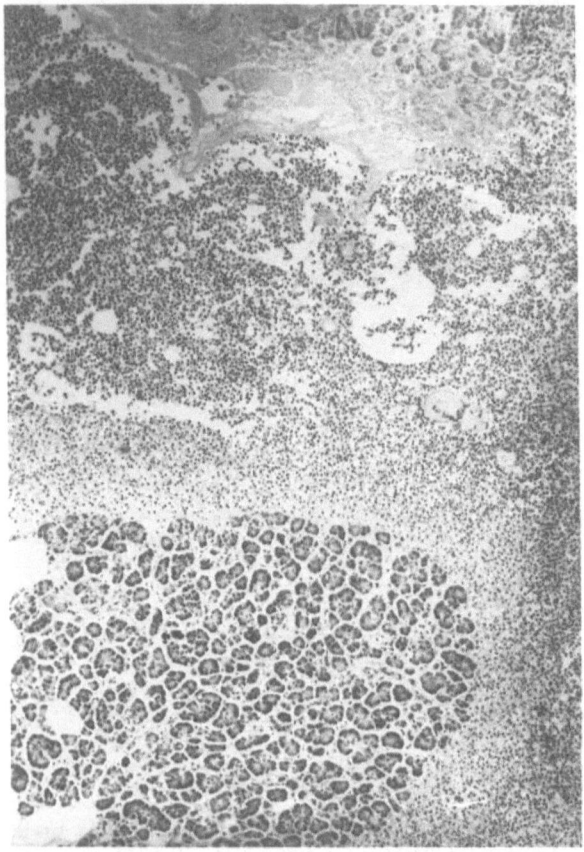

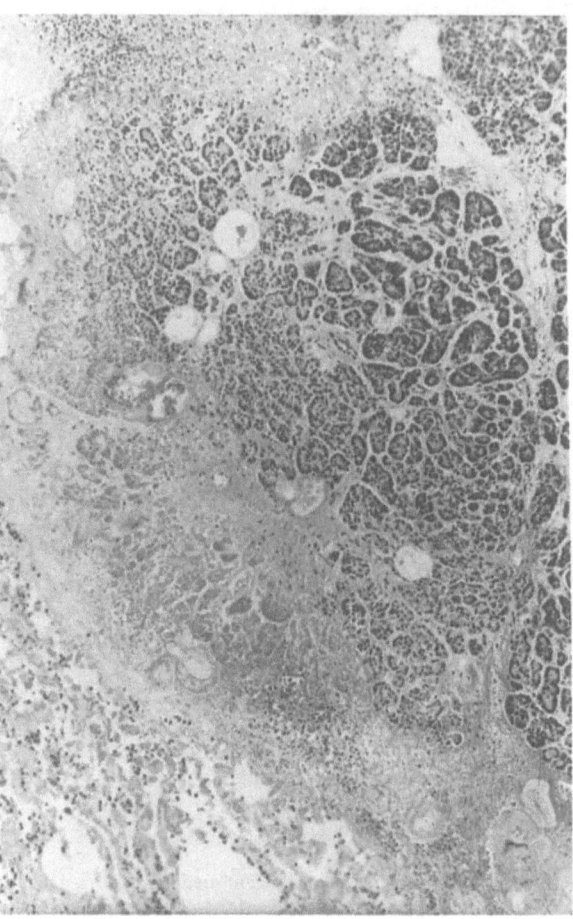

Fig. 12.6. Another area in the pancreas illustrated in Figs 12.1–12.5. There is well-marked fat necrosis and leucocytic infiltration of the interstitial tissues, with relatively undamaged glandular tissue. H&E, × 60

Fig. 12.8. In a different part of the pancreas illustrated in Fig. 12.7, there is interstitial inflammation with early necrosis of the adjacent glandular tissue. H&E, × 60

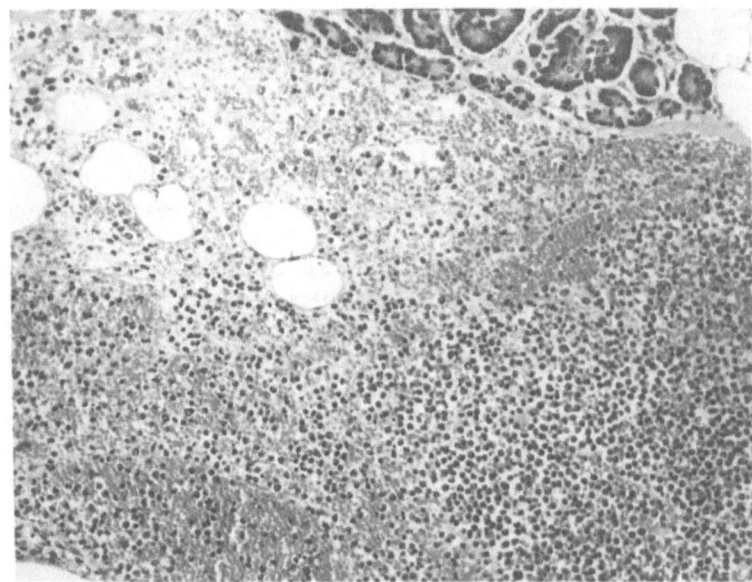

Fig. 12.7. A view, with higher magnification, of the polymorphonuclear leucocytic infiltration shown in Fig. 12.6. H&E, × 150

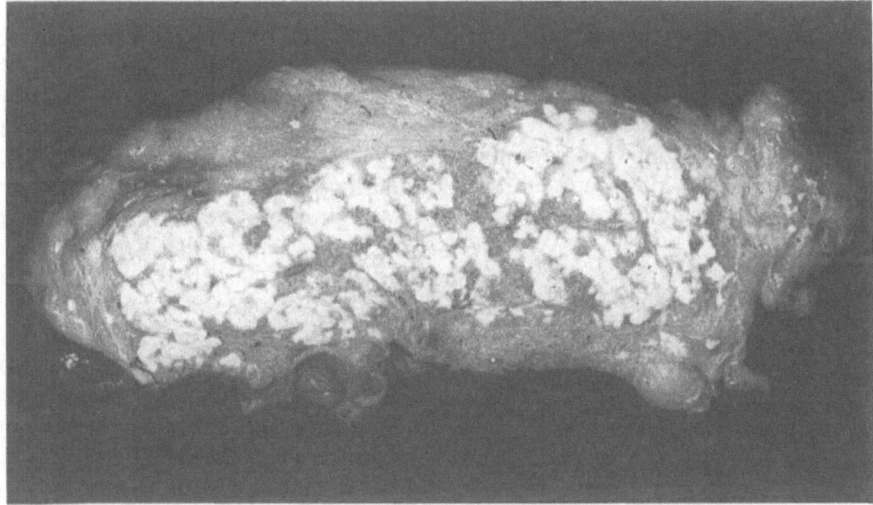

Fig. 12.9. Macroscopic view of the pancreas from a hypothermic patient. White areas of fat necrosis are marked, but haemorrhage is absent.

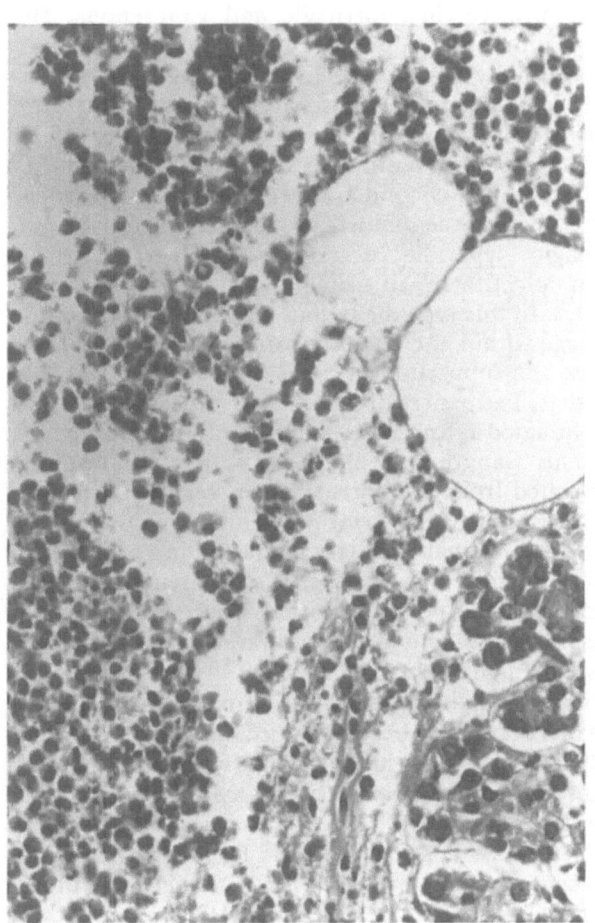

Fig. 12.10. Leucocytic infiltration of the interstitial tissue in the pancreas shown in Fig. 12.9. H&E, × 375

Histological Evidence of Initiating Factors in Man

It has been pointed out many times that pancreatitis is not a single disease with a single cause, and the many different ways in which acute pancreatitis can be produced experimentally, as well as the many aetiological factors that have been noted clinically, all suggest that this is so. Foulis (1980) suggested that it may be possible to differentiate histologically between two types of pancreatitis caused in different ways. Because, as Wharton (1932) has pointed out, each pancreatic lobule receives its arterial blood supply through a single branch from the interlobular arterial plexus, Foulis considered that the part of the lobule that was likely to be most vulnerable to ischaemia would be the part of the periphery furthest from the entrance of the lobular artery. In a review of the necropsy material from 37 cases of acute pancreatitis, he identified a number of different patterns in the distribution of the necrosis. He classified the cases histologically into groups, and, having completed his classification, studied the results in the light of the clinical histories of the patients.

He concluded that there were two initiating mechanisms in acute pancreatitis. The first mechanism was inflammation of the ducts, with subsequent necrosis of the pancreatic parenchyma surrounding the excretory ducts; such cases were associated with a history of alcohol abuse or with cholelithiasis. The second initiating mechanism was ischaemia, which led to necrosis confined to the microcirculatory periphery of the pancreatic lobule. Such cases were usually secondary to some form of shock, either septic or cardiac in origin. Mixed patterns were present in a number of examples, and Foulis considered that abnormality due to either mechanism might progress through a final common pathway of vascular damage to widespread pancreatic necrosis. Heatley (1990) provides support for Foulis' findings.

Age and Sex

Acute pancreatitis may occur in patients of any age, but it is rare in childhood and becomes more common in people over the age of 50 years (Parkash 1972). Men tend to be more commonly affected when there is an association with alcoholism; in women there is most likely to be an association with biliary disease. In reviewing the distribution of age and sex in pancreatitis, Dürr (1979) was able to refer to an example of pancreatitis in an unborn foetus and to report on 188 occurrences of the disease in children; he discussed the possible reasons for the very different ratios between the sexes that have been published by different workers. The clinical aspects of acute pancreatitis in the upper age groups have been the subject of a study by Hoffman et al. (1959). Fan et al. (1988) were able to substantiate earlier reports that the death rate is higher in elderly patients with acute pancreatitis, but, when death due to concomitant diseases is excluded, age ceases to be a risk factor for mortality.

Pancreatitis in childhood is unusual, but does occur. Ziegler et al. (1988) were able to report 49 patients. Of these, the cause was traumatic in 16, with road traffic accidents and child abuse predominating. Biliary disease was present in another 16, of whom six had pigment gallstones associated with sickle cell anaemia; six had systemic diseases, eight had ductal anomalies and three were idiopathic.

Morbid Anatomy

Singer, in his *Short History of Medicine*, published in 1928, expressed the opinion that, "The task of naked-eye pathological anatomy, effectively begun by Morgagni, was effectively completed by Karl Rokitansky of Vienna (1804–78)." Neither Morgagni nor Rokitansky, however, appear to have had any significant experience of acute inflammation of the

pancreas. Rokitansky, for example, dealt with inflammation of the pancreas along with inflammation of the salivary glands and, as translated by Edward Sieveking, stated that "inflammation of the pancreas, at all events in the acute form, is very rare", after which he proceeded to describe inflammation of the salivary glands. It was in 1889 that Reginald Heber Fitz, an American who had studied in Vienna with Rokitansky and in Berlin with Virchow, described the clinical and pathological features of acute pancreatitis and established the disease as a well-defined entity. In doing so, as has been pointed out by Major (1948), he performed for pancreatitis that which he had previously performed for acute appendicitis in 1886. Fitz's communication was delivered as the Middleton Goldsmith Lecture for 1889, and it was published soon after that, in three instalments, in the *Boston Medical and Surgical Journal*, under the title, "Acute pancreatitis. A consideration of pancreatic hemorrhage, hemorrhagic, suppurative and gangrenous pancreatitis and disseminated fat necrosis." As was indicated by the title, Fitz recognised three anatomical varieties: suppurative, haemorrhagic and gangrenous. He stated that the suppurative type might be acute, but was usually subacute or chronic, and tended to form abscesses that might discharge their contents into the stomach or duodenum, or open into the cavity of the great omentum to form a large peritoneal abscess. It was comparatively infrequently associated with disseminated fat necrosis. The haemorrhagic type he described as "peracute" or "apoplectiform", it usually proving fatal in 2 to 4 days. In this type the lesions were those of haemorrhage within and near the pancreas, with extension into the subperitoneal tissue, perhaps as far as the pelvis. Peripancreatitis might be expected and disseminated fat necrosis was a common accompaniment. Gangrenous pancreatitis, he said, usually resulted from haemorrhagic pancreatitis but could be secondary to perforating inflammation of the gastrointestinal or biliary tracts and proved fatal in the course of a few weeks. The gangrenous process involved the peripancreatic tissues and produced more or less complete sequestration of the pancreas, which might lie in the omental cavity, soaked in pus, and attached only by a few shreds. Both pus and pancreas might be discharged into the intestine. Splenic thrombophlebitis might occur but hepatic abscesses were rare. Disseminated fat necrosis was frequent.

The classification proposed by Fitz gained wide acceptance, and, by 1910, Opie, in the second edition of his book *Disease of the Pancreas,* could write that acceptance was almost universal.

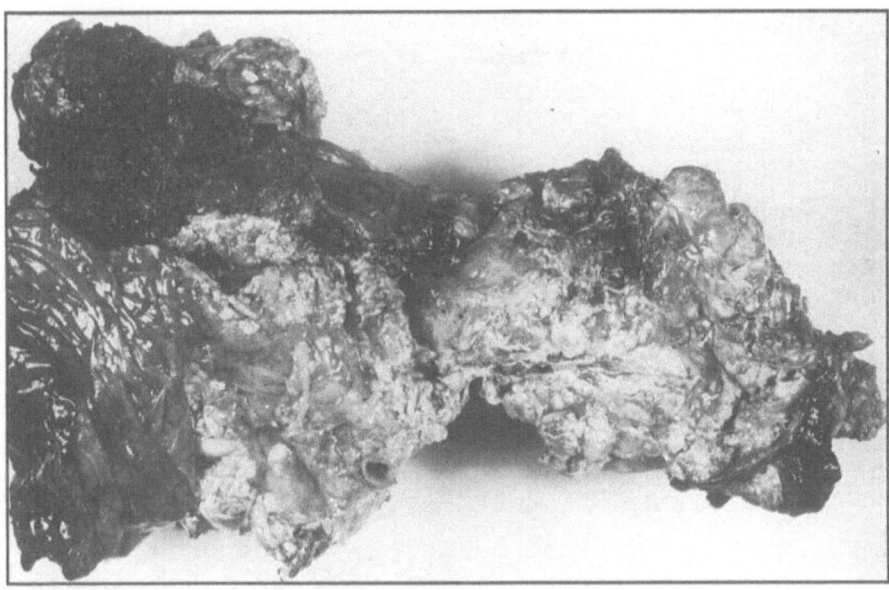

Fig. 12.11. Haemorrhagic pancreatic necrosis that developed in a 46-year-old woman 9 months after she had received a renal transplant. The mucosa of the opened duodenum is on the left, attached to the head of the pancreas. A haematoma covers the upper border of the pancreas and is most abundant above the head of the pancreas and the attached portion of duodenum. White areas of necrosis are present in the glandular tissue of all parts of the pancreas. Symptoms of pancreatitis had been present for 6 days before her death.

Opie's own work on pancreatitis has been mentioned already in relation to the reflux of bile in the pathogenesis of pancreatitis, and it was he who emphasised that, in haemorrhagic pancreatitis, the inflammation was in fact necrosis. Opie's description of the lesions of acute haemorrhagic pancreatitis has scarcely been improved upon by more recent writers.

He recognised that the appearance of the pancreas varied with the duration of the disease and that if there was survival for 2 weeks or longer the haemorrhagic appearances became those of gangrene. If a patient died within a few days of the onset of symptoms, the pancreas was very much enlarged, very firm and usually covered with clotted blood that had become blackish-red. The lesser sac of the peritoneum contained blood-stained fluid and the peripancreatic tissues were often infiltrated with blood. He said that fat necrosis always accompanied haemorrhagic necrosis of the pancreas. He emphasised also that the organ was rarely affected in its entirety, and that sharply defined areas of relatively normal parenchyma persisted and contrasted sharply with the red, reddish-brown or reddish-black necrotic tissue. Appearances of that type are illustrated in Figs 12.1 and 12.11 of the present work. Microscopically, he described the transition from

necrotic to apparently normal tissue as abrupt, with leucocytic margination and exudation of fibrin that might be trivial. He said that in the areas of damage, the glandular tissue, interstitial connective tissue and walls of blood vessels became necrotic, although for a time the outlines of the architecture remained recognisable. The relatively intact tissue in contact with the necrotic zone contained capillaries in which there was hyaline thrombosis. Microscopic appearances similar to those described by Opie are illustrated in Figs 12.12–12.15.

In describing the stage of gangrene, Opie relied mainly on the descriptions given by Fitz, and stated that at the end of the second week of the disease the pancreas formed a soft, black, friable mass with the lesser omental cavity filled with chocolate-coloured fluid containing large bluish-black clots, amongst which, in some cases, the glandular remnants might lie free, or almost free. Disseminated fat necrosis was usually conspicuous.

In more modern studies of the morbid anatomy and histopathology of acute pancreatitis, for example those of Roberts et al. (1950), Thal et al. (1957a), White (1966) and Baggenstoss (1973), there seems to be some degree of agreement that there are two main anatomical forms: acute interstitial pancreatitis, in which haemorrhage is not a feature, and

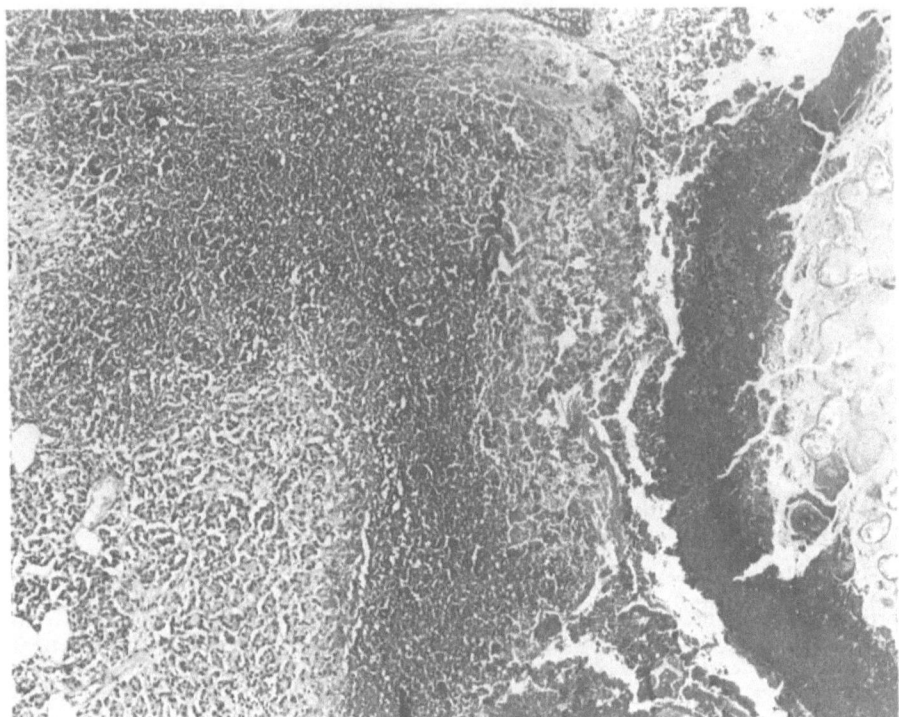

Fig. 12.12. The microscopic appearance of part of the pancreas illustrated in Fig. 12.11. Fat necrosis, to the right, is separated by a zone of extravasated blood from necrotic glandular tissue. Recognisable pancreatic tissue is present in the lower left corner. H&E, × 60

acute pancreatic necrosis, in which haemorrhage may be marked. Either type may be fatal, though the latter is considerably more dangerous.

Acute Interstitial Pancreatitis

The clinical illness associated with this type of pancreatitis may be as catastrophic as that associated with acute haemorrhagic pancreatitis. It was found by Thal and his colleagues that fatal cases did not survive long enough to develop the later sequelae that may follow acute haemorrhagic pancreatitis. The longest survival in their six such patients was 9 days. These workers found that the usual macroscopic appearance of the gland was that it was swollen and pale, with peripancreatic fat necrosis, and that on the cut surface the lobules were separated by oedematous interstitial tissue, while in some cases purulent material was seen to exude from the duct; in one case there were multiple small abscesses.

Microscopically, there was diffuse acute inflammatory infiltration in all their specimens, with polymorphonuclear leucocytes in the interstitial tissue, oedema and fibrinous exudate. In some, there were microscopic abscesses, while in four of

the six, the ducts contained polymorphonuclear leucocytes and cellular debris. There was also focal or diffuse dilatation of ductules that suggested the probable presence of obstructive lesions of the ducts, although the areas of squamous metaplasia of the epithelium of the ducts, thought by Rich and Duff (1936) to be important, were not found. Although there was leucocytic migration in and around the walls of veins and venules, thrombosis of vessels and acute necrotising arteritis were not found. This important difference from acute haemorrhagic pancreatitis, in which arteritis and thrombotic lesions are conspicuous, has been confirmed by Baggenstoss (1973).

Baggenstoss has pointed out that oedematous pancreatitis that is transient and relatively mild is probably quite common, and is recognised by surgeons as causing swelling of the pancreas that may be associated with fat necrosis in the adjacent tissues (Fig. 12.16). The risks of pancreatic biopsy, however, are such that samples from pancreases are rare, but Elman (1933) obtained microscopic confirmation of acute interstitial pancreatitis, without necrosis, haemorrhage or suppuration, in 37 patients that underwent laparotomy because of misdiagnoses of intestinal obstruction, perforation

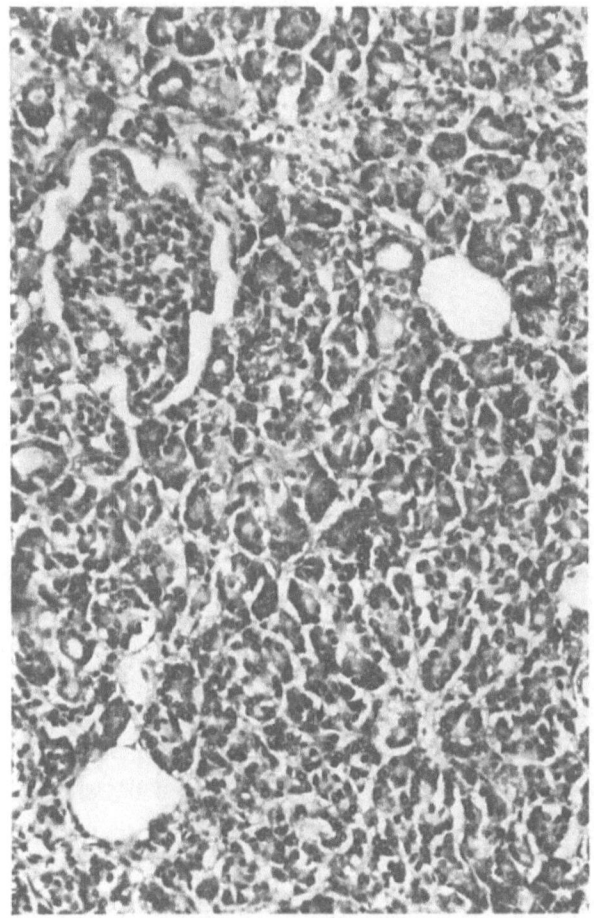

Fig. 12.13. An area of the pancreas illustrated in Fig. 12.11, in which the pancreatic tissue, including an islet, is undamaged. H&E, × 150

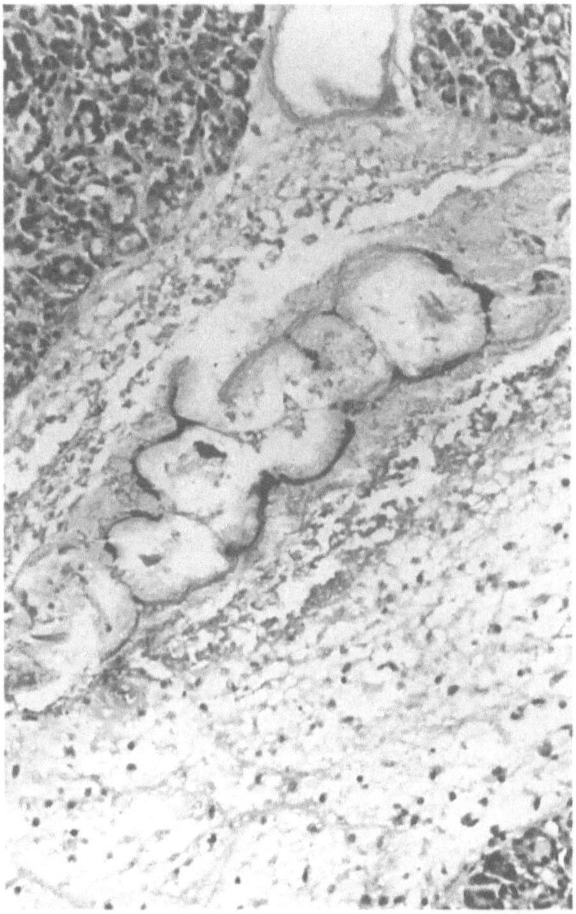

Fig. 12.14. Early calcification in necrotic fat in the pancreas illustrated in Figs 12.11–12.13. There is no necrosis of the adjacent glandular tissue. H&E, × 150

of a viscus, biliary disease or appendicitis. In these, the pancreas was oedematous, swollen and indurated. Most instances of pancreatitis of this type will resolve, though it may leave some residual interstitial focal fibrosis, but, as has been mentioned earlier, there is experimental evidence to show that, if acute oedematous pancreatitis is complicated by vascular lesions, then acute haemorrhagic pancreatitis may be superimposed. Even without the development of acute haemorrhagic necrosis, however, acute interstitial pancreatitis may be rapidly fatal, as recorded by Thal et al. (1957a). In such cases the inflammation is not entirely interstitial and there may be some infiltration of the lobules and acini by granulocytes, but this is less marked than the leucocytic infiltration of the interstitial tissue. In these severe cases, too, microabscesses may develop in association with interstitial fat necrosis, with involvement of the edges of the adjacent glandular

lobules. The pancreatitis of hypothermia is usually of the interstitial type with much fat necrosis, but without haemorrhage.

The pancreatitis that is found incidentally on microscopic examination of the pancreas in subjects who have died of diseases unrelated to the pancreas is usually of the interstitial type, for example those reported by Sachar and Probstein (1954), Evans et al. (1958), Stein and Powers (1958) and Czernobilsky and Mikat (1964). In such pancreases the changes may be quite mild and it is thus not surprising that there was no clinical evidence of pancreatic disease. Moreover, in the majority, the lesions are not acute. Thus, Czernobilsky and Mikat classified only eight of their 43 cases as acute, the others being chronic or healed. Even in those classified as acute, the illustrations are of interstitial oedema with only scanty infiltration by neutrophilic polymorphonuclear leucocytes.

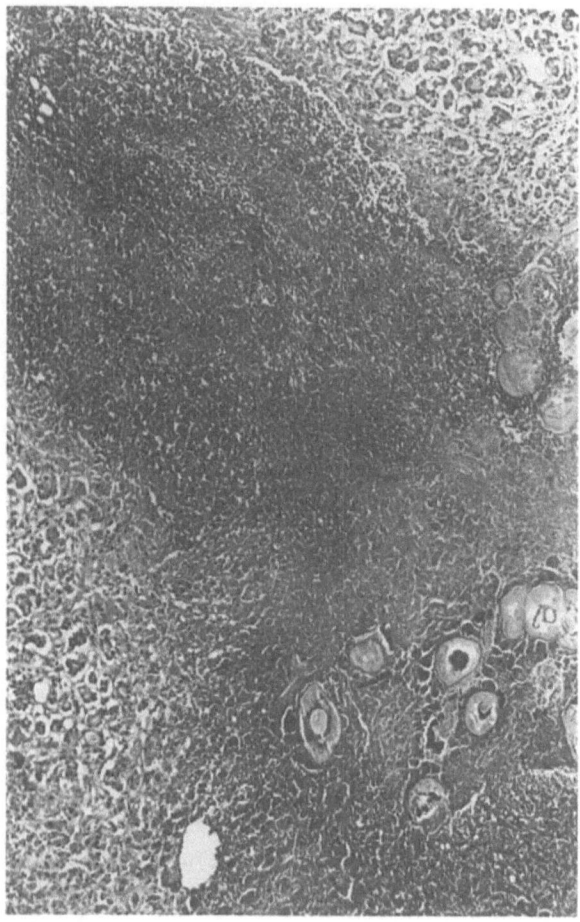

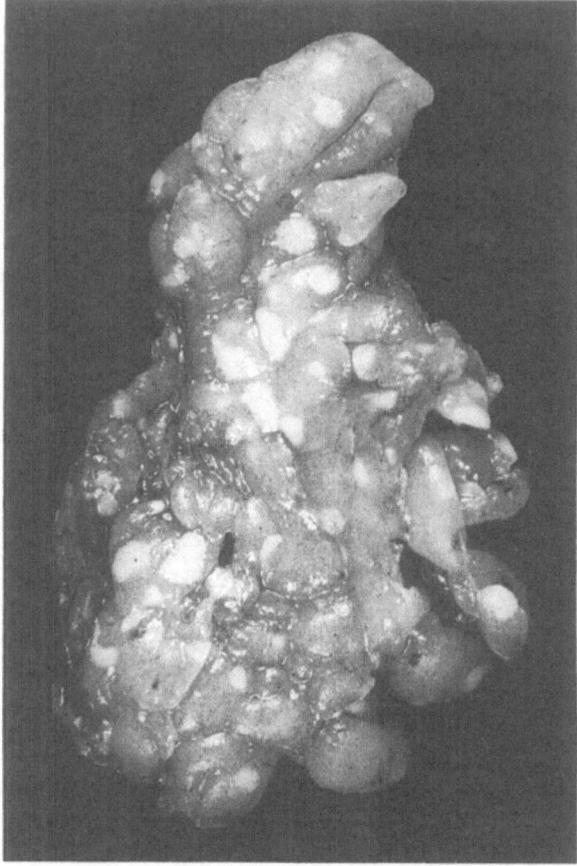

Fig. 12.16. The macroscopic appearance of white opaque areas of fat necrosis in part of the omentum removed during a laparotomy in a patient with acute interstitial pancreatitis.

Fig. 12.15. Another area in the pancreas illustrated in Figs 12.11–12.14. There is necrosis of fat and of the adjacent glandular tissue. H&E, × 60

Acute Haemorrhagic Pancreatitis

The macroscopic appearances have been well described by Opie (1910) and there is little to be added to his description, which was quoted a little earlier. There is swelling and oedema, with, in addition, necrosis of the pancreas and of the adjacent fatty tissue.

Fat Necrosis

Fat necrosis is often said to be pathognomonic, and usually accompanies haemorrhagic necrosis, but some degree of fat necrosis is commonly found post-mortem in the bodies of patients who have died from diseases unrelated to the pancreas. Quite rarely, there may be patches of necrosis in fat at a distance from the pancreas, in the thoracic cavity

(Roberts et al. 1950), for example, or in the subcutaneous tissues (Swerdlow et al. 1960) or the bone marrow (Scarpelli 1956). Small areas of necrosis in the pancreas may be pale, cream-coloured and opaque, or even chalk-like and white, but the larger lesions are haemorrhagic and look red, brown or black. It is often difficult to assess much how of the picture is the result of post-mortem autolysis. Because the clinical picture of eventually fatal pancreatitis may last for several months, at autopsy there may be abscess-like areas of walled-off necrotic material or, if bacterial infection has occurred, there may be true abscesses, from which pyogenic cocci or coliform organisms may be cultured. Fistulous communications between abscesses and adjacent organs may have developed.

It is unusual for the destruction of the pancreas to be complete (Roberts et al. 1950). MacLean (1977), who recorded the appearances at autopsy in three late fatalities following acute pancreatitis, was impressed by the comparative normality of the residual portions of the pancreas. In these cases there was extensive extraperitoneal necrosis of tissue and MacLean suggested that the secretions of the surviving pancreatic tissue, following disruption of the duct system, might have caused progressive enzymatic destruction of the extrapancreatic tissues. It is, however, sometimes surprising how the ducts may survive, even when there has been extensive necrosis of the glandular tissue.

Serous Effusions

Free fluid is usually present in the peritoneal cavity, and pleural effusions may also be present, with or without fat necrosis in the extrapleural tissues of the intercostal regions, as described by Swerdlow et al. (1960). Roberts et al. (1950) found that abdominal effusions that varied in amount from 200 ml to 3000 ml (average 1200 ml) were present in 18 of the 25 cases of the more fulminant type of acute pancreatic necrosis whose autopsy findings they reported, and that fluid was recorded as being absent in only three. The fluid was described as bloody or brown in 13; there was general peritonitis in five. Unilateral or bilateral pleural effusions were found in 17 of the 23 subjects in which the pleural cavities were examined.

Biliary disease with calculi, or a history of removal of biliary calculi, was present in 18 of the 23 subjects on which a complete autopsy had been carried out; in three of these, stones were trapped at the ampulla of Vater.

Gas Formation

There have been reports of the formation of gas within the pancreas during pancreatitis, so-called emphysematous necrotising pancreatitis. Such a patient, in whom gas bubbles were recognised radiologically in the pancreas, was described by Fischer and Geffen (1959), who stated that radiological signs of gas in the pancreas indicate a very poor prognosis. Their patient developed a huge abscess in the lesser sac of the peritoneum, and when this was drained large pieces of necrotic pancreatic tissue were removed. Aerobic and anaerobic cultures of this material yielded no growth. The patient died 16 days after the gas had been demonstrated, but no gas could be recognised post-mortem in the disorganised pancreas. The immediate cause of death was haemoperitoneum from eroded blood vessels.

The radiological recognition of subdiaphragmatic gas in association with acute haemorrhagic pancreatitis has been reported by Fielding and Loughran (1979), but, in their patient, infection by a gas-forming organism appears to have been responsible. Their patient was a 58-year-old man, who had been ill for 3 days with pancreatitis and had subcutaneous discoloration in the flanks due to retroperitoneal haemorrhage (Grey–Turner's sign). Gas was seen in a film of the abdomen, lying under both hemidiaphragms, retroperitoneally and around both the spleen and the gall bladder. Laparotomy was undertaken because perforation of a viscus was suspected, but no perforation was found. There was severe haemorrhagic pancreatitis, with blood-stained fluid in the peritoneal cavity, and gas was heard to escape when the lesser sac of the peritoneum was opened. *Aerobacter aerogenes*, a gas-forming organism, was grown from samples of the blood and peritoneal fluid. After the laparotomy, the patient was treated with intravenous lincomycin and gentamycin, peritoneal lavage and intravenous fluids, but within 2 days he developed radiological signs of a pneumomediastinum with patchy pneumonic consolidation. He died 4 days after the laparotomy. The autopsy confirmed the presence of acute necrotising pancreatitis, with bronchopneumonia and pneumomediastinum. The microscopic appearances of the pancreas are shown in Figs 12.17–12.19.

Microscopic Appearances

The microscopic appearances of the pancreas in acute haemorrhagic pancreatitis differ, because of the very variable duration of the illness when fatal, but, as was first emphasised by Opie, the essential feature is necrosis, with, when survival has been short, a relatively trivial inflammatory reaction. The necrosis involves all components of the pancreas: the fat in the interstitial connective tissue, the fibrous interstitial tissue, the blood vessels in the interstitial tissue, with haemorrhage as a result, and the epithelial tissues, including the islets. Necrosis tends to be most conspicuous in the fat and least conspicuous in the glandular tissue (Figs 12.12, 12.14, 12.15); it may extend within the interstitial tissue around glandular tissue, in which it is limited to the periphery of the lobules. Nerves in the interstitial tissue may be involved. The necrosis is usually patchy and seldom involves the entire gland; the transition from necrotic tissue to normal-looking tissue is abrupt and, sometimes, practically no vital reaction is recognisable, probably because death of the tissue has been recent. In other cases there is a narrow band of fibrinous exudate with polymor-

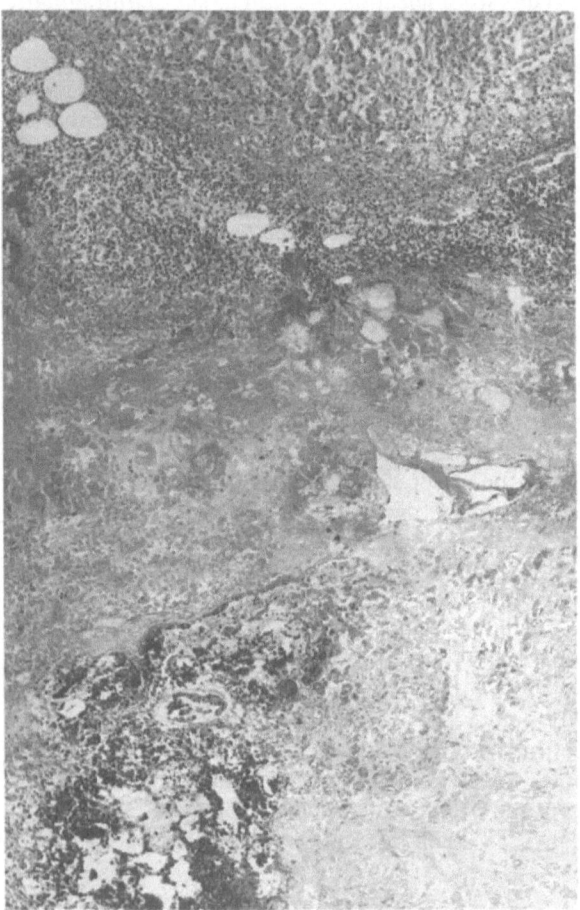

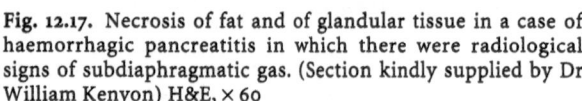

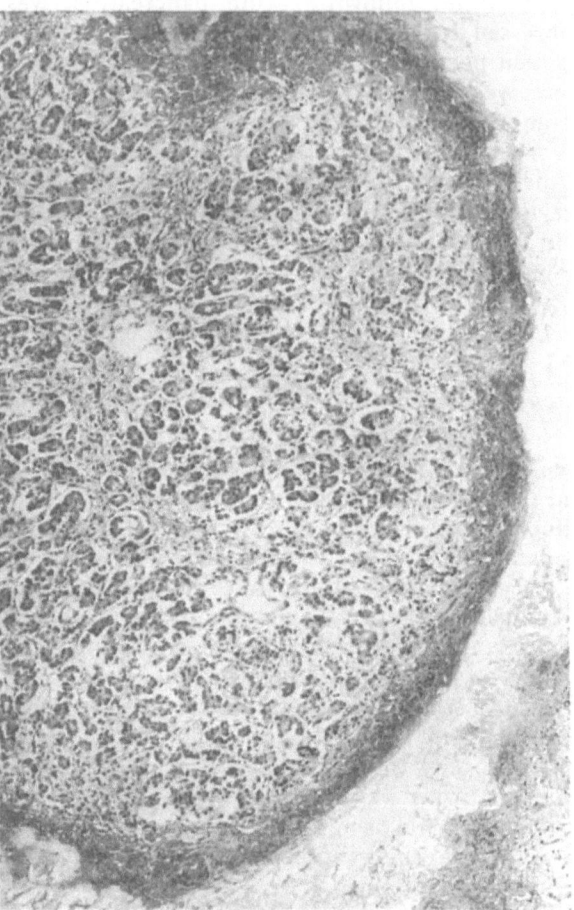

Fig. 12.17. Necrosis of fat and of glandular tissue in a case of haemorrhagic pancreatitis in which there were radiological signs of subdiaphragmatic gas. (Section kindly supplied by Dr William Kenyon) H&E, × 60

Fig. 12.18. Interstitial necrosis and necrosis of the peripheral parts of the glandular lobules in the same case as that illustrated in Fig. 12.17. H&E, × 66

phonuclear leucocytes between the two types of tissue. The amount of inflammatory reaction varies from place to place in different parts of the same pancreas, and in some areas, especially in the interstitial tissues, polymorphonuclear leucocytes may be abundant (Fig. 12.10). The degree of disruption of the necrotic tissue varies, probably with the age of the lesion. In early necrosis, the architecture is retained and cells can be recognised, although their nuclei have disappeared. In necrotic fat, the staining reaction with haematoxylin and eosin becomes basophilic even when the patient has died on the second or third day of illness (Roberts et al. 1950), probably because of deposition of calcium to form calcium soaps, but Baggenstoss (1973) found it difficult to demonstrate calcium histochemically in such tissue. Crystals of fatty acid may be present, sometimes with collections of brown pigment from the digested fat. In the glandular tissue, more so

than in other parts of the pancreas, the areas of necrosis resemble infarcts, and, because arterial and arteriolar branches involved in the necrotising process tend to be blocked by thrombi, areas of true infarction may develop.

The changes in the tissue adjacent to the necrotic areas depend upon the type of necrotic tissue and upon the age of the lesion. Necrotic fatty tissue becomes surrounded first by polymorphonuclear granulocytes, later by foamy macrophages and multinuclear cells, and finally by fibrous tissue (Figs 12.20–12.25).

Necrotic glandular tissue, which may seem at first to provoke no reaction, becomes surrounded by an acidophilic zone of partial necrosis in which there are nuclear remnants mixed with relatively well-preserved polymorphonuclear leucocytes. This zone is recognisable in patients who have survived for a week or less, and it has a distinct resemblance to the

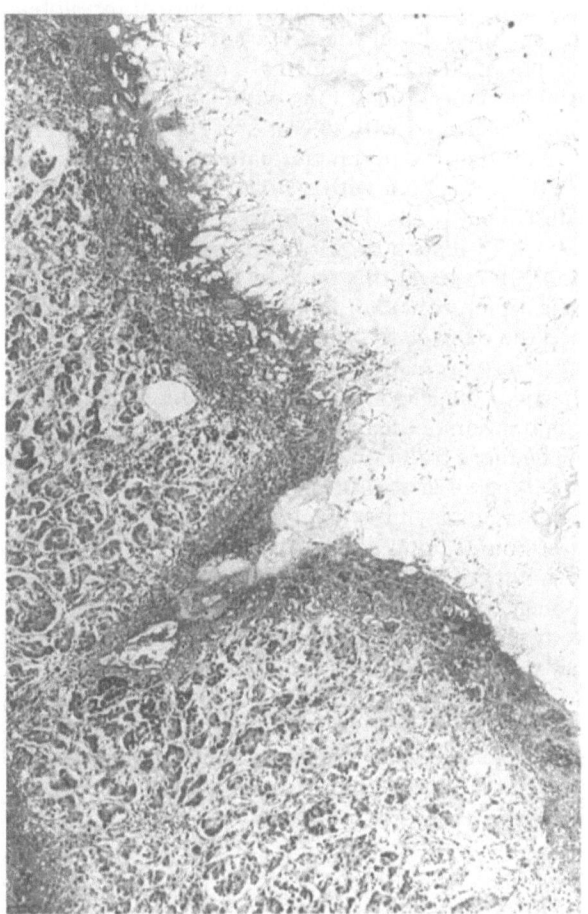

Fig. 12.19. Fat necrosis and perilobular glandular necrosis in the same case as that illustrated in Figs 12.17 and 12.18. H&E, ×60

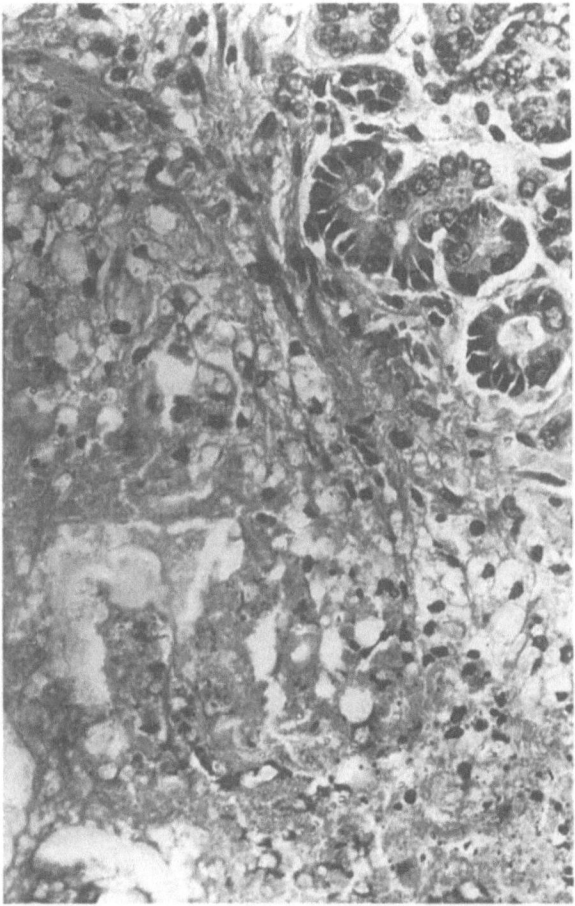

Fig. 12.20. A reaction of foamy phagocytes around an area of fat necrosis in the pancreas in acute pancreatitis. H&E, ×375

floor of a peptic ulcer. When the illness has lasted for over a week, a zone of yellow haematoidin pigment is said by Baggenstoss (1973) to become well marked.

With the passage of time, polymorphonuclear infiltration becomes more marked, especially in the interlobular septa, where some degree of oxygenation has remained, for leucocytes are unable to penetrate completely the ischaemic tissue for any distance. If survival is prolonged for several weeks, sloughs of necrotic gland become surrounded by liquid pus in which secondary bacterial infection may or may not have occurred.

Vascular Damage

The vascular damage that occurs in acute pancreatitis was considered by Rich and Duff (1936) to be an essential step in the pathogenesis of the disease, the haemorrhage being the result of the necrosis of the walls of the arteries and veins. The arterial lesions resemble those of polyarteritis nodosa and they are illustrated in Fig. 12.2. The veins and the smaller blood vessels in affected areas of the pancreas usually contain thrombus (Fig. 12.3). The vascular damage is generally taken to be secondary to the necrotising process in the pancreas, but it is also believed to be important in contributing to the progression of the process.

Although there is a certain resemblance between the arterial lesions of acute haemorrhagic pancreatitis and the necrotising arterial lesions of polyarteritis nodosa, the pancreatic lesions that are sometimes found at autopsy in fatal cases of polyarteritis are usually infarcts, and reports of acute haemorrhagic pancreatitis due to polyarteritis nodosa are rare. It is true that Bocanegra et al.

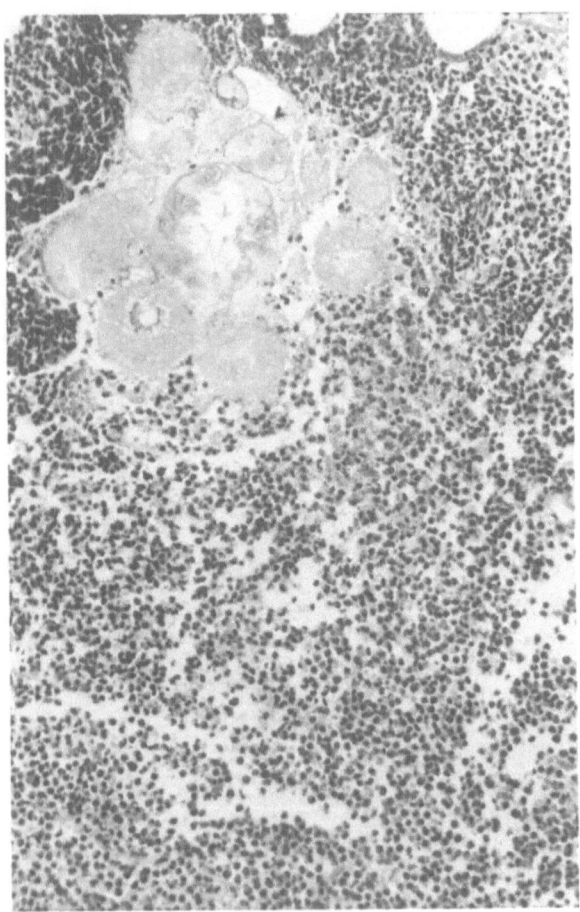

Fig. 12.21. An early abscess forming in acute haemorrhagic necrosis. Necrotic fat is surrounded by pus cells. H&E, × 150

(1980) have reported the development of a pancreatic pseudocyst during the downhill course of a fatal case of the necrotising vasculitis of polyarteritis nodosa, but there was no autopsy to establish the cause of the pseudocyst. In the patient with polyarteritis nodosa reported by Thorne et al. (1980), presentation was with an abrupt onset of pancreatic insufficiency; the pancreatic lesion demonstrated by endoscopic retrograde pancreatography had the appearance of chronic, not of acute, pancreatitis.

Periductal and Perilobular Patterns

Although reflux of bile or duodenal fluid is suspected by many to be important in initiating acute haemorrhagic pancreatitis, lesions of the ducts are inconspicuous microscopically and are scarcely mentioned by some authors. Foulis (1980), however, has described necrosis of the pancreatic

parenchyma in the immediate vicinity of intralobular or interlobular ducts, associated with polymorphonuclear leucocytes and eosinophilic proteinaceous concretions within the ducts, sometimes associated with necrosis of the duct wall. He thought that the periductal pattern of necrosis was usually associated with a history of alcoholism or with cholelithiasis. He also described a perilobular pattern of distribution of the necrosis (Figs 12.18, 12.19). In cases of this type, he correlated the histological picture with a history of shock, and attributed the damage to ischaemia in the areas in which the microcirculation was most vulnerable to the effects of the shock. In some cases he recognised a combination of the two patterns.

The more traditional explanation for the perilobular type of distribution of necrosis is that the advancing enzymes travel with greater ease in the interlobular connective tissue and damage the periphery of the lobules only after they have caused damage to the adjacent interstitial tissue. In sections from the parts of the pancreas that seem, with the naked eye, to be unaffected, it is quite common to find signs of chronic pancreatitis, or of scarring that may be the residue of previous pancreatitis. Squamous metaplasia of the epithelium of the ducts, at one time thought to be important in the aetiology of the disease, is uncommon.

Ultrastructure

The ultrastructure of the pancreatic acini in six patients who had pancreatic resections carried out for acute necrotising pancreatitis was studied by Helin et al. (1980). In one, a man aged 64, the disease was associated with biliary disease; in the remaining five, alcohol was thought to be the aetiological factor. Frankly necrotic areas were avoided and the specimens were selected from areas that were oedematous macroscopically or on light microscopy. Zymogen granules were found to be increased in size and number, with loss or variation of electron density and peripheral dissolution. Increased autophagic activity was indicated by autophagic vacuoles and residual bodies. The acinar lumina were dilated and there was effacement of microvilli and invaginations in the luminal plasma membranes of the acinar cells. Fibrillar material was observed in the acinar lumina and in the interstitium, especially in the areas with severe cellular degeneration. The findings were interpreted as indicating increased activity of the zymogen granules, increased autophagocytosis and penetration of acinar luminal contents into the interstitium.

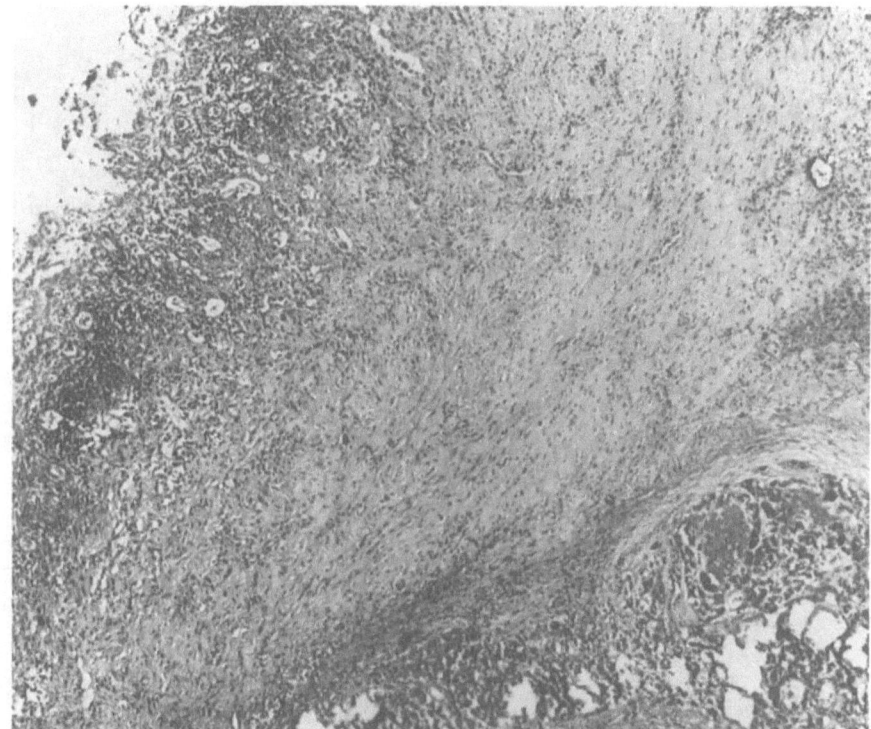

Fig. 12.22. The wall of a chronic abscess of the pancreas in a patient who died 6 months after an attack of acute pancreatitis. There is an inner zone of granulation tissue and an outer fibrous zone, separating the abscess from distorted pancreatic tissue in the lower right corner. H&E, × 60

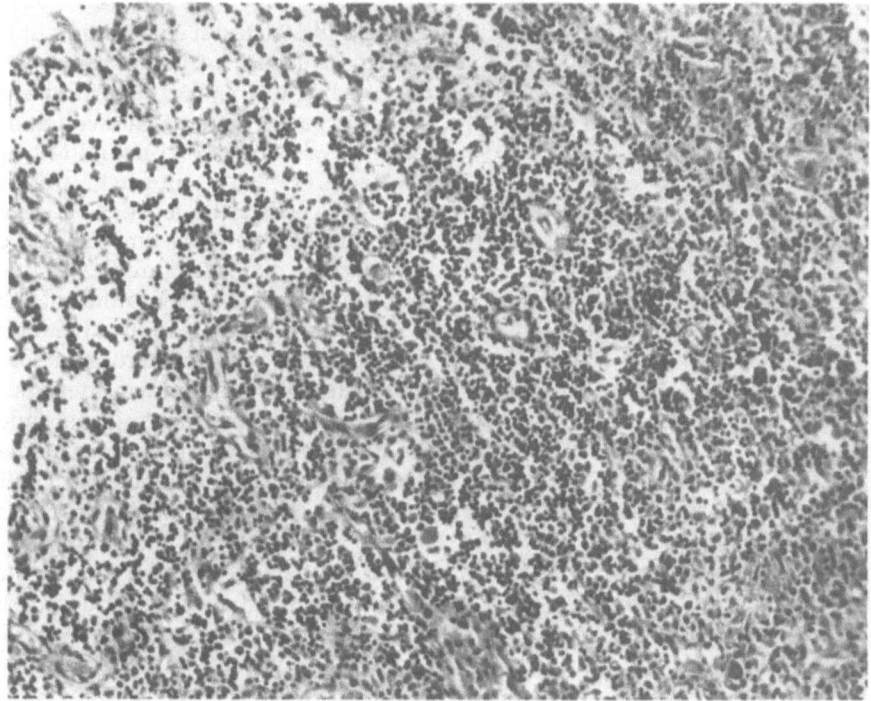

Fig. 12.23. Chronic inflammatory cells in the wall of the abscess illustrated in Fig. 12.22. H&E, × 150

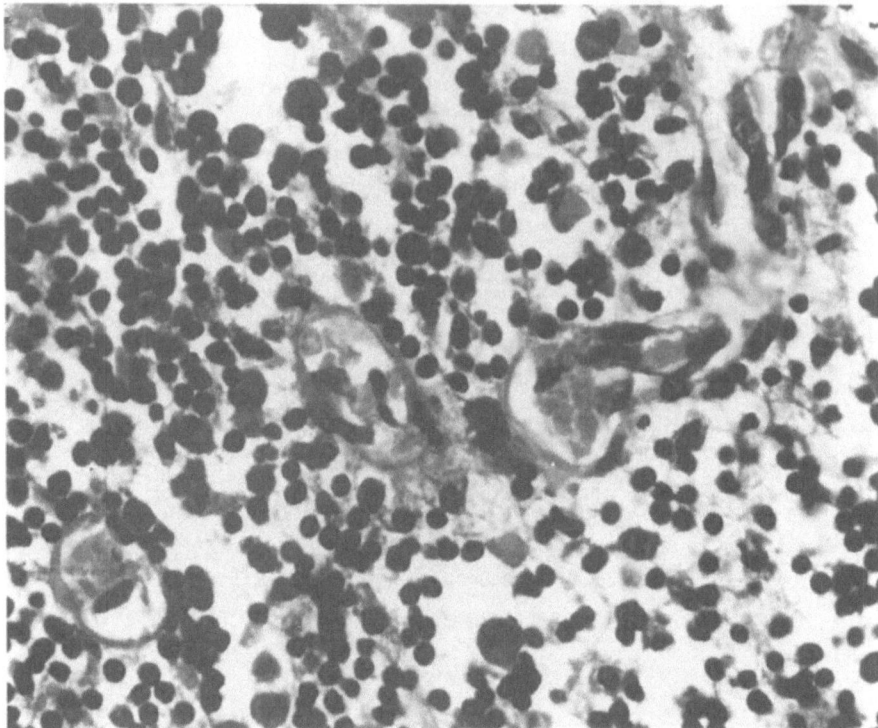

Fig. 12.24. Lymphocytes and plasma cells in the wall of the abscess shown in Figs 12.22 and 12.23. H&E, × 600

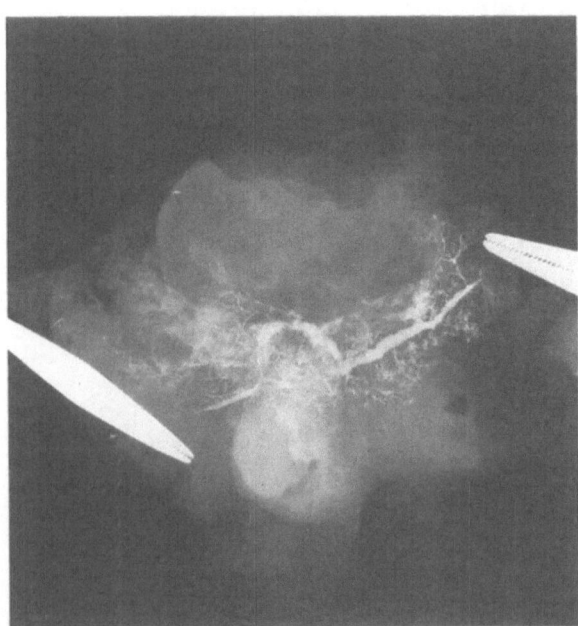

Fig. 12.25. A radiograph of the distorted pancreatic duct after it had been injected with barium, in a pancreas that contained the chronic abscess illustrated in Figs 12.22–12.24.

The ultrastructural changes in human pancreases resected because of acute pancreatitis were also observed by Aho et al. (1982). They examined material from seven patients, and concluded that acinar and fat cells undergo concomitant necrosis in the affected areas, that zymogen granules degenerate in the acinar cells at the border between the necrotic and non-necrotic areas, and that secretory proteins may become displaced into the interstitium outside the acinar lumina. They found that the fat content of damaged fat cells is reduced and that older areas of fat necrosis become surrounded by fibroblasts.

Trapnell (1966) has drawn attention to an important discrepancy between the anatomical changes in the pancreas and mortality in acute pancreatitis. Of the 76 deaths that occurred amongst the patients he studied, 57 (75%) died within the first 2 weeks of the illness, at a time when the pancreatic changes were found, post-mortem, to be predominantly those of oedema with fat necrosis. Haemorrhage was less constant and less marked, and necrosis of the gland was usually absent. In Trapnell's opinion, death occurred at a time when the pancreatic lesions were minimal, and that the cause of death had to be attributed to "irreversible shock", probably because of the liberation of vasoactive substances from the relatively inconspicuously damaged pancreas. From the appearances of the pancreas in his fatal cases, Trapnell formed the opinion that the severity of the pancreatic lesions depended upon the duration of the illness, survival until the third week being necessary for the full picture of necrosis and autodigestion to develop, at which stage death tended to be the result of one of the complications of the disease, such as abscess or haemorrhage.

Non-pancreatic Lesions Attributable to Acute Pancreatitis

In patients with mild interstitial pancreatitis without complications, recovery is the rule, but, as has been stated already, severe interstitial pancreatitis may be rapidly fatal. In haemorrhagic pancreatitis, however, mortality is high, and, according to the publications cited by Nugent and Mobarhan (1973), it has ranged in the past from 50% to 75%. However, by 1978, according to results published by workers between 1976 and 1978, and collected by Dürr (1979), the mortality for acute and relapsing acute pancreatitis was estimated to be between 5.4% and 13%, with an overall mortality of 10.4% for the 1502 cases in seven reported series.

The pathophysiology that causes death is complicated, and includes the effects of haemorrhage into and around the pancreas, together with the liberation of vasoactive peptides by the action of trypsin on precursors in the plasma to cause systemic vasodilatation and increased vascular permeability, with decreased effective blood volume. This leads to shock, with cardiopulmonary, renal and hepatic failure, to which the effects of local and generalised bacterial infection are often added.

Hypocalcaemia and Hypomagnesaemia

Hypocalcaemia as a consequence of acute pancreatitis was first described by Edmondson and Berne in 1944. Their attention was drawn to the potential problem by a patient with acute pancreatitis who developed tetany, despite normal levels of carbon dioxide in the bloodstream. Stimulated by this finding, they monitored total serum calcium in 50 further patients with acute pancreatitis, and found it to be low in 36 of these, at least at some point in the progression of the disease. Three of the 50 patients developed tetany, one with a very low serum calcium indeed; in contrast, another patient with tetany had a serum calcium only marginally below the lower limit of the normal range. Subsequently, Edmondson et al. (1952) confirmed these early findings in a further series of 27 patients, showing that severe hypocalcaemia was associated with extensive fat necrosis; they speculated that the calcium was bound by the saponification of fat, or that it was lost via the bowel. They also demonstrated hypomagnesaemia in four of 20 patients.

Other authors have demonstrated a close correlation between total serum calcium and mortality rate (Feller et al. 1974; Ranson et al. 1974). For example, Feller et al. found no deaths in 75 patients whose total serum calcium remained above 9 mg dl^{-1}, but there were five deaths amongst the 12 individuals whose levels dropped below 7 mg dl^{-1}. Interpretation of these early studies is complicated by the fact that total serum calcium comprises free ionised calcium and albumin-bound calcium. Allam and Imrie (1977) found that serum ionised calcium was normal in most of their eight patients; most hypocalcaemia, they argued, was actually a reflection of hypoalbuminaemia. A previous study by the same group had shown hypoalbuminaemia to be associated with a poor prognosis.

Much of the difficulty has arisen because the majority of laboratories measure only total serum calcium on routine blood samples, and calculate a "corrected" ionised calcium from a knowledge of the serum albumin concentration. Croton et al. (1981) measured ionised calcium directly, with results contradictory to those of Allam and Imrie (1977). They found that low serum calcium occurs frequently in acute pancreatitis, and that it is related to the severity of the disease; the directly measured ionised calcium correlates poorly with a calculated ionised calcium in the first 24 hours of an attack of acute pancreatitis, but correlates well thereafter. Whatever the merits of the various viewpoints on serum calcium and outcome, tetany is known to indicate a a very poor prognosis. Jones (1985) was able to report an exceptional case, distinguished not only by the patient's survival, but also by the fact that tetany was amongst the presenting complaints.

Parathyroid hormone and calcitonin levels rise in acute pancreatitis, but not to levels greater than those seen in patients stressed by other severe disease (Drew et al. 1978). Hypomagnesaemia may inhibit both the release of parathyroid hormone and its peripheral action (Drew et al. 1978), as well as cause tetany independently of hypocalcaemia.

Renal Failure

Renal failure is a well-recognised feature af acute pancreatitis (Carey 1979), and, of 41 newly diagnosed patients with acute pancreatitis reviewed by Gordon and Calne (1972), six had developed acute renal failure, all within 2 weeks of the onset of the illness; of the six, three died. Gordon and Calne were unable to explain the acute renal failure, and pointed out that none of their patients had had any episodes of hypotension. Gupta (1971) found mesangial widening and capillary basement membrane thickening in most of the patients in his series, with tubular necrosis and vacuolar degeneration in a smaller number. Frost et al. (1990) confirmed that acute renal failure complicating acute pancreatitis has a poor prognosis; of 14 patients requiring dialysis, ten died. Indeed, their review of the literature suggested that the mortality from this complication had not improved over the previous four decades.

Brandes et al. (1989) described a patient with a pancreatic abscess that extended into the right pararenal space, leading initially to hydronephrosis, and subsequently to pyelonephritis. They were able to find reports of six other patients in which hydronephrosis complicated acute pancreatitis, but none of these had pyelonephritis as well.

Pulmonary Failure

Respiratory failure is a well-recognised problem in patients with acute pancreatitis, and in 1977, McKenna et al. were able to identify a number of possible contributory causes:

1. Aspiration, the risk of which is increased by the nasogastric suction that is commonly necessary
2. Fluid overload, which may be aggravated by the action of a myocardial depressant factor that has been demonstrated experimentally by Lefer et al. (1971)
3. Hypotension, which is common in acute pancreatitis
4. Embolism by fat, or thrombi from diffuse intravascular coagulation
5. The effects of altered pulmonary capillary permeability induced by histamines, kinins and complement-derived anaphylatoxins
6. Agglutinin reactions to the leucocytes in the transfusions of whole blood that are often necessary

Murphy et al. (1980) studied the pathophysiology of 14 patients who had acute pancreatitis, and who had no previous cardiorespiratory disease. Gas exchange and shunt measurements were performed,

and the main defect found was a left-to-right shunt. In general, these patients were not breathless, so there was no mechanical obstruction to the airways, and pulmonary oedema was not common. They concluded that they were observing "possibly another variant" of the adult respiratory distress syndrome (ARDS). Lankisch et al. (1983) studied 36 cases at autopsy, and found the pulmonary changes to resemble those of "shock lung", a synonym, of course, for ARDS. In the early phase, they found interstitial and intra-alveolar oedema, dilated lymphatics and capillary congestion, with leucocyte margination and adherence. Following this was a phase of hyaline microthrombi and intra-alveolar haemorrhage, leading on to typical hyaline membranes and proliferation of type II pneumocytes. Lankisch et al. (1983) suggested various possible mechanisms, and placed particular emphasis on blood-borne mediators from the site of pancreatic inflammation. Possible mediators included histamine, trypsin, phospholipase A, triglycerides and activated complement. Experimental evidence using the rat as a model suggests that phospholipase A_2 causes an accumulation of platelet activating factor within the lung, leading the authors to speculate that this is an important mechanism (Zhou et al. 1992). Guice et al. (1989), however, provided evidence that activated complement may be important, leading to neutrophil activation within the pulmonary vasculature, with damage mediated by oxygen-derived free radicals.

In addition to changes within the lungs, there may sometimes be pleural effusions, or an effusion in only one of the pleural cavities. The fluid is usually brown or blood-tinged, and the average volume in either pleural cavity was 425 ml in 17 cases of acute pancreatic necrosis found by Roberts et al. (1950) to have pleural effusions at autopsy. Occasionally either pleural cavity might contain as much as 1500 ml of fluid. Pleural effusions are usually associated with peritoneal effusions and, in acute pancreatitis, the effusions are attributed to the effects of lymphatic communications between the cavities.

Cardiac Abnormalities

Acute pancreatitis may cause electrocardiographic changes (Barbezot and Waterworth 1978), though no anatomical changes have been found. Patients, nevertheless, sometimes develop poor cardiac output during an attack of acute pancreatitis, a feature associated with a poor prognosis (Bank et al. 1983). Lefer et al. (1971) believed that this was due to an unidentified myocardial depressant factor; more recently, Chardavoyne et al. (1989) have suggested that reactive oxygen metabolites may be involved. They demonstrated a progressive decline in the cardiac index in dogs with experimental acute pancreatitis, and showed that this decline occurred less quickly if the levels of oxygen free radicals were reduced by pretreatment with catalase or superoxide dismutase.

Pericardial effusion is a rare complication of pancreatitis and tends to be associated with pleural effusions (Mitchell 1964); it may cause cardiac tamponade (Lipson and Stephenson 1971).

Abnormalities of the Nervous System

A number of neurological abnormalities can be observed in acute pancreatitis, related to hypoxaemia or electrolyte disturbances; complications of associated disorders, such as the delirium tremens of alcohol withdrawal may also become evident. On occasion, cerebral fat embolism may also complicate the picture (Johnson and Tong 1977).

In the central nervous system, lesions associated with acute haemorrhagic pancreatitis have been reported by various authors; such lesions are believed to be responsible for the clinical syndrome of pancreatic encephalopathy. This condition has been reviewed by Pallis and Lewis (1974), who have summarised the clinical and pathological features of three of the published cases that they considered to be true examples of pancreatic encephalopathy. In such subjects, the lesions tended to be more marked in the brain stem, especially in the pons. In one, there was massive pontine demyelination with relative preservation of the neuronal elements; in another, there were multiple small areas of axonal and myelin destruction, with some neuronal loss in the central pons; while in the third, there was central pontine softening with myelin and axonal loss and neuronal changes. All three also had foci of necrosis or loss of myelin in the cerebellum and in the cerebral hemispheres. The lesions are suspected to be due to the action of lipases and proteolytic enzymes liberated into the circulation from the damaged pancreas. Pallis and Lewis were of the opinion that pancreatic encephalopathy may be more common than is generally recognised, but they emphasise that, when encephalopathic symptoms develop in patients with pancreatitis, it is necessary to exclude delirium tremens, cerebral disturbance due to shock, renal failure, hyperosmolarity, hypokalaemia, and either hypercalcaemia or hypocalcaemia.

Gross et al. (1988) described a peripheral neuropathy in four patients with acute pancreatitis, though they pointed out that factors other than the pancreatitis itself might have contributed to the axonal damage they demonstrated with electrophysiological tests. All the patients had needed parenteral nutrition, during which they might have developed hypovitaminosis, and all had been treated with metronidazole, which occasionally induces peripheral neuropathy. Further, a syndrome of "neuropathy of the severely ill" is recognised; this might have been responsible. Vallat and Vital (1989) described a similar patient, in which the confounding factors can be largely excluded, and support the contention that there is a causative link between acute pancreatitis and peripheral neuropathy.

Multiple Organ Failure

The various systemic complications of acute pancreatitis may occur alone, but two or more are often present in the same patient at the same time. In addition, there is a phenomenon of multiple organ failure that occurs in 5%–27% of patients (Warshaw and Jin 1985), which is distinct from a summation of the complications in single organs. Multiple organ failure complicates serious diseases other than pancreatitis, such as septicaemia, and is a frequent cause of prolonged admission to intensive care units. In acute pancreatitis, it is more likely to become established if one of the various types of pus-harbouring collections is present, and is characterised by a hypermetabolic sequence that is difficult to interrupt therapeutically. Encephalopathic confusion is often an early sign, and may be rapidly followed by ARDS and renal failure with tubular necrosis. Cardiac failure may also occur, and finally there is hepatic failure accompanied by severe coagulopathy, rapidly leading to death (McFadden 1991).

Ophthalmic Abnormalities

Ophthalmic changes in association with acute pancreatitis are said to be infrequent, though Wells et al. (1990) suggest that they are often overlooked because other symptoms predominate the clinical picture, or because many clinicians are unaware of the phenomenon. Purtscher's retinopathy may occur. This has been shown by Inkeles and Walsh (1975), who used fluorescent angiography, to be due to arteriolar obstruction. They suggested that the obstruction of the retinal arterioles might be due to fat embolism caused by the hyperlipidaemia that occurs during acute pancreatitis. Subsequent work by Jacob et al. (1981) has produced evidence in favour of emboli of a different type as the cause of the retinopathy. Their patient became suddenly blind durng an episode of acute alcoholic pancreatitis and had the fundoscopic appearances of Purtscher's retinopathy. Jacob et al. proposed that aggregated granulocytes had embolised the retinal arterioles, for they found that plasma samples from eight of 12 patients with acute pancreatitis caused granulocyte aggregation in vitro. They went on to demonstrate that the aggregant was an activated fragment of the complement system, derived from C5 by the action of trypsin, and suggested that proteases from the inflamed pancreas might have initiated the process that caused the retinopathy in their patient, and in those previously reported.

Abnormal Blood Coagulation

Various abnormalities of coagulation may occur during acute pancreatitis (Carey 1979), and hypercoagulability has long been recognised (Shinowara et al. 1963). Murphy et al. (1977) found hyperfibrinogenaemia and raised fibrin degradation products in 18 of 25 patients with acute pancreatitis, one of whom also had thrombocytopenia, completing the picture of disseminated intravascular coagulation (DIC). Various other authors have also described DIC (Pitchumoni et al. 1988), but, in general, thrombocytopenia is rare in acute pancreatitis. Intravascular coagulation and thromboembolism contribute susbstantially to the complications of acute pancreatitis.

Subcutaneous Oedema

Subcutaneous oedema during pancreatitis has been reported by Howard et al. (1963), who suggested that increased capillary permeability with loss of protein into the tissues, because of the release of an active peptide from the pancreas, had been responsible. Their observations on the turnover of albumin in their patient seemed to indicate that the lowered serum albumin that coincided with the oedema was not the result of leakage from the bowel.

Fat Necrosis

The foci of fat necrosis that accompany disease or injury of the pancreas have been the subject of much experimental investigation. The work up to 1979 has been reviewed by Lee and Howard (1979). Areas of fat necrosis have been found in association with various forms of pancreatitis in man, with trauma of the pancreas and with some carcinomas,

especially when it is a well-differentiated carcinoma of acinar cells. Fat necrosis has also accompanied experimentally induced pancreatitis in animals. The damage to the fatty tissues is presumed to be due to the escape of lipase and co-lipase from the abnormal pancreas, but there are uncertainties about the exact mechanism that leads to fat necrosis. In pancreatitis, the fat in the interstitial tissue appears to be the most vulnerable component of the pancreas and the adjacent fatty tissue is commonly involved, with areas of whitish-yellow opacity in the fat of the retroperitoneum, the omentum and the mesentery, especially towards the root of the mesentery. Much less commonly there is also peripheral or disseminated fat necrosis, sometimes referred to as metastatic fat necrosis.

The occurrence of fat necrosis, especially disseminated fat necrosis, in pancreatitis, is inconstant and does not seem to correlate at all well with the severity of the disease. It is true that fat necrosis has been caused experimentally by the induction of acute pancreatitis in rats (Storck 1971) and by the injection of canine lipase combined with canine co-lipase into the peritoneal cavities of mice (Lee et al. 1979), but disseminated fat necrosis may occur in human patients in the absence of pancreatitis, as in the syndromes of Weber–Christian panniculitis and systemic Weber–Christian disease (Milner and Mitchinson 1965). Foci of fat necrosis in the vicinity of the pancreas are commonplace after death in people who have died of disease unrelated to the pancreas.

Lesions of bone in acute pancreatitis are usually confined to the marrow and are the results of fat necrosis. Such lesions were found by Scarpelli (1956) in seven of 67 subjects with acute pancreatitis, but not unless there was either widespread abdominal fat necrosis or extra-abdominal fat necrosis in other fatty tissues. Fat necrosis in the bone marrow was found in all three of Scarpelli's cases in which there was extra-abdominal fat necrosis. If intramedullary fat necrosis has occurred in acute pancreatitis it is sometimes recognisable by conventional radiographs (Immelman et al. 1964), and characteristic appearances may be seen on magnetic resonance imaging (Haller et al. 1989).

Subcutaneous necrosis is a well-recognised complication of acute pancreatitis, and may also accompany pancreatic carcinoma. The lesions resemble erythema nodosum on clinical examination, but histologically there is prominent necrosis with replacement of fatty lobules by ghost cells (Higgins and Ive 1990); this distinguishes the lesion from erythema nodosum and other clinical differential diagnoses, such as allergic vasculitis and Weber–Christian disease. On occasion, there may be acute arthritis as well as subcutaneous necrosis (Saag et al. 1992); acute arthritis may also occur alone. The pathogenesis of arthritis is thought to be another form of fat necrosis, with damage to fat within synovial cells caused by circulating enzymes (Hammond and Tesar 1980). Birefringent calcium deposits may form around globules of necrotic fat, and may be mistaken for the sodium urate crystals of gout (Saag et al. 1992). In general, the arthritis is short-lived, but Hammond and Tesar described a man with acute alcoholic pancreatitis whose arthritis lasted for two and a half years.

Fat Embolism

Guardia et al. (1989) presented the autopsy findings of a woman with very extensive retroperitoneal mesenteric and omental fat necrosis, in whom fat emboli were demonstrated in the capillaries of the lungs, heart and kidneys; there were multiple petechial haemorrhages in the brain. The patient had been treated with an intravenous fat emulsion, but had become hypoxic before this therapy had commenced, and the authors believe the embolic fat must have been derived from the necrotic adipose tissue they found around the pancreas. They found several similar reports in the literature, including one of definite cerebral fat embolism (Johnson and Tong 1977). Interestingly, fat embolism was a feature of one of the patients in Edmondson and Fields' (1942) report, in which the complication of hypocalcaemia was first recorded.

Complications and Sequelae

Pus-Harbouring Collections

Although the clinical courses and morphological changes associated with sepsis in the pancreas vary widely from patient to patient, until recently all were categorised as abscesses by many authors (Bittner et al. 1987), and, only in a minority of the reports reviewed by Lumsden and Bradley (1990), was there a clear distinction into reproducible subgroups. Other authors have generated a bewildering variety of diagnostic categories, which is particularly regrettable because this group of complications is the commonest cause of death in acute pancreatitis; an early report (Miller et al. 1974) found an overall mortality of 53.9% in a series of 69 examples.

The confusion was illustrated by Bassi et al. (1990) who found, when they reviewed the literature, that it was impossible to find precise and consistent meanings for terms such as "peripancreatic sepsis", "phlegmon", "pancreatic abscess", "purulent pancreatitis", and so on. This prompted them to devise a classification of their own, based on a review of 1090 patients in their unit who had required surgery for either acute or chronic pancreatitis. Of these, they selected 108 in whom purulent material had been found during operation. In 79 of these, the pus had been found during or after an attack of acute pancreatitis, and in 29 it had accumulated as a complication of chronic pancreatitis. They divided the collections of pus into two categories: a spreading type in which the pus was mixed with necrotic retroperitoneal slough and was not localised by walls or boundaries, and a localised form with more or less distinct walls. In both kinds, the collections were usually multiple. When the clinical histories were compared with the lesions it was found that the spreading type of lesion had been present in 90% of the patients in whom early operation and debridement of the pancreas had been necessary, while 80% of the patients in whom an operation became necessary only after an interval had the localised type. They suggested the use of the following terms for such lesions: "infected pancreatic necrosis", "infected pancreatic pseudocyst" and "pancreatic abscess". They advised that such lesions should be distinguished from uninfected pancreatic necrosis, sterile effusions and uninfected pseudocysts. This classification closely resembles an earlier one proposed by Bittner and colleagues in 1987.

Pancreatic abscesses are particularly liable to be multilocular and complex, extending from the pancreas into adjacent structures. Abscesses may form in the anterior and posterior pararenal spaces, and the lesser sac. From the lesser sac exudate may spread into the subphrenic space, and along the paracolic gutters as far as the pelvis. Other sites that may be involved include the abdominal wall, either pleural space, the posterior mediastinum and the scrotum (Bjornson 1991), or even the bronchial tree (Steedman et al. 1967). External rupture readily leads to generalised peritonitis (Kaushik et al. 1984). The accumulation of pus in the lesser sac may compress the duodenum and common bile duct, as well as displace and compress organs such as the spleen, jejunum or transverse colon. The behaviour of an abscess is determined to some extent by the region of the pancreas that has undergone necrosis. Thus, an abscess originating in the head is likely to affect the duodenum and the superior mesenteric vessels, one arising in the body may compress the jejunum and displace the stomach, while one originating in the tail may displace the stomach, spleen and transverse colon. Erosion of major blood vessels, as in other stages of the evolution of acute or chronic pancreatitis, may lead to fatal haemorrhage.

A wide variety of fistulae have been reported, including pancreatocolic, enterocutaneous, duodenal and gastropancreatic types (Lumsden and Bradley 1990).

Gas formation in abscesses of the pancreas is not usually recognisable during surgery or autopsy, but it can be demonstrated by conventional radiography (Woodard et al. 1981) or computed tomography (Mendez and Isikoff 1979); ultrasonography is less reliable.

The routes whereby necrotising pancreatitis becomes infected are not clearly established, though the gastrointestinal and biliary tract are probable sources in most patients; haematogenous spread during bacteraemia is another possible route (Widdison et al. 1990; Bjornson 1991). Infections are often polymicrobial, supporting the suggestion of a gastrointestinal origin (Holden et al. 1976). The risk of developing superinfection is related to the severity of the underlying pancreatitis (Becker et al. 1984), as is the risk of a fatal outcome once infection is established (Malangoni et al. 1986). Apart from a high incidence of superinfection in post-operative pancreatitis, the cause appears to have little effect on the likelihood of developing infection (Ranson and Spencer 1977).

When a pancreatic abscess has lasted for more than a few weeks, the granulation tissue of its wall develops the characteristics of subacute or chronic inflammation, with many fibroblasts, amongst which the inflammatory cells are mainly lymphocytes and plasma cells. The wall of an abscess that was found at autopsy 6 months after an attack of acute pancreatitis is illustrated in Figs 12.22–12.24. The patient was a woman aged 73, who had acute pancreatitis towards the end of April 1972. She was treated conservatively and was able to leave hospital early in May 1972. She was readmitted in late October of the same year with steatorrhoea and hypoproteinaemia. In hospital she developed ilio-femoral venous thrombosis and died of pulmonary embolism. At autopsy, the additional findings were that the abdominal cavity contained several hundred millilitres of clear yellow fluid; similar fluid was found in the left pleural cavity. The gall bladder contained stones but the common bile duct was normal. Foci of fat necrosis were present in the omentum, the epiploic fat, and the indurated retroperitoneal fatty tissue down to the level of the pelvic brim. The transverse colon was attached by adhesions to the head of the pancreas and the pancreas was largely replaced by abscess cavities, the largest of which was in the head and measured 3 cm in diameter. Culture of the pus in the pancreatic abscesses yielded a mixed growth of coliform organisms: *Klebsiella* species and *Proteus* species. In spite of the destruction of much of the pancreas, the main duct was relatively well preserved, though distorted. Fig. 12.25 illustrates the radiological appearances of the duct after it had been injected with barium.

Pseudocysts

A pseudocyst is a collection of fluid in the vicinity of the pancreas and the most common site is the lesser sac of the peritoneum, where inflammatory adhesions tend to localise uninfected enzyme-containing fluid that has escaped from the pancreas following damage to the gland. The development of a pseudocyst may complicate acute pancreatitis, chronic pancreatitis or trauma. Earlier accounts pay little attention to the difference in pathogenesis and outcome associated with the various underlying conditions, despite the fact that frequency of complications, liability to spontaneous resolution etc. are related to such factors (Williams and Fabian 1992). A recently proposed classification (D'Edigio and Schein 1991) divides pseudocysts into postnecrotic type I, which is associated with acute pancreatitis, post-necrotic type II, which follows an acute exacerbation of chronic pancreatitis, and a retention type, associated with distortion and dilatation of the pancreatic duct in chronic pancreatitis. The retention type often has connections with the pancreatic duct system, whereas the post-necrotic types generally do not.

It takes 2, 3 or 4 weeks, or even longer, for a pseudocyst to form. Having formed, the progress of a pseudocyst may be towards eventual spontaneous resolution (Trapnell 1971; Bradley and Clements 1975), or the contents of the cyst may become infected with conversion of the cyst into an abscess. The walls of a pseudocyst, even in the absence of infection, are of granulation tissue and the appearances are quite nonspecific (Figs. 12.26–12.29). Where pancreatic tissue forms the wall, the microscopic appearances may be reminiscent of those of an area of the pancreas that has been eroded by a peptic ulcer of the duodenum (Figs 12.30, 12.31). When confronted with a biopsy of the wall of a pseudocyst, the pathologist has to report that the appearances are compatible with those of the wall of a pseudocyst, without being able to give a more definite diagnosis. The vascularity of the wall is very marked, and haemorrhage into the cyst may occur, not only from the cyst wall, but also because large arteries, such as the splenic or pancreaticoduodenal vessels, may become eroded by the digestive enzymes within the cyst, with the formation of a small

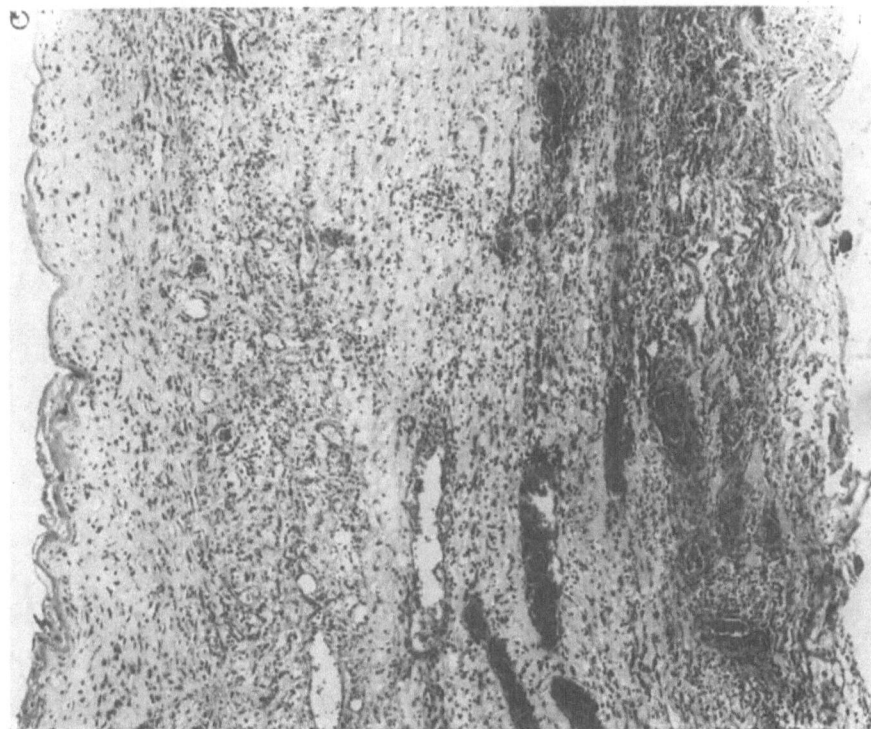

Fig. 12.26. The wall of a pancreatic pseudocyst. The more vascular, somewhat concave, surface of the wall is the inner aspect. H&E, × 53

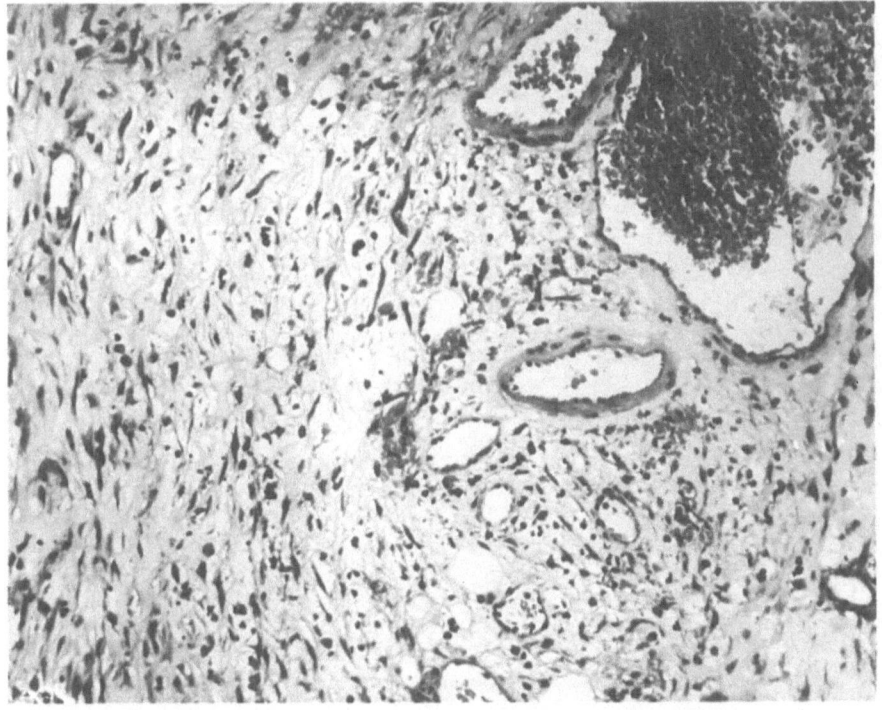

Fig. 12.27. The very vascular, cellular fibrous tissue of which most of the wall of the pseudocyst is composed. H&E, × 135

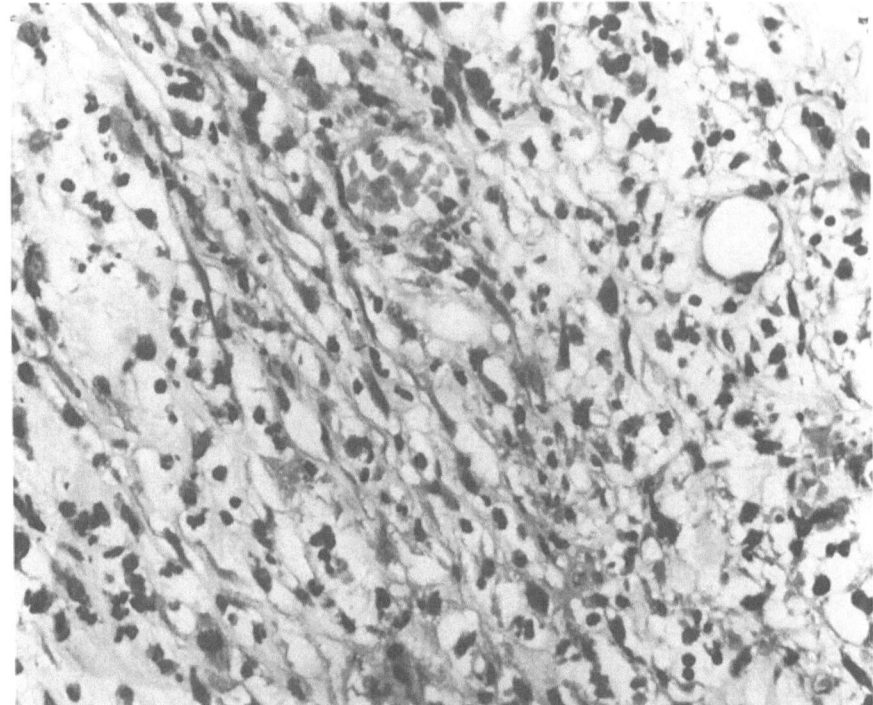

Fig. 12.28. Another part of the wall of the pseudocyst; in which subacute inflammatory cells are present between the fibroblasts. H&E, ×330

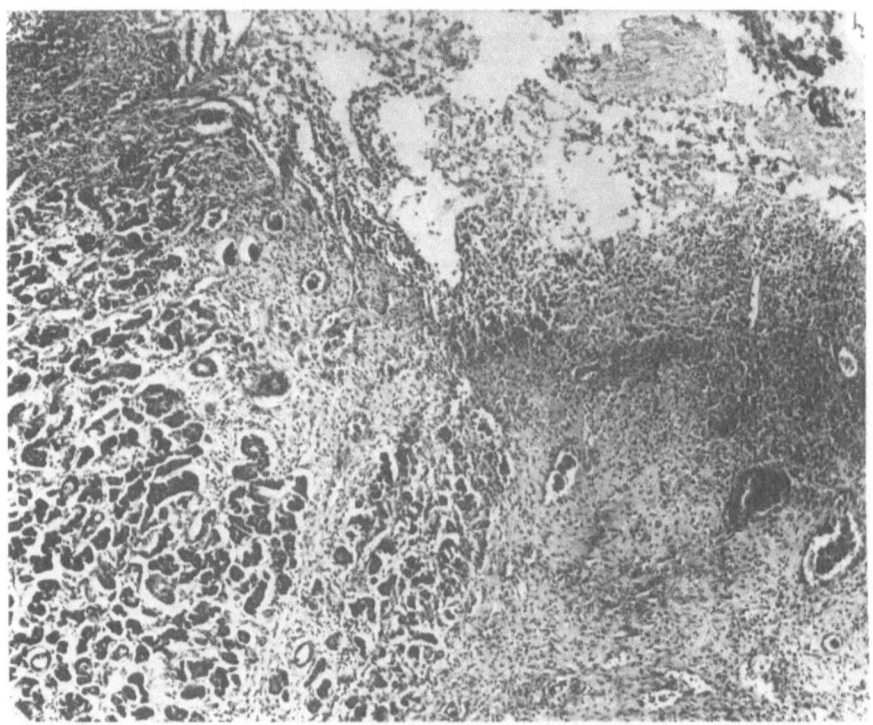

Fig. 12.29. Pancreatic tissue forming part of the wall of the pseudocyst. The appearances resemble those seen when a duodenal ulcer erodes the pancreas. H&E, ×60

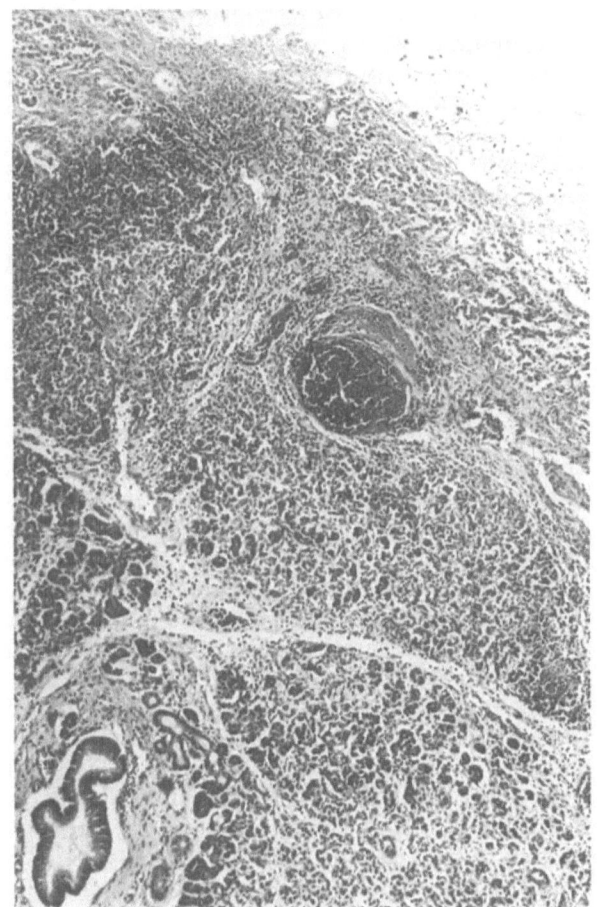

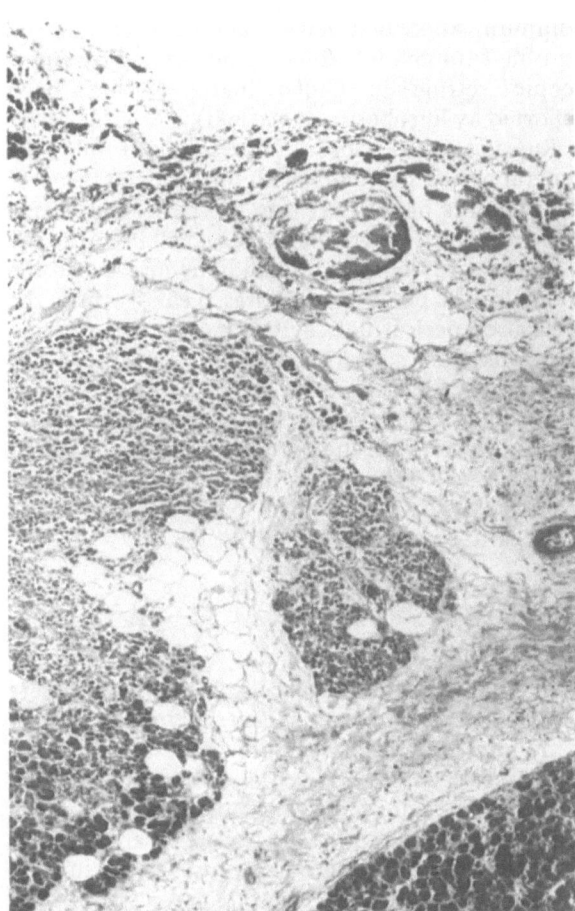

Fig. 12.30. Thrombus in a vessel in the pancreatic tissue that is being eroded by the pseudocyst. H&E, × 60

Fig. 12.31. Pancreatic tissue in the floor of a duodenal ulcer that involved the pancreas. The appearances resemble those in the parts of the pseudocyst that involved the pancreas. H&E, × 60

aneurysm that ruptures to cause catastrophic haemorrhage. A pseudocyst into which fatal haemorrhage occurred is illustrated in Fig. 12.26. If external drainage is not carried out, the haemorrhage may take place into the stomach or duodenum.

Pancreatic pseudocyst formation is an uncommon complication of acute pancreatitis, occurring in about 5% of patients (White 1966). In the series of 41 cases described by D'Edigio and Schein (1991), the lesions associated with acute pancreatitis ranged in diameter from 2 cm to 25 cm, with an average of 8.9 cm, which is considerably larger than the average diameter of pseudocysts in chronic pancreatitis. Pseudocysts may present clinically as abdominal masses, and may displace other abdominal organs in a variety of ways (Judd et al. 1931; Jordan 1960; White 1966; Grace and Jordan 1976).

According to Judd and his colleagues, the pseudocyst usually tends to bulge forwards below the stomach between the leaves of the transverse meso-

colon, being covered anteriorly by the omentum, or, less commonly, the bulging forward may be between the stomach and the liver, behind the stomach displacing it forwards, or, very rarely, it may be in a downward direction retroperitoneally behind the root of the mesentery.

If a pseudocyst continues to enlarge, it may compress the gastric pylorus and the duodenum or, less commonly, the common bile duct, or, uncommonly, the portal vein or colon (Grace and Jordan 1976).

Rupture of a pseudocyst may occur into the general peritoneal cavity, or into an adjacent hollow organ, to cause an internal fistula. The published cases of rupture of pancreatic cysts up to 1960 were reviewed by Hanna (1960), who found that rupture into the peritoneal cavity was the commonest, having occurred in 23 of the 47 ruptures. Rupture into the stomach, duodenum, colon or elsewhere in the alimentary tract occurred less commonly. Hanna's review, however, included cystic neoplasms of the pancreas as well as pseudocysts. A fistulous communication between a pancreatic pseudocyst and the common bile duct, demonstrated by endoscopic retrograde cholangiography, has been reported by Ellenbogen et al. (1981).

Rupture of a pancreatic pseudocyst into the general peritoneal cavity, with the sudden release of the contents of the cyst into the peritoneum may cause a surgical emergency, but a small leak into the peritoneal cavity may be insidious and cause the condition of pancreatic ascites. Leakage into the pleural or pericardial cavities may occur, causing effusions that contain pancreatic enzymes. The development of pancreatic ascites, with or without effusions in other serous cavities, is usually associated, however, with the pseudocysts of insidious or unsuspected pancreatitis (Ingram and Sheiner 1980), rather than with those that may follow acute pancreatitis.

Haemorrhage

Haemorrhage tends to complicate the most severe cases of acute pancreatitis, especially when laparotomy and drainage procedures have been carried out, either at an early stage of the illness, or when an abscess or pseudocyst has been drained. If drainage has been carried out, the blood may escape through the drainage tubes or through sinuses to the surface. Even without drainage, acute pancreatitis may be complicated by severe haematemesis (Trapnell 1971), or by haematemesis and melaena (Howard 1960b). Haemorrhage was the commoneset cause of death in the series of fatal cases of acute pancreatitis collected by Howard, and seemed to be particularly liable to complicate post-operative pancreatitis. Characteristically, the bleeding occurred between the second and fourth week of the illness. In patients who have died of haemorrhage, the pathologist may not be able to identify the exact source of the haemorrhage even when abundant fresh blood is present in the alimentary canal, but, in others, the erosion of the portal, splenic or superior mesenteric veins may be recognisable. Occasionally, vascular damage may be diffuse or widespread, and several vessels may be involved (Stroud et al. 1981). The formation of aneurysms, with rupture and arterial haemorrhage, may also complicate either acute or chronic pancreatitis. Such aneurysms have been demonstrated in the walls of the gastroduodenal and pancreaticoduodenal arteries by Eckhauser et al. (1980), using selective mesenteric arteriography during life. The splenic artery seems more liable to be damaged, with aneurysm formation and haemorrhage, in chronic, rather than acute, pancreatitis.

There may also be other causes of gastrointestinal bleeding in pancreatitis, and attention has been drawn to these by Marks et al. (1967). These include acute gastric erosions, bleeding from mucosal vessels in which congestion has been induced by contiguous pancreatitis, splenic vein obstruction by pancreatic compression, and the Mallory–Weiss syndrome. Chronic peptic ulceration or gastric or ampullary carcinoma may be present as well as pancreatitis, and in alcoholism there may be bleeding from gastritis or from oesophageal varices due to alcoholic cirrhosis of the liver.

Thrombosis

Thrombosis of both veins and arteries may complicate acute pancreatitis. Splenic vein thrombosis was present in 13.1% of autopsy cases in one large series (Renner et al. 1985). Splenic vein thrombosis is associated with particularly high levels of serum amylase (Rogers and Klatt 1989), and may lead to the further complication of portal hypertension and variceal bleeding (Little and Moossa 1981).

Thal et al. (1957a), and many others, have found venous and arterial thrombosis in the vicinity of the pancreas in autopsy material from fatal cases of acute pancreatitis. Infarction of organs, however, as the result of such thrombosis is unusual, although several reports have appeared. In 1965, Sheikh reported a patient in which duodenal ischaemia complicated acute pancreatitis in a child. He attributed the ischaemia to thrombosis of the gastroduodenal artery. Infarction of the small intestine as a complication of acute pancreatitis has also been described by Collins et al. (1968), who attributed the ischaemia of the bowel to fat necrosis in the mesentery, and a similar mechanism, in which both arteries and veins in the mesentery related to a segment of jejunum had been occluded by thrombosis induced by fat necrosis in the adjacent sigmoid mesocolon, has been described by Griffiths and Brown (1970). Scholefield et al. (1988) described a case of gastric and splenic infarction due to venous thrombosis, associated with ischaemia of the abdominal wall. It is the colon, however, that appears to be most vulnerable to damage as a result of acute pancreatitis and, with the ten cases in their own series, Abcarian et al. (1979) found that 75 had been reported up to that time. The colonic lesions included pseudo-obstruction, necrosis, haemorrhage, fistula and ischaemic colitis. Necrosis and haemorrhage were usually associated with pancreatic abscesses or pseudocysts, and were attributed to the effects of direct pressure upon blood vessels. The transverse colon and splenic flexure were the areas most likely to be affected by inflammatory masses in the body or tail of the pancreas. A year later, Nottle (1980) reported a case of almost total colonic infarction due to acute pancreatitis that had caused thrombosis of the right colic, middle colic and left colic arteries. The clinical clue was the passage of bright red blood from the rectum, and a rapid deterioration in the patient's condition. Aldridge et al. (1989) recorded another case of almost total colonic necrosis, and noted that, of another 22 patients who required pancreatic resection and/or debridement, nine had necrosis or perforation of the colon. Histological examination suggested that the mechanism was infarction in four of the ten colonic resection specimens, and direct spread of inflammation from the pancreas in six.

Obstruction of the Colon

The colon may become obstructed by external compression from an inflammatory mass (Miln and Barclay 1952; Mair et al. 1976), which may then resolve spontaneously. There may also be more persistent strictures, of which Dürr (1979) was able to refer to 38 published cases. Mair et al. suggested that such strictures are caused by external fibrosis, but Carboni et al. (1982) pointed out that 84% of the strictures occur at the splenic flexure (i.e. at the watershed between the areas of supply of the middle and left colonic arteries), and propose that some or all are ischaemic in origin.

Duodenal Obstruction

Duodenal obstruction due to primary involvement of the intestine by the adjacent inflammatory process in the pancreas has been discussed by Bradley and Clements (1981), who found nine occurrences of the condition during a 3-year study of 878 patients with pancreatitis. In four patients, the obstruction developed during moderately severe pancreatitis, and resolution took place in the course of 3 weeks in all four patients. Only one patient was explored surgically; there was marked duodenal oedema with a haematoma within the wall. In the remaining five patients, the process was more chronic, and inflammation, muscle destruction and extensive fibrosis were found on duodenal biopsy.

Necrosis of the Common Bile Duct

The intrapancreatic portion of the common bile duct is obviously at risk when necrotising pancre-atitis involves the head of the pancreas, but damage to the duct, with escape of bile, is a distinctly uncommon complication of acute pancreatitis. Patients, such as that of Zaslow (1953), have been reported, and other examples of this complication have been cited by Howard (1960c), and by Baggenstoss (1973). Obstruction of the common bile duct is more likely to occur in chronic pancreatitis than in acute pancreatitis.

Disturbances of Carbohydrate Metabolism

Many patients with acute pancreatitis develop minor transient hyperglycaemia and glycosuria, and a few go on to mild but permanent diabetes mellitus. (Pitchumoni et al. 1988). Eriksson et al. (1992) showed that diabetes mellitus is very common in those who are treated with partial or total pancreatectomy, but over one-quarter of those who survive fulminating pancreatitis without surgery also develop acute pancreatitis. More severe hyperglycaemia is one of the poor prognostic signs of acute pancreatitis (Ranson et al. 1974). Hypoglycaemia may also occur in the early stages of acute pancreatitis. Pre-existing diabetes mellitus worsens the course of acute pancreatitis, and diabetics are over-represented in autopsy populations (Renner et al. 1985).

Long-Term Sequelae

In the UK, there was recurrence of acute pancreatitis in 133 of 430 individuals who survived a first attack (Trapnell and Duncan 1975), and in over 50% of 389 patients in the USA (Satiani and Stone 1979). Nevertheless, it is generally held to be uncommon for acute pancreatitis to leave important degrees of scarring, and Sarles et al. (1979) insisted that it is exceptional for there to be sufficient cicatricial fibrosis for chronic pancreatitis to follow. Klöppel and Maillet (1992) hold rather different views, and recently put forward a hypothesis that interstitial fat necrosis and haemorrhage induce perilobular fibrosis as healing takes place; in turn, the perilobular fibrosis is thought to cause stenoses and dilatations of the interlobular ducts, which hamper the normal flow of pancreatic secretions. Stasis of pancreatic secretions permits protein plugs to precipitate and calcify, and chronic pancreatitis is then established. Klöppel and Maillet suggested that this sequence of events can only take place if there is intrapancreatic necrosis, which condition is relatively unusual, compared with peripancreatic necrosis. This, they believe, is why only few cases of acute pancreatitis progress to chronic pancreatitis.

Death and Undetected Acute Pancreatitis

The overall mortality from acute pancreatitis is low: Puolakkainen et al. (1986) recorded a death rate of 2.3% for all clinically detected cases, and 22% for the small subgroup with acute haemorrhagic pancreatitis. Of those who die, over 90% do so after the first attack. Mortality rates based on clinical and biochemical diagnoses may be underestimates, because a considerable proportion of fatal cases of acute pancreatitis are not correctly identified until autopsy. Wilson et al. (1988) studied deaths in patients with acute pancreatitis over a period of 11 years; of a total of 126, 53 (42%) had been undeteced until autopsy. Of these 53, only 36 had presented atypically; in the substantial majority, acute pancreatitis was sufficiently severe and widespread to have cause or contributed to death. Post-operative acute pancreatitis was particularly likely to be missed. Lankisch et al. (1991) studied post-mortem reports on 43 patients, of whom 13 had been undiagnosed until autopsy; of these, eight had probably had acute pancreatitis on admission to hospital. Lankisch et al. (1991) found that non-diagnostic or normal levels of serum amylase are inappropriately believed to rule out acute pancreatitis, and further investigations are thus abandoned prematurely. In their review of the literature, they find that the proportion of cases of fatal acute pancreatitis that go undetected before death ranges from 6.6% to 86.0%.

Some patients with acute necrotising pancreatitis die so quickly that there is no time for clinical investigation, and Williams (1954) was able to report five patients where death had occurred rapidly or instantly outside hospital. In only one of these, an elderly woman with recent pulmonary embolism, was there any additional factor that might cause any doubt that pancreatitis was the cause of death; in another of Williams' cases, a young man died very soon after demonstrating his apparent fitness by successfully running to catch a bus. Wilson et al. (1988) comment that more cases of fatal acute pancreatitis will go undetected if the autopsy rate continues its generalised decline.

References

Abcarian H, Eftaiha M, Kraft AR, Nyhus LM (1979) Colonic complications of acute pancreatitis. Arch Surg 114: 995–1001

Ackerman LV (1942) Acute pancreatitis following blood transfusion. Arch Pathol 34: 1065–1069

Acosta JM, Ledesma CL (1974) Gallstone migration as a cause of acute pancreatitis. N Engl J Med 290: 484–487

Acosta JM, Rossi R, Ledesma CL (1977) The usefulness of stool screening for diagnosing cholelithiasis in acute pancreatitis. Am J Dig Dis 22: 168–172

Acosta JM, Pellegrini CA, Skinner DB (1980) Etiology and pathogenesis of acute biliary pancreatitis. Surgery 88: 118–125

Aho HJ, Nevalainen TJ, Havia VT, Heinonen RJ, Aho AJ (1982) Human acute pancreatitis: a light and electron microscopic study. Acta Pathol Microbiol Immunol Scand [A] 90: 367–373

Aldridge MC, Francis ND, Glazer G, Dudley HAF (1989) Colonic complications of severe acute pancreatitis. Br J Surg 76: 362–367

Allam BF, Imrie CW (1977) Serum ionized calcium in acute pancreatitis. Br J Surg 64: 665–668

Amorosi EL, Ultmann JE (1966) Thrombotic thrombocytopenic purpura: report of 16 cases and review of the literature Medicine 45: 139–159

Anderson MC, Schiller WR (1968) Microcirculatory dynamics in the normal and inflamed pancreas. Am J Surg 115: 118–127

Archbald E (1919) The experimental production of pancreatitis in animals as a result of the resistance of the common duct sphincter. Surg Gynecol Obstet 28: 529–545

Armstrong CP, Taylor TV (1986) Pancreatic duct reflux and acute gallstone pancreatitis. Ann Surg 204: 59–64

Armstrong CP, Taylor TV, Torrance HB (1984) Bile and bacteria in acute gallstone pancreatitis [editorial]. Br J Surg 71: 1001

Armstrong CP, Taylor TV, Jeacock J, Lucas S (1985) The biliary tract in patients with acute gallstone pancreatitis. Br J Surg 72: 551–555

Axelsson L, Bergerfeldt M, Bjork P, Olsson R, Olsson K (1990) Release of immunoreactive canine leukocyte elastase normally and in endotoxin and pancreatic shock. Scand J Clin Lab Invest 50: 35–42

Baer L, Neu HC (1966) Intravascular clotting and acute pancreatitis in primary hyperparathyroidism. Ann Intern Med 64: 1062–1065

Baggenstoss AH (1973) Pathology of pancreatitis. In: Gambill EE (ed) Pancreatitis. Mosby, St Louis, pp 179–212

Balldin G, Genell S, Ohlsson K (1989) Pancreatic abscess: formation, diagnostic procedures and treatment. Dig Dis Sci 7: 104–112

Banerjee AK, Patel KJ, Grainger SL (1989) Drug-induced acute pancreatitis: a critical review. Med Toxicol Adverse Drug Exp 4: 186–198

Bank S, Wise L, Gerstein M (1983) Risk factors in acute pancreatitis. Am J Gastroenterol 78: 637–640

Banks PA, Janowitz HD (1969) Some metabolic aspects of exocrine pancreatic disease. Gastroenterology 56: 601–617

Banks PA, Bradley EL, Dreiling DA et al. (1985) Classification of pancreatitis - Cambridge and Marseilles. Gastroenterology 89: 928–930

Barbezot GO, Waterworth MW (1978) Atrial fibrillation in acute pancreatitis. S Afr Med J 53: 554–555

Barrett PVD, Thier SO (1963) Meningitis and pancreatitis associated with sulphamethizole. N Engl J Med 268: 36–37

Bassi C, Vesentini S, Nifosi F et al. (1990) Pancreatic abscess and other pus-harboring collections related to pancreatitis: a review of 108 cases. World J Surg 14: 505–512

Batalden PB, Van Dyne BJ, Cloyd J (1979) Pancreatitis associated with valproic acid therapy. Pediatrics 64: 520–522

Beck IT, Kahn DS, Solymar J, McKenna RD, Zylberszac B (1964) The role of pancreatic enzymes in the pathogenesis of acute pancreatitis: III. Comparison of the pathologic and biochemical changes in the canine pancreas on intraductal injection with bile and with trypsin. Gastroenterology 46: 531–542

Becker JM, Pemberton JH, DiMagno EP, Ilstrup DM, McIlrath DC, Dozois RR (1984) Prognostic factors in pancreatic abscess. Surgery 96: 455–460

Beger HG, Bittner R, Block S, Büchler M (1986) Bacterial contamination of pancreatic necrosis: a prospective clinical study.

Gastroenterology 91: 433–438

Benbow EW (1988) Simultaneous acute inflammation in entopic and ectopic pancreas. J Clin Pathol 41: 430–434

Bencosme SA, Lazarus SS (1956) The pancreas of cortisone-treated rabbits: a pathogenic study. Arch Pathol 62: 285–295

Bess MA, Edis AJ, Van Heerden JA (1980) Hyperparathyroidism and pancreatitis: chance or a causal association? JAMA 243: 246–247

Bittner R, Block S, Büchler M, Beger HG (1987) Pancreatic abscess and infected pancreatic necrosis: different local septic complications in acute pancreatitis. Dig Dis Sci 32: 1082–1087

Bjornson HS (1991) Pancreatic "abscess": diagnosis and management. Pancreas 6 Suppl: S31–S36

Bliss WR, Sibley JA (1969) The Shwartzman phenomenon and acute hemorrhagic pancreatitis (in dogs). Am J Surg 117: 711–714

Block MA, Wakim KG, Baggenstoss AH (1954) Experimental studies concerning factors in the pathogenesis of acute pancreatitis. Surg Gynecol Obstet 99: 83–90

Block MB, Genant HK, Kirsner JB (1970) Pancreatitis as an adverse reaction to salicylazosulfapyridine. N Engl J Med 282: 380–382

Bocanegra T, Vasey FB, Espinoza LR, Germain BF (1980) Pancreatic pseudocyst: a complication of necrotizing vasculitis (polyarteritis nodosa). Arch Intern Med 140: 1359–1361

Bourke JB, Mead GM, McIllmurray MB, Langman MJS (1978) Drug-associated primary acute pancreatitis. Lancet i: 706–708

Bradley EL, Clements JL (1975) Spontaneous resolution of pancreatic pseudocysts. Am J Surg 129: 23–28

Bradley EL, Clements JL (1981) Idiopathic duodenal obstruction: an unappreciated complication of pancreatitis. Ann Surg 193: 638–648

Braganza JM (1991a) Toxicology of the pancreas. In: Braganza JM (ed) The pathogenesis of pancreatitis. Manchester University Press, Manchester, pp 66–85

Braganza JM (1991b) Evolution of pancreatitis. In: Braganza JM (ed) The pathogenesis of pancreatitis. Manchester University Press, Manchester, pp 19–33

Braganza JM, Jolley JE, Lee WR (1986) Occupational volatile chemicals and pancreatitis: a link? Int J Pancreatol 1: 9–19

Brandes JC, Campbell DA, Kleinman JG (1989) Pyelonephritis complicating relapsing acute pancreatitis. Am J Nephrol 9: 241–243

Brazer SR, Medoff JR (1988) Sulfonamide-induced pancreatitis. Pancreas 3: 583–586

Bunin N, Meyer WH, Christensen M, Pratt CB (1985) Pancreatitis following cisplatin: a case report. Cancer Treat Rep 69: 236–237

Camfield PR, Bagnell P, Camfield CS, Tibbles JAR (1979) Pancreatitis due to valproic acid. Lancet i: 1198–1199

Caos A (1989) Biliary pancreatitis and jaundice associated with obstructed peripapillary duodenal diverticulum. Am J Gastroenterol 84: 982–983

Carboni M, Negro P, Tuscano D, de Bernardinis G, Flati D, Flati G (1982) Secondary colonic lesions in acute pancreatitis. In: Hollender LF (ed) Controversies in acute pancreatitis. Springer-Verlag, Berlin, pp 302–315

Carey LC (1979) Extra-abdominal manifestations of acute pancreatitis. Surgery 86: 337–342

Carone AF, Liebow AA (1957) Acute pancreatic lesions in patients with ACTH and adrenal corticoids. N Engl J Med 257: 690–697

Chardavoyne R, Asher A, Bank S, Stein TA, Wise L (1989) Role of reactive oxygen metabolites in early cardiopulmonary changes of acute hemorrhagic pancreatitis. Dig Dis Sci 34: 1581–1584

Chiari H (1896) Ueber Selbstverdauung des menschlichen Pankreas. Z Heilkunde 17: 69–96

Collins JJ, Peterson LM, Wilson RE (1968) Small intestinal infarction as a complication of acute pancreatitis. Ann Surg 167: 433–436

Cooper RG, Macaulay MB (1982) Pentochlorophenol pancreatitis [letter]. Lancet i: 517

Cope O, Culver PJ, Mixter CG, Nardi GL (1957) Pancreatitis, a diagnostic clue to hyperparathyriodism. Ann Surg 145: 857–863

Cornish AL, McClellan JT, Johnson DH (1965) Effects of chlorothiazide on the pancreas. N Engl J Med 261: 673–675

Croton RS, Warren RA, Stott A, Roberts NB (1981) Ionized calcium in acute pancreatitis and its relationships with total calcium and serum lipase. Br J Surg 68: 241–244

Creutzfeldt W, Schmidt H (1970) Aetiology and pathogenesis of pancreatitis (current concepts). Scand J Gastroenterol 6: 47–62

Czernobilsky B, Mikat KW (1964) The diagnostic significance of interstitial pancreatitis found at autopsy. Am J Clin Pathol 41: 33–43

Davidoff F, Tishler S, Rosoff C (1973) Marked hyperlipidemia and pancreatitis associated with oral contraceptive therapy. N Engl J Med 289: 552–555

Davies M, Klimiuk PS, Adams PH, Lumb GA, Large DM, Anderson DC (1981) Familial hypocalciuric hypercalcaemia and acute pancreatitis. Br Med J i: 1023–1025

Dazai Y, Katoh I, Hara Y, Yoshida R, Kurihara K (1991) Two cases of adult T-cell leukemia associated with acute pancreatitis due to hypercalcemia. Am J Med 90: 251–254

D'Edigio A, Schein M (1991) Pancreatic pseudocysts: a proposed classification and its management implications. Br J Surg 78: 981–984

Denny-Brown D, Sciarra D (1945) Changes in the central nervous system in acute porphyria. Brain 68: 1–16

De Waele B, Smitz J, Willems G (1989) Recurrent pancreatitis secondary to hypercalcaemia following vitamin D poisoning. Pancreas 4: 378–380

Dickson AP, O'Neill J, Imrie CW (1984) Hyperlipidaemia, alcohol abuse and acute pancreatitis. Br J Surg 71: 685–688

Dion YM, Morin J, Fraser W (1992) Extracorporeal lithotripsy of gallstones: clinical experience with 170 patients. Can J Surg 35: 145–150

DiVittorio G, Wees S, Koopman WJ, Ball GV (1983) Pancreatitis in systemic lupus erythematosus [abstract]. Arthritis Rheum 25 (Suppl): S6

Drew SI, Joffe B, Vinik A, Seftel H, Singer F (1978) The first 24 hours of acute pancreatitis. Am J Med 64: 795–803

Duguid H, Simpson RG, Stowers JM (1961) Accidental hypothermia. Lancet ii: 1213–1219

Duncan N (1948) Pancreatitis due to ascariasis [letter]. Br Med J i: 905

Dürr GH-K (1979) Acute pancreatitis. In: Howat HT, Sarles H (eds) The exocrine pancreas. Saunders, London, pp 352–401

Durrington PN, Cairns SA (1982) Acute pancreatitis: a complication of beta blockade. Br Med J 284: 1016

Eaker EY, Toskes PP (1989) Systemic lupus erythematosus presenting initially with acute pancreatitis and a review of the literature. Am J Med Sci 297: 38–41

Eckhauser FE, Stanley JC, Zelenock GB, Borlaza GS, Freier DT, Lindenauer SM (1980) Gastroduodenal and pancreaticoduodenal artery aneurysms: a complication of pancreatitis causing spontaneous gastrointestinal hemorrhage. Surgery 88: 335–344

Edmondson HA, Berne CJ (1944) Calcium changes in acute pancreatic necrosis. Surg Gynecol Obstet 79: 240–244

Edmonson MA, Fields IA (1942) Relation of calcium and lipids to acute pancreatic necrosis. Arch Intern Med 59: 177–190

Edmondson HA, Berne CJ, Homann RE, Wertman M (1952) Calcium, potassium, magnesium and amylase disturbances in acute pancreatitis. Am J Med 12: 34–42

Ellenbogen KA, Cameron JL, Cocco AE, Gayler BW, Hutcheon DF (1981) Fistulous communication of a pseudocyst with the common bile duct: demonstration by endoscopic retrograde cholangiography. Johns Hopkins Med J 149: 110–111

Elman R (1933) Acute interstitial pancreatitis: clinical study of 37 cases showing edema, swelling and induration of the pancreas but without necrosis, hemorrhage, or suppuration. Surg Gynecol Obstet 57:291–309

Elmore MF, Roggs JD (1981) Tetracycline-induced pancreatitis. Gastroenterology 81:1134–1136

Eriksson J, Doepel M, Widén E et al. (1992) Pancreatic surgery, not pancreatitis, is the primary cause of diabetes after acute fulminant pancreatitis. Gut 33:843–847

Evans DB, Slapak M (1975) Pancreatitis in the hard water syndrome. Br Med J iii:748

Evans HW, Gross JB, Baggenstoss AH (1958) Acute and subacute interstitial pancreatitis. Gastroenterology 35:457–464

Fan ST, Choi TK, Lai CS, Wong T (1988) Influence of age on the mortality from acute pancreatitis. Br J Surg 75:463–466

Feiner H (1976) Pancreatitis after cardiac surgery: a morphologic study. Am J Surg 131:684–688

Feller JH, Brown RA, MacLaren Toussaint GP, Thompson AG (1974) Changing methods in the treatment of severe pancreatitis. Am J Surg 127:196–201

Fernandez-del Castillo C, Harringer W, Warshaw AL et al. (1991) Risk factors for pancreatic cellular injury after cardiopulmonary bypass. N Engl J Med 325:382–387

Fielding JA, Loughran CF (1979) Subdiaphragmatic gas in a case of acute pancreatitis. Br J Radiol 52:665–667

Fischer MG, Geffen A (1959) Emphysematous necrotizing pancreatitis. Arch Surg 79:567–569

Fitz RH (1889) Acute pancreatitis. Boston Med Surg J 120:181–187, 205–207, 229–235

Flexner S (1901) Experimental pancreatitis. Johns Hopkins Hosp Rep 9:743–771

Foster ME, Powell DEB (1975) Pancreatitis, multiple infarcts and oral contraception. Postgrad Med J 51:667–669

Foulis AK (1980) Histological evidence of initiating factors in acute necrotising pancreatitis in man. J Clin Pathol 33:1125–1131

Foulis AK (1982) Morphological study of the relation between accidental hypothermia and acute pancreatitis. J Clin Pathol 35:1244–1248

Foulis AK (1984) Acute pancreatitis. Rec Adv Histopathol 12:188–196

Fredrickson DS, Levy RI, Lees RS (1967) Fat transport in lipoproteins: an integrated approach to mechanisms and disorders. N Engl J Med 276:34–44, 94–103, 148–156, 215–225, 273–281

Frick TW, Hailemariam S, Heitz PU, Largiader F, Goodale R (1990) Acute hypercalcaemia induces acinar cell necrosis and intraductal protein precipitates in the pancreas of cats and guinea pigs. Gastroenterology 98:1675–1681

Frick TW, Fryd DS, Goodale RL, Simmons RL, Sutherland DER, Najarian JS (1991) Lack of association between azathioprine and acute pancreatitis in renal transplantation patients. Lancet 337:251–252

Frost L, Pedersen RS, Ostgaard SE, Hansen HE (1990) Prognosis in acute pancreatitis complicated by acute renal failure requiring dialysis. Scand J Urol Nephrol 24:257–260

Gafter U, Mandel EM, Har-Zahar L, Weiss S (1976) Acute pancreatitis secondary to hypercalcaemia. Occurrence in a patient with breast carcinoma. JAMA 235:2004–2005

Gambill EE (1971) Pancreatitis associated with pancreatic carcinoma: a study of 26 cases. Mayo Clin Proc 46:174–177

Gambill EE (1973) Etiology and mechanisms of pancreatitis. In: Gambill EE (ed) Pancreatitis. Mosby, St Louis, pp 50–82

Gambill EE, Baggenstoss AH, Van Patter WG, Power MH (1948) Acute hemorrhagic pancreatitis: study of a patient having disseminate fat necrosis, hypocalcemia, hypopotassemia, uremia, diabetes mellitus, ascites, and bilateral hydrothorax. Gastroenterology 11:371–381

Gaultier M, Fournier E, Gervais P, Bodin F (1964) Encephalopathie pancreatique survenue au decours d'une intoxication oxycar-

bonee. Presse Med 72:3263–3265

Geokas MC (1968) The role of elastase in acute pancreatitis: III. The destructive capacity of elastase on pancreatic tissue in vivo and in vitro. Arch Pathol 1968:135–141

Glazer G (1988) Classification and definitions in acute and chronic pancreatitis. In: Glazer G, Ranson JHC (eds) Acute pancreatitis. Baillière Tindall, London, pp 37–50

Gmaz-Nikulin E, Nikulin A, Plamenac P, Hegewald G, Gaon D (1981) Pancreatic lesions in shock and their significance. J Pathol 135:223–236

Gordon D, Calne RY (1972) Renal failure in acute pancreatitis. Br Med J iii:801–802

Grace RR, Jordan PH (1976) Unsolved problems of pancreatic pseudocysts. Ann Surg 184:16–21

Gregg JA (1977) Detection of bacterial infection of the pancreatic ducts in patients with pancreatitis and pancreatic cancer during retrograde cholangiopancreatography. Gastroenterology 73:1005–1007

Griffiths RW, Brown PW (1970) Jejunal infarction as a complication of pancreatitis. Gastroenterology 58:709–712

Gross JB (1973) Hereditary pancreatitis. In: Gambill EE (ed) Pancreatitis. Mosby, St Louis, pp 109–114

Gross MLP, Fowler CJ, Ho R, Russell RCG, Harrison MJG (1988) Peripheral neuropathy complicating pancreatitis and major pancreatic surgery. J Neurol Neurosurg Psychiatry 51:1341–1344

Guardia SN, Bilbao JN, Murray D, Warren RE, Sweet J (1989) Fat embolism in acute pancreatitis. Arch Pathol Lab Med 113:503–506

Guice KS, Oldham KT, Caty MG, Johnson KJ, Ward PA (1989) Neutrophil-dependent, oxygen-radical mediated lung injury associated with acute pancreatitis. Ann Surg 210:740–747

Gupta RK (1971) Immunohistochemical study of glomerular lesions in acute pancreatitis. Arch Pathol 92:267–272

Guzmán S, Nervi F, Llanos O, León P, Valdivieso V (1985) Impaired lipid clearance in patients with previous acute pancreatitis. Gut 26:888–891

Gyr K, Heitz PU, Belinger C (1984) Pancreatitis. In: Klöppel G, Heitz PU (eds) Pancreatic pathology. Churchill Livingstone, Edinburgh, pp 44–72

Haas GS, Warshaw AL, Daggett WM, Aretz HT (1985) Acute pancreatitis after cardiopulmonary bypass. Am J Surg 149:508–515

Haller J, Greenway G, Resnick D, Kindynis P, Kang HS (1989) Intraosseous fat necrosis associated with acute pancreatitis: MR imaging. Radiology 173:193–195

Hammond J, Tesar J (1980) Pancreatitis-associated arthritis: sequential study of synovial fluid abnormalities. JAMA 244:694–696

Hanna AW (1960) Rupture of pancreatic cysts. Br J Surg 47:495–498

Hardaway R, McKay D (1959) Production of acute hemorrhagic pancreatitis in dogs by means of an episode of intravascular clotting in the pancreas. Surgery 45:557–561

Hardaway R (1962) The role of intravascular clotting in the etiology of shock. Ann Surg 155:325–338

Hardaway R, Burne WH, Geever EF, Burns JW, Mock HP (1962) Studies on the role of intravascular coagulation in irreversible hemorrhagic shock. Ann Surg 155:241–250

Hart CC (1989) Aerosolized pentamidine and pancreatitis [letter]. Ann Intern Med 111:691

Heatley MK (1990) Acute pancreatitis: the correlation between pathogenesis and histological findings at autopsy. Med Sci Law 30:153–158

Helin H, Mero M, Markkula H, Helin M (1980) Pancreatic acinar ultrastructure in human acute pancreatitis. Virchows Arch [A] 387:259–270

Herskovic T, Keating FR, Gross JB (1967) Coexistent pancreatitis and hyperparathyroidism: observations on 15 cases [abstract]. Gastroenterology 52:1093

Higgins E, Ive FA (1990) Subcutaneous fat necrosis in pancreatic disease. Br J Surg 77:532-533

Hoffman E, Perez E, Somera V (1959) Acute pancreatitis in the upper age groups. Gastroenterology 36:675-685

Hochgelerent EL, David DS (1974) Acute pancreatitis secondary to calcium infusion in a dialysis patient. Arch Surg 108:218-219

Holden JL, Berne TV, Rosoff L (1976) Pancreatic abscess following acute pancreatitis. Arch Surg 111:858-861

Hollender LF, Lehnert P, Wanke M, in collaboration with Nagel M (1983) Acute pancreatitis: an interdisciplinary synopsis. Urban and Schwarzenberg, Munich, pp 25-50

Houssin D, Castaing D, Lemoine J, Bismith H (1983) Microlithiasis of the gallbladder. Surg Gynecol Obstet 157:20-24

Howard JM (1960a) Pancreatitis associated with gallstones. In: Howard JM, Jordan GL (eds) Surgical diseases of the pancreas. Lippincott, Philadelphia, pp 169-189

Howard JM (1960b) The causes of death from acute pancreatitis. In: Howard JM, Jordan GL (eds) Surgical diseases of the pancreas. Lippincott, Philadelphia, pp 159-168

Howard JM (1960c) The pathology of pancreatitis. In: Howard JM, Jordan GL (eds) Surgical diseases of the pancreas. Lippincott, Philadelphia, pp 102-115

Howard P, Duff RS, Owen G, Baker WT (1963) Oedema associated with pancreatitis. Lancet ii:707-708

Immelman EJ, Banks S, Krige H, Marks IN (1964) Roentgenologic and clinical features of intramedullary fat necrosis in bones in acute and chronic pancreatitis. Am J Med 36:96-105

Inkeles DM, Walsh JB (1975) Retinal fat emboli: a sequel to acute pancreatitis. Am J Ophthalmol 80:935-938

Ingram DM, Sheiner HJ (1980) Massive pancreatic serous effusions. Aust N Z J Surg 50:137-140

Ivy AC, Gibbs GE (1952) Pancreatitis: a review. Surgery 31:614-642

Izsak EM, Shike M, Roulet M, Jeejeebhoy KN (1980) Pancreatitis in association with hypercalcaemia in patients receiving total parenteral nutrition. Gastroenterology 79:555-558

Jackson B, Files JC, Morrison FS, Scott-Conner CEH (1989) Thrombotic thrombocytopenic purpura and pancreatitis. Am J Gastroenterol 84:667-669

Jacob HS, Goldstein IM, Shapiro I, Craddock PR, Hammerschmidt DE, Weissmann G (1981) Sudden blindness in acute pancreatitis. Arch Intern Med 141:134-136

Jalovaara P, Apaja M (1978) Alcohol and acute pancreatitis: an experimental study in the rat. Scand J Gastroenterol 13:703-709

Johnson DA, Tong NT (1977) Pancreatic encephalopathy. South Med J 70:165-167

Johnston DH, Cornish AL (1959) Acute pancreatitis in patients receiving chlorothiazide. JAMA 170:2054-2056

Jones PA (1985) Survival after profound hypocalcaemia with tetany complicating severe haemorrhagic acute pancreatitis. Postgrad Med J 61:43-45

Jones PE, Oelbaum MH (1975) Frusemide-induced pancreatitis. Br Med J i:133-134

Jordan GL (1960) Pancreatic cysts. In: Howard JM, Jordan GL (eds) Surgical diseases of the pancreas. Lippincott, Philadelphia, pp 283-320

Judd ES, Mattson H, Mahorner HR (1931) Pancreatic cysts: a report of 47 cases. Arch Surg 22:838-849

Kattwinkel J, Lapey A, di Sant'Agnese PA, Edwards WA, Huffy MP (1973) Hereditary pancreatitis: three new kindreds and a critical review of the literature. Pediatrics 51:55-69

Kaushik SP, Vohra R, Verma GR, Kaushik S, Sabharwal A (1984) Pancreatic abscess: a review of 17 cases. Br J Surg 71:141-143

Kawanishi H, Rudolph E, Bull FE (1973) Azathioprine-induced acute pancreatitis [letter]. N Engl J Med 289:357

Keddie NC, Corson JG (1966) Acute pancreatitis: a clinical survey. Postgrad Med 42:234-239

Kelly TR (1984) Gallstone pancreatitis: local predisposing factors. Ann Surg 200:479-484

Keynes WM (1980) A non-pancreatic source of the proteolytic-enzyme amidase and bacteriology in experimental acute pancreatitis. Ann Surg 191:187-199

Keynes WM (1981) Experimental acute pancreatitis. In: Keynes WM, Keith RG (eds) The pancreas. Heinemann, London, pp 269-284

Keynes M (1988) Heretical thoughts on the pathogenesis of acute pancreatitis. Gut 29:1413-1423

Kishimoto W, Nakao A, Takagi H, Hayakawa T (1989) Acute pancreatitis after transcatheter arterial embolization (TAE) for hepatocellular carcinoma. Am J Gastroenterol 84:1396-1399

Klatskin G, Gordon M (1952) Relationship between relapsing pancreatitis and essential hyperlipemia. Am J Med 12:3-23

Klöppel G, Maillet B (1992) The morphologic basis for the evolution of acute pancreatitis into chronic pancreatitis. Virchows Arch [A] 420:1-4

Kobza K, Gyr K, Neuhaus K, Gudat F (1976) Acute intermittent porphyria with relapsing acute pancreatitis and unconjugated hyperbilirubinemia without overt hemolysis. Gastroenterology 71:494-496

Kristensen BO, Skov J, Peterslund NS (1980) Furosemide-induced increases in serum isoamylases. Br Med J ii:978

Kumar S, Schnadig VJ, MacGregor MG (1989) Fatal acute pancreatitis associated with pentamidine therapy. Am J Gastroenterol 84:451-453

Kunelis CT, Peters JL, Edmondson HA (1965) Fatty liver of pregnancy and its relationship to tetracycline therapy. Am J Med 38:359-377

Kusterer K, Enghofer M, Zendler S, Blochle C, Usadel KH (1991) Microcirculatory changes in sodium taurocholate-induced pancreatitis in rats. Am J Physiol 260:G346-G351

Lancet (1992) Biliary sludge: more than a curiosity [editorial]. 339:1087

Lankisch PG (1988) Pathogenesis of pancreatic inflammation. In: Glazer G, Ranson JHC (eds) Acute pancreatitis. Baillière Tindall, London, pp 182-193

Lankisch PG, Rahlf G, Koop H (1983) Pulmonary complications in fatal acute hemorrhagic pancreatitis. Dig Dis Sci 28:111-116

Lankisch PG, Schirren CA, Kunze E (1991) Undetected fatal acute pancreatitis: why is the disease so frequently overlooked? Am J Gastroenterol 86:322-326

Lee PC, Howard JM (1979) Fat necrosis. Surg Gynecol Obstet 148:785-789

Lee PC, Nakashima Y, Appert HE, Howard JM (1979) Lipase and colipase in canine pancreatic juice as etiological factors in fat necrosis. Surg Gynecol Obstet 148:39-44

Lee SP, Nicholls JF, Park HZ (1992) Biliary sludge as a cause of acute pancreatitis. N Engl J Med 326:589-593

Leeson PM, Fourman P (1966) Acute pancreatitis from vitamin D poisoning in a patient with parathyroid deficiency. Lancet i:1185-1186

Lefer AM, Glen TM, O'Neill TJ, Lovat WL, Geissinger WT, Wangensteen SL (1971) Inotrophic influence of endogenous peptides in experimental hemorrhagic pancreatitis. Surgery 69:220-228

Lipson JD, Stephenson HE (1971) Pancreatitis complicated by pericardial effusion and cardiac tamponade. Arch Surg 103:414-416

Little AG, Moossa AR (1981) Gastrointestinal hemorrhage from left-sided portal hypertension: an unappreciated complication of pancreatitis. Am J Surg 141:153-158

Longnecker DS (1991) Pathology of pancreatitis. In: Braganza JM (ed) The pathogenesis of pancreatitis. Manchester University Press, Manchester, pp 3-18

Lumsden A, Bradley EL (1990) Secondary pancreatic infections. Surg Gynecol Obstet 170:459–467

Machado MCC, da Cuhna JEM, Bacchella T, Mott CdeB, Duarte I, Bettarello A (1984) Acute pancreatic necrosis in chronic alcoholic pancreatitis. Dig Dis Sci 29:709–713

Maclean D, Emslie-Smith D (1977) Accidental hypothermia. Blackwell, Oxford, p 404

MacLean N (1977) The role of the surviving pancreas in late fatalities of acute pancreatitis. Br J Surg 64:345–346

McLean R, Martin S, Lam-Po-Tang PRL (1982) Fatal case of L-asparaginase induced pancreatitis. Lancet ii:1401–1402

Mair WSJ, McMahon MJ, Goliger JC (1976) Stenosis of the colon in acute pancreatitis. Gut 17:692–695

Major RH (1948) Classic descriptions of disease, 3rd edn. Blackwell, Oxford, p 654

Malagelada J-R (1986) The pathophysiology of alcoholic pancreatitis. Pancreas 1:270–278

Malangoni MA, Shallcross JC, Seiler JG, Richardson JD, Polk HC (1986) Factors contributing to fatal outcome after treatment of pancreatic abscess. Ann Surg 203:605–613

Mallory A, Kern F (1980) Drug-induced pancreatitis: a critical review. Gastroenterology 78:813–820

Manson RR (1974) Acute pancreatitis secondary to iatrogenic hypercalcemia: implications of hyperalimentation. Arch Surg 108:213–215

Mant AK (1969) Autopsy diagnosis of accidental hypothermia. J Forensic Med 16:126–129

Marks IN, Bank S, Louw JH, Farman J (1967) Peptic ulceration and gastrointestinal bleeding in pancreatitis. Gut 8:253–259

Marx SJ, Attie MF, Levine MA, Spiegel AM, Downs RW, Lasker RD (1981) The hypocalciuric or benign variant of familial hypercalcemia: clinical and biochemical features in fifteen kindreds. Medicine 60:397–412

Matsumoto T, Matsui T, Iida M, Nunoi K, Fujishima M (1989) Acute pancreatitis as a complication of Crohn's disease. Am J Gastroenterol 84:804–807

McConnell RB (1966) The genetics of gastro-intestinal disorders. Oxford University Press, London, pp 170–173

McCutcheon AD (1968) A fresh approach to the pathogenesis of pancreatitis. Gut 9:296–310

McFadden DW (1991) Organ failure and multiple organ system failure in pancreatitis. Pancreas 6 Suppl:S37–S43

McGovern VJ (1971) Shock. In: Sommers SC (ed) Pathology annual, pp 279–298

McKenna JM, Chandrascklar AJ, Skorton D, Craig RM, Cugell DW (1977) The pleuropulmonary complications of pancreatitis. Chest 71:197–204

Mendez G, Isikoff MB (1979) Significance of intrapancreatic gas demonstrated by CT: a review of nine cases. AJR 132:59–62

Menguy RB, Hallenbeck GA, Bollman JL, Grindlay JH (1957) Ductal and vascular factors in etiology of experimentally induced pancreatitis. Arch Surg 74:881–889

Miller RE, Baer JW, Nizin JS, Pascal RR (1985) Hemorrhagic pancreatitis: a complication of transcatheter embolization treated successfully by total pancreatectomy. Am J Surg 149:802–808

Miller TA, Lindenauer M, Frey CF, Stanley JC (1974) Pancreatic abscess. Arch Surg 108:545–551

Miln DC, Barclay THC (1952) Acute colonic obstruction due to pancreatitis. Lancet ii:168–169

Milner RDG, Mitchinson MJ (1965) Systemic Weber–Christian disease. J Clin Pathol 18:150–156

Mitchell CE (1964) Relapsing pancreatitis with recurrent pericardial and pleural effusion. Ann Intern Med 60:1047–1053

Mixter CG, Keynes WM, Cope O (1962) Further experience with pancreatitis as a diagnostic clue to hyperparathyroidism. N Engl J Med 266:265–272

Moss J (1986) Accidental severe hypothermia. Surg Gynecol Obstet 162:501–513

Murphey SA, Josephs AS (1981) Acute pancreatitis associated with pentamidine therapy. Arch Intern Med 141:56–58

Murphy D, Imrie CW, Davidson JF (1977) Haematological abnormalities in acute pancreatitis: a prospective study. Postgrad Med J 53:310–314

Murphy D, Pack AI, Imrie CW (1980) The mechanism of arterial hypoxia occurring in acute pancreatitis. Q J Med 49:151–163

Musa OA, Case RM (1991) Secretory polarity. In: Braganza JM (ed) The pathogenesis of pancreatitis. Manchester University Press, Manchester, pp 34–44

Nagai H, Henrich H, Wünsch P-H, Fischbach W, Mössner J (1989) Role of pancreatic enzymes and their substrates in autodigestion of the pancreas: in vitro studies with isolated rat pancreatic acini. Gastroenterology 96:838–847

Nance FC, Cain JL (1967) Hemorrhagic pancreatitis in germfree dogs. Surg Forum 18:365–367

Neoptolemos JP, Carr-Locke DL, London N, Bailey I, Fossard DP (1988) ERCP findings and the role of endoscopic sphincterotomy in acute gallstone pancreatitis. Br J Surg 75:954–960

Nogueria JR, Freedman MA (1972) Acute pancreatitis as a complication of Imuran therapy in regional enteritis. Gastroenterology 62:1040–1041

Nordback I, Teerenhovi O, Auvinen O (1986) Unifying the terminology of acute pancreatitis [letter]. Lancet i:687

Nottle P (1980) Colonic infarction and pancreatitis: a case report. Aust N Z J Surg 50:184–185

Novis IMS (1923) Partial obstruction of the pancreatic duct by round worms. Br J Surg 10:421

Nugent FW, Mobarhan S (1973) Medical management of acute pancreatitis. In: Carey LC (ed) The pancreas. Mosby, St Louis, pp 153–160

Office of Population Censuses and Surveys (1991) 1990 mortality statistics: cause. England and Wales. (Series DH2 no. 17) HMSO, London

Ogilvie RF (1941) Duodenal diverticula and their complications with particular reference to acute pancreatic necrosis. Br J Surg 28:362–379

Ohlsson K, Genell S (1991) Role of enzyme inhibitors in acute pancreatitis and rationale for their therapeutic use. In: Braganza JM (ed) The pathogenesis of pancreatitis. Manchester University Press, Manchester, pp 198–214

Olsen H (1973) Thrombotic thrombocytopenic purpura as a cause of pancreatitis. Dig Dis Sci 18:238–246

Opie EL (1901) The etiology of acute hemorrhagic pancreatitis. Bull Johns Hopkins Hosp 123:182–188

Opie EL (1910) Disease of the pancreas, 2nd edn. Lippincott, Philadelphia, pp 200–208

Pallis CA, Lewis PD (1974) The neurology of gastrointestinal disease. Saunders, London, pp 192–199

Parkash O (1972) On the anomalous age-dependence of acute pancreatitis. Digestion 5:269–274

Parker WA (1983) Estrogen-induced pancreatitis. Clin Pharm 2:75–79

Parrilla Paricio P, García Olmo D, Pellicer Franco E, Prieto González A, Carrasco González C, Bermejo López J (1990) Gallbladder cholesterolosis: an aetiological factor in acute pancreatitis of uncertain origin. Br J Surg 77:735–736

Payne JE, Tanenberg RJ (1980) Hyperparathyroid crisis and acute necrotizing pancreatitis presenting as diabetic ketoacidosis. Am J Surg 140:698–703

Pellegrini CA, Paloyan D, Acoata JM, Skinner DB (1977) Acute pancreatitis of rare causation. Surg Gynecol Obstet 144:899–902

Peters N, Chalmers TM, Truscott BMcN, Rack JH, Adams PH (1966) Familial hyperparathyroidism. Postgrad Med J 42:228–233

Pfeffer RB, Lazarini-Robertson A, Safadi D, Mixter G, Secoy CF, Hinton JW (1962) Gradations of pancreatitis, edematous through hemorrhagic, experimentally produced by controlled injection of microspheres into blood vessels in dogs. Surgery 51:764-769

Pitchumoni CS, Agarwal N, Jain NK (1988) Systemic complications of acute pancreatitis. Am J Gastroenterol 83:597-606

Popper HL, Necheles H, Russell KC (1978) Transition of pancreatic edema to pancreatic necrosis. Surg Gynecol Obstet 87:79-82

Poulsen HM (1950) Familial lipemia: a new form of liposis showing increase in neutral fats combined with attacks of acute pancreatitis. Acta Med Scand 138:413-420

Prinz RA (1991) Mechanisms of acute pancreatitis: vascular aetiology. Int J Pancreatol 9:31-38

Probstein JG, Joshi RA, Blumenthal H (1957) Atheromatous embolization: an etiology of pancreatitis. Arch Surg 75:566-572

Puolakkainen P, Lempinen M, Schröder T (1986) Fatal pancreatitis: a study of 64 consecutive cases. Acta Chir Scand 152:379-383

Randall PE (1986) Incidence of hypothermia [letter]. Lancet i:275

Randall PE, Heath DF, Little RA (1985) How common is accidental hypothermia? Arch Emerg Med 2:174-175

Rango N (1984) Exposure-related hypothermia in the United States, 1970-79. Am J Public Health 74:1159-1160

Ranson HC, Rifkind KM, Roses DF, Fink SD, Eng K, Localio SA (1974) Objective early identification of severe early pancreatitis. Am J Gastroenterol 61:443-451

Ranson JH, Spencer FC (1977) Prevention, diagnosis and treatment of pancreatic abscess. Surgery 1977:99-106

Rattner DW, Compton CC, Gu ZY, Wilkinson R, Warshaw AL (1989) Bacterial infection is not necessary for lethal necrotizing pancreatitis in mice. Int J Pancreatol 5:99-105

Renner IG, Savage WJ, Pantoja JL, Renner WJ (1985) Death due to acute pancreatitis: a rétrospective analysis of 405 autopsy cases. Dig Dis Sci 30:1005-1015

Reynolds JC, Inman RD, Kimberley RP, Chuong JH, Kovacs JE, Walsh MB (1982) Acute pancreatitis in systemic lupus erythematosus: report of twenty cases and a review of the literature. Medicine 61:25-32

Rich AR, Duff GL (1936) Experimental and pathological studies on the pathogenesis of acute hemorrhagic pancreatitis. Bull Johns Hopkins Hosp 58:212-260

Roberts NJ, Baggenstoss AH, Comfort MW (1950) Acute pancreatic necrosis: a clinicopathologic study. Am J Clin Pathol 20:742-764

Rogers C, Klatt EC (1989) Splenic vein thrombosis in adults with acute pancreatitis. Int J Pancreatol 5:117-121

Rohrmann CA, Surawicz CM, Hutchinson D, Silverstein FE, White TT, Marchioro TL (1981) Diagnosis of hereditary pancreatitis by pancreatography. Gastrointest Endosc 27:168-173

Saag KG, Niemann TH, Warner CA, Naides SJ (1992) Subcutaneous pancreatic fat necrosis associated with acute arthritis. J Rheumatol 19:630-632

Sachar LA, Probstein LG (1954) Terminal acute pancreatitis: an incidental finding at autopsy. Am J Dig Dis 21:52-58

Saint EG (1954) Acute pancreatitis. Med J Aust 2:536-543

Saint EG, Curnow D, Paton R, Stokes JB (1954) Diagnosis of acute porphyria. Br Med J i:1182-1184

Salt WB, Schenker S (1976) Amylase - its clinical significance: a review of the literature. Medicine 55:269-289

Sanfey H, Sarr MG, Bulkley GB, Cameron JL (1986) Oxygen-derived free radicals and acute pancreatitis: a review. Acta Physiol Scand Suppl 548:109-118

Sanford KA, Mayle JE, Dean HA, Greenbaum DS (1988) Metronidazole-associated pancreatitis. Ann Intern Med 109:756-757

Sano ME, Smith LW (1940) Fifty postmortem patients with cancer subjected to local or generalized refrigeration compared to a similar control group of 37 nonrefrigerated patients. J Lab Clin Med 26:443-456

Sarles H (1965) Proposal adopted unanimously by the participants of the Symposium. In: Sarles H (ed) Pancreatitis. Symposium, Marseilles, 25-26 April 1963. Karger, Basel, pp vii-viii

Sarles H, Cros RC, Nicholas R, Durbec JC (1976) Quantity of alcohol consumption and risk of chronic pancreatitis [abstract]. Gut 17:826

Sarles H, Sahel J, Staub JL, Bourry J, Laugier R (1979) Chronic pancreatitis. In: Howat HT, Sarles H (eds) The exocrine pancreas. Saunders, London, pp 402-439

Sarles H, Adler G, Dani R et al. (1989) The pancreatitis classification of Marseilles-Rome 1988. Scand J Gastroenterol 24:641-642

Sarner M, Cotton PB (1984a) Classification of pancreatitis. Gut 25:756-759

Sarner M, Cotton PB (1984b) Definitions of acute and chronic pancreatitis. Clin Gastroenterol 13:865-867

Satiani B, Stone HH (1979) Predictability of present outcome and future recurrence in acute pancreatitis. Arch Surg 114:711-716

Scarpelli DG (1956) Fat necrosis of bone marrow in acute pancreatitis. Am J Pathol 32:1077-1087

Schmidt H, Creutzfeldt W (1969) The possible role of phospholipase A in the pathogenesis of acute pancreatitis. Scand J Gastroenterol 4:39-48

Schmidt H, Creutzfeldt W (1970) Calciphylactic pancreatitis and pancreatitis in hyperparathyroidism. Clin Orthop 69:135-145

Scholefield JH, Goodman AJ, Morgan WP (1988) Abdominal wall and gastric infarction in acute pancreatitis. Pancreas 3:494-496

Schwartz MS, Cappell MS (1989) Pentamidine-associated pancreatitis. Dig Dis Sci 34:1617-1620

Seligson U, Cho JW, Ihre T, Lundh G (1982) Clinical course and autopsy findings in acute and chronic pancreatitis. Acta Chir Scand 148:269-274

Senba M, Nakamura T, Kawai K, Senba MI (1991) HTLV-1 and acute pancreatitis [letter]. Lancet 337:1489

Sheikh H (1965) Duodenal ischaemia complicating acute pancreatitis. Br Med J i:1539-1540

Shinowara GY, Stutman LH, Walters MI, Ruth ME, Walker E (1963) Hypercoagulability in acute pancreatitis. Am J Surg 105:714-719

Sibert JR (1975) A British family with hereditary pancreatitis. Gut 16:81-88

Singer C (1928) A short history of medicine. Clarendon Press, Oxford, p 158

Singer MV, Gyr K, Sarles H (1985) Revised classification of pancreatitis. Gastroenterology 89:683-685

Singleton JW, Law DH, Kelley ML, Mekhjian HS, Sturdivant RAL (1979) National Cooperative Crohn's Disease Study: adverse reactions to study drugs. Gastroenterology 77:870-872

Sitges-Serra A, Alonso M, de Lecea C, Gores PF, Sutherland DER (1988) Pancreatitis and hyperparathyroidism. Br J Surg 75:158-160

Smith LW (1940) Pathologic changes observed in human tissues subjected to subcritical temperatures. Arch Pathol 30:424-438

Smyth CJ (1940) Etiology af acute hemorrhagic pancreatitis with special reference to the vascular factors. An analysis of autopsies. Arch Pathol 30:651-669

Steedman RA, Doering R, Carter R (1967) Pancreatic abscess. Surg Gynecol Obstet 125:757-762

Steer ML, Meldolesi J (1988) Pathogenesis of acute pancreatitis. Annu Rev Med 39:95-105

Steer ML, Meldolesi J, Figarella C (1984) Pancreatitis: the role of lysosomes. Dig Dis Sci 29:934-938

Stein AA, Powers SR (1958) Terminal pancreatitis. Arch Pathol 65:445-448

Steinberg WM (1992) Acute pancreatitis – never leave a stone unturned. N Engl J Med 326 : 635–637

Stenvinkel P, Alvestrand A (1988) Loop diuretic-induced pancreatitis with rechallenge in a patient with malignant hypertension and renal insufficiency. Acta Med Scand 224 : 89–91

Storck G (1971) Fat necrosis in acute pancreatitis: morphological and chemical studies in the rat. Acta Chir Scand 417 : 1–36

Stroud WH, Cullom JW, Anderson MC (1981) Hemorrhagic complications of severe pancreatitis. Surgery 90 : 657–665

Swerdlow AB, Berman ME, Gibbel MI, Valaitis J (1960) Subcutaneous fat necrosis associated with acute pancreatitis. JAMA 173 : 765–769

Thal A, Brackney E (1954) Acute hemorrhagic pancreatic necrosis produced by local Shwartzman reaction. Experimental study on pancreatitis. JAMA 155 : 569–574

Thal A, Molestina JE (1955) Studies on pancreatitis: III. Fulminating hemorrhagic pancreatitis produced by means of staphylococcal toxin. Arch Pathol 60 : 212–220

Thal A, Perry JF, Egner W (1957a) A clinical and morphologic study of forty-two cases of fatal acute pancreatitis. Surg Gynecol Obstet 105 : 191–202

Thal A, Tansathithaya P, Egner W (1957b) An experimental study of bacterial pancreatitis. Surg Gynecol Obstet 103 : 459–468

Thorne JC, Bookman AA, Stevens H (1980) A case of polyarteritis presenting as abrupt onset of pancreatic insufficiency. J Rheumatol 7 : 583–586

Tilney NI, Bailey GL, Morgan AP (1973) Sequential system failure after rupture of abdominal aortic aneurysm. Ann Surg 178 : 117–122

Trapnell JE (1966) The natural history and prognosis of acute pancreatitis. Ann R Coll Surg Engl 38 : 265–287

Trapnell JE (1971) Complications of acute pancreatitis. Ann R Coll Surg Engl 49 : 361–372

Trapnell JE, Duncan EHL (1975) Patterns of incidence in acute pancreatitis. Br Med J ii : 179–183

Uden S, Blower AL, Taylor TV, Benbow E, McMahon RFT, Braganza JM (1988) Exploration of a role for activated leucocytes in fatal pancreatitis [abstract]. J Pathol 155 : 351

Vallat JM, Vital C (1989) Peripheral neuropathy complicating pancreatitis [letter]. J Neurol Neurosurg Psychiatry 52 : 810

Waldner H (1992) Vascular mechanisms to induce acute pancreatitis. Eur Surg Res 24 (Suppl 1) : 62–67

Warshaw AL, Jin G (1985) Improved survival in 45 patients with pancreatic abscess. Ann Surg 202 : 408–415

Warshaw AL, O'Hara PJ (1978) Susceptibility of the pancreas to ischaemic injury in shock. Ann Surg 188 : 197–201

Wells AD, McDonnell PJ, Burnard KG (1990) Purtscher's retinopathy in acute pancreatitis. Br J Surg 77 : 820

Whalley PJ, Adams RH, Combes B (1964) Tetracycline toxicity in pregnancy, liver and pancreatic dysfunction. JAMA 189 : 357–362

Wharton GK (1932) The blood supply of the pancreas with special reference to that of the islands of Langerhans. Anat Rec 53 : 55–76

Whipple GH (1907) Pancreatitis and focal necrosis. Bull Johns Hopkins Hosp 18 : 391–396

White TT (1966) Pancreatitis. Edward Arnold, London, pp 87–88

White TT, Morgan A, Hopton D (1970) Postoperative pancreatitis: a study of seventy cases. Am J Surg 120 : 132–137

Widdison AL, Karanjia ND, Reber HA (1990) Route(s) of spread of bacteria to the pancreas in acute necrotizing pancreatitis [abstract]. Pancreas 5 : 736

Willemer S, Dombrowski H, Adler G, Bussmann JF, Arnold R (1992) Recurrent acute pancreatitis and intraluminal duodenal diverticulum. Pancreas 7 : 257–261

Williams G (1954) Acute pancreatic necrosis as a cause of sudden death. Br Med J i : 1184–1185

Williams KJ, Fabian TC (1992) Pancreatic pseudocyst: recommendations for operative and nonoperative management. Am Surg 58 : 199–205

Wilson C, Imrie CW (1986) Occult pancreatic cancer with recurrent acute pancreatitis. Postgrad Med J 62 : 765–767

Wilson C, Imrie CW, Carter DC (1988) Fatal acute pancreatitis. Gut 29 : 782–788

Woodard S, Kelvin FM, Rice RP, Thompson WM (1981) Pancreatic abscess: importance of conventional radiology. AJR 136 : 871–878

Zaslow J (1953) Acute pancreatitis with necrosis and perforation of the common bile duct. Arch Surg 67 : 47–51

Zhou W, McCollum MO, Levine BA, Olson MS (1992) Role of platelet-activating factor in pancreatitis-associated acute lung injury in the rat. Am J Pathol 140 : 971–979

Ziegler DW, Long JA, Philippart AI, Klein MD (1988) Pancreatitis in childhood: experience with 49 patients. Ann Surg 207 : 257–261

13 Non-infective Chronic Pancreatitis

Following an international conference in 1963 (Sarles 1965), it was agreed that pancreatitis should be classified as: (1) acute pancreatitis; (2) relapsing acute pancreatitis; (3) chronic pancreatitis with acute exacerbations; and (4) chronic pancreatitis. In subsequent clinical practice, however, it was found almost impossible to distinguish between recurrences of acute pancreatitis and acute episodes in the course of chronic pancreatitis. Thus, at a second international conference (Gyr et al. 1984), the classification was simplified to: (1) acute pancreatitis and (2) chronic pancreatitis. In chronic pancreatitis the damage in the gland progresses whether there are acute exacerbations or not, whereas, in acute pancreatitis, with or without relapses, the damage can be arrested and further attacks prevented if a cause can be found and removed; gallstones are an example of such a cause.

In chronic pancreatitis, the main lesions, as summed up by Heitz and Klöppel during the symposium in 1984, are lobular scarring of the parenchyma, with frequent dilatations of small ducts due to downstream strictures of these ducts, protein plugs that may or may not be calcified in the ducts, frequent abnormalities of the epithelium lining the ducts, fibrous replacement of the exocrine parenchyma, and infiltration by cells typical of chronic inflammation with relative preservation of the endocrine tissue until late in the disease.

Obstructive chronic pancreatitis is a morphologically distinct form of chronic pancreatitis in which there is dilatation of the ductal system behind an occlusion of a major duct. There is diffuse atrophy of the acinar parenchyma with widespread perilobular fibrosis, but without disruption of the lobules until late in the disease. Calculi and protein plugs are usually absent.

Clinical Effects of Chronic Pancreatitis

In most patients with chronic pancreatitis there is recurrent or persistent abdominal pain, and although the diagnosis includes the word "chronic", it was pointed out by Comfort et al. (1946) that the symptoms tend to be "vigorous, sometimes violent. They rarely are mild or vague." The attacks of abdominal pain are usually severe and prolonged. It is also believed that, even between clinical exacerbations, the damage in the pancreas will progress until such a loss of pancreatic function is reached that steatorrhoea develops, with undigested meat fibres in the faeces; sooner or later diabetes mellitus supervenes. Although the pain is usually incapacitating there have been cases in which all the pathological features of chronic pancreatitis have been found unexpectedly in the absence of any history of pain. Old age alone seems to cause some of the fibrotic changes of chronic pancreatitis (Schmitz-Moorman et al. (1984) and even calcification (Nagai and Ohtsubo 1984).

Classification of Chronic Pancreatitis

Chronic pancreatitis can be subdivided into:

Alcoholic chronic pancreatitis
Nutritional (tropical) pancreatitis
Obstructive chronic pancreatitis
Metabolic chronic pancreatitis
Hereditary chronic pancreatitis
Pancreatitis associated with pancreatic malformations
Auto-immune chronic pancreatitis
Idiopathic chronic pancreatitis

Alcoholic Chronic Pancreatitis

This type of chronic pancreatitis, in which the pathological changes are characteristic, has long been recognised by Professor Henri Sarles of Marseilles to be common in the South of France and to be associated with the heavy consumption of alcoholic beverages. The clinical and histopathological features of this disease have been the subject of many publications by Professor Sarles with various colleagues, and a review of much of this work was published by Sarles et al. in 1979, while the results of further work were reviewed by Sarles et al. in 1980, and again by Sarles in 1986. He found that there were radiological signs of pancreatic stones in about half the patients on presentation, while in the remainder, calcifications became recognisable on plain radiographs of the abdomen during the following 2 years. This convinced Sarles and his group that all the patients had chronic calcifying pancreatitis.

The disease is predominantly one of men (H. Sarles et al. 1965), and during the first attack of pain it may be impossible to differentiate clinically between acute pancreatitis, the onset of alcoholic chronic pancreatitis, or other types of chronic pancreatitis. Sarles et al. (1980), claimed that a marked elevation of the level of the iron-binding protein, lactoferrin, in pancreatic juice obtained endoscopically will distinguish chronic calcifying pancreatitis from other types. They did not find similar hypersecretion of lactoferrin in patients with recurrent acute pancreatitis, or in alcoholics without pancre-

atic lesions, or in juice obtained from patients with pancreatic cancer. They concluded that the finding was specific for the diagnosis of chronic calcifying pancreatitis. Lactoferrin was also found to be increased in the zymogen granules of the acinic cells of certain acini in chronic calcifying pancreatitis; this increase became more marked as the disease progressed (Sarles 1986). This assay had not, however, gained general acceptance in clinical practice by 1986 (Di Magno and Clain 1986).

Alcoholic Consumption

The relationship between the development of chronic calcifying pancreatitis and the amount of alcohol consumed has been investigated by Sarles and his colleagues (1980), who found that in the West, Japan and South America, there is a strict correlation between the mean daily amount of alcohol consumed and the logarithm of the risk of developing chronic calcifying pancreatitis, and that even small amounts of alcohol, such as 1–20 g per day, increase the risk. There are, of course, certain individuals, as has been mentioned in relation to acute pancreatitis, whose pancreases seem to be particularly vulnerable to injury by alcohol. In such people there is reported to be a preponderance of blood group O (Marks et al. 1973), but the genetic significance of the studies of the HLA groups A1 and BW40 in relation to chronic pancreatitis suggested by Gosselin et al. (1978), Betuel et al. (1980) and Gullo et al. (1982) has not been confirmed by Chevallier et al. (1982). The mean consumption of alcohol before the first symptoms of chronic calcifying pancreatitis develop has been calculated by Sarles et al. (1979) to be between 150 g and 175 g of ethanol per day for about 18 years for men and about 11 years for women. In the alcoholic beverages commonly available in Britain such daily consumption might represent about a bottle of spirits or at least eight pints of beer (Stockwel and Stirling 1989).

The effects of diet are less important in the developed countries, but there is a positive linear correlation between the logarithm of the relative risk of developing chronic calcifying pancreatitis and the consumption of protein, but the effect of protein is much weaker than the effect of alcohol (Sarles 1986). Sarles has also found that, as far as fat is concerned, the lowest risk is linked to the average fat consumption (80–100 g day $^{-1}$); a higher risk is associated with low fat diets, and the highest risk with high fat diets. The effects of alcohol, protein, and fat consumption are additive.

The earliest changes in the structure of the gland in calcifying chronic pancreatitis can not be recognised by routine microscopy of the pancreas, but morphometric comparisons with normal controls (Sarles 1986) have shown an increase in the overall size of the acinar cells, with enlargement of their nuclei, nucleoli, endoplasmic reticulum and Golgi apparatus. Such enlargement has been interpreted as indicating increased function, possibly with modifications of the composition of the secretion produced.

The further stages in the pathogenesis of the disease have been studied by Nakamura et al. (1972) by three-dimensional reconstruction of the pancreatic ducts. They cut serial sections from ten pancreases that had been removed surgically because of alcoholic calcifying chronic pancreatitis and compared the findings with those from two pancreases in which chronic pancreatitis had been caused by obstruction of the main duct by a small carcinoma, and with the findings in a similarly sectioned normal pancreas.

As a result of these studies, they concluded that in alcoholic chronic calcifying pancreatitis the earliest lesion was the formation of precipitates of protein within small ducts. The precipitates formed plugs that evolved into calculi by the addition of calcium. The distribution of the plugs was characteristically patchy and a plugged duct might be surrounded by normal ducts. The acini that discharged their secretion into an obstructed duct were usually abnormal but were not invariably so. However, pathological acini were always associated with abnormal ducts and it was concluded that the lesions of the ducts led to the lesions of the parenchyma. The epithelium of the plugged ducts was usually abnormal, but was sometimes, presumably in early lesions, normal. The ductal epithelium gradually became atrophic and surrounding fibrosis led to permanent narrowing or complete obstruction, as a result of which certain lobules became cut off from the duct system. Such lobules might atrophy and disappear, or dilate to form cysts, leaving a picture of isolated groups of acini and rounded cavities lined by cuboidal cells, some of which could be identified by their ultrastructure as being modified acinar cells while others were altered ductal epithelial cells. The vicinity of the damaged lobules and ducts became infiltrated by lymphocytes; such infiltration could be recognised to have replaced the ductal structure that had initiated the lesion.

The authors were impressed by the patchy and irregular distribution of the lesions in alcoholic chronic pancreatitis and by the contrast that became apparent when these lesions were compared with those of the two cases of chronic obstructive pancreatitis. In the latter, the obstruction having been in the main duct near the ampulla, the lesions were uniformly distributed throughout the whole pancreas, without the alternating stenosis and dilatation of the ducts and the protein plugs that were conspicuous in the alcoholic specimens.

The late effects of alcoholic chronic calcifying pancreatitis are to leave a pancreas that is usually enlarged, but, in material obtained at autopsy, as distinct from specimens removed surgically, the gland may be atrophic. An atrophic gland is thought to represent the final stage in the evolution of the disease. Such an atrophic pancreas is illustrated in Fig. 13.1 and a less atrophic gland is shown in Fig. 13.2. The pancreas usually feels nodular and dilatation of the ducts may or may not be present. Dilatation of the whole duct system is not characteristic of chronic calcifying pancreatitis, but, if calculi reach the main duct, the effects of chronic obstructive pancreatitis may be added to the picture. A pancreas with atrophy of the parenchyma, lithiasis and dilatation of the ducts has been illustrated by Baggenstoss (1973). In early cases the only signs of pancreatic disease may be foci of fat necrosis. In advanced cases there may be adhesions to adjacent organs, to the spleen, for example, as in Fig. 13.2. Small cysts with a smooth lining to their walls, within the glandular tissue, as in Fig. 13.1, are usually retention cysts due to stenosis of ducts; larger cysts with an irregular necrotic lining, as in Fig. 13.2, are pseudocysts and may extend beyond the margins of the pancreas. Pseudocysts that are the result of fat necrosis may be adjacent to the pancreas in the retroperitoneal or mesenteric fat.

The plugs that obstruct the ducts are not recognisable macroscopically and may not be sufficiently calcified to be opaque radiologically (Figs 13.3–13.6). The earliest stages of the accumulation of calcium within such plugs are shown in Figs 13.7 and 13.8.

According to Sarles et al. (1979) calcifications are nearly always intraductal and consist of calcium carbonate and protein material in varying proportions. A badly damaged pancreas may, however, also contain some areas of parenchymal calcification (Fig. 13.9). Whatever the distribution of the calcification within the pancreas, there is much evidence, for example the findings of Owens and Howard (1958), that there is a close association between clinical radiological evidence of calcification in the pancreas and chronic alcoholism, at least in the USA and Western Europe. No such association is clearly recognisable, in spite of the similarity of the pancreatic lesions, in the types of pancreatic calcification that are common in parts of Africa, Indonesia and India.

The importance of obstructive lesions in the tributaries of the main ducts in chronic alcoholic

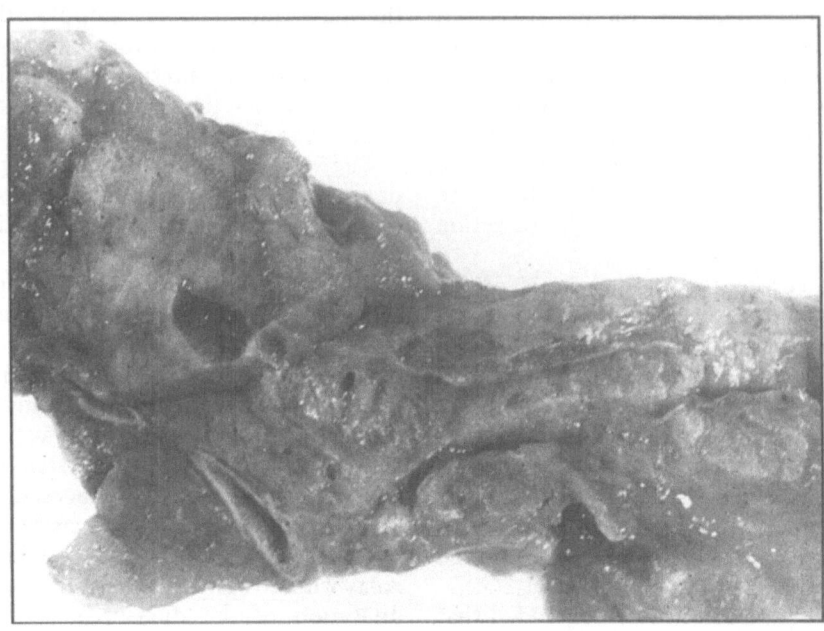

Fig. 13.1. The macroscopic appearance of an atrophic-looking pancreas in which a small retention cyst is associated with moderate dilatation of the duct. The patient was an alcoholic man aged 49, who died of a suicidal overdose of paracetamol. (Courtesy of Dr A.R. Williams)

pancreatitis, as studied by serial endoscopic pancreatography, has been noted by Nagata et al. (1981). Such findings provide confirmation for the conclusions reached by Nakamura et al. (1972) by pathological methods. A marked contrast between the clinical effects of multiple obstructive lesions in small ducts in chronic alcoholic pancreatitis and the effects of obstruction of the main ducts is suggested by the promising results in the relief of pain in chronic alcoholic pancreatitis that have been obtained by deliberate obstruction of the main pancreatic duct (Little et al. 1979; Roesch and Gebhardt 1981). Such relief may be because obstruction of the main duct completes the functional failure of the

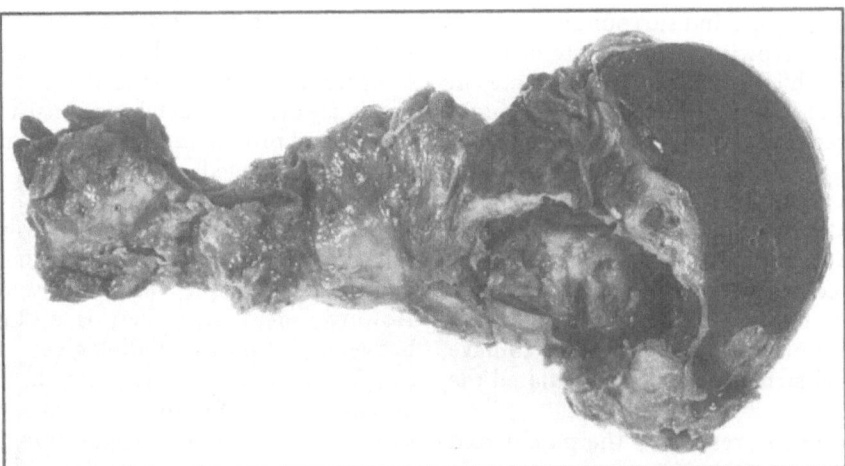

Fig. 13.2. The macroscopic appearance of the pancreas and spleen from a man aged 37, who died of lobar pneumonia. He had drunk 6–8 pints of beer a day for many years, and, in the period before his death, a bottle of sherry each day. The pancreas felt fibrotic and a pseudocyst can be seen between the tail of the pancreas and the hilum of the spleen. A small subcapsular infarct is present near the lower pole of the spleen. There was no recognisable communication between the pseudocyst and the duct system of the pancreas. (Courtesy of Dr William Taylor)

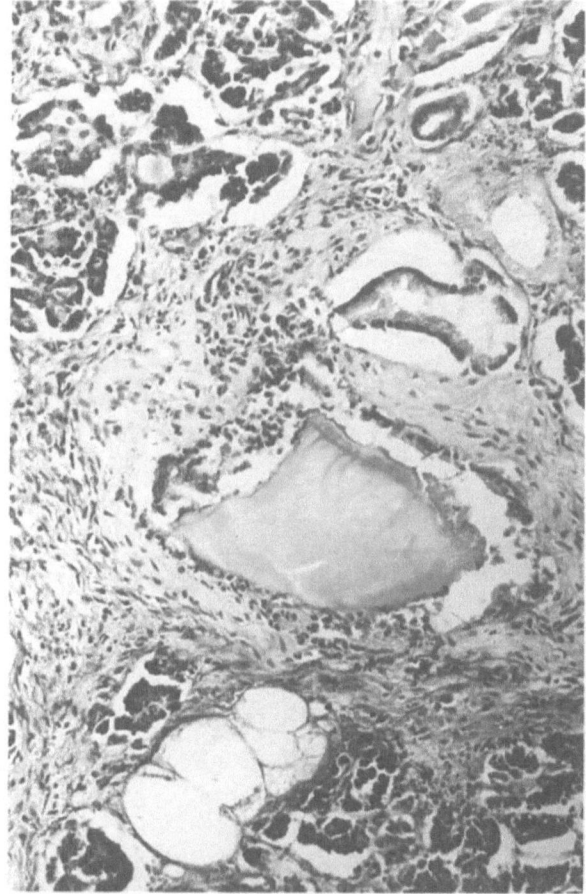

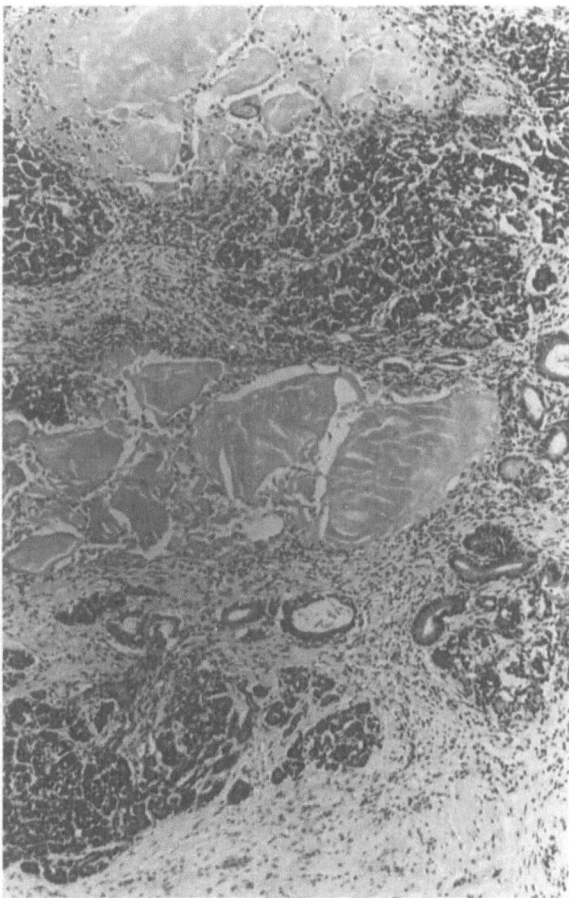

Fig. 13.3. A small duct is filled with hyaline secretion that was strongly eosinophilic. An epithelial lining remains in part of the wall of the duct, but, where the plug of secretion is still in contact with the wall, the lining epithelial cells have been replaced by chronic inflammatory cells. There is periductal fibrosis and oedema. The specimen was obtained from a man aged 68, who had been obliged to use a wheelchair because of old poliomyelitis. He died of bronchopneumonia, but an autopsy was ordered by the coroner because there was a long history of heavy drinking. H&E, × 150

Fig. 13.4. Hyaline secretion with a characteristically fragmented appearance. The walls of the duct within which the secretion has accumulated have disintegrated. The section is from the pancreas illustrated macroscopically in Fig. 13.2. H&E, × 60

pancreas; Ammann et al. (1973) noted that, when a pancreas affected by chronic alcoholic pancreatitis has lost all function, the originally severe pain may disappear. Their experience was that the average time necessary for this to happen was 6.6 years.

An analysis of the relationship between pain and recognisable lesions of the nerves in the pancreas was carried out by Bockman et al. (1988) in 18 patients with chronic alcoholic pancreatitis in whom duodenum-preserving resection of the head of the pancreas had been carried out for the relief of pain. They found that the mean diameter of the nerves in these patients was significantly greater than the diameter of the nerves in controls, and that the

mean area of tissue served per nerve was significantly less than in controls. Foci of inflammatory cells were prominent in some specimens, but it was only occasionally that such foci were associated with nerves or ganglia (Figs 13.10–13.12), and in such cases the invasion of the nerve tissue was not massive. Neural elements without inflammatory infiltration also existed. Ultrastructurally, however, there was evidence of oedema in the nerve bundles and the alterations seen in the perineural sheaths suggested that they no longer provided a barrier between the surrounding connective tissue and the internal neural components. The authors concluded that in chronic pancreatitis the nerves are retained

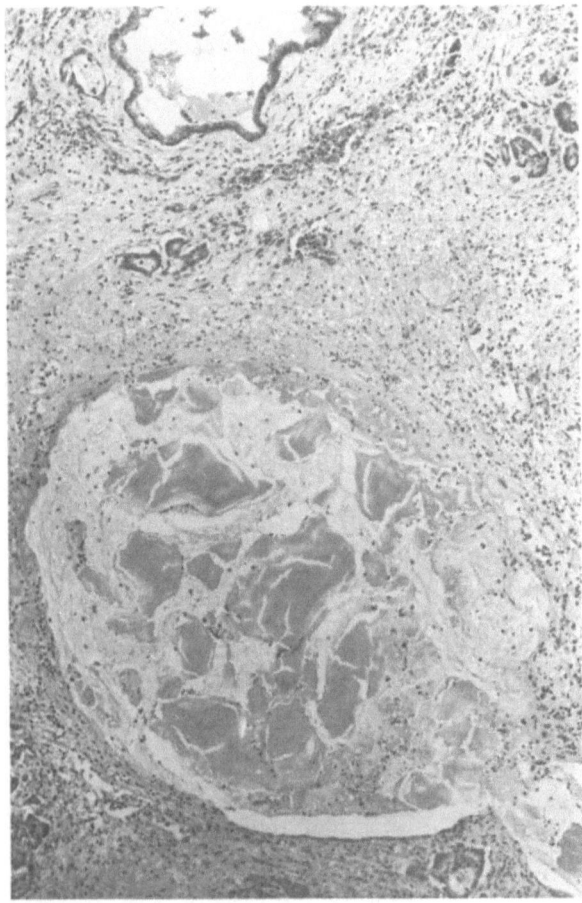

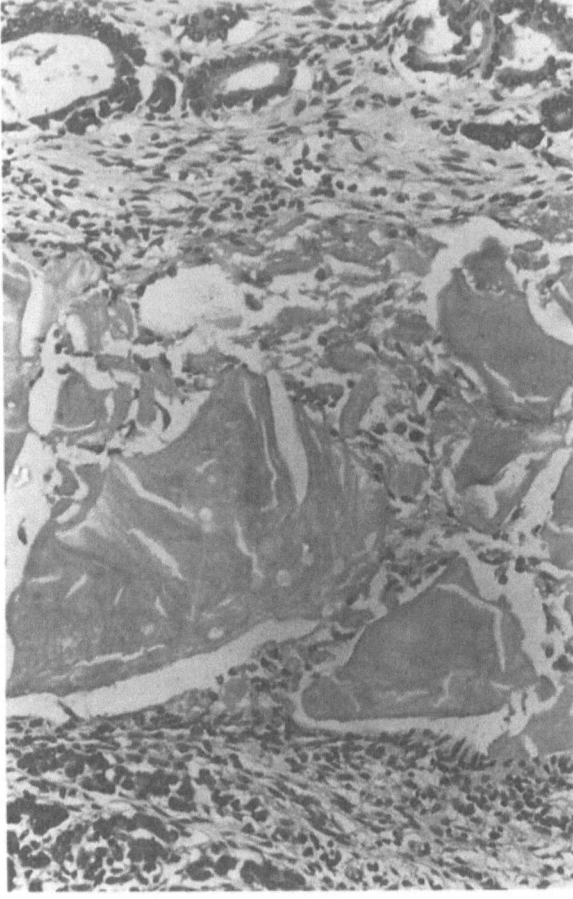

Fig. 13.5. Hyaline secretion, with crazy-paving-like clefts and fractures, within a duct whose wall has largely been replaced by inflammatory fibrous tissue. Adjacent glandular tissue is atrophic and fibrotic. (Courtesy of Dr A.R. Williams) H&E, × 60

Fig. 13.6. Secretion that was strongly eosinophilic, and in which there are clefts, appears to be undergoing organisation by fibrous tissue that has extended from the fibrous tissue that replaces the normal wall of the duct. The section is from the pancreas illustrated in Fig. 13.2. H&E, × 150

preferentially, while the pancreatic parenchyma undergoes degeneration and fibrous replacement. They felt that the increased diameter of the nerves in chronic pancreatitis argued against the pain of the disease being due to constriction of the nerves by fibrosis.

Nutritional (Tropical) Pancreatitis

Because the lesions of the pancreas associated with malnutrition tend to be found in tropical countries they are usually taken to be tropical diseases. However, lesions that seem to be identical to those found in Africa, South East Asia and Jamaica have been found in Europe during conditions of famine (Véghelyi et al. 1950).

Kwashiorkor

The pancreatic lesions of kwashiorkor, the syndrome of protein-calorie malnutrition in young children in tropical Africa, the West Indies and Thailand, are those that have been studied most thoroughly, and although, without treatment, there is eventual fibrous replacement of the organ, the basic lesion is atrophy of the glandular tissue with practically no histological signs of inflammation.

The essential pathology of kwashiorkor was described by Davies in 1948, and the results of further observations were published by Trowell et al. in their book about the disease in 1954. In kwashiorkor the most conspicuous abnormality at autopsy is severe fatty change in the liver, but Trowell and his colleagues came to the conclusion that atrophic

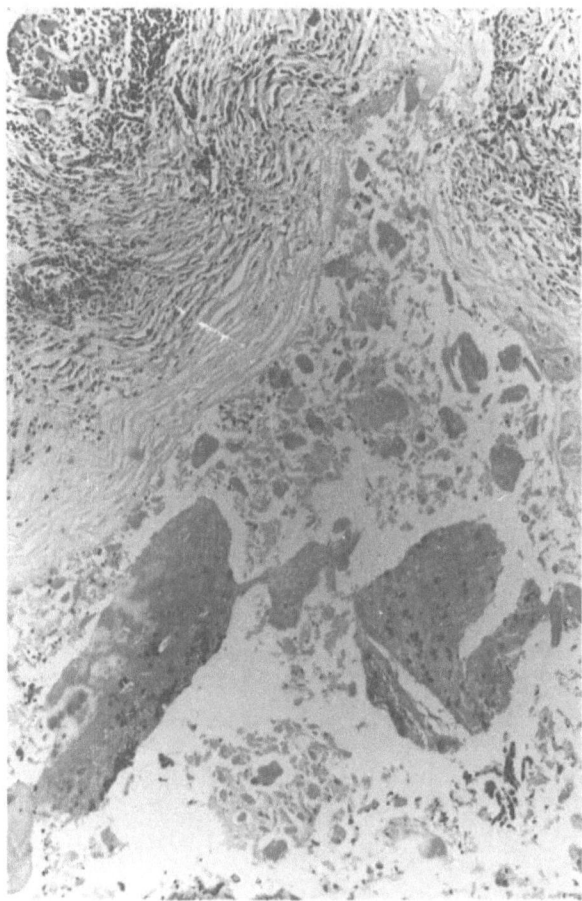
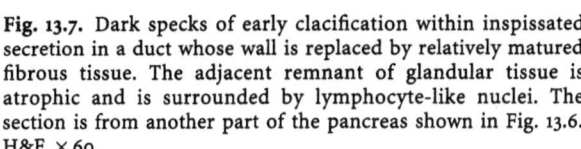
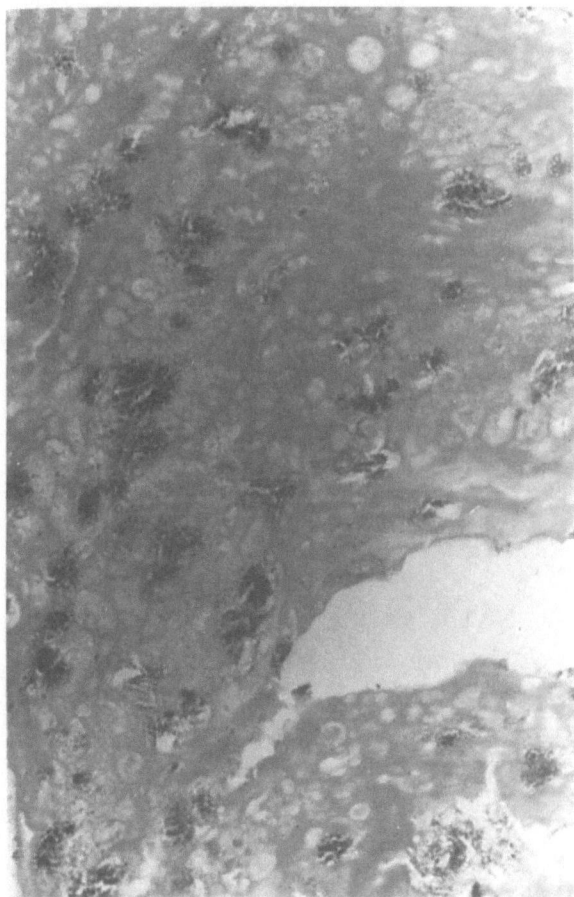

Fig. 13.7. Dark specks of early clacification within inspissated secretion in a duct whose wall is replaced by relatively matured fibrous tissue. The adjacent remnant of glandular tissue is atrophic and is surrounded by lymphocyte-like nuclei. The section is from another part of the pancreas shown in Fig. 13.6. H&E, × 60

Fig. 13.8. A higher magnification of the areas of calcification shown in Fig. 13.7. H&E, × 375

changes in the acinar cells of the pancreas are the most constant and persistent lesion in the disease. Similar, but less important, changes occur in all cells that normally produce large amounts of secretion, and probably, to some extent, in many other types of cell throughout the body. At autopsy, the pancreas is said to be small and to be affected relatively slowly by autolysis. A definite sclerosis that can be recognised by palpation is uncommon in children but is frequent in adults. Microscopically, the secreting cells of the acini are found to have shrunk and to have lost their secretory granules, the cells being reduced to little more than nuclei with a thin rim of surrounding cytoplasm. Some time after the atrophy of the acinar cells has become established, there is an increase in the amount of fibrous tissue in the pancreas, especially around the acinar cells. The increase is slow and irregular but, in older children, the fibrosis is diffuse and the acini may have disappeared from wide areas. In the earlier stages there may seem to have been hypertrophy and some hyperplasia of the islets, but later the islets tend to disappear. There are no important changes in the ducts in uncomplicated kwashiorkor. The process may be arrested and complete restoration of function can be obtained by appropriate dietary therapy with administration of protein (Barbezat and Hansen 1968), but a certain amount of fibrosis tends to persist despite clinical improvement (Trowell et al. 1954), and advanced atrophy and fibrosis may be irreversible.

An electron microscopic study of pancreatic changes in 14 children who had died in Thailand with untreated kwashiorkor was carried out by

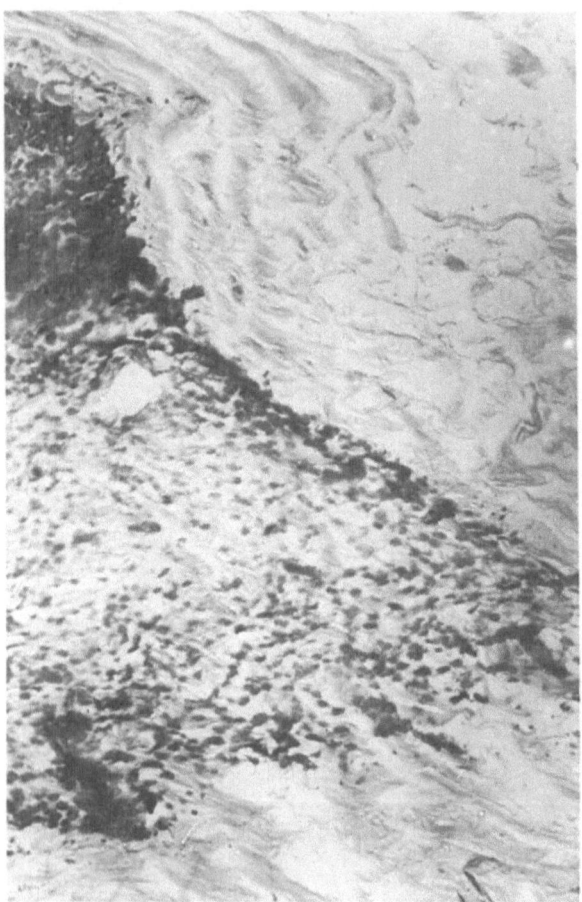

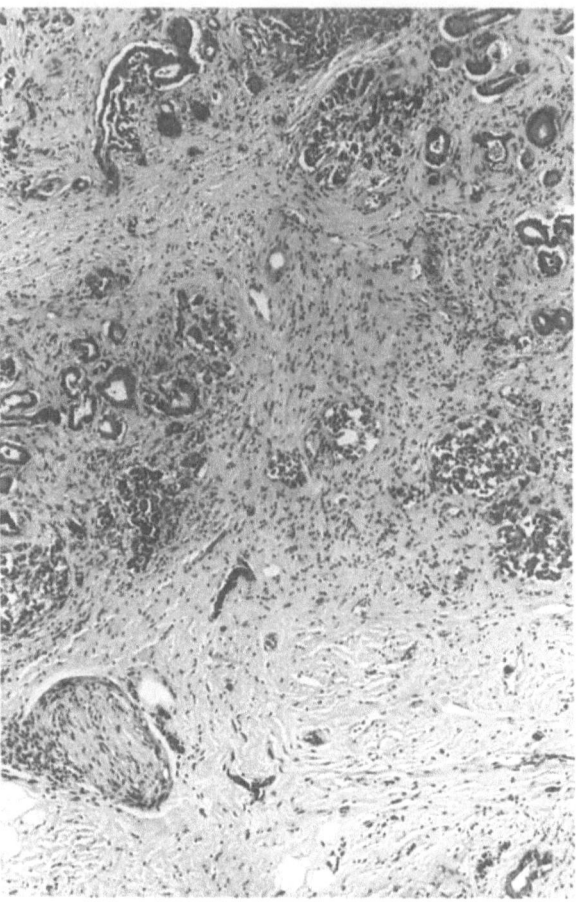

Fig. 13.9. Calcification in hyaline fibrous tissue in the pancreas illustrated macroscopically in Figs 13.30 and 13.31. H&E, × 150

Fig. 13.10. Dense fibrosis with acinar atrophy and partial destruction of islets. Destruction of ducts is less marked. A nerve is embedded in the fibrous tissue. A case of alcoholic pancreatitis. H&E, × 60

Blackburn and Vinijchaikul (1969). They described alterations in the organisation of the endoplasmic reticulum of the acinar cells, in which cytoplasmic matrix and segments of reticular membranes were sequestered within cisternal spaces. They interpreted this as the specific mechanism by which the cytoplasmic atrophy was produced.

Calcifying Pancreatitis in the Tropics

Radiological signs of calcification in the pancreas, usually in association with diabetes mellitus, were noted in Javanese adults by Zuidema (1959), who attributed the condition to malnutrition; a similar disease of adults was found to be relatively common in Uganda by Shaper (1960, 1964). In 1960, Shaper described the lesions of the pancreas in seven such

cases. All had various degrees of fibrosis, which in the earlier stages was perilobular and periductal, while in the more advanced stages, interacinar fibrosis had caused obliteration of the lobule, leaving only residual isolated areas of glandular tissue. Infiltration by fat was well marked in three. Signs of inflammation were trivial or absent. The islets of Langerhans were usually hard to find and those present were either hypertrophic or seemed hydropic or fibrotic. Calcification, which had been recognisable radiologically during life, was entirely within the ducts and several pancreases had eosinophilic material in the acini or larger ducts. Such changes are very reminiscent of those of the chronic calcifying pancreatitis of alcoholism and, in about half the 36 African patients in the group of cases published by Shaper in 1964, there was a history of episodic heavy drinking. Shaper thought that the course of the disease was similar to that of

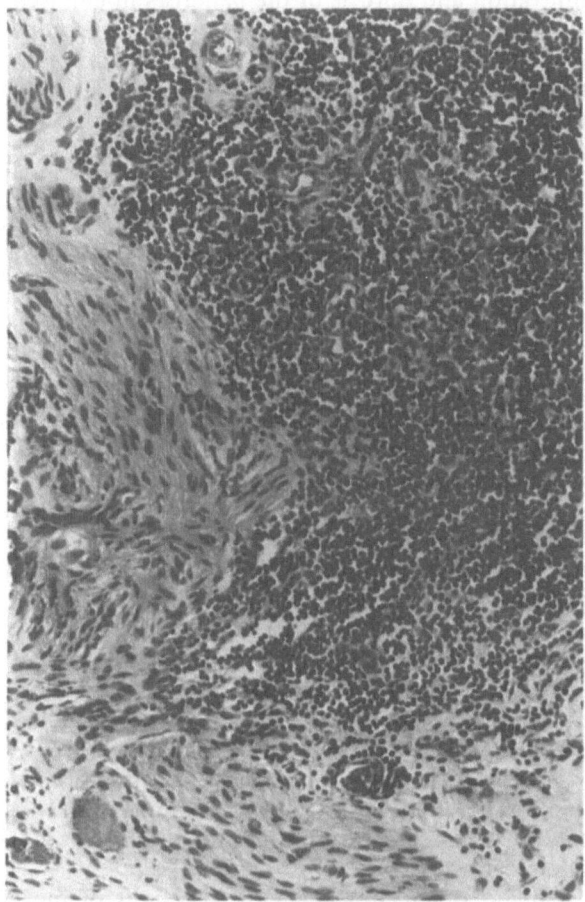

Fig. 13.11. A nerve cell and nerve fibres with an adjacent clump of lymphocytes in alcoholic pancreatitis. H&E, × 150

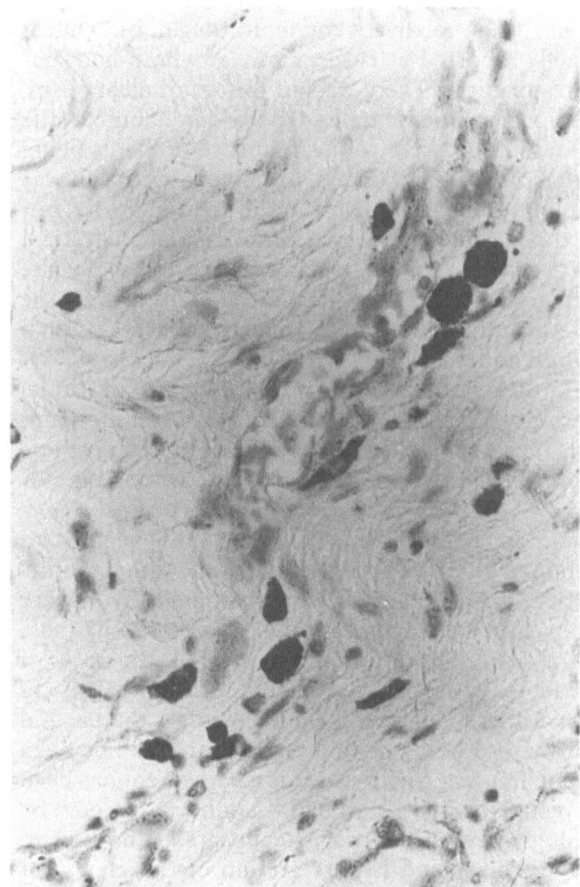

Fig. 13.12. Haemosiderin-filled phagocytes in dense fibrous tissue in the pancreas in alcoholic pancreatitis. Perls' stain, × 375

alcoholic pancreatitis in other countries, but he differentiated between episodes of heavy drinking and chronic alcoholism. He expressed the opinion that, as the disease occurred against a background of low protein–high carbohydrate nutrition, nutritional imbalance might make the pancreas particularly susceptible to the effects of alcohol, or other unknown factors, which might initiate progressive and irreversible pancreatic damage. He did not regard the disease as alcoholic pancreatitis and pointed out that Zuidema's (1959) Indonesian subjects with pancreatic calcification, all of whom had been living on diets that were very low in protein, had not taken alcohol at all.

Additional material for pathological study was obtained in Uganda by Banwell et al. (1967), in their study of the malabsorption syndrome that was common in that country. Pancreatic tissue was obtained at necropsy on eight of their subjects, and four pancreatic biopsies were also available.

Macroscopically, the gland was usually nodular. It felt hard, and calcareous nodules were often palpable, mainly in the head. In three, fat necrosis was recognisable and there was extensive fatty infiltration in two others, in one of which no acinar tissue could be identified with certainty. Two of the glands were smaller than normal. Microscopically, there was extensive fibrosis that was mainly interlobular, but was also intralobular and even interacinar. The acinar tissue was atrophic and disorganised, with loss of the lobular pattern. The atrophic acini occurred in isolated areas separated by fibrous tissue. Zymogen granules were rarely seen. The main pancreatic ducts and the ductules were frequently dilated and, in four specimens, laminated mucus was present within the ducts. In two cases this had begun to calcify. There was no metaplasia of the epithelium of the ducts. Lymphocytes and plasma cells infiltrated the fibrous tissue. There were haemosiderin deposits in one specimen.

In Western Nigeria, too, pancreatic calcification seems to be relatively common; Olurin and Olurin (1969) reported 45 cases, many of whom had diabetes mellitus. There was no history of alcoholism, and males and females were both liable to the disease. Most were young adults, 30 of the 45 being either 20 years old or less. Protein malnutrition was thought to be responsible in the great majority, but in three, calcified ova of *Schistosoma haematobium* were present in the pancreas as well as in the urinary tract; in one, ova were present also in the liver, pulmonary blood vessels and abdominal lymph nodes.

In the state of Kerala in the south of India, chronic calcifying pancreatitis is very common and was found in 5.47% of autopsy cases by Geevarghese (1968). This state was created in 1956 with the intention of uniting groups of people who spoke a common language, but, up to 1988, these people had retained their various religious and other habits (Miller 1988). In general, however, their diet is very poor in protein and most of Geevarghese's patients were total abstainers from alcohol. In 16% of patients with chronic calcifying pancreatitis in India, there is bilateral enlargement of the parotid salivary glands, but this association has not been noted in other countries. This enlargement has been investigated by Alapatt and Ananthachari (1967) by sialography and biopsy; it appears to be due to hypertrophy and hypersecretion of the glandular tissue.

It has been suggested by Pitchumoni and Thomas (1973) that protein malnutrition alone may not be responsible for the high incidence of pancreatic calcification with diabetes mellitus in the state of Kerala. Cassava and the tapioca derived from it are important in the diet of the people of this state, and Pitchumoni and Thomas suspect that the removal of the toxic juice of the cassava may sometimes be incomplete, as shortage of fuel may lead to reduction of the prolonged boiling necessary to destroy the toxins. Thus, traces of the cyanogenic glucosides may remain to injure pancreases that have been made vulnerable by protein malnutrition. Cassava pancreatitis is now becoming recognised in Western Europe in patients that have migrated from cassava-consuming areas (Assan et al. 1984).

The effects upon the pancreas that have been induced in animals by diets deficient in trace elements such as zinc, selenium and copper have not been recognised as being of importance in human disease.

Deficiency of vitamins seems also to be of little importance in relation to pancreatic disease in man, but Pitchumoni et al. (1986) refer to a report of fatty infiltration and fibrosis of the pancreas in children who had died of pellagra. Cystic spaces, squamous epithelial metaplasia with keratinisation, and polymorphonuclear leucocytic infiltration were all marked in the pancreas of the baby with vitamin A deficiency reported by Wilson and Du Bois in 1923.

Chronic Obstructive Pancreatitis

Obstruction of the pancreatic ducts has long been recognised to be important as a cause of chronic pancreatitis and Opie (1902, 1910) described the effects of the obstruction as leading to chronic interstitial pancreatitis of the interlobular type, as distinct from the interacinar type that he found in association with cirrhosis of the liver, arteriosclerosis and haemochromatosis. He stated that in interlobular chronic interstitial pancreatitis the process exaggerated the lobulation of the gland, which was normally obscure, and that wide bands of sclerotic tissue could be seen with the naked eye to separate groups of lobules. The gland was hard and dense, with a nodular or granular surface. One of his illustrations shows pancreatic tissue in which acinar tissue has been largely replaced by fibrous tissue. Islets, however, are conspicuous in the fibrous tissue. The one duct in the illustration is lined by columnar mucus-secreting epithelium and is not conspicuously dilated.

Opie's conclusions seem, in the light of more recent studies, to be an oversimplification, and it is now recognised that stenosis of ducts within the gland may develop during chronic pancreatitis, as has been described in chronic calcifying pancreatitis, with important secondary effects in the further progress of the lesions. In obstruction of the main duct, too, episodes of more or less acute inflammation are liable to occur and to leave signs of damage, while in long-standing chronic or chronic relapsing pancreatitis, calculi may form within large ducts and add their obstructive effects to the subsequent progress of the disease. Within Opie's lifetime the preservation of the islets he had noted was exploited by Banting and Best (1921–1922) in the experiments that led to the discovery of insulin, but, in more recent animal experiments by Yeo et al. (1989), it has been shown that, in chronic pancreatitis induced by obstruction of the pancreatic duct, there is deficiency of circulating insulin and intolerance of glucose at a stage when the islets are histologically and ultrastructurally intact.

In the studies in which the effects of chronic obstruction of the main duct by a small carcinoma were compared with those of alcoholic chronic cal-

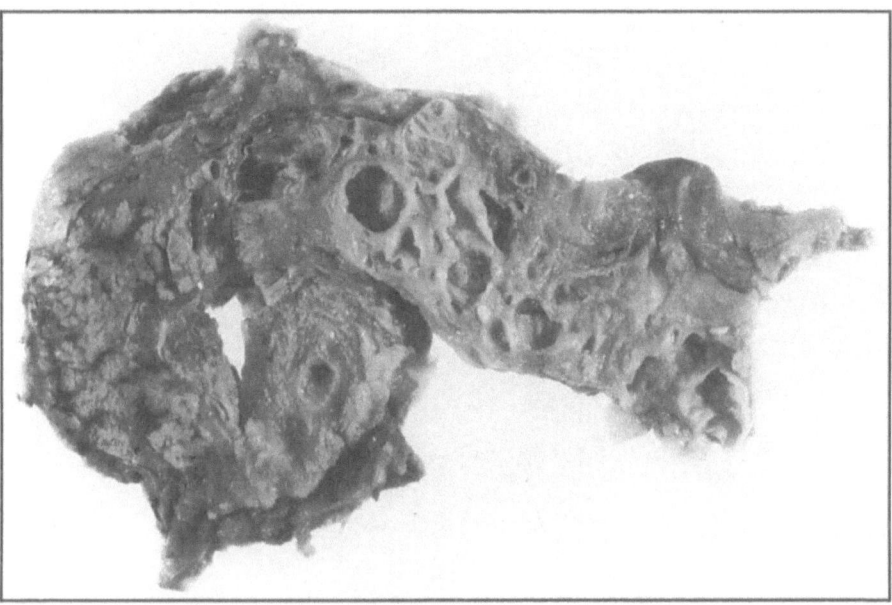

Fig. 13.13. Chronic obstructive pancreatitis associated with a diverticulum of the second part of the duodenum near the duodenal papilla. Dilatation of the ducts is most marked in the body and tail of the pancreas.

cifying pancreatitis by Nakamura et al. (1972), the uniformity of the effects throughout the pancreas, especially the dilatation of the whole system of ducts, has been emphasised by these authors. They found that such uniformity contrasted with the focal nature of the areas of damage in the case of alcoholic pancreatitis.

The most common cause of obstruction of the main pancreatic duct is carcinoma, either of the head of the pancreas, or of the duodenal papilla or ampulla of Vater. Such obstruction is liable to be associated with pancreatitis and, as judged by microscopic examination of material, significant pancreatitis was present in 26 of 255 patients with pancreatic or ampullay carcinoma (Gambill 1971), while clinical evidence of pancreatitis had been present in 31% of these cases.

Other causes of obstruction of the major pancreatic ducts include the condition of pancreas divisum that is discussed on pp. 30–31, 294. Lambert et al. (1987) recorded three cases of pancreas divisum as the cause of chronic obstructive pancreatitis in a series of 14 patients with chronic pancreatitis who they treated by pancreatectomy. Their series also included one in which chronic obstructive pancreatitis had been caused by a choledochal cyst.

A diverticulum of the second part of the duodenum, though often without clinical effect, may, as has been pointed out by Ogilvie (1940–1941), obstruct the pancreatic duct, with or without

obstruction also of the common bile duct. In the pancreas, the result is dilatation of the pancreatic duct system, with gradual atrophy of the pancreatic parenchyma and fibrous replacement of the acini, but with relative preservation of the islets. Signs of inflammation consist mainly of clumps of lymphocytes and more diffuse scattered lymphocyte-like nuclei throughout the fibrous tissue. This, combined with dilatation of the duct, is illustrated in Fig. 13.13. The macroscopically obvious dilatation of the main ducts in this case is illustrated in Fig. 13.14; the microscopic appearance is shown in Fig. 13.15.

The importance of calculi in the main pancreatic duct as a cause of obstructive pancreatitis is less clear, for clinical evidence of chronic or recurring pancreatitis is often present for months or years before calculi can be recognised radiologically. Calculi are said (Rohrmann et al. 1981) to be particularly characteristic of hereditary pancreatitis, but their effect upon the progress of the disease is not clear, although it seems likely that the effects of obstruction by the calculi will be added to the poorly understood pathology of hereditary pancreatitis.

In communities in which ascariasis is common and in animals, especially cats (Appleby 1981), chronic pancreatitis may be associated with obstruction of the pancreatic duct by parasites. A fluke, *Eurytrema procyonis*, seems to have a special affinity of the pancreatic ducts; it has not been found in the biliary ducts. The adult fluke was first

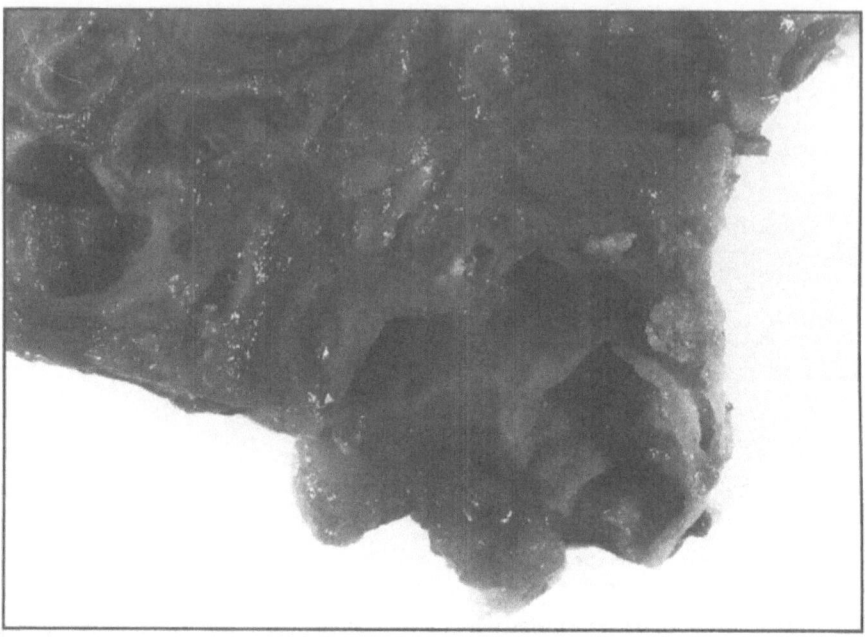

Fig. 13.14. A slightly magnified view of the dilated ducts near the tail of the pancreas shown in Fig. 13.13. Gritty white calcified material is attached to the walls of some of the ducts.

recognised in the pancreatic ducts of racoons, but it has since been identified in 10.7% of a sample of 290 domestic cats from around St Louis, MO. It causes ductal obstruction and chronic pancreatitis, with fibrosis and atrophy of the gland (Fox et al. 1981), but does not cause clinical evidence of pancreatic failure.

Metabolic Chronic Pancreatitis

According to the definitions of acute and chronic pancreatitis agreed at Marseilles in 1984 (Gyr et al. 1984), the attacks of pancreatitis that may complicate certain abnormalities of metabolism should be classified as episodes of acute pancreatitis, but, if the abnormality of metabolism remains uncorrected, repeated attacks over many years will cause a pancreas with pathological features of those of chronic pancreatitis.

Hyperlipidaemic Pancreatitis

The episodes of pancreatitis that are liable to occur in people with familial hyperlipidaemia and hyperlipoproteinaemia can be prevented by the control of blood lipids. Information about the pathology of the pancreas in such cases is not available.

Hypercalcaemic Chronic Pancreatitis

The role of hypercalcaemia as a cause of acute pancreatitis has been discussed in Chap. 12. Patients in which pancreatic calcification has coincided with hyperparathyroidism are rare, but parenchymal pancreatic calcification has been reported by Smith and Cooke (1940), while calculi were reported in association with hyperparathyroidism by Martin and Canseco (1947) and Rogers et al. (1947).

Chronic Renal Failure

This too is occasionally associated with chronic pancreatitis, and an example of chronic calcifying pancreatitis in a case of long-standing renal failure is illustrated in Fig. 13.16; the parathyroid glands were not recognised to be enlarged. Two occurrences of chronic pancreatitis in association with chronic renal failure are included among the pre-existing conditions tabulated by Di Magno and Clain (1986) in their review of chronic pancreatitis.

Hereditary Chronic Pancreatitis

The acute pancreatitis that is now well recognised to occur in certain families has been discussed in

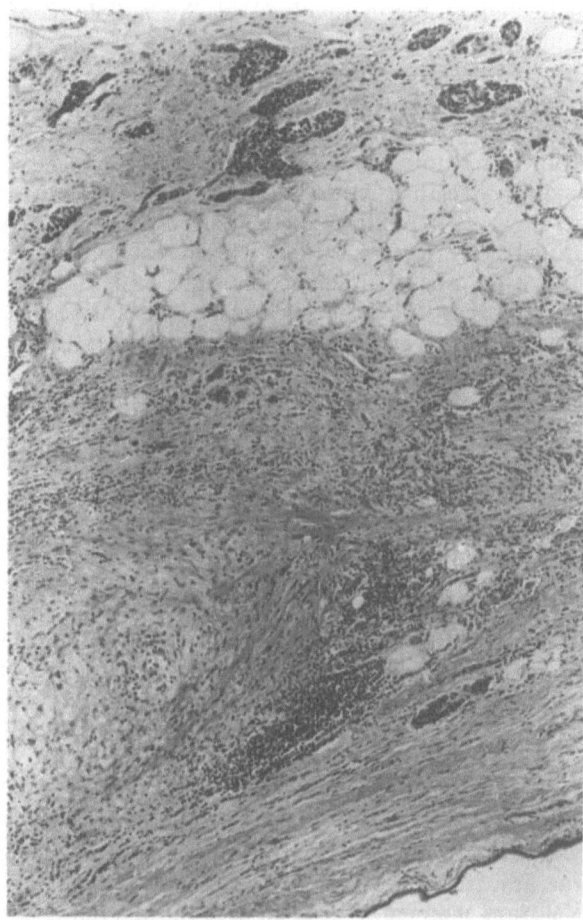

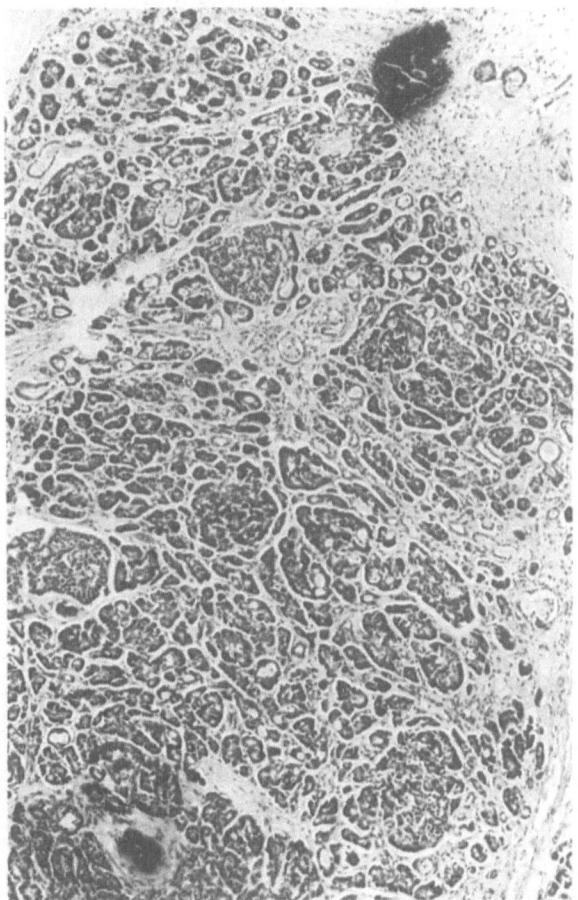

Fig. 13.15. The microscopic appearance of the pancreas illustrated macroscopically in Figs 13.13 and 13.14. Exocrine glandular tissue has disappeared from the vicinity of the dilated duct and has been replaced by fibrous tissue infiltrated by lymphocytes. Islets, however have survived and are embedded in fibrous tissue. H&E, × 60

Fig. 13.16. Calculi within small ducts with interlobular and intralobular fibrosis in the pancreas of a non-alcoholic woman who died of chronic uraemia due to congenital cystic disease of the kidneys. The dilatation of the acini in this section is a feature that is commonly present in the pancreas after death in uraemia. H&E, × 60

Chap. 12. In such families, the attacks tend to begin during childhood, but Sarles has noted familial aggregations of two or three non-alcoholic subjects, in whom symptoms began at an age similar to that at which chronic calcifying pancreatitis becomes recognisable. Sarles also refers to studies, carried out by Chevallier et al. (1982), of the blood groups and HLA antigens in members of two kindreds in whom various members, in different generations, suffered from chronic non-alcoholic pancreatitis. The results led Chevallier et al. to conclude that HLA antigens are not linked with a predisposition to chronic pancreatitis.

In the pancreases from other cases of hereditary pancreatitis that became available for pathological examination the picture was that of a very chronic process, for the disease had usually been present for many years before surgery or necropsy was carried out. The glands were hard and shrunken and there were calculi in the ducts. Microscopically the acinar tissue was almost unrecognisable in a background of fibrous tissue while apparently normal islets were easily seen. These appearances have been illustrated by Kattwinkel et al. (1973). There is nothing in such appearances that is characteristic of the hereditary type of chronic pancreatitis as distinct from other types. In hereditary pancreatitis there can be little doubt that, although individual attacks may heal, the cumulative effects of repeated attacks result in the pathological findings that have been described above. Moreover, the risk of malignancy in the damaged pancreas is high; according to Barkin and Fayne (1986), there is a thirty-fold increase in the incidence of pancreatic carcinoma.

Chronic Pancreatitis Associated with Congenital Abnormalities of the Pancreas

Pancreas Divisum

The repeated attacks of pancreatitis that may be associated with the ductal abnormality of pancreas divisum have been discussed in Chap. 3. Repeated acute attacks may lead eventually to a chronic obstructive pancreatitis. In a series of 14 patients on whom total pancreatectomy with preservation of the duodenum was carried out by Lambert et al. (1987), the cause of the chronic pancreatitis was attributed to pancreas divisum in three, and to another type of ductal abnormality in a fourth. In a larger series of 58 pancreatic resections for chronic pancreatitis, Lowes et al. (1988) found that in eight in which the disease was attributed to obstruction there were two cases of pancreas divisum.

Annular Pancreas

When a previously asymptomatic annular pancreas causes duodenal obstruction in an adult, the cause usually turns out to be inflammation in the abnormal pancreas (Lloyd-Jones et al. 1972). This is borne out in more recent case reports, such as those of Glinsky et al. (1987) and of Rode et al. (1988). In the patient described by Glinsky and his colleagues, however, chronic renal failure due to diabetic nephropathy was also present, the patient having been diabetic since childhood. As was mentioned earlier (p. 292), chronic pancreatitis has occasionally been associated with chronic renal failure, although the significance, if any, of the association is unknown.

Congenitally Short Pancreas

Calcifying chronic pancreatitis in a gland in which only the head region could be identified by ultrasonography and computerised tomography has been described by Bretagne et al. (1987). The authors attributed the pancreatic malformation to partial agenesis.

Auto-immune Chronic Pancreatitis

Immunological factors, especially those that might induce a Schwartzman-type of reaction, have been studied in relation to the aetiology of acute haemorrhagic pancreatitis; thus, it is not surprising that abnormalities of the immune responses have been suspected of being involved in the aetiology of otherwise idiopathic chronic pancreatitis.

In 1960, it was shown by Witebsky et al. that it was possible to induce the formation of pancreas-specific antibodies in rabbits, but, when the sera of rabbits immunised with pooled rabbit pancreas incorporated into Freund adjuvants were tested in vitro against an extract of the antibody-producing animal's own pancreas, there was no reaction, while in vivo no gross or microscopic signs of damage to the pancreas could be produced. The antibodies were regarded as isoantibodies rather than auto-antibodies (Rose et al. 1960).

In the same year, Murray and Thal showed that the sera from most patients with chronic pancreatic disease, or carcinoma of the pancreas, contained antibodies that were specific for the human pancreas. Some of the control sera from patients with other diseases, especially diabetes mellitus, gave occasionally positive reactions. The antibodies were usually isoantibodies but the authors believed that auto-antibodies might sometimes occur and might, in time, lead to chronic pancreatits.

In Sjögren's syndrome, a failure of function of various glands is associated with immunological abnormalities. In 1973 Whaley et al. published a study of the clinical and immunological aspects of a series of cases of Sjögren's syndrome that included two patients in whom chronic pancreatic disease was associated with the syndrome. A little later, Waldram et al. (1975) gave an account of a new syndrome affecting a sister and brother. The components of the syndrome were chronic pancreatitis, sclerosing cholangitis and the Sjögren type of sicca complex. In these patients, the serum immunoglobulins were normal and auto-antibodies were absent, a result in keeping with the finding by Lendrum and Walker (1975) that pancreatic antibody, as detected by the immunofluorescent technique, was usually absent in chronic pancreatitis. Nevertheless, Waldram et al. expressed the opinion that immune mechanisms might be involved, because they found that in both patients there was leucocyte migration inhibition in the presence of an antigen prepared from bile duct epithelium. Further immunological studies by Ludwig et al. (1977) demonstrated that in four of 12 patients with Sjögren's syndrome, and in eight of 31 patients with rheumatoid arthritis, there was antibody that produced diffuse fluorescence of intralobular and interlobular pancreatic duct cells. These workers considered that their demonstration of antibodies to pancreatic duct cells pointed to the involvement of auto-immune mechanisms in the pathogenesis of the subclinical exocrine insufficiency of the pancreas that may exist in Sjögren's syndrome and rheumatoid arthritis.

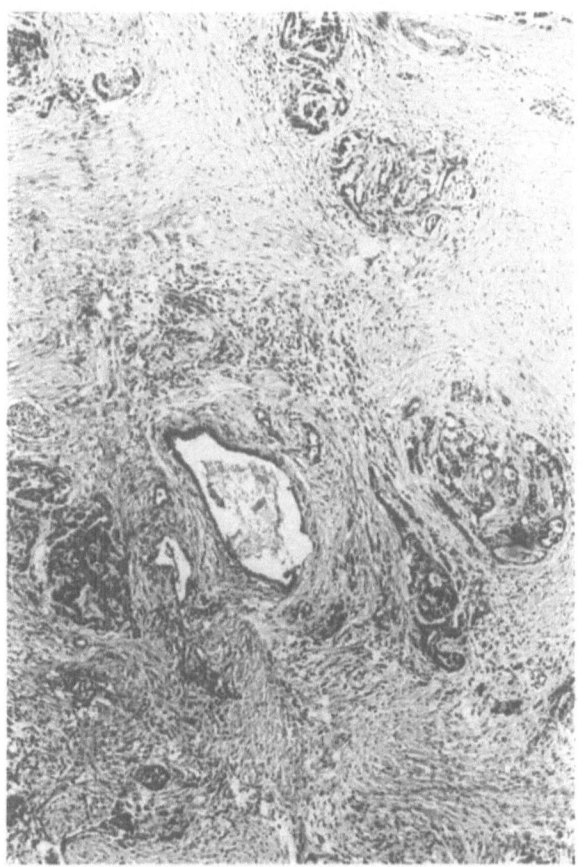

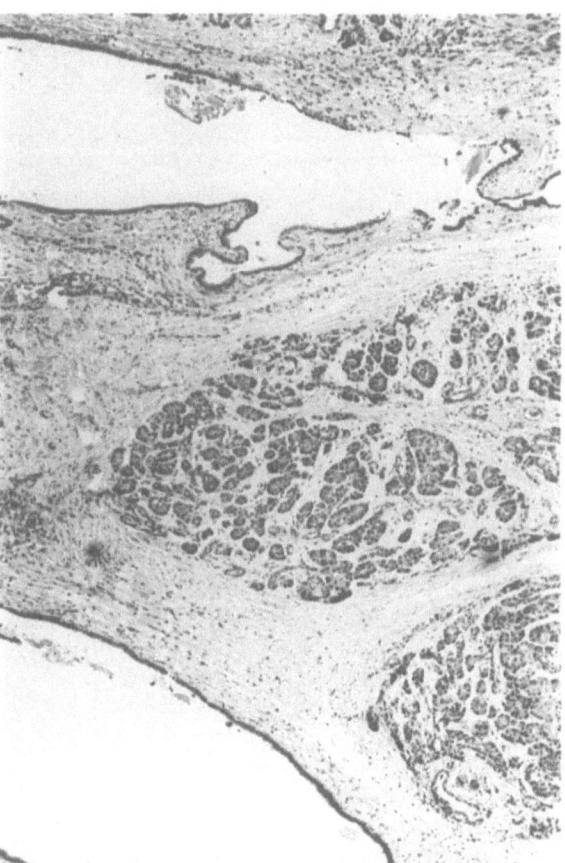

Fig. 13.17. Idiopathic chronic relapsing pancreatitis. Cellular fibrous tissue has replaced much of the parenchyma, but distorted acinar tissue is recognisable. A moderately dilated duct contains a little pale-staining non-laminated secretion. H&E, × 60

Fig. 13.18. Idiopathic chronic relapsing pancreatitis. The disease had been present for 5 years. Dilated ducts that contain little secretion are lined by low atrophic epithelial cells and there is periductal, perilobular and intralobular fibrosis. This is a different area of the pancreas shown in Fig. 13.17. H&E, × 60

In primary biliary cirrhosis, a disease in which a high titre of non-organ-specific mitochondrial antibody is nearly always present, observations by Epstein et al. (1980) indicate that pancreatic secretion is reduced, while Fonseca et al. (1986) have shown that the majority of patients in a group of 33 with primary biliary cirrhosis had raised serum levels of immunoreactive trypsin and pancreatic lipase, a finding the authors took to indicate that damage to the exocrine pancreas was present. In 1992, Jalleh et al. reported that there was aberrant expression of the major histocompatibility complexes in ductular and ductal epithelial cells, together with T-cell infiltration in the pancreases in a series of patients with chronic pancreatitis of varying aetiologies and of differing ages. The authors interpreted these findings as immunohisto-chemical evidence that a component of auto-immunity was present in all these patients, in spite of the differing aetiologies.

Idiopathic Chronic Pancreatitis

In certain cases of chronic pancreatitis, none of the recognised aetiological factors may be present, and yet repeated episodes of severe and incapacitating pancreatitis may occur. Figs 13.17–13.21 illustrate the microscopic lesions of the pancreas in such a situation. The patient was a professional soldier who was 26 years old at the time of his death; he was not addicted to alcohol. During 1964 and 1965, while serving in Germany, he had repeated attacks of pancreatitis, during one of which he had undergone laparotomy, with a subsequent operation for the repair of an incisional hernia. After eight or ten attacks of pancreatitis, he was discharged from the army. In July 1966, cholecystectomy, with exploration of the common bile duct and sphincterotomy, were carried out in a civilian hospital, but the attacks of pain continued. In April 1967, partial pan-

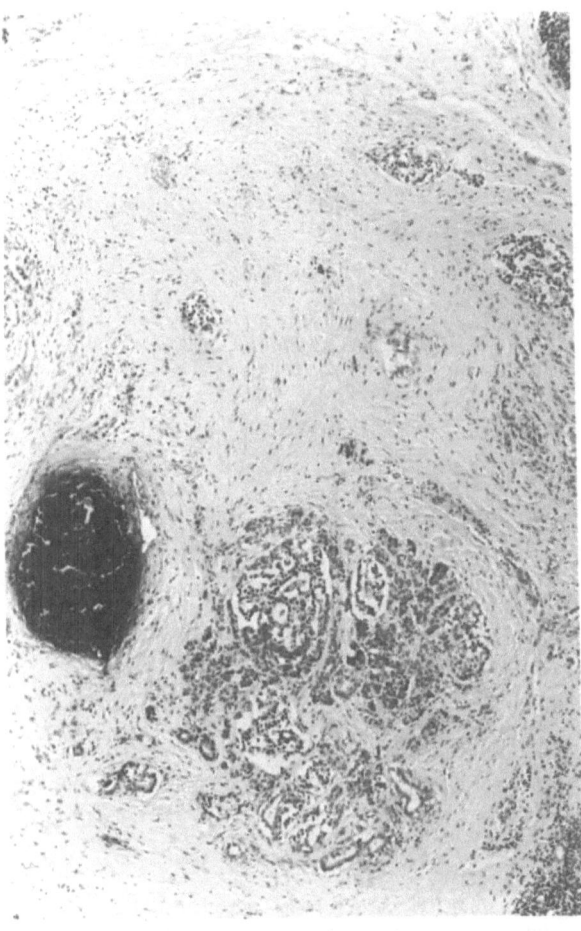

Fig. 13.19. Another part of the pancreas illustrated in Figs 13.17 and 13.18. A small duct, without a recognisable epithelial lining, contains calcified materials, and there is marked interlobular fibrous tissue in which there are clumps of lymphocytes with atrophic islets. The glandular lobule is atrophic and there is intralobular fibrosis. H&E, × 60

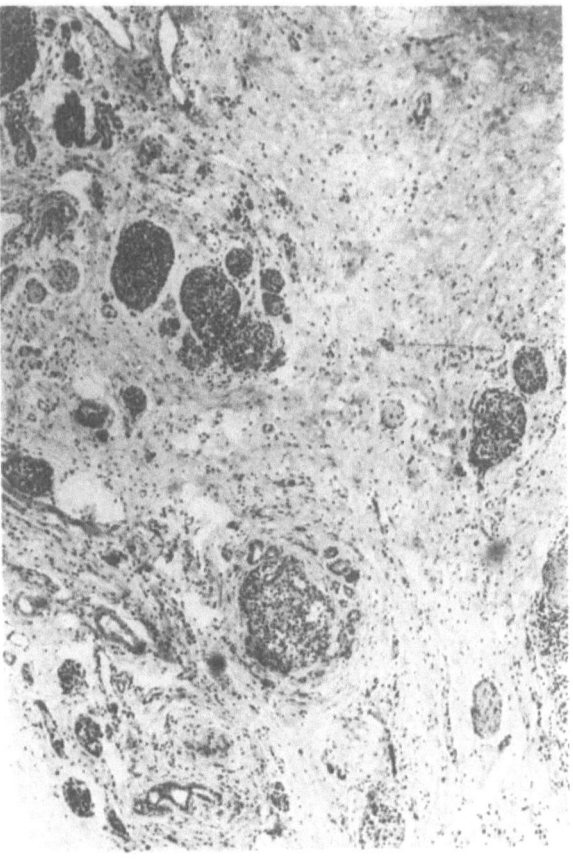

Fig. 13.20. The same pancreas as in Fig. 13.19. In this area, disappearance of the exocrine tissue is almost complete, but groups of islets remain in the fibrous tissue that has replaced the exocrine glandular tissue. H&E, × 60

createctomy with removal of the spleen was carried out with no effect, and in February 1969 subtotal pancreatectomy was undertaken. The operation was complicated by uncontrollable bleeding that led to the patient's death.

In the surgically removed pancreatic tissue, and in the pancreatic remnants found attached to the duodenum at the autopsy, there was extensive interlobular fibrosis, with disappearance of much of the acinar tissue, and interacinar fibrosis; dilatation of ducts was well marked in some places, while in others the ducts contained microscopic concretions. Some slightly dilated ducts contained mucoid secretion, but inspissated eosinophilic secretion within the ducts was not seen. Clumps of lymphocytes were numerous throughout the fibrous tissue and around

nerves. The fibrous tissue contained foci of necrotic fat cells, but no giant cells were found and there were no cholesterol clefts. Islets of Langerhans were conspicuous in parts of the fibrous background from which acinar tissue had disappeared completely.

Pancreatic Calculi and Pancreatic Calcification

At one time pancreatic calculi were believed to be rare (Mayo 1936), but, by 1939, Haggard and Kirtley

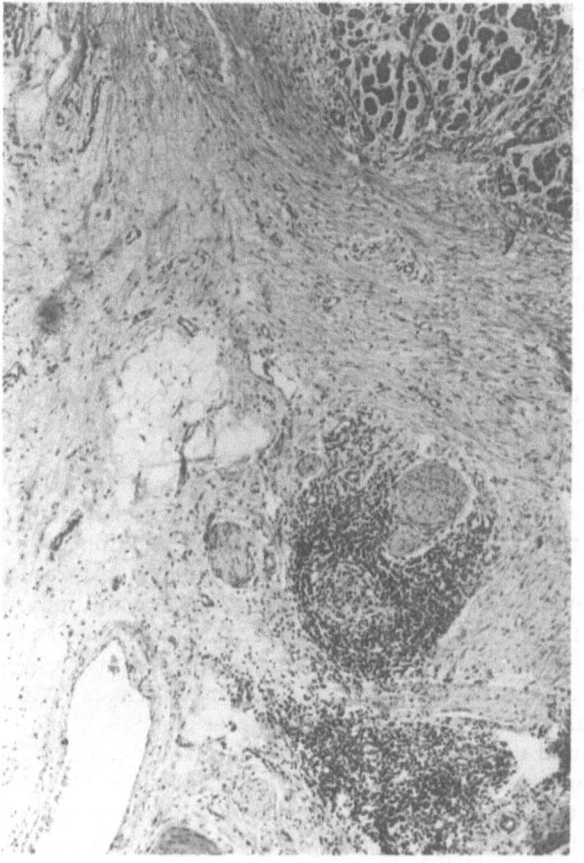

Fig. 13.21. The same pancreas as in Figs 13.17–13.20. There is inter-lobular fibrosis with perineural clumps of lymphocytes and some fat spaces in the fibrous tissue. H&E, × 60

by the elastic van Gieson method they found coarse elastic fibres in the walls of the cavities that had contained stones. The elastic fibres around the stones were similar to those in the walls of the ducts; the authors concluded that the stones had originally been within ducts, where their mechanical effects had caused denudation of the lining of the ducts, and such severe destruction of their walls, that they became unrecognisable except for the remnants of elastic tissue. In all their cases of apparent parenchymal calcification they interpreted the appearances as indicating that the calcified material had originated within ducts.

Parenchymal Calcification

In spite of the conclusion reached by Stobbe et al., as has just been mentioned, it is sometimes difficult to recognise the ductal origin of calcification material, as is illustrated in Fig. 13.9. The results of X-ray crystallographic studies quoted by Baggenstoss (1973) suggest that areas of fat necrosis may undergo calcification by deposition of hydroxyapatite, a phosphate of calcium to which calcium carbonate groups are bonded, whereas intraduct calculi contain calcium carbonate only. Calcification that has not originated within ducts may also occur occasionally in exocrine, or endocrine (Fig. 13.22) neoplasms of the pancreas and in the walls of parasitic cysts within the pancreas.

Composition of Ductal Calculi

Ductal calculi consist mainly of calcium carbonate, which accounts for over 95% of their weight. Their most interesting component, however, is a protein that has become known as stone protein, which received its name because it was first found within pancreatic calculi. It is now known to be one of the normal constituents of pancreatic juice and its function is believed to be to prevent the formation of stones within the pancreatic ducts. The normal amount of stone protein in pure pancreatic juice collected by cannulation of the pancreatic duct has been established, and it has been found that, when the secretion of stone protein is subnormal, calculi are liable to form. When stone protein is completely absent from the pancreatic juice, unusually large stones have been formed (Sarles et al. 1982). It seems that it is only when deficiency of stone protein has allowed calcium carbonate crystals (calcite) to be deposited on the epithelium of the pancreatic ducts that small amounts of stone protein become incorporated into the calculi. Stone

were able to review 65 patients in whom operations had been carried out for pancreatic stones, and could refer to 139 others, some reported in the seventeenth and eighteenth centuries, who had not been treated by operation.

True Calculi Within Ducts

In the past, calcification within the pancreas was usually differentiated into two types: true stones within the ducts, and false stones due to foci of calcification in areas of pancreatic parenchyma damaged by pancreatitis (Haggard and Kirtley 1939; Comfort et al. 1946; Wirts and Snape 1947). More recent work, however, led Stobbe et al. (1970) to the conclusion that pancreatic lithiases always represent calculi that have originated within the ducts. The latter authors based their conclusion upon studies of 43 cases of pancreatic lithiasis, collected from 27 787 autopsies. When they stained their material

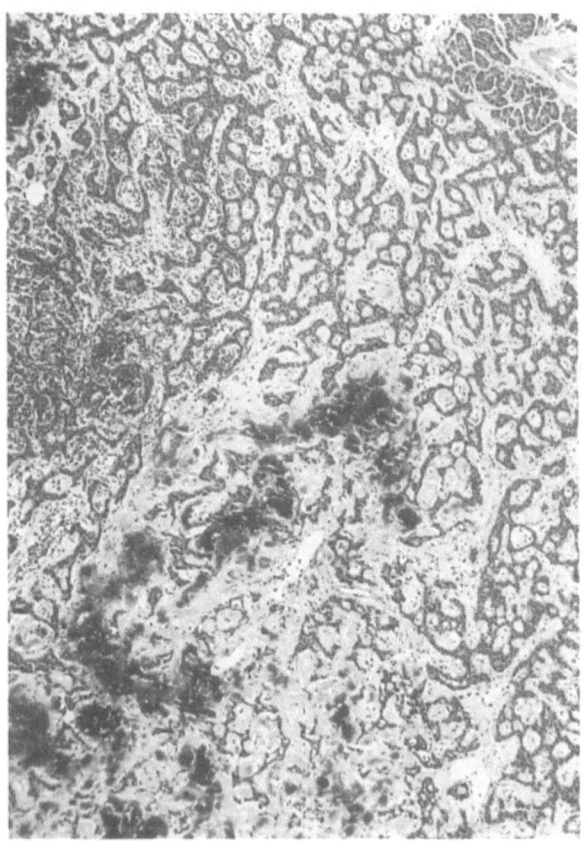

Fig. 13.22. Some of the numerous foci of calcification that were present in a insulin-secreting adenoma of islet cells that had caused hypoglycaemic attacks in a man aged 49 for a year before the tumour was removed. H&E, × 60

protein accounts for only 0.15% of the weight of the stone.

The work on the nature and effects of stone protein by Sarles and his associates, along with the work of others, has been the subject of a number of reviews by Sarles, for example, those in 1984 and 1986. Such work has shown that, in vitro, in conditions that simulate those of pancreatic juice, calcium carbonate, which is normally in a super-saturated solution in pancreatic juice, will be precipitated. The addition of stone protein, however, will prevent the precipitation. In relation to chronic calcifying pancreatitis, Sarles has pointed out that many alcoholics do not develop chronic pancreatitis. Such people have been shown to secrete normal amounts of stone protein, while the alcoholics in whom chronic calcifying pancreatitis has developed secrete stone protein subnormally. He has speculated also that the 5%–7% of patients with hypercalcaemia who develop pancreatitis do so because they secrete less stone protein than the great majority of hypercalcaemic

patients who do not develop pancreatitis. Likewise, in familial pancreatitis and in tropical pancreatitis, it may be that those in the kindred, or those in the community, who develop the disease are those who secrete insufficient stone protein to protect them from calculi. Deficient secretion of stone protein might even be responsible for some of the cases of idiopathic chronic calcifying pancreatitis. The secretion of stone protein has been found to be normal in patients with pancreatic disease other than chronic calcifying pancreatitis.

Stone protein is a glycoprotein, but its carbohydrate component has yet to be determined; it has a molecular weight of 13 500. Its amino acid composition is unusual, with 33 aspartate and 20 glutamate residues. There is no methionine, but there are three phosphorylated residues: two phosphoserines and one phosphothreonine. It has no known enzymatic activity and no immunological cross-reaction with the pancreatic enzymes. It can be detected in the blood by an assay that uses a monoclonal antibody. The level in the blood rises in acute or chronic pancreatitis (Schmiegel et al. 1986). The sequence of secretory pancreatic stone protein messenger RNA has been established by Giorge et al. (1989), who found that its level in those with chronic calcifying pancreatitis was only one-third of that in controls, whereas the levels of trypsinogen, chymotrypsinogen and colipase messenger RNA were not altered. They concluded that secretory stone protein gene expression was specifically reduced in patients with chronic calcifying pancreatitis.

The Development of Calculi

Nakamura et al. (1972) traced the evolution of precipitates of protein within ducts into calculi and demonstrated the damaging effects of the plugging of the ducts upon the unrelated pancreatic parenchyma. The early stages of the deposition of calcified material are illustrated in Figs 13.7 and 13.8. It may take up to 2 years for radiological signs of calcification to develop in patients recognised clinically as having chronic calcifying pancreatitis (Sarles et al. 1980).

The organic component of fully developed stones and its relationship to the crystals of calcium carbonate has been studied by Bockman et al. (1986). These workers decalcified stones removed from the pancreatic ducts of patients in America and France with chronic calcifying pancreatitis, and then used scanning and transmission electron microscopy to examine the sponge-like material that remained. They found that the crystals had been embedded in a heterogeneous gel-like matrix with dense areas of

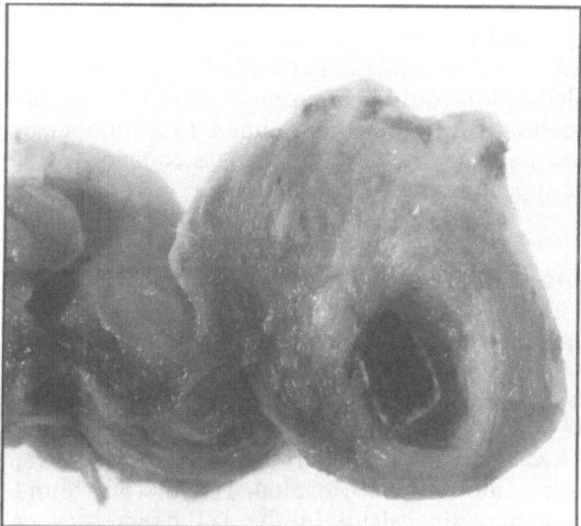

Fig. 13.23. A solitary calculus found near the tail of the pancreas in man aged 75 years, who had died of pulmonary disease and who had not suffered from abdominal symptoms. × 5

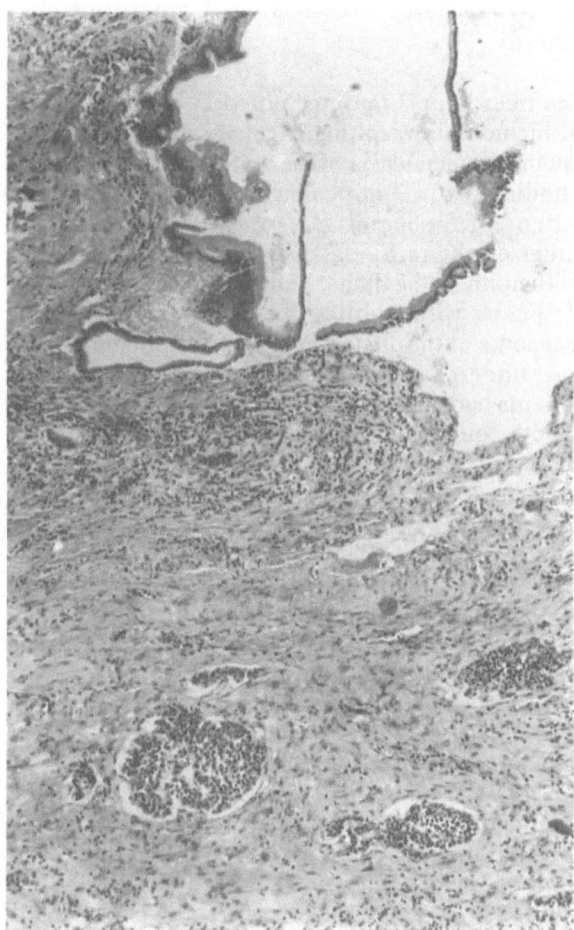

Fig. 13.24. The wall of the cavity that had contained the stone shown in Fig. 13.23. The separation of the ductal epithelium that had lined the cavity is an artefact. Islets remain in the adjacent pancreatic tissue, but the exocrine glandular tissue is replaced by fibrous tissue infiltrated by lymphocytes. H&E, × 60

proteinaceous fibrous material. There were also deposits that resembled fibrin, while altered cellular components accounted for minor portions of the matrix. They considered such appearances to be consistent with the formation of the stones from components of the pancreatic juice that included pancreatic stone protein, glycosaminoglycans, occasional cells and precipitated calcium carbonate.

Further studies (Montalto et al. 1988) of the organic matrix of stones obtained from patients with nutritional chronic pancreatitis in Kerala have shown that such stones, like the stones of alcohol chronic pancreatitis, contained pancreatic stone protein. This suggested to the authors that some pathophysiological links might exist between the apparently different aetiological forms of calcifying pancreatitis.

Single and Multiple Calculi

Pancreatic calculi may be single, and a solitary stone in a small duct (Fig. 13.23) may cause anatomical abnormalities only in its immediate vicinity (Fig. 13.24), without any symptoms. More commonly, however calculi are multiple and are associated with the symptoms and signs of chronic pancreatitis. In such cases, the main duct may contain a relatively large stone near the duodenum, with many small calculi in the ducts in the more distal parts of the pancreas. According to Edmondson et al. (1950) who collected 26 cases of

pancreatic lithiasis from 36 000 autopsies, the commonest site for calculi is in the duct of Wirsung, within 2–4 cm of the ampulla of Vater, perhaps because the calculi became impacted there while being carried towards the duodenum, rather than having been formed at that site. They found that the larger calculi were all situated in the outflow tract of the pancreatic juice; microcalculi within the acini were found only when microscopically detectable calculi were present in the small ducts of the same pancreases. The other microscopic features were those of chronic pancreatitis, with more marked dilatation of the ducts and more marked atrophy of the parenchyma in some parts of the pancreas than was seen in chronic pancreatitis without concretions in the ducts.

Epithelial Metaplasia in Ducts Containing Calculi

The microscopic findings noted by Edmondson et al. included intraepithelial calcification in areas of squamous metaplasia of the epithelium of the ducts, a finding that was not confirmed by the later observations of Stobbe et al. (1970), who commented rather on the rarity of squamous metaplasia in the epithelium of the ducts. They found, instead, in ten of 14 cases with multiple diffuse intraductal calculi, that some of the ducts were lined by epithelium that had undergone goblet cell metaplasia; all ten patients had a history of alcoholism.

Both squamous metaplasia and goblet cell metaplasia are by no means uncommon in ducts that do not contain calculi, (see pp. 21–23), and the association of either type of metaplasia with ductal calculi may well be coincidental. Epithelial injury in the early stages of the formation of calculi has, however, been illustrated by Sarles (1986) in photomicrographs in which it can be seen that calcite crystals have pierced the epithelium of small ducts.

Relationship of Calculi to Pancreatitis

Although in most studies there seems to be a close association between pancreatic concretions and clinically evident chronic pancreatitis, the association is not invariable, especially if the evidence for pancreatic calcification is entirely radiological. Thus Gambill and Pugh (1948), in their study of 39 patients selected solely on radiological evidence of pancreatic calcification, found that, while the symptomatology was commonly that of pancreatitis, a number (about two-fifths) gave no, or an indefinite, history of pancreatitis. Among those with a definite history of pancreatitis, calcification was recognisable in one-fifth on radiographs taken at about 1 year after the onset of pain, but, in another one-fifth, calcification was not discovered until between 11 and 20 years later. They found a high degree of correlation between the extent of pancreatic calcification and the incidence of diabetes and steatorrhoea, complications that developed only in patients with clinically definite pancreatitis.

Somewhat similar results were obtained by Owens and Howard (1958) in their study of the natural history of chronic alcoholism and alcoholic pancreatitis. They concluded that pancreatic calcification was a sequel to chronic alcoholism, characteristically, but not invariably, developing after many years of alcoholic pancreatitis. Radiological detection of the calcification became possible after an interval from the onset of alcoholism that, in their

patients, averaged 15 years. An interval of 6 years separated the onset of relapsing pancreatitis from that of detectable calcification; by the time calcification could be seen radiologically, the pancreatitis had become continuous. In a number of their patients, the onset of diabetes coincided with the appearance of calcification.

Calculi in the Aged

The importance of age, at least in Japan, in relation to pancreatic lithiasis, has been pointed out by Nagai and Ohtsubo (1984). Their study was based on the findings in 418 pancreases from autopsies at the Tokyo Metropolitan Geriatric Hospital and St Luke's International Hospital, Tokyo. They found no pancreatic calculi in the 134 pancreases of patients less than 69 years of age, but in those of 119 patients aged 70–80 years, they found five cases of lithiasis (4.2%), with nine among 117 pancreases from patients aged 80–90 years (7.7%); in pancreases from 48 subjects over 90 years old, there were eight with lithiasis (16.7%).

Most of the stones were scattered throughout the peripheral ducts. Comparison with the clinical histories indicated that such stones in the aged were unassociated with signs or symptoms, and occurred in the absence of a history of alcoholism or hypercalcaemia. Ductal stenosis, squamous metaplasia and the presence of lactoferrin (as demonstrated immunohistologically) in the epithelial lining of the ducts were strongly associated with pancreatic lithiasis in the aged, though the pathogenic sequence remains speculative.

Calculi in Infants Treated with ACTH

In infants who had been treated with adrenocorticotrophic hormone because of infantile spasm, the development of renal and pancreatic calcifications were reported by Hanefeld et al. (1984). There were ten children in their series; pancreatic calcification, together with nephrocalcinosis, was found by ultrasonography in five. No functional impairment of either the kidneys or the pancreas, could, however, be demonstrated.

Size and Shape

Pancreatic calculi tend to be small in comparison with either urinary or biliary calculi, and seldom exceed 1–2 cm in diameter; thus Sarles et al. (1982), whose experience of pancreatic calculi is very exten-

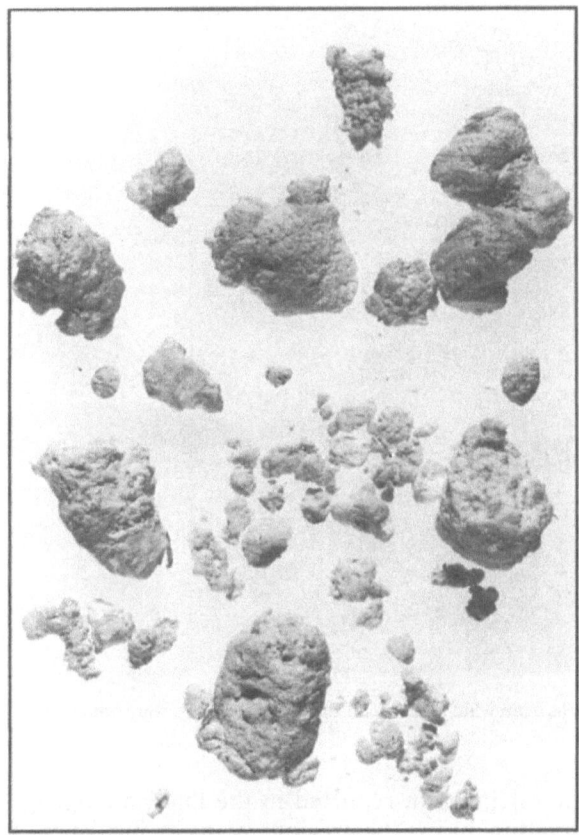

Fig. 13.25. Pancreatic calculi obtained by maceration of the pancreas illustrated in Fig. 13.30. (Courtesy of Mr Tony Russell, Department of Anatomy, University of Liverpool) × 1.5

sive, described calculi that measured 3 × 2 cm as "giant" stones. The shape of pancreatic calculi is rather irregular; they are usually whitish and have rough surfaces to which brownish granules may be attached. Because of their irregular surfaces, the calculi tend to remain attached to the walls of the ducts in which they lie, and may crumble into a coarse off-white powder if they are removed roughly or are cut through accidentally. Examples of pancreatic calculi that were obtained by maceration of pancreases in which calcification had been demonstrated by post-mortem radiography are shown in Figs 13.25–13.28.

In the past, it has been suggested that biliary calculi might make their way into the pancreatic ducts and also that a pancreatic calculus lodged at the duodenal end of the bile duct may be stained with bile pigment and acquire a layer of cholesterol. Reports of such cases were mentioned by Opie (1910), but no recent examples have been found.

In Opie's experience, the obstructive effects of calculi in the main ducts were similar to those of lig-

ation of the pancreatic ducts in experimental animals and resulted in severe sclerosis of the gland, with chronic inflammation of the interlobular type that tended to spare the islets of Langerhans. Such an effect is not, however, invariable, nor was it the most common effect observed by Hepp et al. (1959) in their study of 17 cases of chronic calcifying pancreatitis. The macroscopic lesions they found were of three types. One type corresponded to the sclerotic gland described by Opie, but such a gland was not the commonest in their series, although they found four examples of this lesion. The commonest abnormality, of which they found ten examples, was enlargement of the pancreas with marked dilatation of the duct of Wirsung within a moist, oedematous gland. In the remaining three cases in the series there was deformity of the pancreas by a false cyst, from which communication with the duct of Wirsung could be demonstrated.

Pancreatic Calcification Associated with Carcinoma

There seems to be general agreement that, as far as chronic calcifying pancreatitis is concerned, the calculi within the ducts have not formed because of retention of secretion due to a pre-existing stricture of the duct but, by their presence, they have caused obstruction that leads to progressive damage. Alternatively, when obstruction of the larger ducts has been caused, as is common in carcinoma of the head of the pancreas, stones may occasionally form within the ducts, whose secretion is prevented from reaching the duodenum. As radiologically recognisable calcification seems to require at least a year to develop, it can be only in carcinomas that progress unusually slowly that secretion retained within the ducts can become calcified within the time permitted by the disease. Such cases have, however, been reported, by Leger et al. (1961) for example, and the reports have been reviewed by Guien (1979), who himself found four of this type amongst ten examples of pancreatic calcification associated with carcinoma.

The superimposition of carcinoma upon pre-existing chronic calcifying pancreatitis is also uncommon. The development of carcinoma within a pancreas in which there is heavy radiological calcification may cause decalcification in the area involved by the neoplasm (Tucker and Moore 1963). Nevertheless, there are various reports of chronic calcifying pancreatitis in which carcinoma of the pancreas developed. The most striking of these reports is that of Paulino-Netto et al. (1960), who found that among 24 patients with pancreatic lithiasis there were six

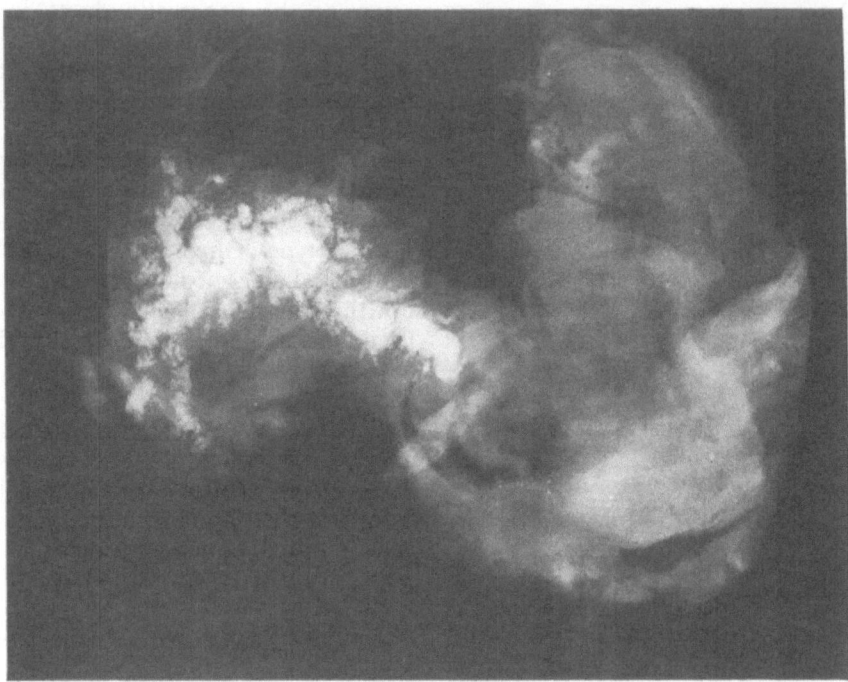

Fig. 13.26. Post-mortem radiograph of the calcification in the pancreas from which the calculi shown in Fig. 13.25. were obtained.

shown at laparotomy to have histologically proved carcinoma of the pancreas. A much lower incidence was found by Johnson and Zintel (1963), who could find no examples among their own cases of chronic calcifying pancreatitis, and could find only 24 pancreatic carcinomas amongst the 677 cases of pancre-

atic calcification reported in the English language literature during the previous years, an incidence of 3.6%. An even lower incidence was found in South African patients by Marks et al. (1968), who had no carcinomas amongst 89 cases of alcoholic-induced pancreatitis with calcification, and only two carcino-

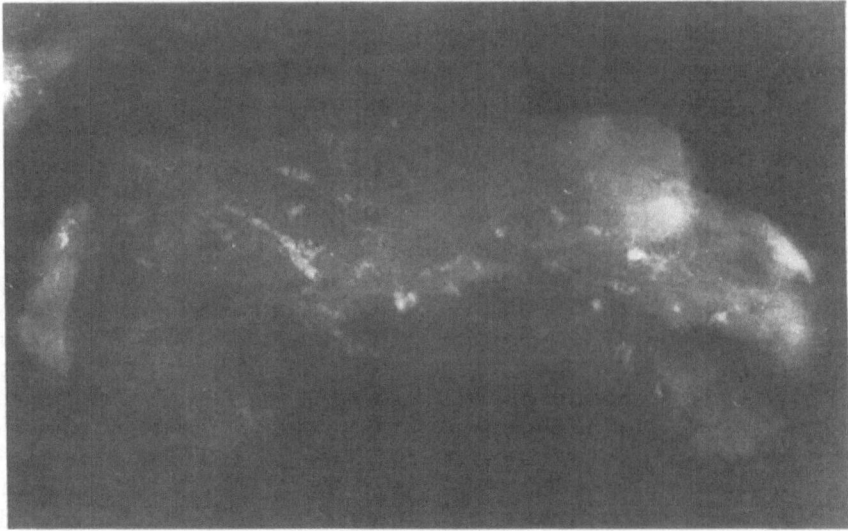

Fig. 13.27. Post-mortem radiograph of a pancreas obtained from a woman aged 73 years, who died of bronchopneumonia that supervened upon chronic bronchitis. Both kidneys were granular and shrunken; there was general arteriosclerosis. No history of alcoholism was obtained.

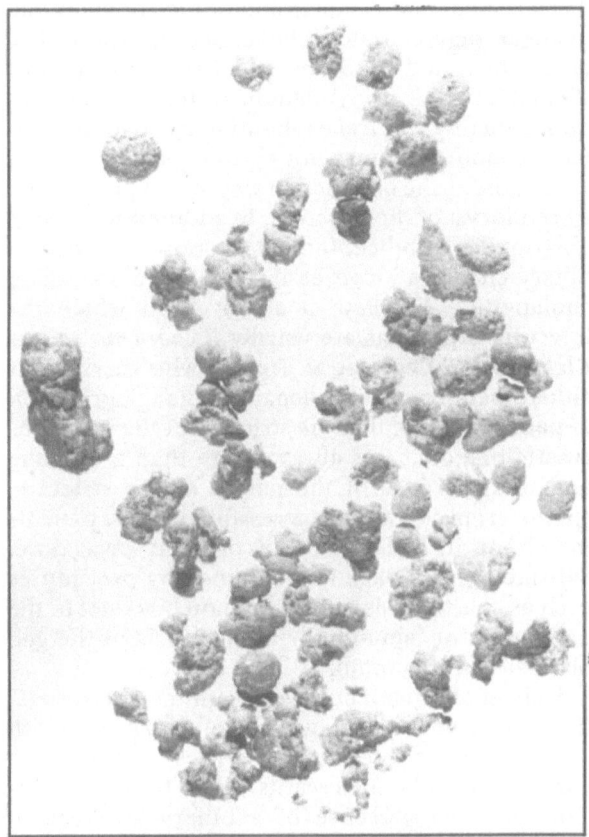

Fig. 13.28. The calculi that were obtained by maceration of the pancreas shown in Fig. 13.27. (Courtesy of Mr Tony Russell, Department of Anatomy, University of Liverpool) × 1.5

mas amongst 224 cases of alcoholic-induced pancreatitis without calcification.

Unlike the chronic calcifying pancreatitis of adults, the hereditary chronic pancreatitis of children that leads to pancreatic calcification in young adults, or even during childhood, seems to carry a substantial risk of pancreatic cancer. Kattwinkel et al. (1973) found that amongst 54 patients with definite or suspected hereditary pancreatitis, eight died of pancreatic carcinoma, while five died from some other abdominal tumour.

A scirrhous adenocarcinoma of the pancreas that appeared to have arisen in a lipomatous pseudohypertrophic pancreas was reported by Salm in 1960; in that pancreas, calcareous material within the ducts formed casts of the ducts.

Calcification in Cystic Lesions of the Pancreas

Both cystadenomas and cystadenocarcinomas of the pancreas may contain small areas of calcification on radiological examination (Guien 1979), but this was found in only one of the 11 cystadenomas in the group of cases collected by Becker et al. (1965). A cystadenocarcinoma of the pancreas in association with long-standing chronic relapsing pancreatitis and pancreatic calcinosis was reported by Dreiling (1959). A pancreatic cyst, the nature of which was not clear, but whose contents included amylase, was reported by Shattock in 1896 to contain a calculus that was diagnosed, by the microscopic appearance of its crystals, as consisting of calcium oxalate.

Hydatid cysts of the pancreas may be found radiologically to have calcification in their walls (Guien 1979), but this sign was not recognisable in the hydatid cysts of the pancreas reported by Anderson and Peebles Brown (1959–1960), and by Kattan (1975).

Calcification of a pancreatic pseudocyst is unusual, but two examples of pseudocysts that were sufficiently calcified to appear as spherical calcified masses in abdominal radiographs have been reported and discussed by Munn et al. (1987).

Calcification in Other Lesions of the Pancreas

Calcification may occur in insulinomas; an example of this is illustrated in Fig. 13.22. Such calcification is said by Guien (1979) to be very rare.

Calcification of the islets of Langerhans may be recognised microscopically in certain cases of type II diabetes (Volk and Wellmann 1977), but this, too, is seldom seen. If there are thrombi in angiomatous malformations that involve the pancreas these may occasionally calcify. Calcification in a glucagonoma is illustrated in Fig. 10.19.

Complications of Chronic Pancreatitis

Biliary Obstruction

It was recognised as long ago as 1904 by Mayo Robson that chronic pancreatitis might be a cause of obstruction of the common bile duct, but the differentiation between chronic pancreatitis and carcinoma of the head of the pancreas during an operation remains difficult; the demonstration of chronic pancreatitis in a biopsy, as is illustrated in Fig. 13.29, does not by any means exclude the presence also of a carcinoma, for the chronic inflammation that surrounds a scirrhous carcinoma is indistinguishable

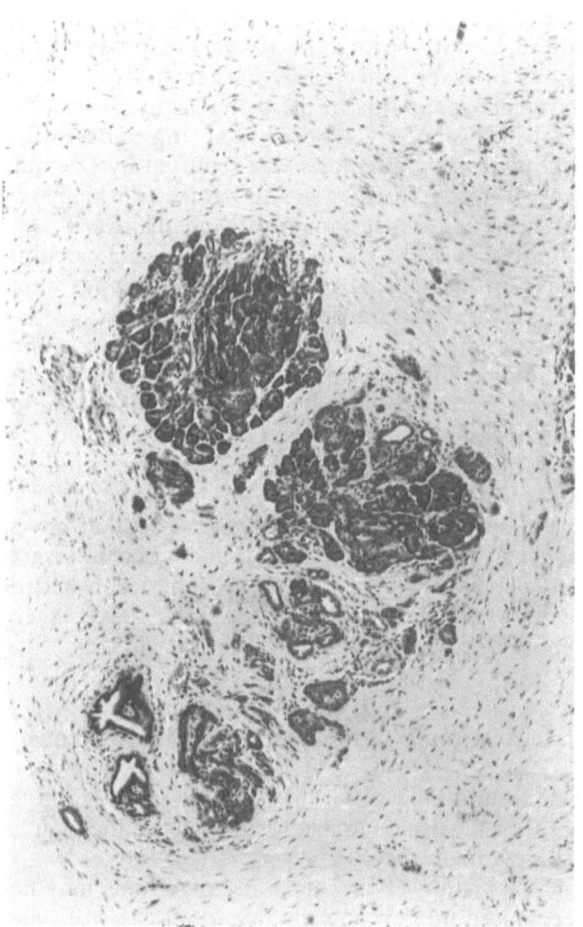

Fig. 13.29. Pancreatic fibrosis in a biopsy of the head of the pancreas in a man with obstructive jaundice. Such fibrosis does not exclude the presence of a carcinoma as the cause of the jaundice, for such appearances are not uncommon in the scirrhous reaction around a pancreatic carcinoma. H&E, × 60

microscopically from chronic pancreatitis unrelated to a carcinoma. A biopsy specimen should, if it is not obviously malignant, always be stained to demonstrate mucin, for, as in the case of linitis plastica, carcinoma cells secreting small globules of mucin may not otherwise be recognised.

Transient jaundice that rarely lasts for more than 10 days may follow an exacerbation of chronic relapsing pancreatitis (Sarles et al. 1979), but jaundice that lasted longer than a month is said by these authors to have occurred in only 3% of the 253 patients with chronic pancreatitis studied in Italy by Gullo et al. (1977). The anatomical cause is usually obstruction of the intrapancreatic portion of the common bile duct by the contraction of fibrous scar tissue. The obstruction is usually partial rather than complete (Warshaw et al. 1976), and the progressive

displacement and compression of the common bile duct, as demonstrated cholangiographically, has been illustrated by Sachs and Partington (1956). Weinstein et al. (1963) demonstrated the obstruction, either by surgical exploration or at autopsy, in ten alcoholic patients with chronic pancreatitis; in four of these, the obstruction was due to pressure by a pseudocyst of the pancreas. In addition to causing obstructive jaundice, the obstruction may lead to biliary cirrhosis (Scott et al. 1977) or to ascending cholangitis (Warshaw et al. 1976), in which the infecting organisms are usually *Escherichia coli* or *Klebsiella*. Yadegar et al. (1980), who carried out either operative or transhepatic cholangiograms on 21 patients, found that the stricture of the intrapancreatic bile duct was always more than 2 cm long and that, because of the length of the stricture, sphincteroplasty was unsuccessful in all the patients in whom it had been the original procedure. Satisfactory drainage was obtained by procedures such as anastomosis of the common bile duct to the duodenum or jejunum, or anastomosis of the gall bladder to the jejunum.

Stahl et al. (1988), however, from their retrospective review of the management of 38 patients with intrapancreatic bile duct strictures secondary to chronic alcoholic pancreatits, came to the conclusion that the presence of a biliary stricture in patients with chronic pancreatitis is not, by itself, and indication for operative intervention.

It has already been mentioned in relation to chronic obstructive pancreatitis that obstruction may be caused by a choledochal cyst, but recurrent pancreatitis may, according to Ng et al. (1987), itself contribute to the development of choledochal cysts.

Hepatic Complications and Associated Lesions

In chronic alcoholic pancreatitis, it might be expected that alcoholic injury to the liver would be associated with the pancreatic damage, but figures for the coincidence of alcoholic cirrhosis of the liver with chronic alcoholic pancreatitis vary greatly. Kirshbaum and Shure (1942–1943), for example, in a study of autopsy material, found fibrosis of the pancreas in 36.2% of 356 American cases of cirrhosis of the liver; cirrhosis was present in half their cases of pancreolithiasis. In France, Sarles and Gerolami-Santandrea (1972) found clinically recognisable cirrhosis of the liver in only 2.3% of 378 patients with chronic pancreatitis. Sarles et al. (1979) have suggested the explanation for such variations may be that, in people vulnerable to chronic alcoholic pancreatitis, cirrhosis of the liver develops more slowly than the pancreatitis. They found that if they based the incidence of alcoholic injury to the liver on the results of liver biopsy on patients with alcoholic pancreatitis, a much higher incidence of cirrhosis and pre-cirrhotic lesions was disclosed. More recently, Wilson et al. (1989) investigated the incidence of hepatobiliary complications in 39 patients in Glasgow, who required surgery because of chronic pancreatitis. All the patients had pre-operative liver biopsy in addition to liver function tests and ultrasonic examination; endoscopic retrograde pancreatography was carried out in 33 and percutaneous transhepatic cholangiography in five. Common bile duct stenosis was found in 16 (62%) of the 26 patients in whom cholangiography was successful. There were features indicating extrahepatic biliary obstruction in the biopsy specimens from 11 patients. Three patients had parenchymal liver disease (cirrhosis, resolving hepatitis and alcoholic hepatitis respectively), while two others had features that suggested previous alcoholic-induced injury.

Other studies of liver biopsy specimens in pancreatitis (Haboubi et al. 1986; Benett et al. 1989) suggest the effects of oxygen-derived free radicals or toxic metabolites formed by the action of free radicals upon tissue components.

Effects of Pseudocysts

The effects of pseudocysts in causing biliary obstruction have already been mentioned, but, when a pseudocyst becomes extrapancreatic, it becomes liable to affect any of the organs with which it may come in contact. The effects of the pseudocysts that may follow acute pancreatitis have been discussed earlier, but, in chronic pancreatitis, they may cause the presenting symptoms of an illness at a stage when the chronic pancreatitis is still unsuspected. The organs that may be involved include the stomach, duodenum, diaphragm and spleen, along with the arteries and veins of the upper abdomen. The effects of a pseudocyst depend upon the region of the pancreas in which the cyst has arisen. In the series of 99 pancreatic pseudocysts investigated by endoscopic retrograde pancreatography in 83 patients by Sugawa and Walt (1979), the cysts were in the head in 51 patients, in the body of the gland in 21, and in the tail in 20. Small cysts within the pancreas do not affect adjacent organs, but, of these 99 cysts, 50 were between 2 cm and 5 cm in diameter, while 29 were more than 5 cm in diameter, and were thus liable to protrude from the surface of the pancreas and to become attached by inflammatory adhesions to neighbouring structures. In four of Sugawa and Walt's patients, a spontaneous orifice between a pseudocyst and the stomach

had formed; in one, there was an opening between a pseudocyst and the duodenum. Fig. 13.2 illustrates a pseudocyst in the tail of the pancreas; the cyst, which was 9 cm in diameter, is attached to the hilum of the spleen and has caused an infarct near the lower pole of the spleen. A small fistula may develop in the wall of a pseudocyst and allow the enzyme-containing contents of the pseudocyst to escape into the pleural or peritoneal cavities, with the development of serous effusions in which there is an abundance of amylase.

Two examples of marked calcification in the walls of pseudocysts have been reported by Munn et al. (1987). In one of these patients there was a history of blunt abdominal trauma 40 years previously; the recent history was of 48 hours of abdominal pain. The cyst was found to contain pus and streptococci when it was removed. In the other patient, there was a history of an episode of severe abdominal pain 9 years before the recent history of 4 days of increasing abdominal pain. The cyst fluid yielded a growth of E. coli. Cystoduodenostomy was followed by an uneventful recovery and an apparent cure on review 24 months later.

Oesophageal obstruction due to the mediastinal extension of a pancreatic pseudocyst has been recorded by Winton et al. (1986). Their patient was a heavy drinker who denied any abdominal pain, but in whose computed tomogram there were signs of chronic inflammation in the body and tail of the pancreas. His dysphagia, which had progressed rapidly to complete oesophageal obstruction, was relieved by posterior cystogastrostomy. A very similar patient was encountered by Woods et al. (1989), in whom normal oesophageal function was also restored by drainage of a pancreatic pseudocyst that had extended into the mediastinum.

The value of preoperative endoscopic retrograde cholangiopancreatography in a series of 40 patients with pancreatic pseudocysts has been described by Nealon et al. (1989). The differentiation of pancreatic pseudocysts from pancreatic necrosis by computed tomography on the same group of patients was discussed by Mainwaring et al. (1989).

An unusual case of chronic obstructive pancreatitis and pseudocyst formation due to obstruction of the middle of the main pancreatic duct by a small carcinoid has been described by Gettenberg et al. (1988).

Serous Effusions

Leakage from a pseudocyst is only one of the causes of the serous effusions that may complicate chronic pancreatitis, for effusions may occur in the absence of a pseudocyst. It may be possible to demonstrate a fistulous communication between the disrupted duct system of the pancreas and the site of the effusion, but the effusion may occur in the absence of any communication between the pancreas and the affected serous cavity.

An example of fistulous communication has been described by Davidson et al. (1979). They described the illness of a 38-year-old black American, who had recurrent pericardial and pleural effusions during a 10-month period. The effusions had a high protein and amylase content, and an operative pancreatogram demonstrated a fistulous communication that ran from the middle region of the pancreas, through the mediastinum, into both pleural spaces, and into the pericardial sac. Surgical detachment of the fistula and Roux-en-Y decompression of the pancreatic duct produced a cure.

A series of 27 patients with internal pancreatic fistulas that caused either ascites or pleural effusions, or both, was reported by Cameron in 1978. He conluded that disruption of the main pancreatic duct could occur without symptoms in an alcoholic patient and cause an internal fistula between the duct and the peritoneal cavity with massive ascites as a result. If the fistula developed in the posterior direction, the pancreatic secretions would track upwards retroperitoneally into the mediastinum and thence into one or both pleural spaces. Amylase in the effusions was always present in large amounts, the content usually being several thousand units; the albumin content was usually about 3 g dl^{-1}. As amylase is not detectable in the ascitic fluid of patients with alcoholic cirrhosis of the liver, the high amylase content of the fluid in pancreatic ascites is of great diagnostic importance in differentiating between these complications of alcoholism; indeed, a high amylase content of a serous effusion would be completely diagnostic of a pancreatic cause in a man. In a woman, such a finding would almost be diagnostic of pancreatic disease, but, in 1979, Cramer and Bruns published a report of their patient with an amylase-producing ovarian neoplasm that caused a pseudo-Meig's syndrome, with amylase-containing pleural fluid.

The condition of massive serous effusion is becoming recognised increasingly to be an almost specific complication of chronic pancreatitis, and, as has been pointed out by Ingram and Sheiner (1980), the difficulty in making the diagnosis is mainly due to the absence of symptoms of pancreatitis, most patients seeming to be suffering only from the effects of the effusion. Once suspected, the diagnosis can be confirmed by demonstrating a greatly raised amylase level in the fluid withdrawn from the effusion. Serum amylase is usually, but not always, elevated. Ingram and Sheiner reported five such patients, four with pleural effusions and one with ascites, the preponderance of pleural effusions tending to confirm the statement by Sarles et al. (1979) that ascites is less common.

In addition to the 94 cases reviewed by Hotz et al. (1977), 26 others have been reported (Ingram and Sheiner 1980; Bedingfield and Anderson 1986; Pottmeyer et al. 1987; Martin et al. 1989), a total of 120. Amongst these, the examples described by Pottmeyer et al. are of interest because eight of the ten had no abdominal symptoms and complained only of the effects of their pleural effusions. In some of the published cases, leakage from a pseudocyst caused the effusion, but the important factor seems to be the disruption of the duct system, with or without a recognisable pseudocyst. In one of the patients reported by Bedingfield and Anderson, for example, there was a pseudocyst in the head of the pancreas, but the cause of a left pleural effusion was found to be a fistulous track that connected the tail of the pancreas with the left pleural cavity. There was a stricture in the proximal part of the pancreatic duct and dilatation of the duct behind the stricture. Disruption of the ducts, sufficient to cause serous effusion, may also be a sequel of acute pancreatitis; trauma of the pancreas is also an important cause. Trauma caused the effusions in 14 of the 85 patients with pancreatic ascites reviewed by Donowitz et al. (1974).

It has already been mentioned that effusions may occur in the absence of any fistulous communication between a pseudocyst, or damaged pancreatic ducts, and the site of the effusion; they may occur in the synovial spaces of joints, such as the ankles or knees. In this type, the effusions are usually associated with disseminated fat necrosis; it is probable that fat necrosis adjacent to the serous lining of the affected cavities provokes an inflammatory reaction that causes the effusion. Inflammatory and granulomatous lesions were found in a pleural biopsy by Potts et al. (1975) in a patient with chronic pancreatitis with subcutaneous fat necrosis and polyserositis; the serous effusions in this syndrome resemble the effusions caused by a fistula in having a high content of amylase.

Bronchobiliary Fistula

This unusual complication of alcoholic chronic pancreatitis was reported by Genell et al. in 1987. Hepatic and subphrenic sepsis, superimposed upon hepatic biliary obstruction caused by chronic alcoholic pancreatitis, led to the development of the fistula.

Effects of Chronic Pancreatitis upon Blood Vessels

The fibrous tissue that replaces so much of the glandular tissue of the pancreas is liable to involve also the structures in contact with the pancreas. The structures vulnerable to such involvement include the common bile duct, where involvement has already been discussed, the splenic and portal veins, the splenic and pancreaticoduodenal arteries, the spleen, and the splenic flexure of the colon. Partial obstruction of the abdominal lymphatic vessels was demonstrated by lymphangiography by J.-C. Sarles et al. (1965) in 10% of patients with chronic pancreatitis.

The intimate anatomical association of the splenic vein with the pancreas seems to make it particularly liable to the effects of pancreatic disease, either by compression or by thrombosis, which commonly extends to the portal vein, a vein itself liable to be involved directly by pancreatic disease. The result is that portal hypertension develops, with varices from which alimentary haemorrhage may occur. Although such patients may be alcoholic, cirrhosis of the liver may be absent and the portal hypertension is then entirely of the extrahepatic type (Turrill and Mikkelsen 1969; Keith et al. 1982; Nishiyama et al. 1986). One of the hereditary pancreatitis kindreds studied by McElroy and Christiansen (1972) had a special tendency for the pancreatitis to be complicated by thrombosis of the splenic or portal veins. Sarles et al. (1979) found that haematemesis and melaena occurred in 9% of their patients with chronic pancreatitis.

Before the introduction of angiography, chronic pancreatitis was scarcely recognised as an important cause of damage to the splenic and pancreaticoduodenal arteries. Thus, in 1964 Kelley et al. were able to find over 300 reports of splenic artery aneurysms, and could refer to five cases of aneurysm of the pancreaticoduodenal arteries as well as their own; but none of these aneurysms was attributed to chronic pancreatitis. It is true that in 1956 Hendrick reported an aneurysm of the pancreaticoduodenal artery in a patient in whom there had been recurrent attacks of pancreatitis, but Hendrick believed that the aneurysm, which was 4 cm long and 6 cm in diameter, had compressed the neck of the pancreas to cause the attacks of pancreatitis and was not a result of the pancreatitis. Excision of the aneurysm relieved the patient's symptoms.

In 1967, however, Kadell and Riley drew attention to the serious gastrointestinal bleeding that is common in patients with chronic pancreatitis, and, although incidental gastrointestinal disease such as peptic ucler was often responsible, they were able to demonstrate angiographically, in two patients, that pancreatic pseudocysts had caused erosion of the splenic artery. Other reports of arterial aneurysms due to pancreatitis, with or without pseudocysts, include that of Boijsen et al. (1969), one of whose patients was a man aged 51 with chronic pancreatitis, who had a 16 mm wide, angiographically demonstrated splenic arterial aneurysm, which they believed had penetrated the pancreas to reach the pancreatic duct. In 1969, an aneurysm of the gastroduodenal artery associated with chronic pancreatitis was found angiographically by Abrams et al. In 1975, Harris et al. recognised an aneurysm of the pancreaticoduodenal artery angiographically; there was displacement of the head of the pancreas, consistent with the effects of a pancreatic pseudocyst. They were able, at autopsy, to confirm the presence of a pseudocyst in the head of the pancreas. They found that an aneurysm in the posterior wall of the pseudocyst had caused both chronic and acute haemorrhage. There was a fistulous communication between the pseudocyst and the duodenum. In two other patients with chronic pancreatitis, both of whom were alcoholics, they demonstrated an aneurysm of the dorsal pancreatic artery in one, and aneurysms at the junction of the posterior and inferior pancreaticoduodenal arteries and of the transverse pancreatic artery in the other, by angiography of the coeliac and superior mesenteric arteries.

Other reports of angiographically discovered aneurysms due to pancreatitis followed (White et al. 1976; Walter et al. 1977; Corbeau et al. 1978; Bivins et al. 1978; Lung et al. 1980; Thakker et al. 1983), and information about these lesions began to accummulate. Thus it seems that aneurysms of branches of the peripancreatic arteries are a relatively common feature of chronic pancreatitis; they were found in seven of 72 cases investigated angiographically by White et al. They are not a feature of carcinoma of the pancreas; there were no aneurysms in the arteriograms of 84 patients with carcinoma of the pancreas reviewed by these workers. Angiographically demonstrated aneurysms may thus be important in differentiating between chronic pancreatitis and carcinoma of the pancreas, for both can cause encasement of the vessels and obstruction of the splenic or superior mesenteric veins. However, the presence of an aneurysm is valuable evidence in favour of a diagnosis of chronic pancreatitis. Continuing damage to the wall of an aneurysm by the digestive enzymes of the pancreas may cause rupture with massive haemorrhage, usually into the alimentary tract, but also through surgical drain sites, or fistulas. The haemorrhage may also be into the peritoneal cavity or into a pseudocyst. A rare type of haemorrhage, in which an aneurysm of the splenic artery or one of its branches ruptures into the pancreatic duct system to cause

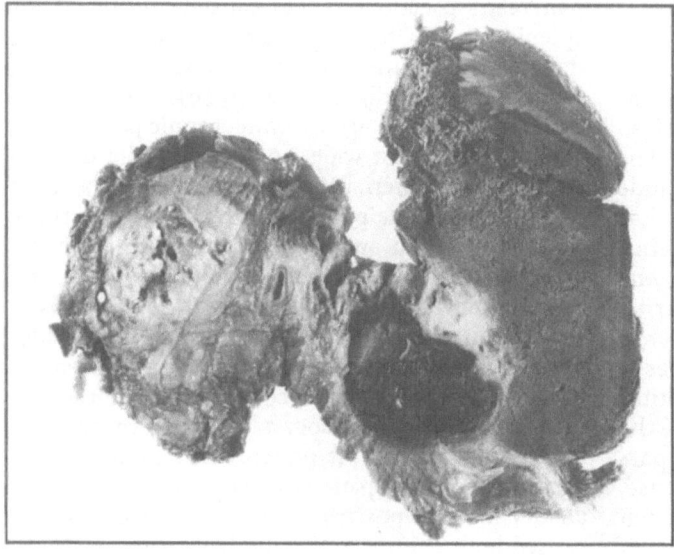

Fig. 13.30. A coronal section through the spleen, pancreas and an aneurysm of the splenic artery. The pancreas was extensively calcified, and calcified material had ulcerated through the peritoneum at the root of the mesentery. The specimen was obtained from a man aged 59, who was not an alcoholic. He had complained of upper abdominal pain and was being investigated in hospital when he collapsed and died. The aneurysm of the splenic artery occupied the tail of the pancreas and the hilum of the spleen. It contained 300 g of blood clot and had ruptured into the peritoneal cavity, which contained over 2 litres of fluid blood.

bleeding from the duodenal papilla, has been described by several groups of workers (Corbeau et al. 1978; Bivins et al. 1978; Lung et al. 1980; Harper et al. 1984). A large aneurysm of the splenic artery that complicated chronic calcifying pancreatitis is illustrated in Figs 13.30 and 13.31. The aneurysm eventually ruptured and caused a fatal intraperitoneal haemorrhage.

Urinary Effects

What was claimed to be the first published example of bilateral necrosis and obliteration of the ureters

was reported by Meller et al. (1988). Their patient was a black man aged 45, whose pancreatic pseudocyst was drained through the posterior wall of the stomach. He appeared to recover but 6 months later he became anuric because of bilateral ureteric obstruction, attributed by the authors to the effects of the pseudocyst.

Splenic Complications

Spontaneous, or almost spontaneous, rupture of the spleen as a result of chronic pancreatitis has been reported by Gardner and Preston (1961). They gave

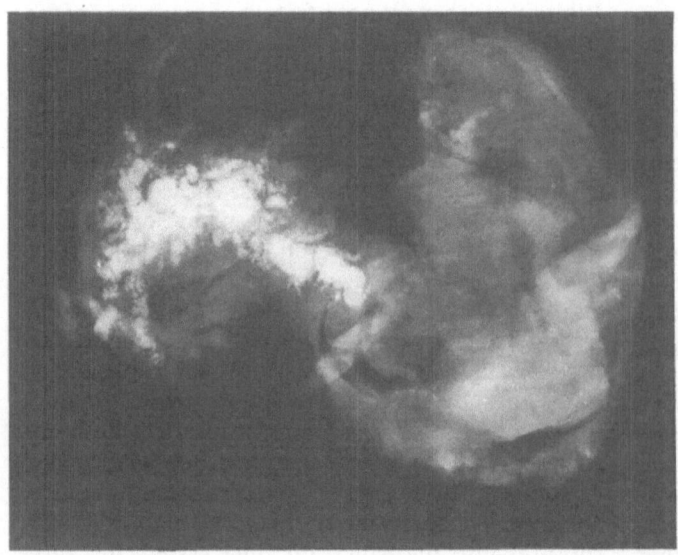

Fig. 13.31. This is a radiograph of the specimen shown in Fig. 13.30. There is extensive calcification of the pancreas. Microscopically, after decalcification, islets were numerous in inflammatory fibrous tissue, but exocrine glandular tissue was almost unrecognisable. The man's fasting blood sugar had been normal.

an account of two patients, and suggested that fibrous fixation of the hilum of the spleen by the adjacent pancreatitis might make the spleen vulnerable to rupture by trivial trauma. They referred to two previous reports of rupture of the spleen after pancreatitis. Rupture of the spleen with haemoperitoneum has also been encountered as a rare complication of chronic pancreatitis by Moreaux and Bismuth (1969), while splenic necrosis attributable to an aneurysm of the splenic artery has been reported by Blery et al. (1973). An infarct of the spleen in association with a pseudocyst that is adhering to the spleen is illustrated in Fig. 13.2.

Fat Necrosis

In discussing the fat necrosis that may accompany acute pancreatitis, it was pointed out that the degree of necrosis does not seem to be related to the severity or acuteness of the pancreatitis. Fat necrosis, including disseminated fat necrosis, may accompany pancreatitis that is mild and chronic, and almost without symptoms directly related to the pancreas. Fat necrosis with panniculitis can, of course (as was mentioned in relation to acute pancreatitis), also occur in the absence of pancreatic disease, either as the localised type of mesenteric panniculitis described by Ogden et al. (1965), or as the subcutaneous panniculitis of Weber–Christian disease. Pancreatic enzymes cannot be recognised in most cases of Weber–Christian disease, but Förström and Winkelmann (1975) described a patient with acute, generalised panniculitis, in which both amylase and lipase activity could be demonstrated in specimens from the lesions of the skin. The patient had an increased urinary amylase level and some elevation of lipase in the serum; a secretin test caused an eightfold elevation of urinary amylase, with some elevation of lipase and amylase levels in the serum, but with normal results from a study of the fluid obtained by duodenal drainage. The pancreas was found at the autopsy to be normal, both macroscopically and microscopically. It is thus evident that the relationship between subcutaneous fat necrosis and pancreatic disease is not a simple one, and, as has been suggested by Potts et al. (1975), immunological factors are probably involved as well as the effects of circulating pancreatic lipase. The type of subcutaneous fat necrosis associated with pancreatic disease has been studied by Hughes et al. (1975), who described painless or painful subcutaneous nodules on the legs, buttocks or trunk that were associated with either pancreatitis or carcinoma of pancreas. The pancreatic disease might have been causing no symptoms other

than the subcutaneous nodules, but arthritis, particularly of the ankles, was commonly present as well. Gastrointestinal symptoms could be entirely absent. These authors believed that the microscopic appearances of the nodules were sufficiently characteristic to be pathognomonic of pancreatic disease, the essential feature being "ghost-like" cells, with thick shadowy walls and no nuclei, in the foci of necrosis in the subcutaneous fat (see Figs 13.32, 13.33) Deposits of calcium occurred within and about the necrotic fat cells with the "ghost-like" appearance.

The syndrome of subcutaneous fat necrosis in pancreatic disease may include polyserositis (Potts et al. 1975). These authors reviewed all the reports of this rare syndrome published in the English language literature up to 1975. In support of their argument that the non-pancreatic lesions might be mediated by immune processes, they pointed out that the syndrome might include eosinophilic leucocytosis, and that a vasculitis could be demonstrated in biopsies taken before the foci of necrosis had developed. They also showed that immunoglobulin G (IgG) and C_3 could be demonstrated by the immunofluorescent technique in the pleura, while there were reduced levels of total haemolytic complement in the serum and pleural and pericardial effusions. High amylase levels may be present in the effusions. In the early subcutaneous lesions in the patient they studied there was prominent perivascular lymphocytic infiltration that was interpreted originally as erythema nodosum, but which was found in a biopsy 6 days later to have progressed to fat necrosis with ghost cells. In a pleural biopsy there were "acute inflammatory changes with granulomas" and on the pericardial surface, in specimens obtained after death, there was vascular fibrous tissue with inflammatory cells. The cause of death was bronchopneumonia with recent pulmonary thromboemboli and pulmonary infarction; the head of the pancreas contained an irregular pseudocyst $3 \times 4 \times 2$ cm, with adjacent omental and mesenteric fat necrosis. The patient had had an effusion into the left knee joint, with 200 white blood cells per ml in the aspirated fluid; whose viscosity was normal and which did not contain crystals; the synovial membrane of the knee was not examined after death.

During the clinical course of chronic pancreatitis with subcutaneous fat necrosis the cutaneous nodules may break down and discharge a sterile oily or thick brownish substance (Sarles et al. 1979), as may occur in liquefying nodular panniculitis, a condition taken by Hoyos et al. (1966) to be a variant of Weber–Christian disease. It is said, also by Sarles et al., that effective surgical treatment of the pancreatic component of the syndrome has led to rapid arrest of the fat necrosis, and they refer to cases,

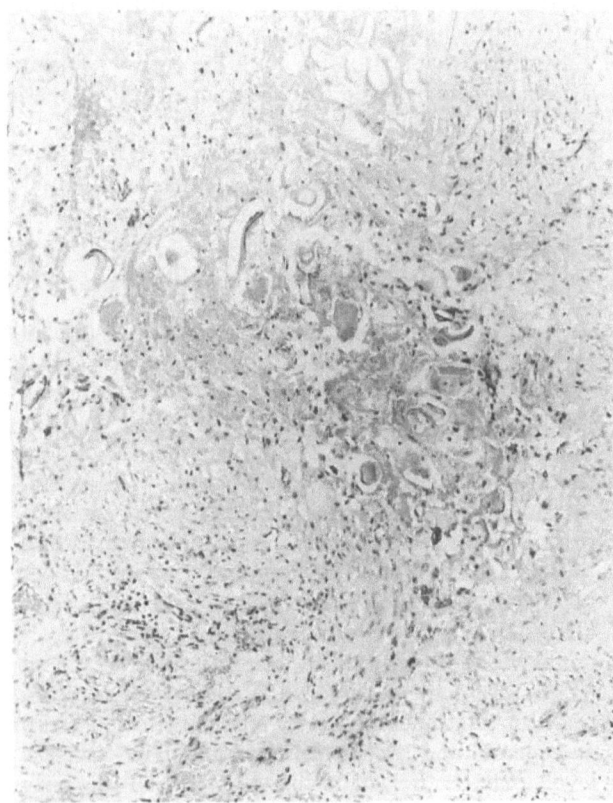

Fig. 13.32. "Ghost-like" cells in an area of fat necrosis that presented as an ulcer of the leg in a patient with chronic alcoholic pancreatitis. (Courtesy of Dr A.H. Clarke) H&E, ×150

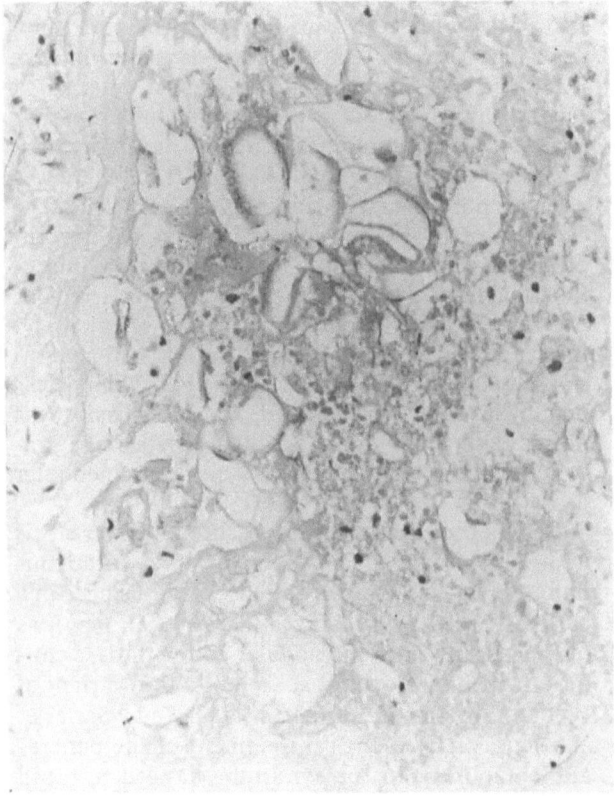

Fig. 13.33. A higher magnification of the "ghost-like" cells in Fig. 13.32. (Courtesy of Dr A.H. Clarke) H&E, ×375

published in the French literature, in which this has occurred.

Polyserositis with intraperitoneal, retroperitoneal and intrathoracic fat necrosis with much granulomatous and fibrotic reaction may complicate chronic pancreatitis in the absence of subcutaneous fat necrosis as is illustrated by the following case history.

The patient was a woman who was aged 44 at the time of her death. When she was admitted to hospital in April 1960 she had been dyspnoeic, tired and anaemic for the previous 18 months. No history of alcoholism was obtained. Hard masses were palpable in the upper abdomen and laparotomy was carried out early in May 1960. Only dense fibrous masses between the loops of the small intestine were found; in biopsy specimens the fibrosis was found to be associated with foci of fat necrosis. The pancreas was not recognised to be abnormal, and was not sampled for microscopic examination. The abdomen was closed. At the beginning of June 1960 the patient was found to have diabetes mellitus but exocrine pancreatic disease was not suspected. The illness was mainly one of respiratory difficulty and the patient died of respiratory and cardiac failure on 15th December 1960. Subcutaneous fat necrosis had not been a feature of the illness.

The post-mortem examination was carried out on the day of death, when widespread fibrosis was found to involve the pleural cavities, peritoneal cavity, pericardium and retroperitoneum. Foci of fat necrosis were recognisable in the dense white fibrous tissue that bound the loops of the intestine together and to the abdominal wall, liver and spleen. The pancreas was very hard, and was surrounded by fibrous tissue that extended into the substance of the gland. A pseudocyst, 15 cm in diameter, located in the root of the mesentery, contained whitish turbid fluid, and a smaller cyst, 3 cm in diameter, was present in the fibrous wall of the main cyst. Retroperitoneal fibrosis extended as far as the pelvis and involved the adrenal glands; it had caused some ureteric obstruction in the pelvic cavity and there was mild bilateral hydronephrosis. The right pleural cavity was obliterated by greatly thickened pleural surfaces that were so bound together that the lung had to be dissected out extrapleurally. There was fibrous thickening also of the left pleural surfaces, but the pleural cavity was only partially obliterated and the remaining space contained 150 ml of clear straw-coloured fluid. There was patchy thickening of the visceral pericardium. The right ventricle was enlarged. The pulmonary arterial branches contained numerous thromboemboli. No other abnormalities were found apart from congestion of the liver and subcutaneous oedema of the legs and

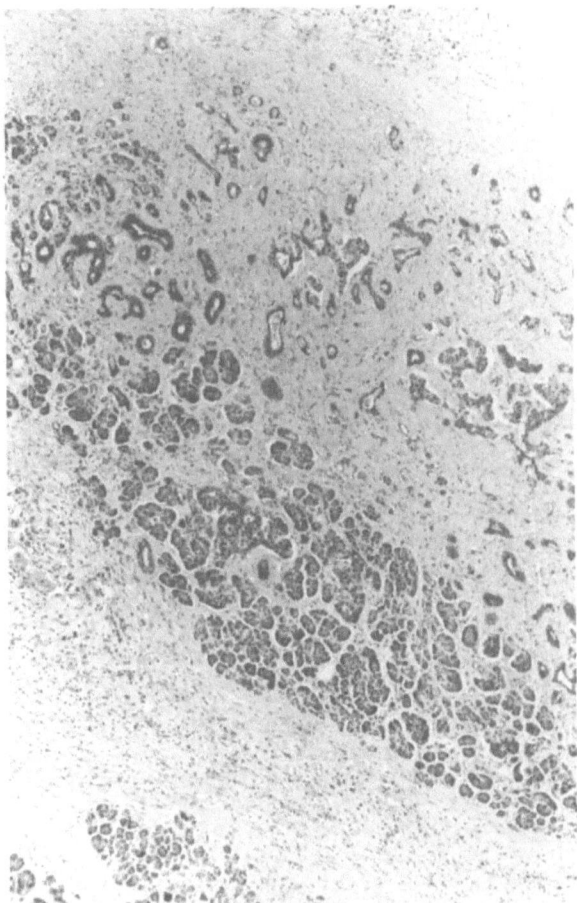

Fig. 13.34. The microscopic appearance of the pancreas of the case with fat necrosis described in the text. Islets are unrecognisable and there is advanced replacement of the exocrine glandular tissue by inflammatory fibrous tissue. H&E, × 60

sacral region. The biliary tract was normal. The joints had caused no symptoms during life and the synovial membranes of the joints were not examined during the autopsy.The microscopic appearance of the pancreas, the wall of the pseudocyst and the granulomatous and fibrous changes associated with fat necrosis in the serous cavities and retroperitoneal regions are shown in Figs 13.34–13.37. There is some resemblance to the cases mentioned by Sarles et al. (1979) in which chronic pancreatitis was complicated by retroperitoneal fibrosis.

Skeletal Lesions

The evidence for intramedullary fat necrosis in chronic pancreatitis is mainly radiological. Immelman et al. (1964) described multiple osteolytic

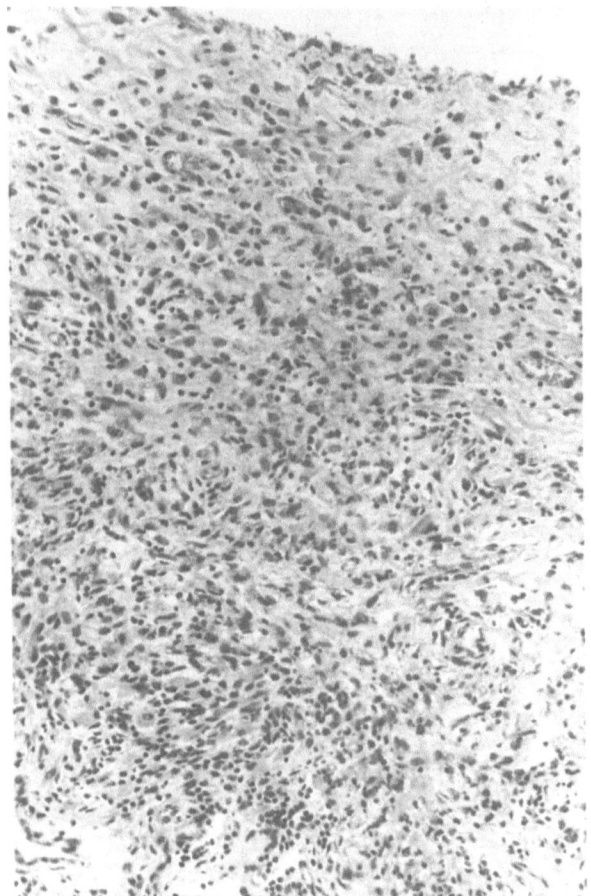

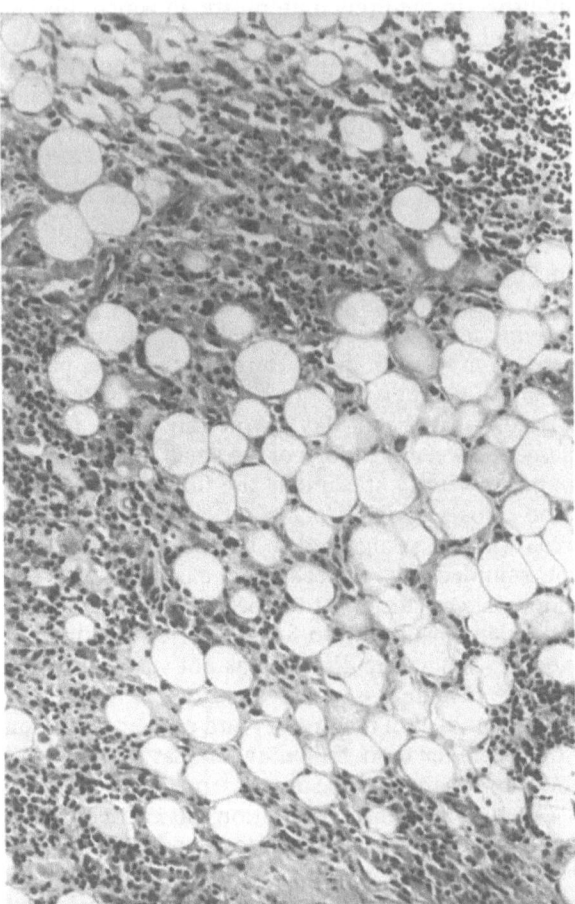

Fig. 13.35. The inflammatory fibrous tissue that formed the wall of an extrapancreatic pseudocyst in the root of the mesentery. H&E, × 150

Fig. 13.36. The granulomatous reaction to fat necrosis in the vicinity of the adrenal glands in the case of chronic pancreatitis described in the text. H&E, × 150

lesions and periosteal reaction in a patient with acute pancreatitis, and calcified intramedullary lesions in two patients with chronic calcifying pancreatitis. The appearances were interpreted as acute intramedullary fat necrosis in the patient with acute pancreatitis and chronic intramedullary fat necrosis in those with chronic pancreatitis. A year later Gerle et al. (1965) described osseous radiological changes in six patients in whom the clinical diagnosis of chronic alcoholic pancreatitis was firmly established. The changes consisted of intramedullary calcific deposits, or aseptic necrosis of the femoral and humeral heads, or combinations of these lesions. In one there were widespread osteolytic defects of the humeri. The aseptic necrosis was attributed to thrombosis of end arteries. Histological confirmation of the presence of fat necrosis with surrounding calcification was obtained by Bank et al. (1966), by biopsies from the

radiological lesions of both femora in a patient with alcohol-induced chronic relapsing pancreatitis.

According to Guien (1979), the osteolytic lesions of chronic pancreatitis may disappear after many months but in advanced disease, the lesions of the head of the femur or humerus may progress to fragmentation and compression of the head of the bone, as in degenerative osteoarthritis. The incidence of radiological lesions of the skeleton in chronic pancreatitis is 6% (Guien 1979).

Pulmonary Emphysema

There are several possible relationships between pulmonary emphysema and pancreatitis. Current ideas about the pathogenesis of emphysema revolve about the protease–antiprotease hypothesis, which states that pulmonary interstitial elastin is broken

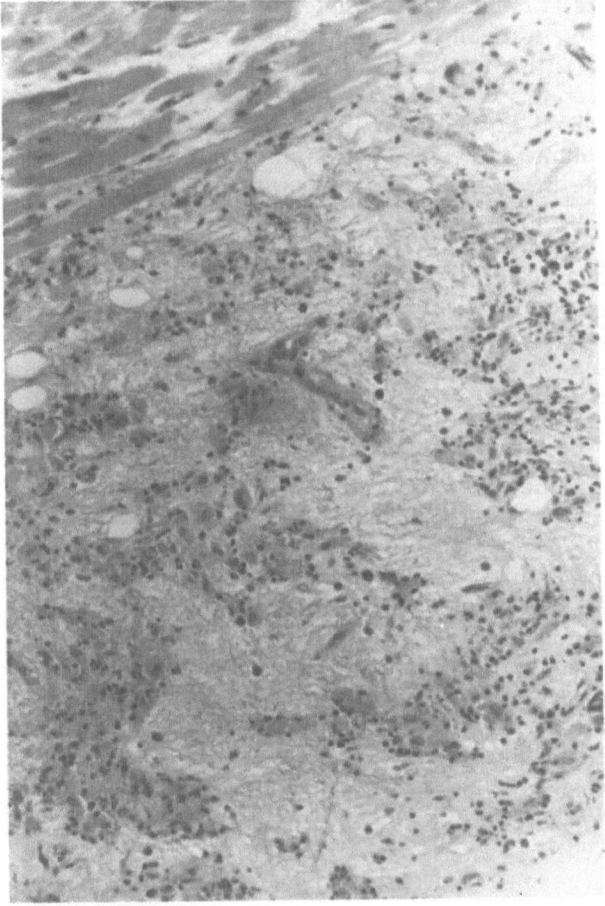

Fig. 13.37. A granulomatous reaction, attributable to fat necrosis, in the epicardial fat. The process does not involve the adjacent myocardium. H&E, × 150

down when an imbalance exists between elastase released from alveolar leucocytes and a serum inhibitor. This inhibitor is a product of the liver, and is usually called alpha₁ antitrypsin. This name is based on the first of its actions to be discovered, though the detection of other in vitro actions has led to a preference for the alternative name of alpha₁ proteinase inhibitor. Brantly et al. (1988) suggest that this title misrepresents the molecule's biological actions, and that the term alpha₁ antitrypsin should be retained because of its familiarity. The protease–antiprotease imbalance hypothesis arose from the observation that individuals who have a deficiency of circulating alpha₁ antitrypsin activity have a high risk of developing panacinar emphysema. Smoking exacerbates the danger by activating alveolar phagocytes, inducing them to release their complement of elastase (Hutchinson 1988).

The pancreas also produces an elastase; indeed, it is this enzyme that is used in most experimental models of emphysema, which can be induced if the enzyme is administered by intratracheal injection, as an aerosol or even by intraperitoneal instillation. Some have therefore suggested that emphysema might follow acute pancreatitis, though attempts to confirm this hypothesis in experimental animals by intravenous infusion of pancreatic elastase have failed (Schuyler et al. 1978). The animals either develop fatal pulmonary haemorrhage or suffer only a temporary drop in pulmonary elastic recoil; the morphological lesion of emphysema cannot be reproduced. Clinical evidence is also inconclusive, and is limited to case reports such as that of Ogilvie et al. (1972), who described a patient in whom the rapid development of basal emphysema coincided with the development of chronic relapsing pancreatitis, with pseudocysts, that caused a marked elevation of pancreatic enzymes in the blood for at least 18 months.

There is a second possible link, for it has been suggested that alpha₁ antitrypsin deficiency renders the pancreas more vulnerable to injury by toxic agents such as alcohol. Novis et al. (1975) showed that the phenotype PiMZ was over-represented in patients with chronic pancreatitis, and Mihas and Hirschowitz (1976) showed that such patients had a low circulating alpha₁ antitrypsin activity. However, a more recent study (Braxel et al. 1982) failed to confirm any association.

The third link is even more tenuous, and arises because alpha₁ antitrypsin deficiency is associated with a panniculitis indistinguishable from that occurring with pancreatitis and pancreatic carcinoma, with both conditions sometimes being described as Weber–Christian disease (Pittelkow et al. 1988). Förström and Winkelmann (1975) described a patient with an acute generalised panniculitis without pancreatitis, in whom they were able to demonstrate amylase and lipase in the skin; unfortunately, they did not measure serum alpha₁ antitrypsin activity.

Islet Cell Tumour

A neuroendocrine islet cell tumour that produced gastrin and ACTH in a patient with calcifying chronic pancreatitis has been reported by Allison et al. (1985).

Late Effects

It is to be hoped that the preceding pages of this chapter will have made it clear that chronic pancreatitis, as indicated by fibrous replacement of the pancreatic parenchyma, with or without calcification, may be the end-stage of several different processes. By the time the end-stage has been reached it is often impossible to assess accurately from the morphology of the gland what the earlier stages may have been, but the type of functional impairment seems to relate, at least to some extent, to the aetiology of the chronic pancreatitis. Thus in kwashiorkor the administration of the appropriate diet is said to produce a complete restoration of pancreatic function, while in the adult form of chronic pancreatitis, as it occurs in tropical Africa and in parts of India, diabetes mellitus is a common effect. However, in tropical Africa an adult type of chronic pancreatitis may present instead as intestinal malabsorption.

In Europe, diabetes is said (Sarles et al. 1979) to complicate chronic pancreatitis in about a third of cases while there is impaired glucose tolerance in another third. The incidence of malabsorption is rather more difficult to assess because, in the absence of pain, malabsorption can be compensated for by an increased intake of protein and fat. Absorption of fat-soluble vitamins is impaired (Braunstein 1961; Rambaud et al. 1970; Prost et al. 1975) and osteomalacia may result from inadequate absorption of vitamin D. There is evidence, too, that there may also be defective absorption of the water-soluble vitamin B_{12} (Henderson et al. 1972) but clinical effects of B_{12} deficiency are rare in chronic pancreatitis.

In the assessment of impaired pancreatic function in chronic pancreatitis by tests that involve the collection of pancreatic secretions from the duodenum it is important to distinguish between the effects of the obstruction of the pancreatic ducts by calculi or strictures and the effects of the destruction of the glandular tissue. To do this, various workers have attempted to assess the relationship between pancreatic exocrine function and the morphology of the pancreatic ducts as ascertained by endoscopic retrograde pancreatography. An example of such work is that of Braganza et al. (1982). They investigated 45 patients with chronic pancreatitis by endoscopic retrograde pancreatography, and the secretin–pancreozymin test combined with serum amylase and lipase levels during the test. Their subjects were 20 patients with alcoholic pancreatitis, four with obstructive pancreatitis due to pancreas divisum or vaterian stenosis, and 21 whose pancreatitis seemed to be idiopathic. Each was assessed as having either advanced or minimal pancreatic changes. They found that in those with advanced disease, when the main pancreatic duct – though dilated and with an occasional stricture – was without calculi, the

secretin–pancreozymin test remained normal. If there were one or two intraductal calculi, there was a fall in the output of bicarbonate but the other secretory constituents remained normal. With more calculi in the ducts, there was a reduction of the volume and concentration of bicarbonate, while in the most advanced cases, with many intraductal calculi and paraductal cysts, there was also a fall in enzyme output. Five of the patients in the last group had steatorrhoea at the time of the study, as well as a profoundly depressed output of enzymes. No correlation was found between the length of the remaining duct and the volume of secretions, peak bicarbonate concentration, post-secretin bicarbonate output, or post-pancreozymin trypsin output.

In the patients with advanced disease, with obstructed ducts but without intraductal calculi, the findings suggested pancreatic cancer rather than chronic pancreatitis.

Carcinoma of the pancreas has been noted as a late sequel of chronic pancreatitis, especially when the pancreatitis is associated with calcification (Paulino-Netto et al. 1960). Calcification commonly develops in the hereditary type of chronic pancreatitis and the risk that carcinoma may become superimposed was pointed out by Logan et al. (1968). This risk has been confirmed by Kattwinkel et al. (1973) and emphasised by Barkin and Fayne (1986).

References

Abrams RM, Kulkarni AV, Beranbaum ER, Santos JS (1969) Aneurysm of the gastroduodenal artery. Br J Radiol 42:384–385

Alapatt JL, Ananthachari MD (1967) A preliminary study of the structure and function of enlarged parotid glands in chronic relapsing pancreatitis by sialography and biopsy methods. Gut 8:42–45

Allison MC, Renfrew CC, Webb WJS, Chappell ME, Pounder RE (1985) Neuroendocrine islet cell tumour producing gastrin and ACTH in a patient with calcifying chronic pancreatitis. Gut 26:426–428

Ammann RW, Hammer B, Fumagalli I (1973) Chronic pancreatitis in Zurich, 1963–1972: clinical findings and follow-up studies of 102 cases. Digestion 9:404–415

Anderson GS, Peebles Brown DA (1959–1960) A case of hydatid cyst of the pancreas. Br J Surg 47:147–149

Appleby EC (1981) Exocrine pancreatic disease. Cited in Cullen GA (1981) Report of meeting of Section of Comparative Medicine. J R Soc Med 74:315–316

Assan R, Boukersi H, Clauser E (1984) Cassava pancreatitis in Western Europe [letter]. Lancet ii:1278

Baggenstoss AH (1973) Pathology of pancreatitis. In: Gambill EE (ed) Pancreatitis. Mosby, St Louis, pp 179–212

Bank S, Marks IN, Farman J, Immelman EJ (1966) Further observations on calcified intramedullary bone lesions in chronic pancreatitis. Gastroenterology 51:224–230

Banting FG, Best CH (1921–1922) The internal secretions of the pancreas. J Lab Clin Med 7:250–266

Banwell JG, Hutt MRS, Leonard PJ et al. (1967) Exocrine pancreatic disease and malabsorption syndrome in tropical Africa. Gut 8:388–401

Barbezat GO, Hansen JDL (1968) The exocrine pancreas and protein calorie malnutrition. Pediatrics (New York) 42:77–92

Barkin JS, Fayne SD (1986) Chronic pancreatitis: update 1986. Mt Sinai J Med 53:404–408

Becker WF, Welsh RA, Pratt HS (1965) Cystadenoma and cystadenocarcinoma of the pancreas. Ann Surg 161:845–863

Bedingfield JA, Anderson MC (1986) Pancreatopleural fistula. Pancreas 1:283–290

Benett I, Sath B, Haboubi NY, Braganza JM (1989) Sclerosing cholangitis with hepatic microvesicular steatosis in cystic fibrosis and chronic pancreatitis. J Clin Pathol 42:466–469

Betuel H, Selman M, Vachon A (1980) Pancréatites chroniques. Liaisons avec les antigènes HLA. Nouvelle Presse Med 9:42

Bivins BA, Sachatello CR, Chuang VP, Brady P (1978) Hemosuccus pancreaticus (hemoductal pancreatitis): gastrointestinal hemorrhage due to rupture of a splenic artery aneurysm into the pancreatic duct. Arch Surg 113:751–753

Blackburn WR, Vinijchaikul K (1969) The pancreas in kwashiorkor: an electron microscopic study. Lab Invest 20:305–318

Blery M, Coulboy J, Graux J-C, Bismuth H (1973) Nécrose de la ratte au cours de la pancréatite chronique. Nouvelle Presse Med 2:915–917

Bockman DE, Kennedy RH, Multingner L, DeCaro A, Sarles H (1986) Fine structure of the organic matrix of human pancreatic stones. Pancreas 1:204–210

Bockman DE, Buchler M, Malfertheiner P, Beger HG (1988) Analysis of nerves in chronic pancreatitis. Gastroenterology 94:1459–1469

Boijsen E, Göthlin J, Hallbröök T, Sandblom P (1969) Preoperative angiographic diagnosis of bleeding aneurysms of abdominal visceral arteries. Radiology 93:781–791

Braganza JM, Hunt LP, Warwick F (1982) Relationship between pancreatic exocrine function and ductal morphology in chronic pancreatitis. Gastroenterology 82:1341–1347

Brantly M, Nukiwa T, Crystal RG (1988) Molecular basis of alpha-1-antitrypsin deficiency. Am J Med 84 (Suppl 6A):13–31

Braunstein H (1961) Tocopherol deficiency in adults with chronic pancreatitis. Gastroenterology 40:224–231

Braxel C, Versieck J, Lemey G, Vanballenberghe L, Barbier F (1982) Alpha-1-antitrypsin in pancreatitis. Digestion 23:93–96

Bretagne J-F, Darnault P, Rasul JL et al. (1987) Calcifying pancreatitis of a congenital short pancreas: a case report with successful endoscopic papillotomy. Am J Gastroenterol 82:1314–1317

Cameron JL (1978) Chronic pancreatic ascites and pancreatic pleural effusions. Gastroenterology 74:134–140

Chevallier B, Cavelier B, Martin J-P, Rivat-Péran L, Signoret C, Colin R (1982) Pancréatite chronique familiale: étude génétique dans deux familles. Gastroenterol Clin Biol 6:596–597

Comfort MW, Gambill EE, Baggenstoss AH (1946) Chronic relapsing pancreatitis. A study of twenty-nine cases without associated disease of the biliary or gastrointestinal tract. Gastroenterology 6:239–285, 376–408

Corbeau A, Sahel J, Fraissinet R, Courjaret P, Burelle H, Clement JP (1978) Pancreatic duct hemorrhage: diagnosis by angiography. J Radiol Electrol Med Nucl 59:275–278

Cramer SF, Bruns DE ((1979) Amylase-producing ovarian neoplasm with pseudo-Meig's syndrome and elevated pleural fluid amylase. Cancer 44:1715–1721

Davidson ED, Horney JT, Satter PP (1979) Internal pancreatic fistula to the pericardium and pleura. Surgery 85:478–480

Davies JNP (1948) The essential pathology of kwashiorkor. Lancet

i:317–320

Di Magno E, Clain JE (1986) Chronic pancreatitis. In: Go VLW, Gardner JD, Brooks FP, Di Magno E, Scheele GA (eds) The exocrine pancreas: biology, pathobiology, and disease. Raven Press, New York, pp 541–575

Donowitz M, Kerstein MD, Spiro HM (1974) Pancreatic ascites. Medicine (Baltimore) 53:183–195

Dreiling DA (1959) Cystadenocarcinoma of the pancreas in a patient with long-standing chronic relapsing pancreatitis and pancreatic calcinosis. J Mt Sinai Hosp 26:589–593

Edmondson HA, Bullock WK, Mehl JW (1950) Chronic pancreatitis and lithiasis: II. Pathology and pathogenesis of pancreatic lithiasis. Am J Pathol 26:37–55

Epstein O, Lake-Bakaar G, Mckavanagh S, Sherlock S (1980) Pancreatic hyposecretion in primary biliary cirrhosis (PBC) – a "dry-gland" disease. Gut 21:A448–449

Fonseca V, Epstein O, Katrak A et al. (1986) Serum immunoreactive trypsin and pancreatic lipase in primary biliary cirrhosis. J Clin Pathol 39:638–640

Förström L, Winkelmann RK (1975) Acute generalized panniculitis with amylase and lipase in skin. Arch Dermatol 111:497–502

Fox JN, Mosley JG, Vogler GA, Austin JL, Reber HA (1981) Pancreatic function in domestic cats with pancreatic fluke infection. J Am Vet Assoc 178:58–60

Gambill EE (1971) Pancreatitis associated with pancreatic carcinoma: a study of 26 cases. Mayo Clin Proc 46:174–177

Gambill EE, Pugh DG (1948) Pancreatic calcification: study of clinical and roentgenologic data on thirty-nine cases. Arch Intern Med 81:301–315

Gardner RJ, Preston FW (1961) Rupture of the spleen associated with pancreatitis. JAMA 177:784–785

Geevarghese PJ (1968) Pancreatitis diabetes. Bombay, Popular Prakasham. Cited by Sarles H, Sahel J, Staub JL, Bourry J, Laugier R (1979) Chronic pancreatitis. In: Howat HT, Sarles H (eds) The exocrine pancreas. Saunders, London, pp 402–439

Genell SN, Fork F-T, Jiborn H (1987) Bronchobiliary fistula in chronic pancreatitis. Acta Chir Scand 153:473–475

Gerle RD, Walker LA, Achord JL, Weens HS (1965) Osseous changes in chronic pancreatitis. Radiology 85:330–337

Gettenberg G, Zimbalist E, Marini C (1988) Chronic pancreatitis and pseudocyst formation secondary to carcinoid tumour of the pancreas. Gastroenterology 94:1222–1224

Giorgi D, Bernard J-P, Rouquier S, Iovanna J, Sarles H, Dagorn J-C (1989) Secretory pancreatic stone protein messenger RNA: nucleotide sequence and expression in chronic calcifying pancreatitis. J Clin Invest 84:100–106

Glinsky NH, Lewis JW, Flueck JA, Fried AM (1987) Annular pancreas associated with diffuse chronic pancreatitis. Am J Gastroenterol 82:681–684

Gosselin M, Fauchet R, Genetet B, Gastard J (1978) Les antigènes HLA dans la pancréatite chronique alcoolique. Gastroenterol Clin Biol 2:883–886

Guien C (1979) Radiological examination of the pancreas. In: Howat HT, Sarles H (eds) The exocrine pancreas. Saunders, London, pp 176–226

Gullo L, Costa PL, Labo G (1977) Chronic pancreatitis in Italy: aetiological, clinical and histological observations based on 253 cases. Rendic Gastroenterol 9:97–104

Gullo L, Tabacci PL, Corazza GR, Calanca F, Campione O, Labo G (1982) HLA-B13 and chronic calcific pancreatitis Dig Dis Sci 27:214–216

Gyr KE, Singer MV, Sarles H (eds) (1984) Pancreatitis – concepts and classification. Second International Symposium on the classification of pancreatitis. Marseilles, 28–30 March 1984. Elsevier, Amsterdam, pp XIX–XXV

Haboubi NY, Ali HH, Braganza JM (1986) Altered liver histology in patients with pancreatitis: a clue to etiology? Mt Sinai J Med

53:380–388

Haggard WD, Kirtley JA (1939) Pancreatic calculi: a review of sixty-five operative and one hundred thirty-nine non-operative cases. Ann Surg 109:809–824

Hanefeld F, Sperner J, Rating D, Rausch H, Kaufmann HJ (1984) Renal and pancreatic calcification during treatment of infantile spasms with ACTH [letter]. Lancet i:901

Harper PC, Gamelli RL, Kaye MD (1984) Recurrent haemorrhage into the pancreatic duct from a splenic artery aneurysm. Gastroenterology 87:417–420

Harris RD, Anderson JE, Coel MN (1975) Aneurysms of the small pancreatic arteries: a cause of upper abdominal pain and intestinal bleeding. Radiology 115:17–20

Heitz PU, Klöppel G (1984) Pathomorphologyof pancreatitis. In: Gyr KE, Singer H, Sarles H (eds) Pancreatitis - concepts and classification. Elsevier, Amsterdam, pp 83–85

Henderson JT, Warwick RRG, Simpson JD, Shearman DJC (1972) Does malabsorption of vitamin B_{12} occur in chronic pancreatitis? Lancet ii:241–243

Hendrick JW (1965) Treatment of aneurysm of the pancreaticoduodenal artery by excision. Ann Surg 144:1051–1053

Hepp J, Tourneur R, Moreaux J (1959) Les lésions du pancréas confrontées aux les downées de la pancréatographie dans les pancréatites chroniques calcifiantes. Nouvelle Presse Med 67:1275–1278

Hotz J, Goebell H, Herforth C, Probst M (1977) Massive pancreatic ascites without carcinoma: report of three cases. Digestion 15:200–216

Hoyos N, Shaffer B, Beerman H (1966) Liquefying nodular panniculitis. Arch Dermatol 94:436–439

Hughes PSH, Apisarnthanarax P, Mullins F (1975) Sub-cutaneous fat necrosis associated with pancreatic disease. Arch Dermatol 111:506–510

Hutchinson DCS (1988) Natural history of alpha-1-protease inhibitor deficiency. Am J Med 84 (Suppl 6A):3–12

Immelman EJ, Banks S, Krige H, Marks IN (1964) Roentgenologic and clinical features of intramedullary fat necrosis in bones in acute and chronic pancreatitis. Am J Med 36:96–105

Ingram DM, Sheiner HJ (1980) Massive pancreatic serous effusions. Aust N Z J Surg 50:137–140

Jalleh RP, Gilbertson JA, Williamson RCN, Foster CS (1992) Immunohistochemical evidence for autoimmunity in chronic pancreatitis [abstract]. J Pathol 167 (Suppl):104A

Johnson JR, Zintel HA (1963) Pancreatic calcification and cancer of the pancreas. Surg Gynecol Obstet 117:585–588

Kadell BM, Riley JM (1967) Major arterial involvement by pancreatic pseudocysts. AJR 99:632–635

Kattan YB (1975) Hydatid cysts in pancreas. Br Med J iv:729–730

Kattwinkel J, Lapry A, di Sant'Agnese PA, Edwards WA, Hufty MP (1973) Hereditary pancreatitis: three new kindreds and a critical review of the literature. Pediatrics 51:55–69

Keith RG, Mustard RA, Saibil EA (1982) Gastric variceal bleeding due to occlusion of splenic vein in pancreatic disease. Can J Surg 25:301–304

Kelley HG, Knoernschild HE, Marable SA (1964) Aneurysms of the pancreaticoduodenal arteries. Am J Surg 107:644–646

Kirshbaum JD, Shure N (1942–1943) Alcoholic cirrhosis of the liver: a clinical and pathologic study of 356 fatal cases selected from 12 267 cases. J Lab Clin Med 28:721–731

Lambert MA, Linehan JP, Russell RCG (1987) Duodenum-preserving total pancreatectomy for end stage chronic pancreatitis. Br J Surg 74:35–39

Leger L, Detrie P, Guyet-Rousset P (1961) Cancer et lithiase du pancréas. Nouvelle Presse Med 69:386–388

Lendrum R, Walker G (1975) Serum antibodies in human pancreatic disease. Gut 16:365–371

Little JM, Stephen M, Hogg J (1979) Duct obstruction with an acrylate glue for treatment of chronic alcoholic pancreatitis.

Lancet ii:557–558

Lloyd-Jones W, Mountain JE, Warred KW (1972) Annular pancreas in the adult. Ann Surg 176:163–170

Logan A, Schlicke CP, Manning GB (1968) Familial pancreatitis. Am J Surg 115:112–117

Lowes JR, Rode J, Lees WR, Russell RC, Cotton PB (1988) Obstructive pancreatitis: unusual causes of chronic pancreatitis. Br J Surg 75:1129–1133

Ludwig H, Schernthaner G, Scherak O, Kolarz G (1977) Antibodies to pancreatic duct cells in Sjögren's syndrome and rheumatoid arthritis. Gut 18:311–315

Lung JA, Schow PD, Knight L (1980) Splenic artery aneurysm–pancreatic duct fistula. Am J Surg 139:430–431

Mainwaring R, Kern J, Schenk WG, Rudolf LE (1989) Differentiating pancreatic pseudocyst and pancreatic necrosis using computerized tomography. Ann Surg 209:562–568

Marks IN, Bank S, Louw JH (1968) Diagnosis and management of pancreatitis. In: Glass GBJ (ed) Progress in gastroenterology, vol 1. Grune and Stratton, New York, pp 412–472

Marks IN, Bank S, Louw JH (1973) Chronic pancreatitis in the Western Cape. Digestion 9:447–453

Martin A, Canseco JD (1947) Pancreatic calculosis. JAMA 135:1055–1060

Martin FM, Rossi RL, Munson JL, ReMine SG, Braasch JW (1989) Management of pancreatic fistulas. Arch Surg 124:571–573

Mayo JG (1936) Pancreatic calculi. Proc Mayo Clinic 11:456–457

McElroy R, Christiansen PA (1972) Hereditary pancreatitis in a kinship associated with portal vein thrombosis. Am J Med 52:228–241

Meller S, Stone NN, Waxman JS, Goodman A (1988) Bilateral ureteral necrosis and obliteration secondary to a pancreatic pseudocyst. J Urol 140:1523–1525

Mihas AA, Hirschowitz BI (1976) Alpha-1-antitrypsin and chronic pancreatitis. Lancet ii:1032–1033

Miller P (1988) Kerala, jewel of India's Malabar coast. Nat Geogr Mag 173:592–617

Montalto G, Multigner L, Sarles H, DeCaro A (1988) Organic matrix of pancreatic stones associated with nutritional pancreatitis. Pancreas 3:263–268

Moreaux J, Bismuth H (1969) Les complications splenique des pancréatites chroniques. A propos de 5 observations. Nouvelle Presse Med 77:1467–1471

Munn J, Altergolt R, Prinz RA (1987) Calcified pancreatic pseudocysts. Surgery 101:511–513

Murray MJ, Thal AP (1960) The clinical significance of circulating pancreatic antibodies. Ann Intern Med 53:548–555

Nagai H, Ohtsubo K (1984) Pancreatic lithiasis in the aged. Gastroenterology 86:331–338

Nagata A, Homma T, Tamai K et al. (1981) A study of chronic pancreatitis by serial endoscopic pancreatography. Gastroenterology 81:884–891

Nakamura K, Sarles H, Payan H (1972) Three dimensional reconstruction of the pancreatic ducts in chronic pancreatitis. Gastroenterology 62:942–949

Nealon WH, Townsend CM, Thompson JC (1989) Preoperative endoscopic retrograde cholangiopancreatography (ERCP) in patients with pancreatic pseudocyst associated with resolving acute and chronic pancreatitis. Ann Surg 209:532–540

Ng WD, Chan YT, Fung H (1987) Recurrent pancreatitis contributing to choledochal cyst formation. Br J Surg 74:206–208

Nishiyama T, Iwoa N, Myose H et al. (1986) Splenic vein thrombosis as a consequence of chronic pancreatitis: a study of three cases. Am J Gastroenterol 81:1193–1198

Novis BH, Bank S, Young GO, Marks IN (1975) Chronic pancreatitis and alpha-1-antitrypsin. Lancet ii:748–749

Ogden WW, Bradburn DM, Rives JD (1965) Mesenteric panniculitis: review of 27 cases. Ann Surg 161:864–875

Ogilvie CM, Parry EW, Murray GH (1972) Pancreatitis and basal emphyema. Br Med J iv: 610–611

Ogilvie RF (1940–1941) Duodenal diverticula and their complications with particular reference to acute pancreatic necrosis. Br J Surg 28: 362–379

Olurin EO, Olurin O (1969) Pancreatic calcification: a report of 45 cases. Br Med J iv: 534–539

Opie EL (1902) The causes and varieties of chronic interstitial pancreatitis. Am J Med Sci 123: 845–868

Opie EL (1910) Disease of the pancreas, 2nd edn. Lippincott, Philadelphia, p 258

Owens JL, Howard JM (1958) Pancreatic calcification: a late sequel in the natural history of chronic alcoholism and alcoholic pancreatitis. Ann Surg 147: 326–338

Paulino-Netto A, Dreiling DA, Baronofsky ID (1960) The relationship between pancreatic calcification and cancer of the pancreas. Ann Surg 151: 530–537

Pitchumoni CS, Thomas EL (1973) Chronic cassava toxicity: possible relationship to chronic pancreatic disease in malnourished populations. Lancet ii: 1397–1398

Pitchumoni CS, Scheele G, Lee PC, Lebenthal E (1986) Effects of nutrition on the exocrine pancreas. In: Go VLW, Gardner JD, Brooks FP, Lebenthal E, Di Magno EP, Scheele GA (eds) The exocrine pancreas: biology, pathobiology, and diseases. Raven Press, New York, pp 387–406

Pittelkow MR, Smith KC, Su WDP (1988) Alpha-1-antitrypsin deficiency and panniculitis: perspectives on disease relationship and replacement therapy. Am J Med 84 (Suppl 6A): 80–86

Pottmeyer EW, Frey CF, Matsuno S (1987) Pancreaticopleural fistulas. Arch Surg 122: 648–654

Potts DE, Mass MF, Iseman MD (1975) Syndrome of pancreatic disease, subcutaneous fat necrosis and polyserositis. Am J Med 58: 417–423

Prost A, Hanniche M, Bordier P, Miravet L, de Sèze S, Rambaud JC (1975) Ostéomalacie et pancréatite chronique associées. Cinq observations. Nouvelle Presse Med 4: 1561–1567

Rambaud JCL, Bordier PH, Rautureau M et al (1970) Ostéomalacie pancréatite chronique et syndrome l'anse stagnante. Nouvelle Presse Med 78: 835–839

Robson AWM (1904) The pathology and surgery of certain diseases of the pancreas. Lancet i: 845–854

Rode J, Dowsett J, Russell RCG (1988) The annular pancreas derives from the ventral primordium [abstract]. J Pathol 155: 351A

Roesch W, Gebhardt C (1981) Endoscopic duct obstruction in severe chronic pancreatitis. Gastrointest Endosc 27: 49–51

Rogers HM, Keating FR, Morlock CG, Barker NW (1947) Primary hypertrophy and hyperplasia of the parathyroid glands associated with duodenal ulcer. Arch Intern Med 79: 307–321

Rohrmann CA, Surawicz CM, Hutchinson D, Silverstein FE, White TT, Marchioro TL (1981) The diagnosis of hereditary pancreatitis by pancreatography. Gastrointest Endosc 27: 168–173

Rose NR, Metzgar RS, Witebsky E (1960) Studies on organ specificity: XI. Iso-antigens of rabbit pancreas. J Immunol 85: 575–587

Sachs M, Partington P (1956) Cholangiographic diagnosis of pancreatitis. AJR 76: 32–38

Salm R (1960) Scirrhous adenocarcinoma arising in a lipomatous pseudohypertrophic pancreas. J Pathol Bacteriol 79: 47–52

Sarles H (ed) (1965) Pancreatitis. Symposium, Marseilles, 25–26 April 1963. Karger, Basel, pp 1–20

Sarles H (1984) Epidemiology and physiopathology of chronic pancreatitis and the role of pancreatic stone protein. Clin Gastroenterol 13: 895–912

Sarles H (1986) Chronic pancreatitis: etiology and pathophysiology. In: Go VLW, Gardner JD, Brooks FP, Lebenthal E, Di Magno FP, Scheele GA (eds) The exocrine pancreas: biology, pathobiology and diseases. Raven Press, New York, pp 527–540

Sarles H, Gerolami-Santandrea A (1972) Chronic pancreatitis. Clin Gastroenterol 1: 167–193

Sarles H, Sarles J-C, Camatte R et al. (1965) Observations on 205 confirmed cases of acute pancreatitis, recurring pancreatitis, and chronic pancreatitis. Gut 6: 545–559

Sarles H, Sahel J, Staub JL, Bourry J, Laugier R (1979) Chronic pancreatitis. In: Howat HT, Sarles H (eds) The exocrine pancreas. Saunders, London, pp 402–439

Sarles H, Figarella C, Tiscornia O et al. (1980) Chronic calcifying pancreatitis (CCP): mechanism of formation of the lesions. New data and critical study. In: Fitzgerald RJ, Morrison AB (eds) The pancreas. Williams and Wilkins, Baltimore, pp 48–66

Sarles H, De Caro A, Multigner L, Martin E (1982) Giant pancreatic stones in teetotal women due to the absence of the "stone protein". Lancet ii: 714–715

Sarles J-C, Pietri H, Sarles H (1965) La lymphographie dans les pancréatites. Nouvelle Presse Med 73: 2885–2888

Schmiegel W-H, Burchert M, Kalthoff H et al. (1986) Pancreatic stone protein in serum of patients with pancreatitis. Lancet ii: 686–687

Schmitz-Moorman P, Himmelmann GW, Brandes H-J et al. (1984) Quantative assessment of pancreatitis-like lesions in humans without pancreatic disease. In: Gyr KE, Singer MV, Sarles H (eds) Pancreatitis - concepts and classification. Elsevier, Amsterdam, pp 83–85

Schuyler MR, Rynbrandt DJ, Kleinerman J (1978) Physiologic and morphologic observations of the effects of intravenous elastase on the lung. Am Rev Respir Dis 117: 97–102

Scott J, Summerfield JA, Elias E, Dick R, Sherlock S (1977) Chronic pancreatitis: a cause of cholestasis. Gut 18: 196–201

Shaper AG (1960) Chronic pancreatic disease and protein malnutrition. Lancet i: 1223–1224

Shaper AG (1964) Aetiology of chronic pancreatic fibrosis with calcification. Br Med J i: 1607–1609

Shattock SG (1896) Calculi of calcium oxalate from pancreatic cyst. Br Med J i: 1034–1035

Smith FB, Cooke RT (1940) Acute fatal hyperparathyroidism. Lancet ii: 650–651

Stahl TJ, Allen MO'C, Ansel HJ, Vennes JA (1988) Partial biliary obstruction caused by chronic pancreatitis. Ann Surg 207: 26–32

Stobbe KC, Re Mine WH, Baggenstoss AH (1970) Pancreatic lithiasis. Surg Gynecol Obstet 131: 1090–1099

Stockwell T, Stirling L (1989) Estimating alcohol content of drinks: common errors in applying the unit system. Br Med J 298: 571–572

Sugawa C, Walt AJ (1979) Endoscopic retrograde pancreatography in the surgery of pancreatic pseudocysts. Surgery 86: 639–647

Thakker RV, Gajjar B, Wilkins RA, Levi AJ (1983) Embolisation of gastroduodenal artery aneurysm caused by chronic pancreatitis. Gut 24: 1094–1098

Trowell HC, Davies JNP, Dean RFA (1954) Kwashiorkor. Arnold, London, pp 122–162

Tucker DH, Moore IB (1963) Vanishing pancreatic calcification in chronic pancreatitis: a sign of pancreatic carcinoma. N Engl J Med 268: 31–33

Turrill FL, Mikkelsen WP (1969) Sinistral (left-sided) extrahepatic portal hypertension. Arch Surg 99: 365–368

Véghelyi PV, Kemény TT, Pozsonyi J, Sòs J (1950) Dietary lesions of the pancreas. Am J Dis Child 79: 658–665

Volk W, Wellmann KF (1977) Idiopathic diabetes. In: Volk BW, Wellmann KF (eds) The diabetic pancreas. Baillière Tindall, London, pp 231–260

Waldram R, Kopelman H, Tsantoulas D, Williams R (1975) Chronic pancreatitis, sclerosing cholangitis, and sicca complex in two siblings. Lancet i: 550–552

Walter JF, Chuang VP, Bookstein JJ, Reuter SR, Cho KJ, Pulmano CM (1977) Angiography of massive hemorrhage secondary to pancreatic disease. Radiology 124:337–342

Warshaw AL, Schapiro RH, Ferruci JT, Galdabini JJ (1976) Persistent obstructive jaundice, cholangitis, and biliary cirrhosis due to common bile duct stenosis in chronic pancreatitis. Gastroenterology 70:562–567

Weinstein BR, Korn RJ, Zimmerman HJ (1963) Obstructive jaundice as a complication of pancreatitis. Ann Intern Med 58:245–258

Whaley K, Webb J, McAvoy B et al. (1973) Pancreatic disease and Sjögren's syndrome. Q J Med N Ser 42:513–548

White AF, Baum S, Buranasiri S (1976) Aneurysms secondary to pancreatitis. AJR 127:393–396

Wilson C, Auld CD, Schlinkert R et al. (1989) Hepatobiliary complications in chronic pancreatitis. Gut 30:520–527

Wilson JR, Du Bois RO (1923) Report of a fatal case of keratomalacia in an infant, with postmortem examination. Am J Dis Child 26:431–446

Winton TL, Birchard R, Nguyen KT, Taguchi K (1986) Esophageal obstruction secondary to a mediastinal pancreatic pseudocyst. Can J Surg 29:376–377

Wirts WJ, Snape WJ (1947) Disseminated calcification of the pancreas: subacute and chronic pancreatitis. Am J Med Sci 213:290–299

Witebsky E, Rose NR, Nadel H (1960) Studies on organ specificity: X. The serologic specificity of pancreas extracts. J Immunol 85:568–574

Woods CA, Foutch PG, Waring JP, Sanowski RA (1989) Pancreatic pseudocyst as a cause for secondary achalasia. Gastroenterology 96:235–239

Yadegar J, Williams RA, Passaro E, Wilson SE (1980) Common duct stricture from chronic pancreatitis. Arch Surg 115:582–586

Yeo CJ, Bastidas JA, Schmieg RE et al. (1989) Pancreatic structure and glucose tolerance in a longitudinal study of experimental pancreatitis-induced diabetes. Ann Surg 210:150–158

Zuidema PJ (1959) Cirrhosis and disseminated calcification of the pancreas in patients with malnutrition. Trop Geogr Med 11:70–74

14 Bacterial, Granulomatous, Viral and Parasitic Lesions of the Pancreas

Pancreatic Abscess

Primary bacterial inflammation of the pancreas is rare, but if acute pancreatitis has caused necrosis of a part of the pancreas, or if a pseudocyst has been formed, bacterial infection may convert the necrotic tissue or the pseudocyst into an abscess. The origin of the organisms, and the route by which they reach the pancreas, may vary from patient to patient, and may included blood-borne infection, lymphatic or direct spread from the colon or infection from the biliary tract. Direct penetration of the wall of the transverse colon by its normal bacterial flora is the most probable route; intestinal organisms are those that are most commonly identified in pus from pancreatic abscesses. A mixture of organisms was present in 13 of the 32 pancreatic abscesses studied by Altemeier and Alexander (1963). No staphylococcal infection was present in the pancreatic abscesses reported by Evans (1969), but staphylococci were found in 12 of Altemeier and Alexander's cases, and in eight of the 60 positive bacterial cultures obtained from pancreatic abscesses by Bolooki et al. (1968). The source of these infections may not have been the intestine. *Candida albicans* has been reported as the cause of abscesses of the pancreas by various authors. Such reports have been reviewed by Richter et al. (1982), who added two patients of their own, in which *C. albicans*, without accompanying bacteria, was isolated from the pus drained from abscesses that had complicated acute pancreatitis. One of the patients recovered after antifungal chemotherapy, but the other, who was treated with antibiotics but received no antifungal therapy, died after a fulminating illness during which there were repeated episodes of haemorrhage from the abscess cavity.

Salmonella Infections

Before there was any specific therapy for typhoid fever, suppurative parotitis was a well-known complication of this disease, but pancreatitis appears to have been a very rare complication. A few reports of single cases, published in French journals, and in a Polish journal, are referred to by Russell et al. (1976), who reported the case history of a woman with typhoid fever in whom enzyme studies indicated that the pancreas was inflamed. The authors were uncertain whether the pancreatitis had contributed significantly to the patient's symptoms, all of which could have been attributed to uncomplicated typhoid fever, but they suggested that, as pancreatic enzyme studies are not ordinarily carried out in typhoid fever, unsuspected pancreatic inflammation may be responsible for the persistent abdominal discomfort experienced by some patients. Pancreatitis, as indicated by abdominal pain, a computed tomographic scan of the abdomen, and raised serum pancreatic enzyme levels, has been reported by Hearne et al. (1989) during the course of typhoid fever. In their patient there was also biochemical evidence of typhoid hepatitis.

A pancreatic abscess from which *Salmonella typhi* was cultured was reported by Kune and Coster (1972). Their patient was a woman, aged 47, in

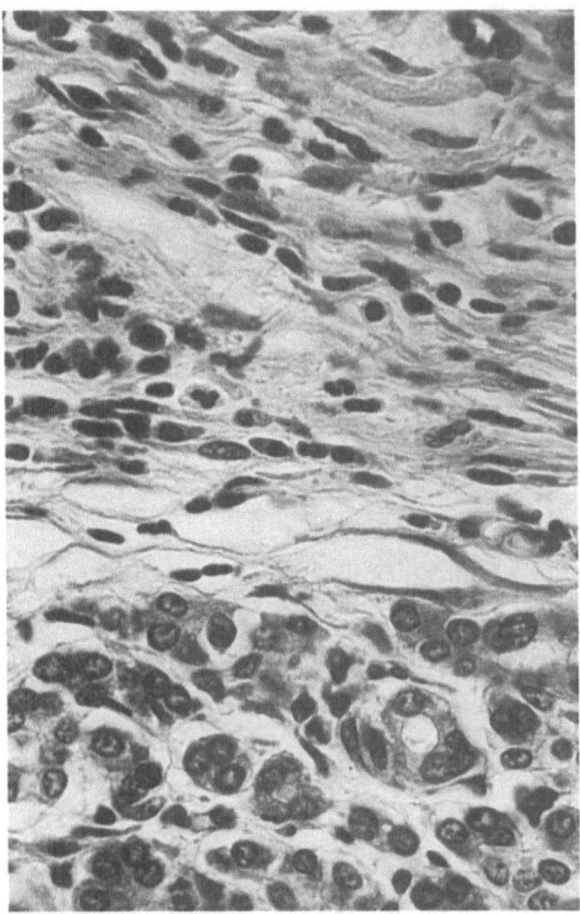

Fig. 14.1. Interstitial pancreatitis in a fatal case of *S. typhimurium* colitis. The interstitial tissue looks oedematous and is infiltrated by plasma cells with occasional polymorphonuclear cells. (Courtesy of Dr J.F. Boyd, Ruckhill Hospital, Glasgow) H&E, × 600

ascended the ducts; it was attributed by the author to bacterial (endotoxic) shock (Fig. 14.1).

Mild to moderate pancreatitis, as indicated by raised serum amylase and lipase, was diagnosed by Renner et al. (1991) in several of 16 patients with *S. typhimurium* enteritis and in 22 of 31 patients with *S. enteritidis* enteritis. Such a high frequency of concomitant pancreatitis was certainly not the experience of Murphy et al. (1991), who found a slightly elevated serum amylase level in only one of their many patients with salmonella infection.

Yersiniosis as a Possible Cause of Pancreatitis

Primary yersiniosis usually occurs as an acute abdominal disturbance, which may be followed 1–3 weeks later by a reactive phase in which skin rashes with pains in muscles and joints may be important symptoms. Lindholdt and Hansen (1985) reported the case of a young woman who had symptoms that suggested acute appendicitis, but whose appendix was uninflamed when it was removed, although the terminal ileum was noted during the appendicectomy to be hyperaemic. Five days later, the patient developed acute pancreatitis with marked elevation of the serum amylase and ultrasonic enlargement of the pancreas. At this time, stool culture yielded *Yersinia enterocolitica* type 3 and the yersinia agglutinin titres rose from 300 to 12 800. An uncharacteristic rash appeared on the extensor surfaces of her limbs and the authors made the suggestion that her pancreatitis might be a manifestation of the reactive phase of yersiniosis. The patient made a slow recovery after conservative treatment of her pancreatitis combined with tetracycline therapy. The authors referred to two previously reported patients in whom acute pancreatitis had coincided with the reactive phase of yersinosis.

whom severe acute pancreatitis was complicated by a pancreatic abscess that was drained 17 days after the onset of the illness. The gall bladder, which contained stones, was removed during the operation to drain the abscess. *S. typhi* was grown from the gallstones as well as from the pus and necrotic material from the abscess. The authors suggested that their patient was a chronic typhoid carrier who harboured typhoid bacilli in her biliary tract, and developed acute pancreatitis due to reflux of salmonella-containing bile, with the later development of a typhoid abscess in the necrotic pancreatic tissue.

What has been described as "a subtle diffuse acute interstitial pancreatitis" has been reported by Boyd (1969) in association with colitis due to *S. typhimurium*. This was found in four fatal cases and did not appear to be due to infection that had

Acute Pancreatitis Associated with *Campylobacter* Infection

Gallagher et al. (1981) reported a patient in whom acute pancreatitis coincided with infection by *Campylobacter coli/jejuni*. A young woman was thought to have appendicitis, but her symptoms included lower right-sided backache. At operation, the appendix and the lower abdominal organs looked normal. Her pain continued after the appendix had been removed, she was febrile and there was marked elevation of the serum amylase. Stool cultures grew *C. coli/jejuni* and there was a rise in serum complement-fixing antibody to these organisms. The patient recovered spontaneously.

Two years later, Pitkänen et al. (1983) reported that 11 hospital patients in their series of 188 with campylobacter enteritis, had pancreatitis as indicated by elevated serum amylase or lipase values.

Acute Haemorrhagic Pancreatitis Complicating Legionnaire's Disease

An example of this complication has been reported by Bollaert et al. (1986).

Syphilitic Pancreatitis

Acquired syphilis of the pancreas was rare even before effective anti-syphilitic treatment became available. Thus Schlesinger, writing in 1898, could refer only to a few examples of the condition that had been published up to that time. He referred, for example, to syphilitic induration of the pancreas with gummata in a 43-year-old man, which had been published by Schlagenhaufen in 1895, and stated that Petersen had found only one diseased pancreas in a series of 88 autopsies upon subjects with tertiary syphilis. Simmonds (1921) undertook an investigation into the question of whether syphilitic disease of the pancreas might be important in the aetiology of diabetes mellitus. Among 300 cases of diabetes that came to autopsy he found only three in which residual damage in the pancreas might have been the result of syphilis.

A more recent case of syphilis of the pancreas was described by Stürmer and Becker (1987) in their study of 34 cases of granulomatous pancreatitis. The patient was a 36-year-old man who had his pancreas resected by the Whipple procedure because an ultrasonic examination had shown an echo-poor space-occupying lesion, 4.5–5.0 cm in diameter, in the gland, and a percutaneous fine needle biopsy had failed to indicate a diagnosis. The man had had recurrent diffuse upper abdominal pain with severe diarrhoea and he had high-grade cholestasis. On histological examination, there was dense perilobu-

lar and intralobular fibrosis in the head of the gland, with numerous granulomas of epithelioid cells and giant cells of the Langhans type. Some of the granulomas were closely related to segmentally narrowed arteries and arterioles. The surrounding fibrous tissue was sparsely infiltrated by round cells and numerous plasma cells, and there was a peripheral margin of densely packed fibroblasts. Granulomas were also found in the mucosa of the body of the stomach and in the submucosa of the duodenal bulb. The histological diagnosis of tertiary syphilitic pancreatitis was confirmed by positive specific serological tests.

In congenital syphilis, the pancreas is involved in about 20% of affected newborns (Hurst 1934). The pancreatic lesions are of little clinical importance in that they are found in stillborn infants, or in premature babies that die soon after birth, and are only a component of a general disease that involves many organs, of which bones, lungs, spleen and liver are more commonly affected than the pancreas. The pancreatic lesions of congenital syphilis were recognised first by Birch-Hirschfeld in 1875. He found that the pancreas was affected in 13 of 23 cases of congenital syphilis, an unusually high incidence, for Opie (1900–1901) found pancreatic lesions in only 29 of 124 syphilitic newborn infants. Schlesinger (1898) made a detailed study of six cases and described a diffuse interstitial pancreatitis in which inflammatory fibrous tissue infiltrated the interlobular and interacinar areas, penetrating in some places between the cells of the acini. He believed that the increase of the interstitial tissue originated about the blood vessels, the arteries in particular being affected by a syphilitic periarteritis, indicated by lymphocytic infiltration of their adventitial coats. The increase of interstitial tissues was associated with atrophy of the acinar cells and loss of the periacinar capillary network, but without atrophy of the islets of Langerhans.

The apparent preservation of the islets aroused the interest of Opie (1900–1901), who himself described the pancreatic lesions in two babies who had died of neonatal congenital syphilis. In one, in addition to atrophy and fibrous replacement of the acini, there was marked infiltration by plasma cells and eosinophils, while in the other, though interstitial tissue was more abundant, and the parenchymatous elements more scattered, lymphocytes were scanty and plasma cells and eosinophils almost absent. The second infant was somewhat more mature, being 10 cm longer than the first, and Opie suggested that the process in its pancreas was more advanced and less active. A feature of both babies was the presence of numerous islets of Langerhans surrounded by newly formed stroma.

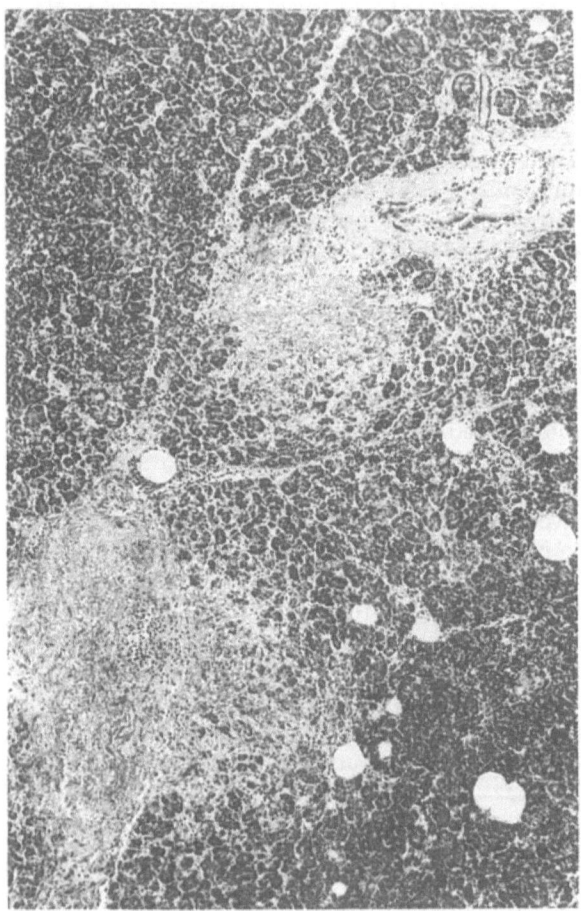

Fig. 14.2. Necrotic miliary tubercles in the pancreas in generalised miliary tuberculosis. H&E, × 60

The islets of Langerhans in congenital syphilis of the pancreas received special study by Pearce (1903), who mentioned incidentally that, in one of the ten specimens in his collection, miliary gummata were present in the pancreas. Gummata, apparently the usual manifestation of acquired syphilis in the pancreas, are most unusual in congenital syphilitic pancreatitis (Schlesinger 1898; Raeburn 1951). Raeburn described a congenital gumma of the pancreas in a premature infant, delivered during the 32nd week of pregnancy, who died on the seventh day after birth in spite of treatment with penicillin. The head of the pancreas contained a hard fibrous mass, 2.5 cm in diameter, spherical and adhering to the duodenum. On section, the mass contained loculi of necrotic, semi-purulent greenish-white material. The body and tail of the pancreas were fibrotic. Raeburn's short communication contains both macroscopic and microscopic illustrations of the lesion. His description states that the areas of necrosis were surrounded by a cellular reaction that included neutrophil leucocytes mixed with plasma cells, lymphocytes, and occasional small multinucleated cells. The process was walled off by dense collagenous tissue in which there were a few miliary gummata and scanty glandular elements. Numerous spirochaetes were demonstrated at the periphery of the necrotic zone.

A more recent example of congenital syphilitic pancreatitis is illustrated by Wigglesworth (1984), who described a foetus of 27 weeks' gestation; there was conspicuous increase in the interacinar connective tissue, with separation of the acini into groups, and infiltration by lymphocytes, plasma cells and macrophages.

Tuberculosis

The pancreas appears to be relatively resistant to tuberculosis and many appear almost unaffected when there is advanced tuberculous disease of the adjacent mesenteric lymph nodes or peritoneum. In generalised miliary tuberculosis, too, when the disease has been disseminated by the blood stream, it seems that is is only occasionally that tubercle bacilli can establish themselves in the pancreas and cause lesions. Thus, Auerbach (1944) found miliary tuberculous foci in the pancreas in only 14 of 297 cases of generalised miliary tuberculosis, an incidence of 4.7%. Small necrotic tubercles in the pancreas of a woman who died of disseminated miliary tuberculosis are illustrated in Figs 14.2–14.4. Although acid-fast bacilli were abundant in the lesions of many of the other organs, no bacilli were found in Ziehl–Neelsen preparations of the pancreas.

A tuberculous abscess of the pancreas has been described by Stambler et al. (1982), who undertook a computer-directed search of the world literature for the previous 15 years and could find no reports of a similar localised tuberculous pancreatic abscess, although they were able to find case reports of tuberculosis of the pancreas that had caused pancreatic and biliary obstruction, or either acute or chronic pancreatitis.

In spite of such rarity, a number of other cases of tuberculous abscess of the pancreas have since been reported, for example by Crowson et al. (1984), de Miguel et al. (1985), Kitai et al. (1987) and Ibrahim et al. (1987). The accounts of such cases indicate that this unusual type of tuberculosis is liable to occur in communities where tuberculosis is still common, and that clinical resemblances to a pyogenic type of

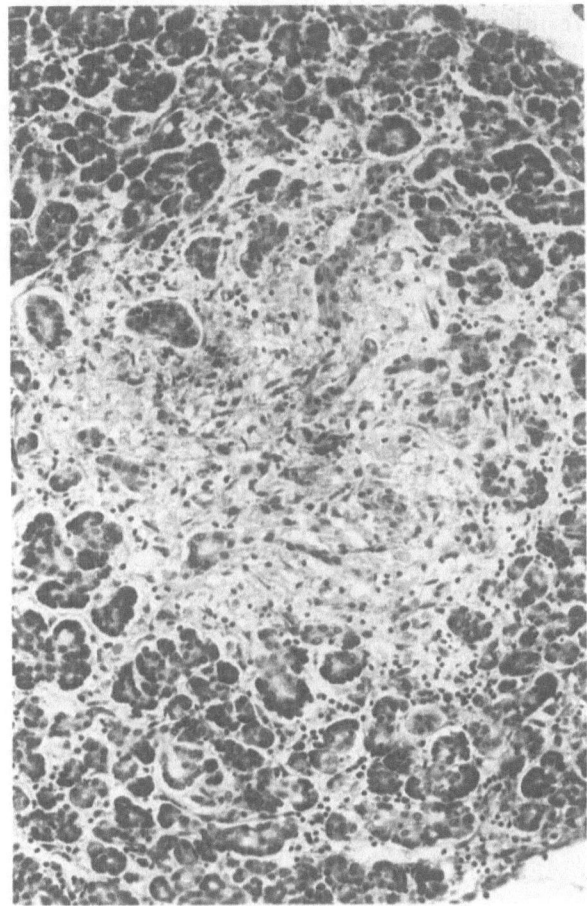

Fig. 14.3. A miliary tubercle without necrosis in the pancreas shown in Fig. 14.2. H&E, × 150

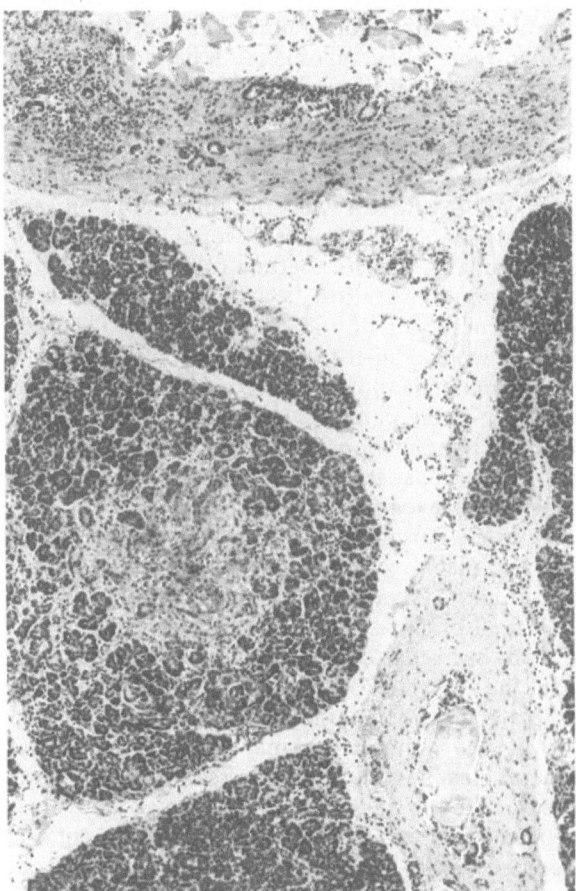

Fig. 14.4. Non-specific chronic inflammatory infiltration of the interstitial tissues associated with a miliary tubercle in the acinar tissue in the pancreas shown in Figs 14.2 and 14.3. The infiltration is most marked around the ducts, which contain inspissated secretion. H&E, × 60

abscess, or to carcinoma of the pancreas, may delay recognition of the true nature of the condition and the initiation of antituberculous therapy. The patient described by Crook and Johnson (1988), was an American Indian woman aged 73, who died of the adult type of respiratory distress syndrome following a cholecystectomy. Disseminated tuberculosis with a purulent pancreatic tuberculous abscess, 4 cm in diameter, had been quite unsuspected until an autopsy had been carried out. The recognition of a tuberculous abscess of the pancreas by its computed tomographic appearances has been described by Berson et al. (1989). Their patient was a Peruvian man whose tuberculous infection was associated with the acquired immune deficiency syndrome (AIDS). More recently (1991), Zeiderman et al. described an 81-year-old man, in whom fibrotic tuberculosis of the pancreas and right adrenal gland

simulated carcinoma of the pancreas, the true nature of a mass in the pancreas being recognised only microscopically following necropsy.

Sarcoidosis

As in tuberculosis, involvement of the pancreas in sarcoidosis occurs only occasionally, and is found incidentally at autopsy in subjects whose clinical histories give no hint of pancreatic disease. The lesions of Boeck's sarcoid were recognised first in the pancreas by Nickerson in 1937. The pancreas was involved in only one of the six cases examined postmortem in his series. The granulomas were relatively rare and solitary and were found in the inter-acinous and intraacinous fibrous tissue. There was no involvement of acini or islets. A patient, in whom symptoms were attributed to sarcoidosis of the pancreas, was followed clinically for 18 months by Curran and Curran (1950). They believed that the pancreatic lesions, which were demonstrated by biopsy of the pancreas, were the only lesions present in their patient, a 48-year-old woman. She became asymptomatic with no therapy other than pancreatic enzyme substitution. In 1954, Ryrie gave a short account of a patient with sarcoidosis of the pancreas. A woman aged 52 had a laparotomy because of obstructive jaundice. There was a hard mass in the head of the pancreas and enlargement of the adjacent lymph nodes. Sarcoid granulomas were found in a biopsy from one of the nodes. The jaundice was relieved by cholecystduodenostomy, but diabetes mellitus developed 1 month after the operation, and insulin was required to control the hyperglycaemia and ketosis. The author could find no reports of other patients in whom pancreatic sarcoidosis had caused diabetes.

In the study of sarcoidosis by Longcope and Freiman (1952), which included 30 autopsies carried out at the Johns Hopkins and Massachusetts General Hospitals, along with a review of the literature, they found an incidence of pancreatic involvement in 6% of 92 cases. Pancreatic involvement was reported as an incidental finding by Tsou et al. (1980), and in 1981 Maher et al. described non-caseating granulomas of the pancreas, probably due to sarcoidosis, causing partial obstruction of the common bile duct in a 59-year-old white man. At laparotomy, there was dilatation of the biliary tract, and the head of the pancreas was enlarged and firm and contained firm white nodules 1–2 cm in diameter. Several enlarged greyish nodular lymph nodes were present in the greater omentum, and an operative cholangiogram demonstrated a long smooth stricture of the common bile duct, while microscopic examination of biopsies of the pancreas and lymph nodes contained epithelioid granulomas. Stains and cultures for acid-fast bacilli and fungi were negative, as were serological and cutaneous sensitivity tests for fungal infection and tuberculosis. Complete resolution of the narrowing of the distal common bile duct was found to have taken place after steroid therapy for 37 days.

In 1983, Friedman and Weinstein described painful granulomatous infiltration of the pancreas, which improved with steroid therapy, in a patient with well-documented sarcoidosis. Steroid therapy also relieved the acute episodes of pancreatitis that occurred in the two patients with sarcoidosis reported by McCormick et al. (1985).

In their study of 34 cases of granulomatous pancreatitis, Stürmer and Becker (1987) gave an account of two with sarcoidosis, in which there was involvement of the pancreas along with lesions in other organs. In one of these, the pancreatic lesions simulated a neoplasm and the granulomas were found only after pancreatic resection had been carried out. In the other, a man known to have sarcoidosis, the granulomas were found in lymph nodes and the pancreas after the pancreas had been removed because of alcoholic chronic pancreatitis.

Pancreatic sarcoidosis causing ultrasonic and computed tomographic images that simulated pancreatic malignancy, was reported by Sagalow et al. in 1988. The patient, a woman aged 28, who had had acute upper abdominal pain, became asymptomatic after a laparotomy during which biopsy of the pancreas was carried out.

Actinomycosis

Cope (1938, 1949) does not mention involvement of the pancreas in the various types of visceral disease that may occur in actinomycosis.

Fungal Lesions

Even when there is widely disseminated fungal disease, with involvement of many viscera, it is quite unusual for the pancreas to be involved. Baker (1942), in his autopsy study of four fatal cases of North American blastomycosis, found no pancreatic lesions, although there were abscesses and other inflammatory lesions in many organs. It is true that pancreatic lesions may occur in coccidioidomycosis, but pancreatic involvement is relatively uncommon. The pancreas was macroscopically abnormal in only one of the 50 fatal cases of the disease studied by Forbus and Bestebreurtje (1946), and fungal lesions were found in the pancreas in only eight when the organs were examined microscopically. Although some of these cases had a clinical history that included nausea and vomiting, abdominal pain was usually absent.

In generalised cryptococcosis, pancreatic lesions may occur but they are of little clinical importance. Cox and Tolhurst (1946), in a review of ten published cases of generalised cryptococcosis, could find a record of pancreatic involvement in only three. Generalised cryptococcal infection is, of course, rare because it can usually develop only when the immune responses have been impaired by disease of the reticuloendothelial system or by the effects of radiation or chemotherapy. It is thus surprising that, since AIDS has become recognised, with the opportunistic infections that may be superimposed upon it, only two examples of cryptococcal involvement of the pancreas in AIDS have been recorded (Bricaire et al. 1988). Such lesions seem, moreover, unlikely to have had clinical significance. In histoplasmosis too, although there may be tuberculoid lesions with necrosis in the lungs, liver, spleen, kidneys and adrenal glands, along with ulcerating lesions in the intestines, mouth and larynx, pancreatic lesions are inconspicuous and probably unimportant. Goodwin et al. (1980), for example, mention that in 28 cases of disseminated histoplasmosis that came to autopsy there were only two in which small clusters of parasite-filled phagocytic cells were present in the connective tissue of the pancreas.

Infection by *C. albicans* was referred to at the beginning of this chapter as a cause of pancreatic abscesses following acute pancreatitis; candidiasis has become notorious as a complication of the chemotherapy of leukaemias and lymphomas, and other solid malignancies.

According to Guice et al. (1987), aspergillosis is second only to candidiasis as a complication of immunosuppression during the chemotherapy of neoplasms. These authors described a case in which disseminated aspergillosis developed in a 63-year-old man whose immunity became suppressed during chemotherapy for a malignant lymphoma. The terminal event was haemorrhagic necrosis of the pancreas. At laparotomy, it was found that both old and fresh blood surrounded the pancreas and that the clot extended into the right retroperitoneum from the pancreas to the iliac crest, and that it had ruptured through the right mesocolon into the peritoneal cavity. There was thrombosis of the right colic artery and vein with infarction of the related area of the colon. The pancreas was haemorrhagic and there was extensive necrosis of the glandular tissue with saponification of the peripancreatic fatty tissue. The necrotic pancreatic tissue was removed, and right hemicolectomy with ileostomy was carried out with drainage of the pancreatic bed and right retroperitoneum. The patient died 3 days later, in spite of antibiotic and supportive therapy. At autopsy, there was massive pulmonary infection by a fungus with the morphology of aspergillus. Arterial thrombi, in which fungal hyphae were demonstrated by the silver methenamine method, were present in the remnants

of the pancreas and similar thrombi containing fungal hyphae were present in many other sites throughout the body. The authors pointed out that, although pulmonary and alimentary lesions due to infection by aspergillus in patients with natural or induced impairment of their immune responses are well known, a patient with the clinical and anatomical features of haemorrhagic pancreatitis due to disseminated aspergillosis had not been reported previously.

In a 10-year review of invasive aspergillosis detected at necropsy, Boon et al. (1991) found involvement of the pancreas in two of 16 cases of haematological malignancy and in two of 12 with liver transplantation. The authors pointed out that they had received high doses of steroid drugs.

Viral Lesions

Varicella-Zoster Pancreatitis

Viral infections that may injure the pancreatic islets have been discussed in Chap. 6. Such infections include the coxsackie B viruses, rubella and varicella-zoster. Occasionally, such viral infections may have some part in initiating acute pancreatitis. Immunosuppression seems to have allowed generalised varicella-zoster infection to develop in a man aged 19, who had received a renal transplant. This man came into contact with zoster, and became acutely ill with symptoms of acute pancreatitis, as well as having the skin lesions of varicella. The patient died, and diffuse haemorrhage into the pancreas was found post-mortem. Microscopically, the pancreas was unfortunately much affected by autolysis. Interstitial haemorrhage could be recognised but there was no leucocytic reaction. Intranuclear inclusions, however, could be seen in some of the nuclei of the acinar cells (Figs 14.5 and 14.6) and viral particles, with the appearances of a herpes-type of virus, were demonstrated in homogenised tissue from the pancreas that was examined by electron microscopy (Fig. 14.7); culture identified the organism as varicella-zoster virus.

Mumps Pancreatitis

Mumps is a generalised viral infection, usually in children, in which painful swelling of the parotid salivary glands is the most usual clinical feature. Less commonly, the submandibular salivary glands

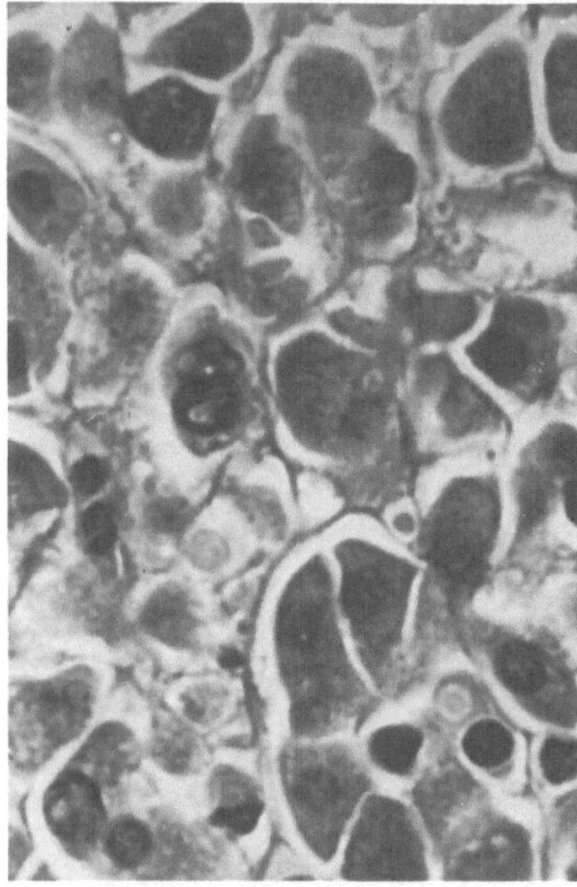

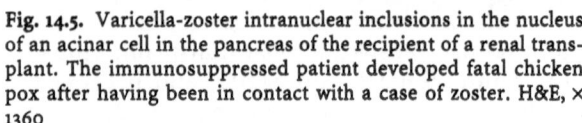

Fig. 14.5. Varicella-zoster intranuclear inclusions in the nucleus of an acinar cell in the pancreas of the recipient of a renal transplant. The immunosuppressed patient developed fatal chicken pox after having been in contact with a case of zoster. H&E, × 1360

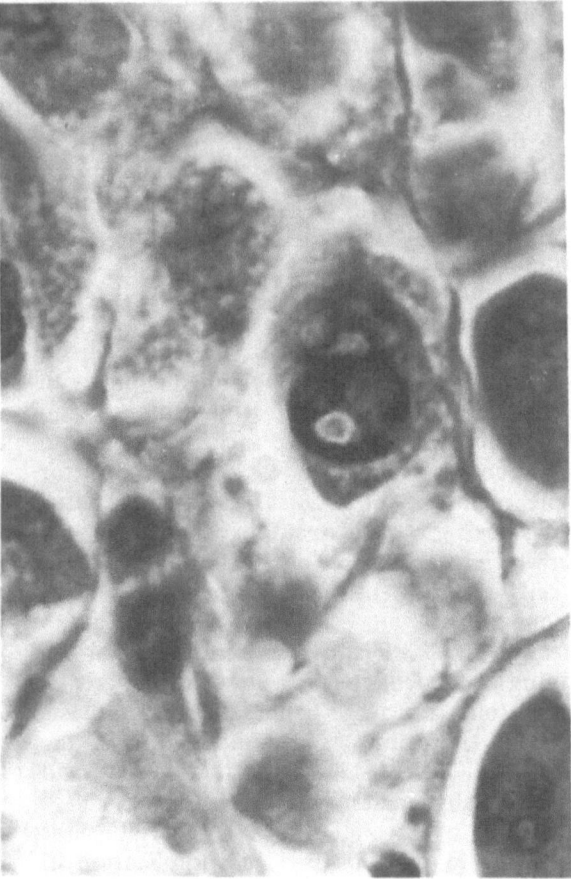

Fig. 14.6. Intranuclear inclusions in the acinar cells of the pancreas shown in Fig. 14.5. H&E, × 2500

may be affected, along with, or instead of, the parotid salivary glands. Less common effects of mumps virus infection include, especially in adults, orchitis, meningoencephalitis, gastroenteritis, subacute thyroiditis, myocarditis and pancreatitis. Moreover, the pancreatitis may occur without associated signs of salivary involvement by the disease. Reports of such occurrence of pancreatitis, in which the diagnosis was a clinical and biochemical one, combined with a rising titre of mumps complement-fixing antibody, have been published by O'Brien et al. (1965), Witte and Schanzer (1968) and Naficy et al. (1973). The patients reported by these authors recovered, but, in 1968, Bostrom gave a pathoanatomical report on a 15-year-old boy, who died suddenly while suffering from mumps. The sudden death was attributed to viral myocarditis. The myocardium was extensively involved, the muscle fibres being separated by oedema in which

there was infiltration by lymphocytes, neutrophils, plasma cells and histiocytes. The salivary glands, especially the parotid glands, were inflamed, as were the right testis and epididymis, and the seminal vesicles. There had been no clinical evidence of pancreatitis. The pancreas seemed normal on examination with the naked eye, but, on microscopic examination, there was mild interstitial inflammation with a few scattered lymphocytes and an occasional polymorphonuclear leucocyte.

Although Bostrom's report does not mention any signs of injury in the pancreatic islets, there has long been a suspicion that damage to the pancreatic islets by the mumps virus may lead to diabetes mellitus. The survey by Jenson et al. (1980) of the pancreases of 250 children who died during fatal viral infections does not include cases of mumps, but McCrae (1963) has reported diabetes mellitus in a child aged 10 months, in whom the onset of the diabetes was

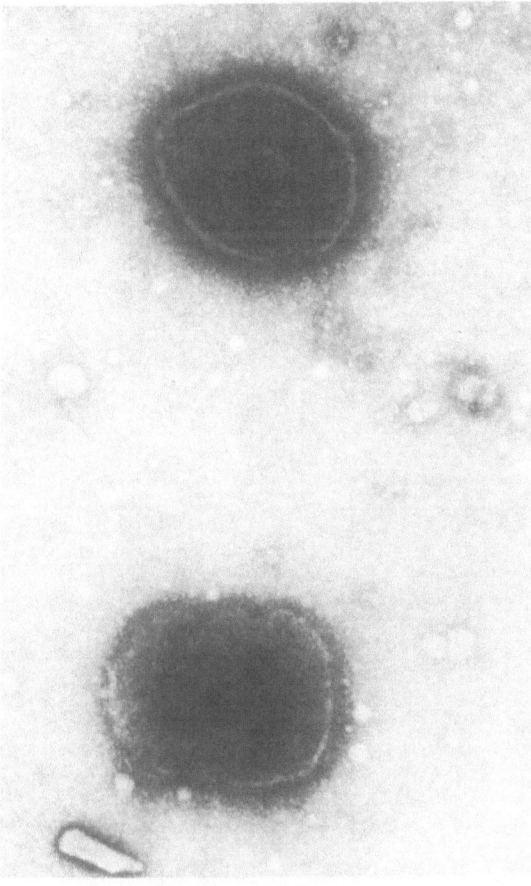

Fig. 14.7. An electron micrograph of a negatively stained sample from the homogenised pancreas shown in Figs 14.5 and 14.6. Two typical enveloped herpes virions are present. (Courtesy of Dr Tony Hart, Department of Medical Microbiology, University of Liverpool) × 77 000

immediately preceded by mumps pancreatitis, as diagnosed clinically and serologically, without involvement of the salivary glands. Another patient, a boy aged 6, who developed diabetes mellitus about 20 days after the onset of mumps, has also been reported by Peig et al. (1981).

The possible importance of viral infection in the aetiology of acute pancreatitis was investigated by Imrie et al. in 1977, by including routine screening for viral infection in the investigation of 116 patients admitted to Glasgow Royal Infirmary because of acute pancreatitis. In five female patients they found significantly rising antibody titres that indicated coxsackie B infection or mumps. In two patients the titres indicted mumps infection only, in one there was evidence of both mumps and coxsackie B, while in two there was evidence of coxsackie B infection without evidence of mumps. In one of those with

evidence of mumps, it seemed likely that biliary disease was also present.

Acute Pancreatitis Due to Infectious Mononucleosis

In 1940, Bernstein suggested that the glycosuria that sometimes occurs during infectious mononucleosis might be due to pancreatic involvement by the disease, and in 1949 Myhre and Nesbitt found elevated lipase and amylase levels in the serum of two of 20 patients with infectious mononucleosis; there were no clinical symptoms or signs of pancreatitis. In 1966, however, Wislocki reported what he believed to be the first reported patient with concurrent infectious mononucleosis and clinically significant acute pancreatitis.

Pancreatitis Due to Infection by Coxsackie B Virus

The damaging effect of certain viruses upon the pancreas has received much study in relation to the aetiology of diabetes. Such work has been reviewed by Craighead (1977), much of which involves the use of viruses that will infect and destroy pancreatic beta cells in mice to cause diabetes. Certain of the viruses that will cause diabetes in mice are also found in the human population. Coxsackie virus B4 is such a virus. In addition to the importance of coxsackie viruses as possible causes of type I diabetes, they have been reported also as having caused acute pancreatitis. In 1973, Ursing reported two adult patients with acute pancreatitis, from whose faeces coxsackie virus B5 was isolated and whose neutralising antibody against the virus showed a four-fold increase. Both recovered, but the father of one of the patients had had acute pancreatitis that developed 16 days before his daughter became ill. No viral studies, however, were done on the father, who developed a pancreatic abscess, was operated upon, and died during the post-operative period.

The prospective study of the possible importance of coxsackie B virus infection in 116 patients with acute pancreatitis, carried out by Imrie et al. in 1977, has already been mentioned. Their serological findings indicated that coxsackie B virus may have been of aetiological importance in three patients, one of whom also had evidence of infection by mumps. A similar study of paired acute and convalescent serum samples from 27 patients with acute pancreatitis was carried out in Leeds by Freeman and McMahon in 1978. They found evidence of infection by coxsackie viruses group B in three patients.

Pancreatitis Associated with *Mycoplasma pneumoniae* Infection

The work of Freeman and McMahon on the association of viral agents with acute pancreatitis included a search for serological evidence of infection by *Mycoplasma pneumoniae*; evidence of such infection was found in no less than nine of their 27 patients. They did not use any direct method that might detect *M. pneumoniae* in the pancreas in any of these patients.

Pancreatic Involvement in Cytomegalic Inclusion Disease

Although the virus of cytomegalic inclusion disease was originally associated with lesions of the salivary glands, generalised forms of the infection are now commonly diagnosed, usually in neonates, young children or adults whose immune defences have been impaired. As might be expected, because of the structural similarities of the salivary glands and the pancreas, the pancreas may be involved (Fig. 14.8). In the study carried out by Smith and Velios in 1950, there was involvement of the pancreas in five of the authors' own 17 patients, while, in the 69 previously reported patients reviewed by Smith and Velios, there was pancreatic involvement in 12. In a series of cases reported by Wyatt et al. (1950), the pancreatic lesions were probably not sufficiently extensive to cause any serious functional disturbance. However, in a report of an adult patient with disseminated cytomegalic inclusion disease, Wyatt et al. (1951) found that in the pancreas there were focal necroses with a polymorphonuclear reaction scattered throughout the parenchyma, in association with an occasional viral inclusion body. In a later report of cytomegalic inclusion disease in adults, Wyatt et al. (1953) again found inclusion bodies in the acinar tissue, and in the islets of Langerhans with, in one, necrotic foci in conjunction with the inclusion-charged parenchymal cells. Wigglesworth (1984) illustrated an infiltration by mononuclear cells in association with the cytomegalic nuclear inclusions in the pancreas in congenital cytomegalovirus infection.

Cytomegalovirus infection is, of course, one of the commoner opportunistic infections in patients with AIDS; it was found, for example, in 25 of the 36 autopsies reported by Welch et al. (1984), often in association with other opportunistic infections. They

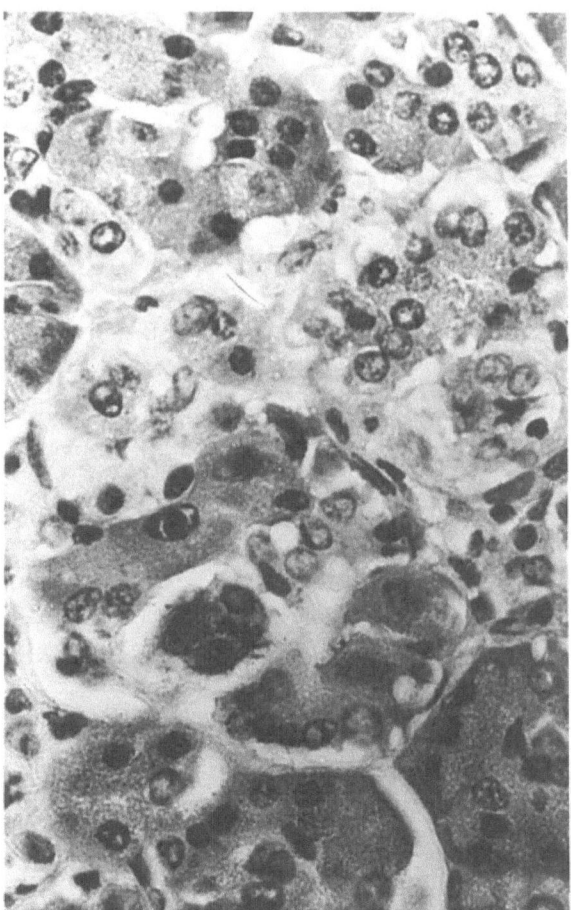

Fig. 14.8. Cytomegalic inclusions in the pancreas of an infant with generalised cytomegalic inclusion disease. (Courtesy of Dr J. Boton, Alder Hey Children's Hospital, Liverpool) H&E, × 600

did not, however, find pancreatic involvement. The pancreas was not abnormal in the series of autopsies upon AIDS sufferers reported by Reichert et al. (1983). By 1985, however, a series of 113 necropsies on cases of AIDS had been collected in Paris and was reported by Bricaire et al. (1988). These workers found ten in which cytomegalic inclusion cells were found in the pancreas. Fig. 14.9 is an illustration of such cells in the pancreas of a fatal case of AIDS. Two cases of cytomegalovirus-associated pancreatic disease in patients with AIDS were reported by Wilcox et al. (1990). In both patients the clinical effects of the pancreatic lesions were overshadowed by more severe AIDS-related conditions and the pancreatic lesions were discovered only at necropsy. In one, foci of necrosis were surrounded by inflammatory cells; ductal, acinar, endothelial and

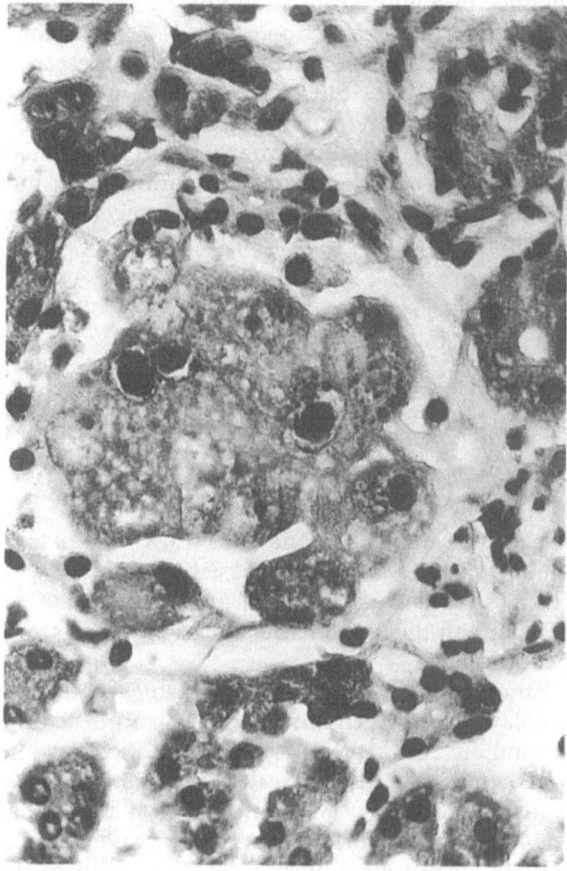

Fig. 14.9. Cytomegalic inclusions in the pancreas of a fatal case of AIDS. (Courtesy of Dr M.S. Kearney) H&E, × 1000

islet cells contained inclusions. In the other, pancreatic fibrosis had caused partial biliary obstruction; inclusions were numerous.

Pancreatic Lesions Attributable to HIV Infection

As patients who have died from the effects of human immunodeficiency virus (HIV) infection have usually required drugs for opportunistic infections, the effects of such drugs may obscure lesions caused directly by the HIV virus. Pentamidine in particular, used to treat pneumonia caused by *Pneumocystis carinii*, has been shown to be toxic to pancreatic islet cells and has also caused haemorrhagic pancreatitis (Zuger et al. 1986). The cutaneous and visceral lesions of Kaposi's sarcoma are,

however, a well-known, although poorly understood, effect of HIV infection. Massive infiltration of the pancreas by Kaposi's sarcoma was found in one of the 13 cases of AIDS in the autopsy series reported briefly by Brivet et al. (1987). In the same series, one had an unsuspected lymphoma in the pancreas, a well recognised complication of impaired immunity.

In the much larger autopsy series of 113 cases of AIDS reported, again very briefly, by Bricaire et al. (1988), almost half had pancreatic lesions. Microscopic pancreatic lesions were present in 54. These included eight in which either Kaposi's sarcoma or lymphoma was found. There were 13 in which the pancreas was affected by opportunistic infections (ten with cytomegalovirus infection, two with cryptococcal infection and one with tuberculosis). The exact significance in relation to the HIV infection of the other microscopic abnormalities is indefinite; such lesions included oedema, ductal metaplasia, fibrosis and vascular lesions.

Chronic pancreatitis with malabsorption in a 3-year-old child, who had persistently raised serum amylases and lipases, was believed by Torre et al. (1987) to be due to the effects of HIV infection upon the pancreas. At autopsy, there was pancreatic fibrosis without calcification. The mother of the child was an intravenous drug user who was HIV antibody positive. The child, who had been negative for HIV antibody at the age of 12 months, had become positive during the next year and died one year after that.

Other authors, Venderell et al. (1987) for example, have described clinical experiences that suggest HIV infection may contribute to the onset of insulin-dependent diabetes mellitus, while others (Zazzo et al. 1987), have reported that 46% of their series of 35 consecutive patients being treated for other aspects of AIDS had laboratory evidence of pancreatitis.

Pancreatic lesions are relatively uncommon as the cause of death in patients who have died from the effects of AIDS. In the ten autopsy cases studied by Reichert et al. (1983), only one had pancreatic disease (involvement by Kaposi's sarcoma and cytomegalovirus infection) but it was not considered to be the main cause of death. In the 36 autopsies reported by Welch et al. (1984) there was one in which death was attributed to acute haemorrhagic pancreatitis; both Kaposi's sarcoma and cytomegalovirus infection were also present. Hui et al. (1984) reported their findings after autopsies on 12 subjects, and found pancreatic involvement by cytomegalovirus infection in one, in whom malignant lymphoma appears to have been the main cause of death. The neoplasm involved lymph nodes, including peripancreatic nodes, spleen, liver and bone marrow.

Pancreatitis in Fulminant Psittacosis

Involvement of the pancreas in psittacosis had not been recognised before 1979, but in that year Byrom et al. reported that there was evidence of pancreatitis in two patients who died of fulminant psittacosis, after presenting with generalised toxaemia and acute renal failure. In one, the blood glucose was abnormally high and serum calcium depressed. At autopsy the abdomen contained serosanguinous fluid and there was no fat necrosis; the pancreas was autolytic. In the other, the serum amylase was raised and the pancreas was congested, but there was no fat necrosis. It might be questioned whether the pancreatic injury was attributable to any specific effect upon the pancreas that the chlamydial infection may have had, or whether the pancreatic effects were non-specific and associated with the circulatory collapse that had been so marked in both patients.

Protozoal Infection and Pancreatic Disease

Coccidiosis is a common cause of disease in domestic and other animals, and one genus of these sporozoan parasites, *Cryptosporidium*, may cause disease in man. In immunologically competent people, the presence of the parasites in the intestinal mucosa causes self-limiting enterocolitis, but, in immunologically compromised people, such as sufferers from AIDS, it causes chronic life-threatening diarrhoea. It is well recognised as one of the opportunistic infections to which patients with AIDS are vulnerable.

In animals, the parasite has been found in the mucosa of the biliary and pancreatic ducts and there has been a report of the development of acute pancreatitis in a young woman who had been suffering from cryptosporidiosis (Hawkins et al. 1987). The patient was a 14-year-old farmer's daughter who had abdominal pain, fever, vomiting and watery diarrhoea. Her faeces contained large numbers of cryptosporidium oocysts. Her symptoms subsided after 4 days, but 3 days after that her abdominal pain recurred more severely. She was admitted to hospital and a diagnosis of acute pancreatitis was established. Abdominal ultrasound indicated that the pancreas was enlarged and that there was ascites. She was treated conservatively and recovered slowly. Cryptosporidium-specific antibody titres obtained by a fluorescent antibody test were consistent with recent infection. Faecal examinations showed reduction and, after a week, disappearance of, the parasites. She developed a pancreatic pseudocyst, 5.5 cm in diameter as determined by ultrasonic scanning but, after 6 weeks, that had almost resolved. The patient remained well, but increased pancreatic echogenicity suggested the possibility of chronic pancreatitis.

Effects of Helminthic Infestation upon the Pancreas

Obstructive lesions of the pancreatic duct predispose to pancreatitis, and Dürr (1979) refers to a publication by Schmieden and Sebening in 1927 in which 50 reported cases of pancreatitis due to invasion of the pancreatic ducts by worms are mentioned.

Pancreatitis of this type is most liable to occur in populations in which alimentary worm infestation is common. Louw et al. (1967), for example, found in South Africa that in their series of 584 patients with acute pancreatitis, 18 were infested with helminths. The large round worm *Ascaris lumbricoides* seems to be the worm most likely to enter the pancreatic ducts. Reports of pancreatitis in association with large round worms within the pancreas include those of Novis (1923), who successfully removed a full-sized living round worm and a partially disintegrated one from the pancreatic duct of a 12-year-old Hindu girl who developed pancreatitis. At laparotomy the pancreas was enlarged and the worms were removed by incising and opening the duct from the head to the tail of the organ. The pancreas was repaired and the patient recovered. During her convalescence several round worms were passed after santonin had been administered.

The development of an upper abdominal abscess in a male child aged 18 months, in association with ascaris infestation, was reported from what was at that time Tanganyika Territory, by Duncan in 1948. The abscess was drained, but the child died. At the post-mortem examination the abscess was found to occupy the whole of the head of the pancreas and to contain the partially digested remains of an adult ascaris. A track extended retroperitoneally into the left and quadrate lobes of the liver, which were destroyed, leaving a cavity that communicated with the surface through the surgical drainage incision at the left costal margin. Although santonin had been administered during the child's illness, with the subsequent passage of two adult ascarides, seven further ascaris worms were found in the small intestine during the autopsy.

More recently, Krige et al. (1987) reported a patient in whom recurrent attacks of pancreatitis were caused by a calcified ascaris in the duct of Wirsung, and, in 1988, Millar et al., in discussing the management of pseudocysts in children in South Africa, found that in five of their 25 patients with a pancreatic pseudocyst there was infestation by ascaris worms.

In India, hepatobiliary and pancreatic ascariasis seems to be relatively common and, working in Kashmir, Khuroo et al. (1990) were able to report their experience of 500 cases collected in slightly over 6 years. Their patients included 31 who presented with pancreatitis; in 16 of these the endoscopic removal of worms from the ampullary orifice relieved the condition.

In countries where infestation by the fluke, *Clonorchis sinensis*, is common, obstruction of the pancreatic duct by the parasite may provoke acute or chronic pancreatitis (Hartley and Douglas 1975), but pancreatitis is by no means an invariable consequence of the entry of flukes into the duct system. In a necropsy study of the pancreatic ducts in 64 subjects with varying degrees of clonorchis infestation of the liver, Chan and Teoh (1967) found worms in the pancreatic ducts in 24. The number of worms in the pancreatic ducts varied from one to 34, with one exceptional case in which there were 114 worms in the main pancreatic duct and its tributaries. When there was heavy infestation of the liver there tended to be heavy infestation also of the pancreatic ducts (ten or more worms). Dilatation of the main pancreatic duct was present in only three cases, in these there was also dilatation of the tributary ducts. Microscopically, there was squamous metaplasia of the ductal epithelium in 14 cases (58.3%), usually in the body and tail portions of the pancreas, where the worms were most often located. Hyperplasia of mucous glands, usually in tributary ducts, was present in 23 of the 24 subjects, and the authors noted that, while squamous metaplasia seemed to be related to heavy infestation of the pancreatic ducts, hyperplasia of the mucous glands was not similarly related. The authors did not mention the finding of the ova of the flukes within the pancreases they studied, and they did not mention any granulomatous reaction that might have been provoked by ova. This is in keeping with the statement by Hou (1955) that the eggs of *C. sinensis* do not stimulate a foreign body giant cell reaction. The absence of a granulomatous reaction to the eggs is surprising as the ova of some other types of fluke, *Schistosoma mansoni* for example, are notoriously liable to provoke a granulomatous and fibrous reaction in organs such as the liver.

A patient with acute pancreatitis attributed to the presence of a *C. sinensis* fluke in the pancreatic duct was described by Shugar and Ryan (1975). It had been 25 years since the patient had lived in an area in which *C. sinensis* infestation was endemic.

A study of the pancreas in infestation by *S. mansoni* was carried out by Mott et al. in 1972. In 20 patients with the hepatosplenic form of Manson's schistosomiasis with portal hypertension, they found functional impairment of the pancreas in 16. As they were treated by splenectomy with splenorenal venous anastomosis, it was possible to obtain a biopsy of the tail of the pancreas during these surgical procedures. In 14 of the 20 patients there were granulomata with fibrosis in the samples from the tails of the pancreases.

The fluke *Eurytrema pancreaticum* is a common parasite of the pancreatic ducts, and rarely of the bile ducts and duodenum, in cattle, buffalo, sheep, goats, and hares in Asia. Less commonly, it is found in camels and in a certain species of monkey, but human infestation is very rare. Ishii et al. (1983) refer to reports of a few human cases whose faeces contained the eggs of this trematode and refer also to a single human occurrence, in which the fluke was found at autopsy, and report a patient of their own. Their patient was a 70-year-old Japanese woman, who died following an operation for gastric cancer. Post-mortem, her pancreatic ducts were found to contain about 15 adult flukes that could be identified as *Eurytrema pancreaticum*. The pancreas appeared to be normal until the ducts were opened; a clump of parasites was then found within a dilated duct at the tail. Microscopically, there was lymphocytic infiltration of the interlobular connective tissue of the adjacent gland, with moderate distension of the inter- and intralobular ductules of the tail by retained secretion. No necrotic or granulomatous lesions were found and there were no eggs within the affected duct or in the parenchyma.

Hydatid Cysts of the Pancreas

People in close contact with dogs that are hosts to the canine tape worm, *Taenia granulosa* (*Taenia echinococcus*) may swallow the eggs excreted by the dogs and become intermediate hosts for the next stage of the worm's life cycle, with the development of hydatid cysts. Hydatid cysts tend to occur in the liver or in various other organs; quite rarely, a hydatid cyst may develop in the pancreas. Because the pancreas is a rare site, cases of hydatid cyst of the pancreas tend to be reported, for example, as by

Anderson and Peebles Brown (1959–1960). The rarity of the pancreas as a site is, however, indicated by the experience of Kattan (1975) in Baghdad. During the years between 1963 and 1975, 780 patients with hydatid disease affecting various tissues and organs were operated upon in one surgical unit; in only two patients was the cyst situated in the pancreas. The mode of presentation of these cysts depended upon the part of the pancreas affected; a cyst in the tail mimicked an enlarged spleen, while one in the head simulated a carcinoma.

Hydatid cysts of the pancreas have also been reported in association with acute pancreatitis (Joske 1955), while Pellegrini et al. (1977) included the rupture of an echinococcal hydatid cyst of the liver into the biliary system among the rare causes of acute pancreatitis that they encountered in a review of 800 patients. Infection of a hydatid cyst of the pancreas caused a pancreatic abscess in the patient reported by Papadimitriou (1987). Drainage of the abscess with removal of the cystic membrane was followed by an external pancreatic fistula, which closed after 3 days of a regimen of somatostatin infusion. Also in 1987, Cosme et al. reported another patient with an infected hydatid cyst of the pancreas that caused a spontaneous fistula into the duodenum.

Strongyloidiasis

In fatal cases of infestation by *Strongyloides stercoralis*, although there may be a granulomatous response in the liver to the presence of the larvae (Poltera and Katsimbura 1974), no pancreatic lesions were mentioned by Poltera and Katsimbura, or by Wilson and Thompson (1964). In the patient reported by Pijls et al. (1986), however, a mass in the head of the pancreas, demonstrated by an echogram of the upper abdomen, caused stenosis of the bile duct and obstructive jaundice. A pancreatic neoplasm was suspected, but, because the patient, a 30-year-old man, had recently returned from India and had larvae of *S. stercoralis* in his faeces he was treated with thiabendazole for 3 days. He recovered so rapidly that the proposed surgical exploration was abandoned. His jaundice disappeared and the ultrasonographic appearances gradually returned to normal. The findings on ultrasonic and laboratory examination were normal 3 years later and the patient felt entirely well.

References

Altemeier WA, Alexander JW (1963) Pancreatic abscess: a study of 32 cases. Arch Surg 87:80–89

Anderson GS, Peebles Brown DA (1959–1960) A case of hydatid cyst of the pancreas. Br J Surg 47:147–149

Auerbach O (1944) Acute generalised miliary tuberculosis. Am J Pathol 20:121–136

Baker RD (1942) Tissue reactions in human blastomycosis: an analysis of tissue from twenty-three cases. Am J Pathol 18:479–489

Bernstein A (1940) Infectious mononucleosis. Medicine 19:85–159

Berson BD, Mendelson DS, Janus CL (1989) Tuberculous abscess of the pancreas in AIDS: CT findings. Mt Sinai J Med 56:297–299

Birch-Hirschfeld FV (1875) Beitrage zur pathologischen Anatomie der hereditaren Syphilis neugeborner, mit besonderer Berucksichtigung einer Veranderung der Bauchspeicheldruse. Arch Heilkunde 16:166–178

Bollaert PE, Maurizi M, Laprevote-Heully MC, Lambert H, Larcan A (1986) Pancréatite aigue nécrotico-hemorrhagique au cours d'une maladie des légionnaires. Presse Med 15:1732

Bolooki H, Jaffe B, Gliedman ML (1968) Pancreatic abscesses and lesser omental sac collections. Surg Gynecol Obstet 126:1301–1308

Boon AP, O'Brien D, Adams DH (1991) 10-year review of invasive aspergillosis detected at necropsy. J Clin Pathol 44:452–454

Bostrom K (1968) Patho-anatomical findings in a case of mumps with pancreatitis, myocarditis, orchitis, epididymitis and seminal vesiculitis. Virchows Arch [A] 344:111–117

Boyd JF (1969) *Salmonella typhimurium*, colitis, and pancreatitis. Lancet ii:901–902

Bricaire F, Marche C, Zoubi D, Saimot AG, Regnier B (1988) HIV and the pancreas. Lancet i:65–66

Brivet F, Coffin B, Bedossa P et al. (1987) Pancreatic lesions in AIDS. Lancet ii:570–571

Byrom NP, Walls J, Mair HJ (1979) Fulminant psittacosis. Lancet i:353–356

Chan PH, Teoh TB (1967) The pathology of *Clonorchis sinensis* infestation of the pancreas. J Pathol Bacteriol 93:185–189

Cope VZ (1938) Actinomycosis. Oxford University Press, London

Cope VZ (1949) Visceral actinomycosis. Br Med J ii:1311–1316

Cosme A, Drive V, Ojeda E, Aramburu V, Irazusta M, Arenas JI (1987) Hydatid cyst of the pancreas with spontaneous fistula to the duodenum. Am J Gastroenterol 82:1311–1313

Cox LB, Tolhurst JC (1946) Human torulosis: a clinical pathological and microbiological study with a report of thirteen cases. Melbourne University Press, Melbourne, p 149

Craighead JE (1977) Viral diabetes. In: Volk BW, Wellmann KF (eds) The diabetic pancreas. Baillière Tindall, London, pp 467–488

Crook LD, Johnson FP (1988) Tuberculosis of the pancreas: a case report. Tubercle 69:148–151

Crowson MC, Perry M, Burden E (1984) Tuberculosis of the pancreas: a rare cause of obstructive jaundice. Br J Surg 71:239

Curran JF, Curran JF (1950) Boeck's sarcoid of the pancreas. Surgery 28:574–578 de Miguel F, Beltran J, Sabas JA, Sadaba F, Santamaria JM, Bustamante V (1985) Tuberculous pancreatic abscess. Br J Surg 72:438

Duncan NA (1948) Pancreatitis due to ascariasis [letter]. Br Med J i:905

Dürr GH-K (1979) Acute pancreatitis. In: Howat HT, Sarles H (eds) The exocrine pancreas. Saunders, London, p 360. Quoting Schmeider V, Sebening W (1927) Chirurgie des Pankreas. Langenbecks Arch Klin Chir 148:319–387

Evans FC (1969) Pancreatic abscess. Am J Surg 117:537–540

Forbus WD, Bestebreurtje AM (1946) Coccidioidomycosis: a study of 95 cases of the disseminated type with special reference to the pathogenesis of the disease. Milit Surg 99:653–719

Freeman R, McMahon MJ (1978) Acute pancreatitis and serological evidence of infection with Mycoplasma pneumoniae. Gut 19:367–370

Friedman HZ, Weinstein RA (1983) Sarcoidosis of the pancreas. Arch Intern Med 143:2182–2183

Gallagher P, Chadwick P, Jones DM, Turner L (1981) Acute pancreatitis associated with campylobacter infection. Br J Surg 68:383

Goodwin RA, Shapiro JL, Thurman GH, Thurman SS, Des Prez RM (1980) Disseminated histoplasmosis: clinical and pathologic correlations. Medicine 59:1–33

Guice KS, Lynch M, Weatherbee L (1987) Invasive aspergillosis: an unusual cause of hemorrhagic pancreatitis. Am J Gastroenterol 82:563–565

Hartley JPR, Douglas AP (1975) A case of clonorchiasis in England. Br Med J iii:575

Hawkins SP, Thomas RP, Teasdale C (1987) Acute pancreatitis: a new finding in cryptosporidium enteritis. Br Med J 294:483–484

Hearne SE, Whigham TE, Brady CE (1989) Pancreatitis and typhoid fever. Am J Med 86:471–473

Hou PC (1955) The pathology of Clonorchis sinensis infestation of the liver. J Pathol Bacteriol 70:53–64

Hui AN, Koss MN, Meyer PR (1984) Necropsy findings in acquired immunodeficiency syndrome: a comparison of premortem diagnosis with postmortem findings. Hum Pathol 15:670–676

Hurst AF (1934) Syphilis of the pancreas. In: Price FW (ed) A textbook of the practice of medicine, 4th edn. Oxford University Press, London, p 720

Ibrahim EM, Al-Sohaibani MO, Al-Suleiman SA, Sattit MB, Al-Mulhim FA, Qaddura F (1987) Tuberculosis of the pancreas: a rare cause of obstructive jaundice and portal hypertension. Trop Gastroenterol 8:167–172

Imrie CW, Ferguson JC, Sommerville RG (1977) Coxsackie and mumps virus infection in a prospective study of acute pancreatitis. Gut 18:53–56

Ishii Y, Koga M, Fugino T et al. (1983) Human infection with the pancreas fluke, Eurytrema pancreaticum. Am J Trop Med Hyg 32:1019–1022

Jenson AB, Rosenberg HS, Notkins AL (1980) Pancreatic islet-cell damage in children with fatal viral infections. Lancet ii:354–358

Joske RA (1955) Aetiological factors in the pancreatitis syndrome. Br Med J ii:1477–1481

Kattan YB (1975) Hydatid cysts in pancreas. Br Med J iv:729–730

Khuroo MS, Zargar SA, Mahajan R (1990) Hepatobiliary and pancreatic ascariasis in India. Lancet i:1503–1506

Kitai JC, Harid AC, Matenga JA (1987) Tuberculosis of the pancreas mimicking carcinoma: report of a case. Cent Afr J Med 33:19–22

Krige JE, Lewis G, Bornman PC (1987) Recurrent pancreatitis caused by a calcified ascaris in the duct of Wirsung. Am J Gastroenterol 82:256–257

Kune GA, Coster D (1972) Typhoid pancreatic abscess. Med J Aust I:417–418

Lindholt J, Hansen PT (1985) Yersiniosis as a possible cause of acute pancreatitis. Acta Chir Scand 151:703

Longcope WT, Freiman DG (1952) A study of sarcoidosis based on a combined investigation of 160 cases including 30 autopsies from the Johns Hopkins Hospital and Massachusetts General Hospital. Medicine 31:1–132

Louw JH, Marks IN, Banks S (1967) The management of severe acute pancreatitis. Postgrad Med J 43:31–44

Maher L, Choi H, Dodds WJ (1981) Noncaseating granulomas of the pancreas: probable sarcoidosis. Am J Gastroenterol 75:222–225

McCormick PA, Malone D, Fitzgerald MX, Fitzgerald O (1985) Pancreatitis in sarcoidosis. Br Med J 290:1472–1473

McCrae WM (1963) Diabetes mellitus following mumps. Lancet i:1300–1301

Millar AJW, Rode H, Stunden RJ, Cywes S (1988) Management of pancreatic pseudocysts in children. J Pediatr Surg 23:122–127

Mott CB, Neves DP, Okumura M, deBrito T, Bettarello A (1972) Histologic and functional alterations of human exocrine pancreas in Manson's schistosomiasis. Am J Dig Dis 17:583–590

Murphy S, Beeching NJ, Rogerson SJ, Harries AD (1991) Pancreatitis associated with salmonella enteritis [letter]. Lancet 338:571

Myhre J, Nesbitt S (1949) Pancreatitis in infectious mononucleosis. J Lab Clin Med 34:1671–1675

Naficy K, Nategh R, Ghadimi H (1973) Mumps pancreatitis without parotitis. Br Med. J i:529

Nickerson DA (1937) Boeck's sarcoid: report of six cases in which autopsies were made. Arch Pathol 24:19–29

Novis JMS (1923) Partial obstruction of the pancreatic duct by round worms. Br J Surg 10:421

O'Brien PK, Smith DS, Galpin OP (1965) Acute pancreatitis and haemolytic anaemia associated with mumps-virus infection. Br Med J ii:1529

Opie EL (1900–1901) On the relation of chronic interstitial pancreatitis to the islets of Langerhans and to diabetes mellitus. J Exp Med 5:397–428

Papadimitriou J (1987) Pancreatic abscess due to infected hydatid disease. Surgery 102:880–882

Pearce RM (1903) The islets of Langerhans in congenital syphilitic pancreatitis. Am Med 6:1020–1021

Peig M, Ercilla G, Millan M, Gomis R (1981) Post-mumps diabetes mellitus [letter]. Lancet i:1007

Pellegrini CA, Paloyan D, Acosta JM, Skinner DB (1977) Acute pancreatitis of rare causation. Surg Gynecol Obstet 144:899–902

Pijls NHJ, Yap SH, Rosenbusch G, Prenen H (1986) Pancreatic mass due to Strongyloides stercoralis infection: an unusual manifestation. Pancreas 1:90–93

Pitkänen T, Pönkä A, Pettersson T, Kosunen TU (1983) Campylobacter enteritis in 188 hospitalized patients. Arch Intern Med 143:215–219

Poltera AA, Katsimbura N (1974) Granulomatous hepatitis due to Strongyloides stercoralis. J Pathol 113:241–246

Raeburn C (1951) Gumma of the pancreas in a premature infant. J Pathol Bacteriol 63:158–159

Reichert CM, O'Leary TJ, Levens DL, Simrell CR, Macher AM (1983) Autopsy pathology in the acquired immune deficiency syndrome. Am J Pathol 112:357–382

Renner F, Nimeth C, Demmelbauer N (1991) High frequency of concomitant pancreatitis in salmonella enteritis [letter]. Lancet 337:1611

Richter JM, Jacoby GA, Schapiro RH, Warshaw AL (1982) Pancreatic abscess due to Candida albicans. Ann Intern Med 97:221–222

Russell J, Forgacs P, Geraci JE (1976) Pancreatitis complicating typhoid fever: report of a case. JAMA 235:753–754

Ryrie DR (1954) Sarcoidosis with obstructive jaundice. Proc R Soc Med 47:879

Sagalow BR, Miller CL, Wechsler RJ (1988) Pancreatic sarcoidosis mimicking pancreatic cancer. J Clin Ultrasound 16:131–134

Schlesinger E (1898) Die Erkrankung des Pancreas bei hereditarer Lues. Virchows Archiv 154:501–528

Shugar RA, Ryan JJ (1975) *Clonorchis sinensis* and pancreatitis twenty-five years after endemic exposure. Am J Gastroenterol 64:400–403

Simmonds M (1921) Diabetes und Syphilis. Arch Dermat Syph 132:235–237

Smith MG, Velios F (1950) Inclusion disease or generalised salivary gland virus infection. Arch Pathol 50:862–884

Stambler JB, Klibaner MI, Bliss CM, La Mont JT (1982) Tuberculous abscess of the pancreas. Gastroenterology 83:922–925.

Stürmer J, Becker V (1987) Granulomatous pancreatitis – granulomas in chronic pancreatitis. Virchows Arch [A] 410:327–338

Torre D, Montanari M, Fiori GP, Dietz A, Sampietro C (1987) HIV and the pancreas [letter]. Lancet ii:1212

Tsou E, Romano MC, Kerwin DM, Soteropoulos GC, Katz S (1980) Sarcoidosis of anterior mediastinal nodes, pancreas, and uterine cervix: three unusual sites in the same patient. Am Rev Respir Dis 122:333–338

Ursing B (1973) Acute pancreatitis in Coxsackie B infection. Br Med J iii:524–525

Venderell J, Nubiola A, Goday A et al. (1987) HIV and the pancreas [letter]. Lancet ii:1212

Welch K, Finkbeiner W, Alpers CE et al. (1984) Autopsy findings in the acquired immune deficiency syndrome. JAMA 252:1152–1159

Wigglesworth JS (1984) Perinatal pathology. Saunders, Philadelphia, p 328

Wilcox CM, Forsmark CE, Grendell JH, Darragh TM, Cello JP (1990) Cytomegalovirus-associated acute pancreatitis disease in patients with acquired immunodeficiency syndrome: report of two patients. Gastroenterology 99:263–267

Wilson S, Thompson AE (1964) A fatal case of strongyloidiasis. J Pathol Bact 87:169–176

Wislocki LC (1966) Acute pancreatitis in infectious mononucleosis. N Engl J Med 275:322–323

Witte CL, Schanzer CB (1968) Pancreatitis due to mumps. JAMA 203:1068–1069

Wyatt JP, Saxton J, Lee RS, Pinkerton H (1950) Generalised cytomegalic inclusion disease. J Pediatr 36:271–294

Wyatt JP, Hemsath FA, Soash MD (1951) Disseminated cytomegalic inclusion disease in an adult, with primary refractory anemia and transfusional siderosis: report of a case. Am J Clin Pathol 21:50–55

Wyatt JP, Simon T, Trubull ML, Evans M (1953) Cytomegalic inclusion pneumonitis in the adult. Am J Clin Pathol 23:353–362

Zazzo J-F, Pichon F, Regnier B (1987) HIV and the pancreas. Lancet ii:1212–1213

Zeiderman MR, Wyman A, Euinton HA, Simms JM, Rogers K (1991) Diagnostic difficulties in patients with a pancreatic mass. Br Med J 302:1395–1396

Zuger A, Wolf BZ, El-Sadr W, Simberkoff MS, Rahal JJ (1986) Pentamidine-associated fatal acute pancreatitis. JAMA 256:2383–2385

Subject Index